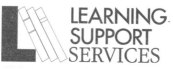

Molecular Biology
of the Neuron

The MOLECULAR AND CELLULAR NEUROBIOLOGY series

Series advisors

G.L. Collingridge, *Department of Anatomy, University of Bristol, Bristol, UK*

R.W. Davies, *IBLS, Division of Molecular Genetics, University of Glasgow, Glasgow, UK*

S.P. Hunt, *Molecular Neurobiology Unit, MRC Centre, Cambridge, UK*

Neurobiology of Alzheimer's Disease
Immune Responses in the Nervous System
Glial Cell Development
Cortical Plasticity: LTP and LTD
Molecular Biology of the Neuron

Molecular Biology of the Neuron

R. Wayne Davies
IBLS, Division of Molecular Genetics, University of Glasgow, Glasgow, UK

Brian J. Morris
IBLS, Division of Neuroscience and Biomedical Systems, University of Glasgow, Glasgow, UK

βIOS
SCIENTIFIC
PUBLISHERS

© **BIOS Scientific Publishers Limited, 1997**

First published, 1997

A CIP catalogue record for this book is available from the British Library.

ISBN 1 859962 40 8

BIOS Scientific Publishers Ltd
9 Newtec Place, Magdalen Road, Oxford OX4 1RE, UK.
Tel. +44 (0) 1865 726286. Fax. +44 (0) 1865 246823

DISTRIBUTORS

Australia and New Zealand
  DA Information Services
  648 Whitehorse Road, Mitcham
  Victoria 3132

India
  Viva Books Private Limited
  4325/3 Ansari Road
  New Delhi 110002

Singapore and South East Asia
  Toppan Company (S) PTE Ltd
  38 Liu Fang Road, Jurong
  Singapore 2262

USA and Canada
  BIOS Scientific Publishers
  PO Box 605, Herndon,
  VA 20172–0605

Typeset by Saxon Graphics Ltd, Derby, UK.
Printed by Information Press Ltd, Oxford, UK.

Contents

Contributors   ix
Abbreviations   xi
Preface   xiv

1 Neuronal genes. *G.J. Stewart and R.W. Davies*   1
    Genes and the future of neuronal molecular biology   1
    Experimental approaches to finding neuronal genes   3
    Using the World Wide Web to find brain-expressed genes   8
    The primary structure of brain-expressed mRNAs   11
    References   18

2 Molecular genetics of nervous and neuromuscular systems.
    H. Jockusch, K.-A. Nave, G. Grenningloh and T. Schmitt-John   21
    Introduction   21
    Developmental neurogenetics: emergence and compartmentalization of
        the nervous system   22
    Pathfinding and guidance of axons   28
    Genetics of cell migration   32
    Neurotrophic factors and their receptors   34
    Genetic control of cell death   37
    Hereditary neurodegenerative diseases: natural and transgenic models   39
    Myelin genetics   42
    Genetics of ion channels and of neuromuscular functions   46
    A glimpse of the genetics of behavior and learning   52
    Neurodegeneration due to aging and infections: genetic factors   55
    Conclusions   58
    References   59
    Further reading   66

3 Neuron-specific gene expression. *A.L. Grant and W. Wisden*   67
    Introduction   67
    Gene silencing   71
    Gene activation via single positive enhancers   74
    Multiple positive and negative elements direct cell type-specific expression
        within the nervous system   75
    Intronic and downstream (3′) regulatory elements in neuronal genes   79
    Locus control regions   80
    Summary   82
    References   82
    Appendix. A description of methods for studying promoters and enhancers of
        neuronal genes   87

4   **The cytoskeleton.** *J. Díaz-Nido and J. Avila*   **95**
    Introduction   95
    Components of the neuronal cytoskeleton   96
    The cytoskeleton in neuronal morphogenesis   106
    The cytoskeleton in neuronal plasticity   112
    The cytoskeleton in intraneuronal transport   113
    The cytoskeleton in neuropathology   116
    References   118

5   **Molecular biology of neurotransmitter release.** *J. Staple and S. Catsicas*   **123**
    Introduction   123
    Modern concepts in neurotransmitter release   125
    Learning and synapses   134
    Concluding remarks   138
    References   138

6   **Voltage-gated ion channels.** *G. Edwards and A.H. Weston*   **145**
    Introduction   145
    General principles   145
    General structure of voltage-sensitive K^+-channels   145
    General structure of voltage-sensitive Ca^{2+}- and K^+-channels   148
    K^+-channels   150
    Ca^{2+} channels   159
    Na^+ channels   165
    Conclusions   171
    References   171

7   **G protein-coupled receptors.** *J.A. Koenig*   **177**
    Introduction   177
    Overall structural features   179
    Receptor–ligand interactions   183
    Receptor–G protein interactions   185
    Regulation of G protein-coupled receptor function   190
    Conclusions   198
    References   199

8   **Molecular biology of neurotransmitter-gated ion channel receptors.**
    T.A. Glencorse and R.W. Davies   **205**
    Introduction   205
    Genes and gene structure   209
    Gene expression   210
    RNA processing   212
    Post-translational modification   214
    Protein structure   216
    Assembly and subcellular localization   223
    Future prospects   224
    References   236

9 **Signaling pathways in neurons: focus on second messengers and
   protein phosphorylation.** *M.R. Boarder*   **241**
   Introduction   241
   The major second messengers and protein phosphorylation cascades   242
   Role of second messenger signaling pathways in neuronal function   256
   References   264

10 **Cell-surface and extracellular matrix glycoproteins implicated in the
   movements of growth cones and neural cells and in synaptogenesis in
   the vertebrate nervous system.** *H. Volkmer and F.G. Rathjen*   **269**
   Introduction   269
   The netrins: chemoattractants and chemorepellents of the ECM   271
   Semaphorins guide axons to their target through repulsion   274
   The tenascins: a family of proteins with complex functions during
      nervous system development   276
   The thrombospondins are implicated in neural cell migration and
      neurite extension   278
   The chondroitin sulfate proteoglycan neurocan   280
   Agrin, an ECM component implicated in synaptogenesis   281
   Multiple functions of the laminin family   283
   The immunoglobulin superfamily   284
   References   289

11 **Genetic control of brain development.** *N.D. Allen, M.J. Skynner, H. Kato
   and J.N. Pratap*   **299**
   Introduction   299
   Segmental development of the vertebrate nervous system   301
   Future prospects   317
   References   318

12 **Neuronal plasticity.** *B.J. Morris*   **323**
   Introduction   323
   Experimental models of neuronal plasticity   323
   Ca^{2+} as the trigger   326
   Rapid, transient plasticity   327
   Slower, sustained plasticity   329
   Unanswered questions   335
   References   335

13 **Neurotrophic factors and the regulation of neuronal survival in the
   developing peripheral nervous system.** *A.M. Davies*   **339**
   Introduction   339
   Neurotrophins   340
   CNTF, LIF, OSM, CT-1 and IL-6   348
   GDNF   350
   References   351

14 **Genetic basis of human neuronal disease.** *M.E.S. Bailey, R.T. Moxley III*
   and K.J. Johnson   **359**
   Introduction   359
   Expanding trinucleotide repeat diseases   360
   Other disease genes with effects mainly on neuronal phenotype   372
   Other disease genes with neuronal phenotypes   382
   References   385

   Index   **395**

Contributors

Allen, N.D. Laboratory of Developmental Neurobiology, The Babraham Institute, Babraham, Cambridge CB2 4AT, UK

Avila, J. Centro de Biología Molecular "Severo Ochoa", Facultad de Ciencias, Universidad Autónoma de Madrid, Madrid E-28049, Spain

Bailey, M.E.S. IBLS, Division of Molecular Genetics, University of Glasgow, Anderson College, 56 Dumbarton Road, Glasgow G11 6NU, UK

Boarder, M.R. Department of Cell Physiology and Pharmacology, PO Box 138, University of Leicester, University Road, Leicester LE2 7RH, UK

Catsicas, S. Glaxo Institute for Molecular Biology S.A., 14 chemin-des-Aulx – CP674, 1228 Plan-les-Ouates, Geneva, Switzerland; and Institut de Biologie Cellulaire et de Morphologie, Université de Lausanne, rue du Bugnon 9, CH-1005 Lausanne, Switzerland

Davies, A.M. School of Biological and Medical Sciences, Bute Medical Building, University of St Andrews, St Andrews, Fife KY16 9TS, UK

Davies, R.W. IBLS, Division of Molecular Genetics, Robertson Building, University of Glasgow, 54 Dumbarton Road, Glasgow G11 6NU, UK

Díaz-Nido, J. Centro de Biología Molecular "Severo Ochoa", Facultad de Ciencias, Universidad Autónoma de Madrid, Madrid E-28049, Spain

Edwards, G. School of Biological Sciences, G38 Stopford Building, University of Manchester, Oxford Road, Manchester M13 9PT, UK

Glencorse, T.A. IBLS, Division of Molecular Genetics, Robertson Building, University of Glasgow, 54 Dumbarton Road, Glasgow G11 6NU, UK

Grant, A.L. MRC Laboratory of Molecular Biology, Hills Road, Cambridge CB2 2QH, UK

Grenningloh, G. Geneva Biomedical Research Institute, Glaxo Wellcome Research and Development S.A., 14 chemin des Aulx, Case postale 674, CH-1228 Plan-les-Ouates, Geneva, Switzerland

Jockusch, H. Developmental Biology Unit, W7, University of Bielefeld, D-33501 Bielefeld, Germany

Johnson, K.J. IBLS, Division of Molecular Genetics, Anderson College, University of Glasgow, 56 Dumbarton Road, Glasgow G11 6NU, UK

Kato, H. Laboratory of Developmental Neurobiology, The Babraham Institute, Babraham, Cambridge CB2 4AT, UK

Koenig, J.A. Department of Pharmacology, University of Cambridge, Tennis Court Road, Cambridge CB2 1QJ, UK

Morris, B.J. IBLS, Division of Neuroscience and Biomedical Systems, West Medical Building, University of Glasgow, Glasgow G12 8QQ, UK

Moxley, R.T. III. Department of Neurology, University of Rochester, 601 Elmwood Avenue, Rochester, NY 19406, USA

Nave, K.-A. Zentrum für Molekularbiologie, Im Neuenheimer Feld 282, D-69120 Heidelberg, Germany

Pratap, J. Laboratory of Developmental Neurobiology, The Babraham Institute, Babraham, Cambridge CB2 4AT, UK

Rathjen, F.G. Max-Delbrück-Centrum für Molekulare Medizin, Robert-Rössle-Strasse 10, 13122 Berlin, Germany

Schmitt-John, T. Developmental Biology Unit, W7, University of Bielefeld, D-33501 Bielefeld, Germany

Skynner, M.J. Laboratory of Developmental Neurobiology, The Babraham Institute, Babraham, Cambridge CB2 4AT, UK

Staple, J. Glaxo Institute for Molecular Biology S.A., 14 chemin-des-Aulx, 1228 Plan-les-Ouates, Geneva, Switzerland; and Institut de Biologie Cellulaire et de Morphologie, Université de Lausanne, rue du Bugnon 9, CH-1005 Lausanne, Switzerland

Stewart, G.J. IBLS, Division of Molecular Genetics, Robertson Building, University of Glasgow, 54 Dumbarton Road, Glasgow G11 6NU, UK

Volkmer, H. Max-Delbrück-Centrum für Molekulare Medizin, Robert-Rössle-Strasse 10, 13122 Berlin, Germany

Weston, A.H. School of Biological Sciences, G.38 Stopford Building, University of Manchester, Oxford Road, Manchester M13 9PT, UK

Wisden, W. MRC Laboratory of Molecular Biology, Hills Road, Cambridge CB2 2QH, UK

Abbreviations

Aβ protein fragment found in β-amyloid and neuritic plaques
A–P anterior–posterior
ABP actin-binding protein
ACh acetylcholine
AChR acetylcholine receptor
AChT acetylcholine transporter
AD Alzheimer's disease
ADF actin depolymerizing factor
ADNFE autosomal dominant nocturnal frontal lobe epilepsy
ALS amyotrophic lateral sclerosis
AMPA D,L-amino-3-hydroxy-5-methyl-4-isoxalone propionic acid
ANP atrial natriuretic peptide
APOE apoprotein E locus
APP amyloid precursor protein
AR androgen receptor
ARF ADP-ribosylation factor
AVED selective vitamin E deficiency
βARK β_2-adrenergic receptor kinase
BDNF brain-derived neurotrophic factor
bHLH basic helix–loop–helix
BMP bone morphogenetic protein
BoNT botulinum neurotoxin
CAM cell adhesion molecule
CaMKII Ca^{2+} calmodulin kinase II
CCK cholecystokinin
ChAT choline acetyltransferase
CIC voltage-gated chloride channel
CJD Creutzfeldt–Jakob disease
CLIP cytoplasmic linker protein
CMT1A Charcot–Marie–Tooth disease 1A
CNS central nervous system
CNTF ciliary neurotrophic factor
CNTFR ciliary neurotrophic factor receptor
COMP cartilage oligomeric matrix protein
cox-2 cyclooxygenase 2
cPLA$_2$ cytosolic phospholipase A$_2$
CRE cAMP-response element
CREB cAMP-response element binding protein
CT-1 cardiotropin-1
CTX conotoxin
D–V dorsal–ventral
DAG diacylglycerol

DBH dopamine-β-hydroxylase
DCC deleted in colorectal cancer (gene)
DHP-R dihydropyridine receptor
DM myotonic dystrophy (dystrophia muscularis)
DMPK myotonic dystrophy kinase/myotonin
DRG dorsal root ganglion
DRPLA dentatorubral-pallidoluysian atrophy
ECM extracellular matrix
EGF epidermal growth factor
EMSA electrophoresis mobility shift assay
ER endoplasmic reticulum
ES cells embryonic stem cells
FALS familial amyotrophic lateral sclerosis
FFI fatal familial insomnia
FGF fibroblast growth factor
FN fibronectin
FRAXA fragile X syndrome
FRDA Friedreich's ataxia
GABA γ-aminobutyric acid
GDNF glia cell line-derived neurotrophic factor
GDNFR glia cell line-derived neurotrophic factor receptor
GluR glutamate receptor
GlyR glycine receptor
GPI glycosyl-phosphatidylinositol
GRK G protein receptor kinase
GSS Gerstmann–Sträussler–Scheinker syndrome
HD Huntington's disease
HH hedgehog
HOX homeobox
HSV herpes simplex virus
5-HT 5-hydroxytryptamine
hyperYPP hyperkalemic periodic paralysis
hypoYPP hypokalemic periodic paralysis
ICE interleukin-1β converting enzyme
IEG immediate-early genes
IFP intermediate filament protein
IgSF immunoglobulin superfamily

IL-6	interleukin-6	NT3	neurotrophin 3
IL-6R	interleukin-6 receptor	OBCAM	opioid-binding cell adhesion molecule
Ins(1,4,5)P$_3$	inositol 1,4,5-triphosphate		
IPL	intraperiod line (of myelin)	OSM	oncostatin-M
KAIN	kainate	P0	protein zero
lacZ	β-galactosidase	PAF	platelet-activating factor
LAMP	limbic system-associated protein	PHF	paired helical filaments
		PKA	protein kinase A
LCR	locus control region	PKC	protein kinase C
LDL	low density lipoprotein	PKG	protein kinase G
LIF	leukemia inhibitory factor	PLA	phospholipase A
LTD	long-term depression	PLC	phospholipase C
LTP	long-term potentiation	PLD	phospholipase D
LV	large vesicles	PLP	proteolipid protein
mAChR	muscarinic acetylcholine receptor	PMP-22	peripheral myelin protein-22
		PNS	peripheral nervous system
MAG	myelin-associated glycoprotein	PPV	plasmalemmal precursor vesicles
MAOA	monoamine oxidase A		
MAOB	monoamine oxidase B	PSA	polysialic acid
MAP	microtubule-associated protein	RAGS	repulsive axonal guidance signal
MAPK	mitogen-activated protein kinase		
		RNP	ribonucleoprotein particle
MARCKS	myristoylated alanine-rich C kinase substrate	RTK	receptor tyrosine kinase
		RTP	receptor-like tyrosine phosphatases
MBP	myelin basic protein		
MCDP	mast cell degranulating peptide	RT-PCR	reverse transcriptase–polymerase chain reaction
MDL	major dense line (of myelin)		
MDLS	Miller–Dieker lissencephaly syndrome	SBMA	spinal and bulbar muscular atrophy
MED	motor endplate disease	SCA	spinocerebellar ataxia
mGluR	metabotropic glutamate receptors	SCG	superior cervical sympathetic ganglion
MJD	Machado–Joseph disease	ScTX	scorpion toxin
MUSK	muscle-specific kinase	SDS-PAGE	sodium dodecyl sulfate–polyacrylamide gel electrophoresis
NAIP	neuronal apoptosis inhibitory protein		
NCAM	neural cell adhesion molecule	SHH	sonic hedgehog
ND	Norrie disease	SHH-C	C-terminal cleavage product of hedgehog protein
NDP	Norrie disease protein		
NF-H	neurofilament triplet protein H	SHH-N	N-terminal cleavage product of hedgehog protein
NF-L	neurofilament triplet protein L		
NF-M	neurofilament triplet protein M	SMA	spinal muscular atrophy
NFT	neurofibrillary tangles	SMN	survival motor neuron (gene)
NgCAM	neuron–glial cell adhesion molecule	SNAP	synaptosomal-associated protein
NGF	nerve growth factor	SNARES	SNAP receptors
NGICR	neurotransmitter-gated ion channel receptors	SOD	superoxide dismutase
		sPLA$_2$	secreted phospholipase A$_2$
NMDA	N-methyl-D-aspartate	SR	splicing regulatory protein
NO	nitric oxide	SV	small vesicles
NrCAM	NgCAM-related cell adhesion molecule	TeNT	tetanus neurotoxin
		TF	transcription factor
NRSE	neuron restrictive silencer element	TGF	transforming growth factor
		TH	tyrosine hydroxylase
NRSF	neuron restrictive silencer factor	TN-C	tenascin-C
NSF	N-ethylmaleimide-sensitive factor	TN-R	tenascin-R
		TN-X	tenascin-X
NT	neurotrophin	TNF	tumor necrosis factor

tPA	tissue plasminogen activator	VAChT	vesicular acetylcholine
Trk	receptor tyrosine kinases		transporter
TSP	thrombospondin	VAMP	vesicle-associated membrane
TSS	transcription start site		protein
α-TTP	α-tocopherol transfer protein	VMAT	vesicular monoamine
TTX	tetrodotoxin		transporters

Preface

The properties of neurons are central to the whole of neuroscience. A proper and detailed understanding of how a particular set of molecules interact to produce neurons and direct their activity and maintenance is fundamental to progress in this important field, and crucial to the development of treatments for neurological diseases. The impact of molecular biology on studies of neuronal function has been gradual but profound, and is set to accelerate dramatically. It is therefore timely to present the state of knowledge of the molecular biology of the neuron. The set of reviews in this volume provide the reader with an overview of neuron molecular biology from genes and gene expression through the molecular systems that determine the excitability of neurons and how this is controlled and transmitted, to the molecules known to play special roles in the development of the nervous system, the survival of neurons, and disease. As well as providing an overview, each chapter has an emphasis that is special to the scientists who wrote it. Although it would have been impossible to describe all of neuron molecular biology in depth in one volume, the overviews provided touch on most aspects and will be extremely valuable to all neuroscientists for whom molecular biology is still foreign territory, while molecular biologists will find new angles to contemplate in the sections that examine certain phenomena in greater detail.

We know an immense amount now about such disparate areas as neurotransmission and axon targeting, due to the rapidly increasing level of definition of molecules involved in these processes; much more than could have been conceived of even 10 years ago. These recent advances, most of which are presented in this book, have been made to a considerable extent using pharmacological tools to define molecular components and biochemical methods to identify them. Increasingly, however, the use of genetic approaches to discover neuronal genes and investigate their functions has become important, particularly since it became clear that a great deal of relevance to human neurons, and even to human brain development and action, could be learnt by studying simpler eukaryotes such as *Drosophila melanogaster* and *Caenorhabditis elegans*, in which genetics can be carried out rapidly and effectively. Yet another new dimension is provided by the Human Genome Project and its associated genome sequencing projects, which are defining new genes at a tremendous rate. In another 10 years we will have the complete genetic blueprint for making a nervous system. Thus the first two chapters by Stewart and R.W. Davies and by Jockusch *et al.* show how neuronal genes are being, and will be, discovered by genetics and molecular biology. Stewart and R.W. Davies also provide a guide to finding neuronal genes on the Internet, list the known completely sequenced genes and show that neuronal transcripts as a class have unique features. Jockusch *et al.* give a comprehensive account of the knowledge of the nervous system that has already been gained by genetic approaches, with many exciting examples, particularly in the area of brain development.

One of the aims of this book is to draw together what is known about basic as well as the more specific molecular biology of the neuron. The molecular account of basic features of neuronal molecular biology that begins with genes and genetics is continued in two chapters by Grant and Wisden, and by Díaz-Nido and Avila, which review how the transcription of neuronal genes is regulated, and the structure and function of the neuronal cytoskeleton, respectively. Transcriptional regulation in neurons has been studied remarkably little, given its key importance in determining specific neuronal phenotypes. Grant and Wisden use examples from the small minority of neuronal genes that have been studied to show some emerging principles underlying the complex patterns of transcription seen in the brain. Other levels of regulation such as RNA editing and alternative splicing are met in other chapters dealing with specific classes of molecules. Díaz-Nido and Avila describe the wide range of molecules involved in the neuronal cytoskeleton, and discuss the part they play in morphogenesis, plasticity and disease. Extracellular matrix molecules are discussed later by Volkmer and Rathjen.

The core of the book is a set of chapters that deals with the molecules involved in the central function of neurons as electrical and chemical signaling devices in the brain. Edwards and Weston describe the molecular and physiological properties of the molecules that play central roles in determining cellular excitability, the voltage-gated ion channels. The transmission of signals between neurons is covered in three chapters that review the molecular understanding of how transmitter molecules are released at synapses, and of the receptor molecules that interact with transmitters to generate responses in the post-synaptic neuron. Many of the molecules that feature in these chapters will be familiar to pharmacologists, clinical and systems neuroscientists; however, the authors have taken a molecular biologist's perspective, which attempts eventually to explain all cell biological phenomena in terms of the properties of amino acid sequences and protein structure. While we are a long way from achieving this for neurons, the reader will find the presentation of these familiar areas different and informative. Staple and Catsicas review the remarkable advances which have been made in understanding the molecular basis of synaptic vesicle docking, fusion and recycling and the involvement of these molecules in synaptic plasticity. Synaptogenesis is discussed in a later chapter by Volkmer and Rathjen. Glencorse and R.W. Davies provide a molecular biologist's view of the regulation, assembly and structure of neurotransmitter-gated ion channel receptors, which provide the molecular basis of fast synaptic transmission. The molecular biology of G protein-coupled receptors is described by Koenig, with particular emphasis on G protein coupling and on regulation of the activity and number of such receptors at the cell surface. Receptor activation results in effects on intracellular signaling pathways in neurons, so this section of the book is completed by a review by Boarder of our knowledge of second messenger pathways and protein phosphorylation in neurons.

The final five chapters present molecular aspects of the development, plasticity, survival and death of neurons. Allen *et al.* describe how genes and proteins define the anteroposterior, dorsoventral and segmental patterning of the neural tube and thus the brain and spinal cord, an area in which dramatic advances are being made. Both Allen *et al.* and Jockusch *et al.* show how important genetic analysis has been in elucidating these fundamental principles of neurobiology. Volkmer and Rathjen address the question of the molecular basis of neuronal connectivity, presenting a review of knowledge of the extracellular and transmembrane molecules involved in growth cone guidance and synaptogenesis. Once connected, neurons retain the ability to remodel their connections in response to inputs. Morris provides a review of the molecular mechanisms known to be involved in plasticity, and a unique review of knowledge of the particular transcription factor and other genes that can be identified as likely to play a part in long-term plastic responses of neurons. Another important component of brain development is the regulation of neuronal survival and death. A.M. Davies reviews the neurotrophic factors and their receptors, and the developmental timing of neurotrophin dependence, with emphasis on the peripheral nervous system.

Neurotrophic factors are also essential to the maintenance and survival of neurons in the adult. Genetic analysis has revealed many other genes that must be functional for the long-term maintenance of an intact human nervous system. In the final chapter, Bailey *et al.* comprehensively review knowledge of the genetic and molecular basis of diseases of the human nervous system. Prion diseases, Alzheimer's disease, oxidative damage diseases and others are covered, with a particular focus on triplet repeat diseases and their molecular mechanisms.

We hope that this volume will provide a molecular perspective on most aspects of neuronal biology for all neuroscientists, provide established neuroscientists with new starting points for further reading and research, and stimulate young neuroscientists to use genetics and molecular biology to solve the many important and exciting scientific problems to be found in the field of neuroscience.

R. Wayne Davies (*Glasgow*)
Brian J. Morris (*Glasgow*)

Neuronal genes

Gregor J. Stewart and R. Wayne Davies

1.1 Genes and the future of neuronal molecular biology

How the nervous system is formed, and how neurons carry out their specialized functions, can only be understood fully when all the proteins that are involved are known and have been studied both individually and within the neuronal context. The information for assembling the nervous system and for co-ordinated neuronal differentiation is in the genes that encode these proteins. The rate of advance of neuronal molecular biology depends entirely on the rate of discovery of the key neuronal proteins, either directly or via the genes. For many years, pharmacological and biochemical approaches were the primary means by which neuronal proteins were identified, because the size and complexity of the mammalian genome made it difficult or impossible to identify neuronal genes directly. Once a neuronal protein was isolated, and its corresponding genomic DNA cloned and sequenced, the rate of discovery frequently increased, because DNA homology-based molecular approaches allow the identification of genes of related sequence and many genes are members of families of related sequences. A striking example of this is provided by the rapid explosion in the discovery of G protein-linked receptors and of subunits of neurotransmitter-gated ion channel receptors once the first protein in each gene family had been laboriously purified, sequenced and reverse translated. Many of the proteins that form the subjects of the chapters of *Molecular Biology of the Neuron* are still those identified directly or indirectly by biochemical approaches.

However, two primary factors have already begun to change how mammalian neuronal genes (and their proteins) are discovered. The first of these is the increasing recognition that genes identified in simpler ('model') organisms as affecting nervous system development or neuronal function will frequently have both sequence and functional homologs in mammalian neurons. For example, virtually all of the genes and proteins that are now central to work on the molecular basis of development of the mammalian nervous system have been identified in other organisms, primarily *Drosophila melanogaster*, with contributions from *Caenorhabditis elegans*. The second factor is the dramatic rate of advance of the Human Genome Project and associated work on other genomes. The first eukaryotic genome, that of the yeast *Saccharomyces cerevisiae*, has already been completely sequenced, revealing an unexpectedly high proportion, over 50%, of genes unknown despite the power of yeast genetics (WWW; http://genome-www.stanford.edu/Saccharomyces/). Even here, genes and proteins relevant to the nervous system can be found, as many proteins involved in intracellular signaling cascades and particularly in cell cycle regulation will have mammalian

Molecular Biology of the Neuron, edited by R.W. Davies and B.J. Morris.
© 1997 BIOS Scientific Publishers Ltd, Oxford.

relatives fulfilling similar functions in neurons and their developmental precursors. Over a quarter of the genome of the nematode *C. elegans* has already been sequenced, and it is projected that this genome will be completely sequenced by the end of 1998. Among vertebrates, there is considerable interest in the puffer fish, *Fugu rubripes*, because its genome is very compact, with about the same number of genes as mammals in one-eighth the amount of DNA. *Fugu* genes show high coding sequence identity with mammalian genes, and regions of conserved synteny between the genomes of *Fugu* and man occur. The predicted gene density is one gene per 6–8 kbp, so that sequence analysis of *Fugu* would provide coding sequence information faster, and simplify the identification and analysis of both coding and noncoding regions. A cosmid-based sequence scanning map of *Fugu* is under construction, and *Fugu* promises to be a useful reference genome (WWW; http://fugu.hgmp.mrc.ac.uk/). The Human Genome Project itself is in transition from genetic map and YAC (and BAC, P1 and cosmid) contig establishment to full scale sequencing. Even using largely pre-genomics approaches, the increasing level of research in human genetics more than doubled the number of genetically mapped human genes between 1990 and 1995 (*Human Genome News*, 1995; *Figure 1.1*). Now that good radiation hybrid sets are available, genetic mapping of human genes has become rapid and simple, limited only by gene identification and manpower. Physical DNA maps of several human chromosomes (e.g. chromosome 19: Ashworth *et al.*, 1995; metric map, FISH map WWW at URL http://llnl-bio.llnl.gov/bbrp/bbrp.homepage.html; YAC maps of all chromosomes at http://www.cephb.fr/ceph-genethon-map.html.) are virtually complete, and sequencing teams capable of delivering the complete sequence of a BAC clone (e.g. 150 kb) in a month (and potentially faster) are already active. It is likely that the sequence of all or most human genes will be available by the year 2005, within 10 years from now.

What this means for the development of molecular biology of the neuron and the

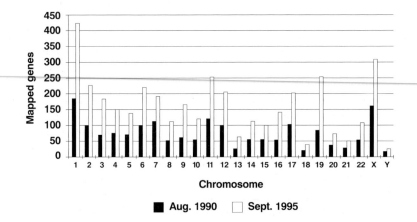

Figure 1.1 Growth of mapped genes, 1990–1995. The number of mapped genes has risen sharply over the past 5 years, from 1772 genes at the inception of the Human Genome Project in 1990 to 3695 genes by 15 September, 1995. Gene distribution depicted here may reflect mapping activity per chromosome rather than relative gene density, which will remain unknown until the majority of genes are mapped. Numbers in this graph do not include genes not yet assigned to chromosomes. (Source: GDB, 1995)

brain, is that the bottleneck of protein or gene identification will be increasingly removed over the next 10 years. All the information for building a neuron and the nervous system will become available, and molecular neuroscientists will focus on the analysis of gene function followed by a synthesis of individual gene functions into a full understanding of the molecular basis of the form and activity of neurons. In the meantime, molecular neuroscientists will continue to make targeted searches for important genes. Here we will outline the approaches that can be taken now to identify new neuronal genes, and also describe how to use the Internet to find out what neuronal genes other scientists are discovering. Since the great majority of neuronal genes have been identified during the last 10 years, and a proportion of them completely characterized, we will also look again with present day data at the proposition made almost 10 years ago (Sutcliffe, 1988), that brain-specific transcripts may have distinct structural characteristics.

1.2 Experimental approaches to finding neuronal genes

1.2.1 Molecular approaches

The great majority of brain-expressed gene sequences in the database are partial cDNA sequences known as expressed sequence tags (ESTs: Adams *et al.*, 1992, 1993; Kato, 1992). ESTs are generated by sequencing into one end of each of a large number of cDNA clones with standard primers from flanking vector sequences. Using fluorescent automated sequencing, the sequence of at least 500 nucleotides can be determined unambiguously. Most EST projects have aimed at finding coding regions within EST sequences as frequently as possible, and have therefore sequenced the 5' ends of oligo-dT primed cDNAs, or used random-primed cDNAs. Messenger RNA populations are, of course, different in each tissue and cell-type. Thus collections of EST sequences, being mRNA based, are representative of the complete set of genes expressed in a given tissue. The brain-derived EST sets in the database will comprise a mixture of neuronal genes, glial genes and a small proportion of genes from other tissues. One of the goals of EST sequencing of standard cDNA libraries is to provide a quantitative molecular description of the expressed gene population in, for example, the brain. When, however, the goal is maximizing the number of different genes encountered, normalized cDNA libraries in which the frequency of the highly expressed cDNA are reduced, are used. Since large numbers of ESTs can be sequenced, many less strongly expressed genes can be discovered in this way, although less efficiently than highly expressed genes. Messenger RNAs with low or localized expression can be discovered more efficiently by prescreening cDNA libraries (Davies *et al.*, 1994), and particularly by analyzing subtracted cDNA libraries (Stewart *et al.*, 1996). Even so, the problem of redundancy will increase as more ESTs are sequenced. One way to deal with this is to obtain oligonucleotide sequence signatures for all new cDNAs before any are sequenced (Milosavljevic *et al.*, 1996).

ESTs can subsequently be mapped back on to the genetic and physical map of the genome to produce a gene expression map of the genome (Khan *et al.*, 1992). This is very important for the co-ordination of genetic maps – made primarily with anonymous sequence variant markers – and the physical map. If ESTs map close to known genetic mutations affecting the tissue from which the original mRNA derived, they provide novel candidate genes for the mutated locus. It can be predicted that mapping only 1000 mouse brain ESTs, if they are randomly distributed, is likely to yield candidates for around 20 of the known neurological mutations of the mouse which have not been assigned to a gene. The same principle applies to discovering the genes in which mutations leading to human hereditary neurological conditions occur. As the number of ESTs, the precision of the map and the number of neurological mutant loci increase, this approach may largely supplant positional cloning, and indeed gene-trapping and other methods of mammalian gene discovery. For example, even with the number of ESTs present in the database (which is a large but nowhere near exhaustive collection), 40% of the genes found by standard analysis of the human 22q11.2 region occurred as ESTs (*Human Genome News*, 1996). It is clear that in the medium term, the integration of genetic and physical maps of man and the mouse provided by EST-based gene expression maps will allow rapid selection of one or a few candidate genes for genetic components of any neurological phenotype.

Given the exponential development of genome projects, the above scenario may not be very far away. However, at present there remains a need for more targeted approaches. The most targeted way to discover genes affecting neuronal function is to use genetics (Section 1.2.2), but considerable effort has also been put into the development of targeted molecular approaches. Since the expression and maintenance of general and specific properties of cells and tissues are determined by the set of proteins expressed, it follows that by comparing the protein or mRNAs present in two different cell types, proteins and genes expressed specifically or more strongly in a given cell type can in principle be identified. Similarly, shifts in the population of genes expressed under different conditions (e.g. before and after ischemia; before or after the induction of long-term potentiation or long-term depression) can also be analyzed to identify genes involved in a particular aspect of neuronal biology. Antibody-based and 2D-protein gel analysis approaches have been used (e.g. in the identification of factors involved in axon targeting; Drescher *et al.*, 1995; Stahl *et al.*, 1990), but the most effective and easiest approaches use cDNA (i.e. mRNA) population differences. Differential screening of cDNA libraries with cDNA probes from two different sources is only effective for relatively highly expressed genes (typically those expressed at 0.5–1% of the total mRNA population). A variant of this is the differential reverse Northern procedure, which has been used to discover genes expressed at moderate to high levels specifically in the hippocampus; this involves using individual cDNAs or small pools as probes on two different mRNA populations as targets in dot blots or Northern transfers.

More recently, polymerase chain reaction (PCR)-based methods of comparing cDNA populations have been developed. In the mRNA differential display method (Liang and Pardee, 1992), different subsets of an mRNA population are produced as cDNA clones using PCR with one primer being oligo-dT dNdN′ (where N and N′ are not T) and the other a random 10-mer. Products that are mRNA population-specific are identified by direct track comparison in polyacrylamide gels, isolated and cloned and/or used to identify corresponding cDNAs. RNA fingerprinting by arbitrarily primed PCR (Welsh *et al.*, 1992) is another rapid method of identifying differentially expressed genes, and this approach has been used successfully to isolate novel brain-specific genes (Dalal *et al.*, 1994). Both of these methods have some disadvantages. They tend to yield false positives (Bauer *et al.*, 1994), tend to be biased towards highly expressed mRNAs (Bertioli *et al.*, 1995), and may not reveal differences if only a few genes are involved (Sompayrac *et al.*, 1995). Another PCR-based technique is representational difference analysis, which was originally designed to distinguish genomic DNA fragments that differ in size or representation between two versions of the same genome (Lisitsyn *et al.*, 1993), but has been applied to discover such differences between cDNA copies of mRNA populations (Hubank and Schatz, 1994). This technique has the real advantage that it does not require the preparation of pure single-stranded cDNAs, or their separation from double-stranded cDNAs as in subtractive hybridization (see below). However, representational difference analysis is more difficult to use, requiring multiple rounds of PCR and subtraction, in order to deal with widely differing levels of otherwise common mRNAs in the original populations, which almost always occur.

The most widely used techniques for the isolation of differentially expressed mRNAs have been variants of subtractive hybridization approaches. The general principle of this approach is that cDNA from an mRNA population containing the mRNAs sought (the tester) is hybridized with a high molar excess of cDNA from an mRNA population lacking the genes of interest (the driver). The tester molecules that hybridize with driver molecules are removed to leave the unhybridized fraction, which is enriched for cDNAs from differentially expressed mRNAs. This approach found early application to the search for brain genes (Rhyner *et al.*, 1986). In recent procedures, the tester and driver cDNAs are prepared as single-stranded molecules using phagemid vectors, and the driver is biotinylated, allowing the removal of all biotin-labeled driver and tester–driver hybrid molecules using avidin-coated magnetic beads or related technology (Duguid *et al.*, 1988; Rubenstein *et al.*, 1990). The remaining tester molecules may be subjected to further rounds of subtractive hybridization, and are then made double-stranded and cloned. This technology has been used to produce several very useful subtracted cDNA libraries from subsets of mammalian brain tissue or stages of brain development. For example, Porteus *et al.* (1992) isolated cDNA clones that are preferentially expressed in the mouse embryonic telencephalon, Swaroop *et al.* (1991) isolated a set of human retina-specific cDNAs, while Savioz and Davies (1995) identified cDNAs that are preferentially expressed in the substantia nigra compared to the cerebellum. An important use of subtracted libraries is as starting points for EST sequencing and genomic mapping since they allow access to mRNAs that are only inefficiently encountered in standard EST sets (Davies *et al.*, 1994; Stewart *et al.*, 1996).

An interesting recent technique called suppression subtractive hybridization (Diatchenko *et al.*, 1996) combines the advantages of PCR-based approaches with the selective power of subtractive hybridization. Suppression subtractive hybridization is based on the suppression PCR technique in which long terminal repeats attached to DNA fragments selectively suppress amplification of those fragments (Siebert *et al.*, 1995), does not require preparation of single-stranded cDNAs or separation of single-stranded and double-stranded cDNAs, and incorporates a normalization step to ameliorate the problem of differences in mRNA abundance. The technique has been used to produce a testis-specific library (Diatchenko *et al.*, 1996), but can easily be used to identify neuron-specific genes.

A different approach to finding important neuronal genes would be to focus on genes encoding a subset of cellular proteins. The most easily distinguished subset, and one that contains many known proteins with unique functions in neuronal development and mature function, is that of secreted proteins. This subset is being accessed by specialized gene-trapping vectors (Skarnes *et al.*, 1992, 1995; Section 1.2.2). An antibody-based screening procedure (signal sequence trap) for cDNA clones that redirect the expression of an export defective receptor to the surface of mammalian cells has been developed (Tashiro *et al.*, 1993). Recently, a molecular selection procedure for mammalian mRNAs encoding a secretion signal sequence has been developed (Klein *et al.*, 1996). Specialized lambda phage vectors are used to make cDNA libraries which can be easily converted to a yeast plasmid library, and which make the extracellular expression of the yeast invertase protein dependent upon the presence of a signal sequence in the mammalian cDNA. Yeast lacking a functional *SUC2* gene that encodes invertase will only grow on sucrose as its sole carbon source if secretable invertase is provided by the cDNA–invertase hybrid. This approach has been used to successfully isolate cDNAs encoding 49 known secreted proteins, and 86 novel secreted proteins from cDNA libraries including libraries made from embryonic rat brain and adult rat pituitary mRNA.

1.2.2 Genetic approaches

Genetics has always been the most effective way to define the molecular components of complex biological systems. A great advantage of genetics is that it can be focused on a particular part of the phenotype (e.g. an aspect of behavior) or a precise aspect of nervous system development, so that the genes discovered are sure to be interesting. Another great advantage is that, if sufficient mutational events are scanned, all genes affecting the phenotype will be discovered, independent of any functional models or preconceptions. Thus in the case of genes involved in Alzheimer's disease, the *APP* amyloid precursor protein gene would certainly have been discovered via the occurrence of the βA4 peptide in amyloid plaques, but the presenilin genes could only have been found using genetics. The limitations of the genetic approach lie in phenotype definition and in gene identification. A great future benefit of the genome projects is that gene identification will no longer be a problem. Many examples of the application of genetics to neuroscience are provided by Jockusch *et al.* (1996).

Once a genetic locus affecting a neurological phenotype in man or rodents has been identified, the corresponding DNA sequence is identified using positional cloning. Positional cloning relies on extensive genetic mapping to define a small region of the genome in which the gene has a high probability of being located. The mouse, and increasingly the rat, genetic systems allow genetic localization to very small regions if sufficient numbers of recombinants are analyzed. In the majority of the mouse genome, 1 cM is approximately equivalent to 1 Mb of DNA, so that localization to a genetic region of 0.1 cM could mean that 100 kb of DNA contain the gene of interest. This can be contained within a single YAC, BAC clone or two overlapping P1 clones. Eventually, complete DNA sequence determination of the region in the mutant and the inbred strain in which it arose may become the standard procedure. Presently, techniques such as exon trapping and cDNA selection or screening are used to find the genes in the region, followed by more limited cDNA sequencing. Positional cloning of human genes is considerably more laborious, because it is not possible to define the genetic map location as precisely as in rodents. Human genetics is, however, extremely important for the discovery of neuronal genes implicated in any dysfunction of the nervous system, because the human phenotype is under much more intense scrutiny through human medicine than that of any other species, the numbers of individuals examined is very large, and certain behavioral phenotypes are easier to recognize (and some may only occur) in man. As the Human Genome Project increasingly provides a physical map, a gene expression map and then actual DNA sequence, much of the labor of positional cloning will be removed. It was noted above that as the density of the EST map increases, mapped ESTs will effectively provide a direct equivalent of positional cloning.

The other increasingly important sources of genetically identified neuronal genes are 'simpler' eukaryotes. It is now apparent that the basic features of body plan development, cell function and differentiation, are extremely similar throughout the Metazoa. *D. melanogaster* and *C. elegans* have powerful experimental genetic systems, and sequence characterization of their genomes is underway. Very large numbers of these organisms can be handled in mutagenesis experiments. This has allowed extensive genetic screens to be designed to search for mutations affecting particular aspects of cell physiology or organismal development. There are many examples in the *Drosophila* literature: one relevant to special aspects of neuronal development is the screen for mutational effects on axon guidance (Seeger *et al.*, 1993) which revealed the novel genes *comm* and *robo*. A particularly important set of technologies are those surrounding P-element transposition in *Drosophila* (reviews: Cooley *et al.*, 1988; Sentry *et al.*, 1994). P-elements are naturally occurring transposons, which have been genetically manipulated so that their mobilization can be controlled, and in some cases reporter gene systems added. P-elements can therefore be used to produce random collections of loss-of-function mutations (Török *et al.*, 1993). Transposon mutagenesis has the great advantage for gene discovery that the inserting element provides a DNA sequence tag for the genomic insertion site. If an *Escherichia coli* origin of replication and a selectable marker are included within the P-element, the genomic sequences flanking the insertion site can easily be cloned by plasmid rescue (Guo *et al.*, 1996). Thus P-element technology links the genetic and physical maps and provides functional (phenotypic) information.

In vertebrates, both extensive genetic screens and integration mutant (transposon-like) screens are being carried out, and will be used more frequently in the future although they will always remain relatively laborious. In the mouse, gene-trap vectors have been developed to allow selection of integration events which hit a transcribed gene (Skarnes *et al.*, 1992). In recent versions this is achieved by placing a visualization marker (*lacZ*) and a selectable marker (*neo*) as a fused coding region downstream of a splice acceptor region in a promoterless construct, so that integration events that pick up a functional splice-donor site in an expressed gene are selected. If this is done in embryonic stem cells, it is then possible to generate mice and breed to investigate the effect of the homozygous insertion mutant. Gene-trap vectors allow direct sequencing of the trapped mRNA via 5′ RACE, give phenotypic information since they usually cause loss-of-function mutation, and can be adapted to allow expression pattern visualization, making them very valuable tools for gene discovery. Gene-trap vectors containing a transmembrane segment coding region upstream of the marker gene allow screening for genes that provide a signal sequence, since this reverses the sequestration of β-galactosidase that occurs with a single upstream transmembrane sequence (Skarnes *et al.*, 1995); in this way secreted and transmembrane protein encoding genes can be found, which are particularly important in nervous system development and function. This approach, however, is too laborious to be used as a screen for a large proportion of the expressed genes in the genome. Vertebrate systems in which a random gene search is to some extent feasible are the zebrafish and certain other fish species such as *Medaka*. Zebrafish genetics is well established, large numbers of the fish can be maintained without exorbitant expense, and the transparent bodies of the fish allow easy visualization of marker gene expression. This has allowed

large-scale screens for mutations affecting particular aspects of development to be initiated (Kuwada, 1995). In the mouse, ethyl-nitrosourea mutagenesis can be used to generate mutations very efficiently, but the breeding and analytical work involved remains
immense. Nevertheless, several large-scale mutagenesis and gene discovery programs are
underway, focusing on particular regions of the mouse genome.

1.3 Using the World Wide Web to find brain-expressed genes

All the above approaches are being used by an increasing number of laboratories, and
the genome projects are advancing rapidly. An ever-increasing avalanche of newly
discovered neuronal genes will be entering the sequence databases. In this section we
will address the question 'how can we find all the brain-expressed mRNAs that have
been deposited in the databases?'. The advent of the Internet has made the searching
of nucleotide databases for specific or related sequences a far less daunting task than
it once appeared. The start point for any nucleotide database search is the NCBI
Entrez nucleotide database search page (http://www3.ncbi.nlm.nih.gov/htbinpost/
Entrez/query?db=n&form=0). The Entrez algorithms (Schuler et al., 1996) allow
searching and retrieval of sequences from the GenBank, EMBL, DDBJ, PIR, PRF
and PDB databases using the search terms described in *Table 1.1*.

In our case, that of searching for sequences that are expressed in the brain, the two
most useful search terms are 'text' and 'organism'. Text term searching allows entries
to be retrieved which contain words which are of relevance to our field of interest,
such as 'brain' and 'neuron', or to refine a search for complete mRNA sequences,
using 'complete' with either 'mRNA', 'cDNA' or 'CDS' (abbreviation for coding
sequence). The text term 'neuron' is an interesting example of one of the quirks in the
Entrez system. Not only does this term find some entries that are neuron-specific
sequences, but it also finds any entry whose citation is in the journal *Neuron* but
which may not necessarily be neuron-specific (381 entries in total). A search using the
term 'neuronal' instead finds 563 entries and avoids picking up the '*Neuron*'-published
nonspecific sequences. Using the 'organism' search term allows large and daunting
lists of entries to be broken down by species and allows cross-species comparisons.

A major caveat with searching the databases is that if the text term you search with
does not occur in a particular database entry, you won't find that entry in your search.
An example, used in this chapter, is the term '3′ UTR'. Not every complete mRNA
sequence entry in the databases explicitly states that the sequence includes all or any
of the 3′ UTR. It may, however, say 'PolyA site at ...', allowing the 3′ UTR to be
deduced. Thus a search with 'PolyA' as the text term would yield a few more entries
than a search with '3′ UTR' alone. Indeed, the term 'complete' as in 'complete
mRNA', does not infer that both the 5′ UTR and 3′ UTR are completely defined and
sequenced; some 'complete' entries contain just the protein coding part of the mRNA.
Thus there are some database entries which include all of the 5′ and 3′ UTRs yet do
not mention this, as well as some entries which have some 5′ or 3′ UTR but not all of
it. The only way to distinguish between these is to refer to the papers cited in the
entry or to contact the authors directly.

1.3.1 Search modes

World Wide Web Entrez allows you to enter terms for searching in several different
ways. In **Selection mode**, when you enter a term, Entrez displays the list of available

Table 1.1. GenBank Entrez search terms

Search term	Definition
Accession	Contains the accession number of the sequence, assigned to the nucleotide or protein record by a sequence database builder.
Author name	Contains the list of authors for a paper in the literature. In the Protein and Nucleotide databases, the authors listed are those of the MEDLINE articles to which a sequence is linked. The format for author names is the last name, followed by a space and the first initial(s), without periods.
Date	Contains the year and month of publication, in the format year/month, e.g. 1984/10. To obtain all of the records published in a given year without regard to month, use the year by itself, e.g. 1984.
E.C. number	A number assigned by the Enzyme Commission to find a particular enzyme.
Feature key	Features of a particular sequence contained in the GenBank entry, e.g. "rep_origin" – origin of replication and "protein_bind" – protein binding site in the DNA sequence.
Gene name	The standard name for a given gene. Greek letters in gene names are spelled out in angle brackets, e.g. <alpha>. If you cannot find a gene using Gene Name, try using the Text term field instead.
Journal title	The name of the journal where the record was published. Journal names are stored in the database in abbreviated form; for instance, the *Journal of Biological Chemistry* is stored as J Biol Chem. If you are not sure how a journal name is abbreviated, use Selection mode to browse the journal titles.
Keyword	Allows you to search using special index terms from a controlled vocabulary associated with the GenBank, EMBL, DDBJ, SwissProt, PIR, PRF, or PDB database.
MEDLINE ID	The MEDLINE Unique Identifier of a given citation.
Properties	Useful for searching particular divisions of GenBank e.g. GenBank division EST. This search term is currently under revision.
Sequence ID	The unique identifier for a given sequence assigned by the NCBI tracking database.
Organism	Contains the scientific and common names for the organisms associated with protein and nucleotide sequences.
Protein name	Contains the name of the protein that this sequence is associated with. The common name of a protein may not be indexed under this field; if you cannot find a particular protein using this field, try Text term.
Substance	Contains the names of any chemicals associated with this record from the Chemical Abstract Service (CAS) registry and the MEDLINE Name of Substance field.
Text term	Includes all of the 'free text' associated with a record, specifically: MEDLINE records: the title and abstract. Protein records: the definition, comment, protein name and protein description. Nucleotide records: the definition, comment, gene name and gene description.

terms for that field, starting at the first term which begins with the characters that you entered. You can then select one or more terms to add to your search. For example, to see the text terms beginning with 'pneum', you would enter 'pneum' in the term box, select 'Text' and 'Selection', then press Accept. Selection Mode thus allows you to browse through the terms in any given field. This can be very useful if you are not sure how something is spelled.

In **Automatic mode,** the term or terms that you enter are immediately added to your search. In addition, with many fields you can enter several terms, separating them by spaces. Entrez will then take each of the terms and place them into your search individually. For instance, if you entered 'central nervous system', the terms 'central', 'nervous', and 'system' would be added to your query. The fields that permit you to enter multiple terms on one line are: Text Word, E.C. Number, Gene, Date and Feature Key.

In **Truncation mode**, Entrez adds all of the terms in the specified search field that begin with the characters you provided into your search, coalescing their records. The truncated term is labeled '{term} ...' in the search. For instance, if you entered 'pneum' in the term box, selected 'Text' field and 'Truncation' mode, then pressed Accept, every text word that began with 'pneum' (pneumonia, pneumonitis, pneumococcus, etc.) would be retrieved and placed into the chosen box under the heading 'pneum ...'. Note that truncations may take a little longer to perform, especially if you enter just a few characters.

1.3.2 Searching the nucleotide databases with sequences

The paragraphs above concern finding groups of sequences related by virtue of their shared origins (i.e. tissue or species). We now turn our attention to discovering sequences that are related by sequence. What this means is comparing a sequence, usually a novel or unknown sequence, with those already deposited in the databases. This can be done as either a nucleotide search using the DNA sequence or a protein search using a conceptual translation of the DNA sequence. We will concern ourselves here with the use of the BLAST (Altschul *et al.*, 1990) facility on the World Wide Web (URL http://www.ncbi.nlm.nih.gov/cgi-bin/BLAST/nph-blast?Jform=0). Other methods of searching such as BLAST via e-mail and via CD-ROM are essentially the same except for the method of sequence submission. For searches of large-scale EST sequencing projects, it is recommended that BLAST via e-mail is used since numerous searches can be submitted and other tasks performed whilst waiting for the results, whereas submission via the World Wide Web is a real-time method where one must wait for the results of one submission (search) before starting the next. Older methods of sequence comparison such as the University of Wisconsin GCG package are not considered here.

There are three BLAST algorithms which are the most useful for general purposes and these are described in the following three paragraphs.

BLASTN compares a given nucleotide sequence with sequences in the following databases:

(i)   **nr** Nonredundant GenBank+EMBL+DDBJ+PDB sequences (but no ESTs or STSs).
(ii) **pdb** PDB nucleotide sequences.
(iii) **vector** Vector subset of GenBank.
(iv) **mito** Database of mitochondrial sequences, Rel. 1.0, July 1995.
(v)   **kabat** Kabat sequences of nucleic acids of immunological interest.
(vi) **epd** Eukaryotic promoter database.
(vii) **month** All new or revised GenBank+EMBL+DDBJ+PDB sequences released in the last 30 days.

BLASTP compares a given protein sequence with protein sequences in the following databases:

(i)   **nr** Non-redundant GenBank CDS translations+PDB+SwissProt+PIR.
(ii) **pdb** PDB protein sequences.
(iii) **kabat** Kabat sequences of proteins of immunological interest.
(iv) **alu** Translations of select *Alu* repeats from REPBASE.
(v)   **month** All new or revised GenBank CDS translation+PDB+SwissProt+PIR sequences released in the last 30 days.
(vi) **SwissProt** SwissProt sequences.

TBLASTX translates a given nucleotide sequence into all six reading frames and compares them to the nucleotide sequences also translated into all six reading frames. TBLASTX uses the following databases:

(i)   **dbest** Nonredundant database of GenBank+EMBL+DDBJ EST Division.
(ii) **dbst** Nonredundant database of GenBank+EMBL+DDBJ STS Division.
(iii) **alu** Select *Alu* repeats from REPBASE.

Note that TBLASTX is the only algorithm which allows searching of the EST and sequence-tagged sites (STS) databases. It is also useful for searching with data of poor quality and for finding more distant relationships between sequences.

There is extensive help documentation available on-line and this will not be repeated here. BLAST automatically filters input sequence for regions of low sequence complexity (e.g. simple sequence repeats) and thus only informative database hits are displayed. Any database entries showing significant sequence similarity to the query sequence can be displayed and saved by following the World Wide Web links attached to the BLAST search results.

The various BLAST searches detailed above are particularly useful for searching with sequence derived from cDNAs and ESTs since the sequence is assumed to come from expressed genes which may or may not have a homolog in the databases, and there are thousands of EST sequences deposited in the databases already. For larger genomic DNA sequences other software can be used to predict whether a gene is present in the sequence by searching for motifs such as promoters, coding regions, splice sites and functional protein motifs; these software tools are reviewed by Fickett (1996).

1.4 The primary structure of brain-expressed mRNAs

In 1988, Sutcliffe analyzed the complete mRNA sequences of 39 brain-expressed genes and made several general conclusions about the structure of brain-expressed mRNAs. Brain-specific mRNAs are longer in total, open reading frame (ORF) and 3′ UTR length than mRNAs which are expressed in the brain, but not specifically; by implication brain-expressed mRNAs are longer on average than mRNAs in other tissues. Brain mRNAs expressed at lower levels were longer still, again in ORF and 3′ UTR length. The actual average lengths found for 30 brain-specific mRNAs were: total mRNA length, 3690 nt; average ORF length, 1569 nt; average 5′ UTR length, 123 nt; average 3′ UTR length, 1303 nt. These special structural characteristics of brain mRNAs, if they are valid, might indicate that mRNA primary and secondary structure is more important in neurons (and glia) than in many other cell types. If so, it would be worthwhile focusing more attention on brain mRNA structure and function than has hitherto been the case. Since 1988 many hundreds more sequences have been deposited in GenBank and related databases, and it is therefore of interest to repeat the analysis on the 'complete' brain-expressed mRNA sequences now available in order to determine if the conclusions hold true.

The nucleotide entries in the GenBank databases are constantly being updated and augmented with new sequences, therefore some of the results of the searches quoted in this chapter may become out of date. However, the general trends quoted will still be valid given the large numbers of sequences already available for analysis.

1.4.1 Beginning the search for brain-expressed mRNAs

The search begins by asking for all the entries containing the word 'brain', yielding 25 901 entries. The majority of these entries are expected to be ESTs deposited as part of the various genome projects (e.g. the WashU-Merck EST Project for human sequences and the WashU-HHMI mouse EST Project) rather than complete mRNAs. This was confirmed when the search was refined using the word 'complete', which yielded only 955 entries. Refining the search further with mRNA gave 805 entries, with CDS 826 and cDNA, 403. What are the 129 entries that do not appear to contain cDNA, mRNA or CDS? A search performed using the Boolean expression 'brain [WORD] & complete [WORD] – mRNA [WORD] – cDNA [WORD] – CDS [WORD]' (i.e. which entries out of the 955 don't contain the words CDS, mRNA or cDNA) yields 65 human immunodeficiency virus (HIV) sequences which were puri-fied from the brains of patients with acquired immunodeficiency syndrome (AIDS)-related neurological disorders, while the remaining 64 entries are 63 mouse ESTs plus rat choline acetyltransferase exon 1 sequence.

Therefore we can safely take the 822 entries found using the CDS refinement as our start point. The analysis of the mRNA sequences was done on a species by species basis to make the analysis less tedious. The results are summarized in *Table 1.2*.

1.4.2 Average length of brain-expressed transcripts

The previous analysis indicated that the average brain-specific transcript was 3690 nucleotides in length and, on average, contained an ORF of 1569 nt. A somewhat wider set including some brain-expressed transcripts not specific to the brain, had an average transcript length of 3243 nt, with an average ORF 1385 nt in length and an average 3' UTR length of 1113 nt. Analysis of the present human brain complete mRNA set for these two parameters gives 2948 nt as the average length of the whole transcript and 1652 for the average length of an ORF. The reduction in the average of the transcript length compared to the earlier data is accounted for entirely by the smaller average 3' UTR length (818 nt) determined in this study. Otherwise the data are consistent. There has not, however, been the increase in average length of known brain transcripts that was predicted in 1988.

A comparative analysis of the human liver mRNA set allows us to examine whether

Table 1.2. Analysis of brain and liver mRNA primary structure

Property	Liver[a]	Human[b]	Mouse[c]	Rat[d]	Bovine[e]	Neuronal[f]
No. of entries	136	277	196	365	61	134
5' UTR average[g,h]	104	205	185	211	172	332
3' UTR average[i]	472	818	525	683	593	716
Transcript length[j]	2134	2948	—	—	—	3782
ORF length	1379	1652	—	—	—	1915

[a] Sequences found via Entrez using the text terms "liver", "complete" and "CDS". The search was further refined using "human" as the organism search term.
[b] Sequences found via Entrez using the text terms "brain", "complete" and "CDS". The search was further refined using "human" as the organism search term.
[c] As (b) but refined using "mouse" as the organism search term.
[d] As (b) but refined using "rat" as the organism search term.
[e] As (b) but refined using "bovine" as the organism search term.
[f] Sequences found via Entrez using the text terms "neuronal", "complete" and "CDS".
[g] All lengths in nucleotides.
[h] Only those sequences with explicit 5' UTR were used to determine the average.
[i] Only those sequences with explicit 3' UTR were used to determine the average.
[j] Only full length transcripts were used to determine the average.

brain mRNAs are larger, on average, than nonbrain transcripts. Liver was chosen because it was expected that there would be a large number of liver sequences in the databases. The search yielded 514 complete liver mRNAs of which 146 were human sequences. Of these, nine incomplete EST sequences were excluded plus one duplicate entry. The remaining 136 sequences were examined for transcript length, ORF size and 5′ and 3′ UTR length. As can be seen from *Table 1.2*, the average value for each parameter is less than that of the brain transcripts. These data show that brain transcripts are larger on average than nonbrain transcripts, with the ORF and particularly the 5′ and 3′ UTRs being relatively longer.

A subset of the 39 sequences, termed 'rarer specifics', which excluded known abundant mRNAs (those encoding major myelins, cytoskeletal proteins, retinal proteins, NSE and S100) was also examined in the 1988 data. It was shown that the rarer specifics had an average transcript length of 4954 nt, an ORF length of 2082 nt, a 5′ UTR length of 224 nt and a 3′ UTR length of 1669 nt. In this study, we regrouped the sequences now available into a more specific set by searching with the words 'neuronal' and 'complete' in order to look at sequences definitely expressed in neurons, some of them specifically. It is expected that the majority of these will not be highly expressed transcripts. The search provided 155 entries, 134 of which were analyzed for transcript length, 5′ UTR, 3′ UTR and ORF size. The 21 entries excluded included duplicate entries, partial exonic sequences, nonneuronal isoforms, vector sequences and five complete genes which contained contradictions between the length of the deduced protein sequence and the combined lengths of the exons. A complete list of the 134 neuronal sequences is given in *Table 1.3* along with the available information for transcript length, 5′ and 3′ UTR and ORF size; the average lengths are included in *Table 1.2*. The average transcript length for these neuronal genes is 3782 nt, which is considerably shorter than the earlier average of 4954 for the 1988 rarer transcripts class, but is indeed considerably longer than the average length of human brain mRNAs of 2948 nt; this difference is due to differences in ORF length (*Table 1.2*). The average ORF size agrees remarkably well with the 1988 data at 1915 nt compared with 2082 nt. The 5′ UTR appears to be, on average, slightly larger than previously determined; 332 nt as compared with 224. The 3′ UTR is significantly shorter on average than in the previous data (716 nt compared with 1669), and this accounts for the majority of the difference in observed transcript lengths. Thus it does seem to be the case that less highly expressed transcripts are longer, primarily due to encoding longer proteins, with somewhat longer 5′ UTRs.

1.4.3 The 5′ and 3′ UTRs

Comparing these results to those of Sutcliffe (1988), it can be seen that the newly determined average length of the 5′ UTR of 205 nt (human sequences) is close to the 224 nt 5′ UTR length of the rarer specific class and greater than the standard brain-specific length of 123 nt found previously, and that genes classed as neuronal have even longer 5′ UTRs at 332 nt. The average 3′ UTR length (818 nt) is significantly smaller than the earlier estimates of 1303 nt for average brain-specific mRNAs and 1669 for rarer specific mRNAs, but still longer than the 3′ UTRs of liver mRNAs. The results presented here are likely to be a more accurate representation of the average sizes of the 5′ and 3′ UTRs of neuronal genes given the larger data set used. The shorter 3′ UTR length is responsible for the shorter overall transcript lengths found here. The previous data also suggested that transcript and 3′ UTR lengths might be

Table 1.3. Neuronal mRNAs

Entry	Transcript[a]	5' UTR[b]	3' UTR[c]	ORF[d]
C. elegans SEM-4 short form	2759	—	—	2147
C. elegans SEM-4 long form	2843	—	—	2234
Mouse Cln3	1639	—	211	1316
Mouse PAF-AH gamma	872	—	—	698
Human potassium channel (Kir3.2)	2507	585	650	1272
Rat preprocortistatin	438	—	—	338
Human palmitoyl protein thioesterase	2279	—	—	920
Rat cannabinoid receptor (CB1)	—	—	—	1422
Mouse astrotactin	6863	—	—	2528
Rat tyrosine phosphatase	2104	—	—	1145
Rat P2X4 ATP-gated channel subunit	1793	—	—	1166
Rat nicotinic acetylcholine receptor subunit β-4	2461	—	947	1487
Mouse nervous system-specific RNA binding protein Mel-N1	2248	—	—	1083
Carassius auratus aldolase C	2061	73	1092	881
Bovine neuronal sodium-dependent glutamate aspartate transporter	3900	—	2130	1629
Human α-7 nicotinic acetylcholine receptor	1977	7	461	1509
Manduca sexta neuronal MNG10	—	—	11	690
Mouse embryonal calcinoma cell FGF 9	777	—	—	626
Rat neuronal cell death-related gene DN-7	2477	—	1692	762
Human protein tyrosine kinase (NET PTK)	3871	—	—	2955
Mouse G-protein-gated potassium channel GIRK4	—	—	—	1260
Rat high affinity glutamate transporter EAAC1	2284	—	519	1572
Human cyclin-dependent kinase 5 activator isoform p39i	1186	—	—	1104
Mus musculus G-protein-coupled potassium channel splice variant mGIRK2A	1998	—	—	1278
D. melanogaster neuron-specific zinc finger trancription factor (scratch)	3084	—	464	1995
D. melanogaster derailed receptor protein tyrosine kinase	3071	348	890	1833
Human zinc finger homeodomain protein	11 893	673	108	11 112
Human retinal nitric oxide synthase (NOS)	4340	—	—	4302
Rat limbic system-associated membrane protein	1238	—	—	1017
Rat neuronal nicotinic acetylcholine receptor-related protein	2895	—	—	1359
Mouse reeler mRNA	4960	—	—	2646
M. musculus myocyte enhancer factor-2A	1839	—	—	1497
Human ELAV-like neuronal protein-2 Hel-N2	2194	—	—	1041
Gallus gallus collapsin-2	2715	—	—	2286
X. laevis neuronal cyclin-dependent kinase 5	1270	—	—	879
Mouse neuronal helix–loop–helix protein NEX-1	1957	—	—	1014
C. elegans neuronal calcium binding protein 2	—	—	—	573
C. elegans neuronal calcium binding protein 1	—	—	—	576
Mouse nicotinic acetylcholine receptor subunit α-7	1848	50	289	1509
Human nicotinic acetylcholine receptor α-4 subunit	2082	—	—	1884
Haemopis marmorata intermediate filament filarin	2095	—	280	1794
Rattus norvegicus neuronal pentraxin precursor	5341	—	—	1299
C. elegans degenerin (deg-1)	2511	32	145	2337
R. norvegicus growth factor (Arc)	3032	—	—	1191
R. norvegicus fos-related antigen 2 (fra-2)	—	—	—	729
Human neuronal nitric oxide synthase (NOS1)	7124	—	—	4305
C. elegans nicotinic acetylcholine receptor α subunit precursor	1921	35	191	1694
Human MAP4	4696	—	—	3459

Table 1.3. (*continued*)

Entry	Transcript[a]	5′ UTR[b]	3′ UTR[c]	ORF[d]
Human neuronal apoptosis inhibitory protein	5414	307	1102	4006
D. melanogaster neurocalcin homolog DrosNCa	5441	305	1400	3606
Bos taurus dopamine and cyclic AMP-regulated neuronal phosphoprotein (DARPP-32)	1691	—	741	609
G. gallus Sox11 transcription factor	1977	363	423	1191
G. gallus Sox2 transcription factor	1355	258	149	948
G. gallus Sox3 transcription factor	1808	185	684	939
Rat protein tyrosine phosphatase PC12-PTP1	2910	—	1109	1239
D. melanogaster ethanolamine kinase	2229	—	—	1488
D. melanogaster (clone 5) ethanolamine kinase	4657	—	—	1554
Pig secreted neuronal and endocrine protein	1236	—	491	624
Mouse voltage-dependent α-1 E calcium channel	9864	602	2443	6819
Human ELAV-like neuronal protein 1 (hel-N1)	2233	584	569	1080
Human high affinity glutamate transporter	1620	—	—	1575
Mouse neuronal intermediate filament protein	3324	72	1737	1515
Mouse brain fatty acid-binding protein (B-FABP)	768	87	282	399
R. norvegicus glypican	1737	—	—	1677
R. norvegicus neuronal calcium sensor (NCS-1)	—	—	—	573
G. gallus neuronal calcium sensor (NCS-1)	—	—	—	573
Zebrafish insulin gene enhancer binding protein	2275	—	1018	1050
Human neuronal kinesin heavy chain	3840	—	—	3099
Homo sapiens voltage-dependent calcium channel α-1E-3 subunit	7089	165	111	6813
H. sapiens voltage-dependent calcium channel α-1E-1 subunit	7032	165	111	6756
M. musculus BALB/c telencephalin precursor	2931	—	137	2754
B. taurus auxilin	4531	131	1666	2733
Rat synaptotagmin III	2096	—	—	1767
C. elegans protein kinase C (PKC1B)	2514	21	346	2124
Rabbit telencephalin	3013	—	—	2739
Rat nicotinic acetylcholine receptor β-2 subunit	2196	—	—	1512
Rat nicotinic acetylcholine receptor α-3 subunit	1858	—	—	1500
B. taurus neurexin I-β	3346	—	—	1314
Human voltage-operated calcium channel α-1 subunit	7110	—	174	6936
R. norvegicus clone 1B426bBMZ neuronal olfactomedin-related ER localized protein	2759	—	—	1458
R. norvegicus clone 1B426bAMZ neuronal olfactomedin-related ER localized protein	2621	—	—	1374
R. norvegicus clone 1B426bBMY neuronal olfactomedin-related ER localized protein	1077	—	—	462
R. norvegicus clone 1B426bAMY neuronal olfactomedin-related ER localized protein	938	—	—	378
R. norvegicus cerebroglycan	2607	—	632	1740
Human sterol carrier protein-2 (SCP-2)	1219	—	704	432
Human sterol carrier protein 2	1500	—	—	870
G. gallus collapsin	3251	—	765	2319
R. rattus protein tyrosine phosphatase	1908	—	678	1104
R. norvegicus transcription factor (Olf-1)	2221	72	436	1713
Rat mRNA for 14–3–3 protein η-subtype	1689	—	—	741
Mouse mRNA for nitric oxide synthase	4388	—	—	4290
D. melanogaster cell adhesion molecule encoding	3726	—	—	3036
Human neurofibromin (NF1)	9026	—	—	8520
X. laevis mRNA for A5-protein	3800	—	—	2784
X. laevis neuronal intermediate filament protein	2290	—	—	1413
X. laevis low molecular weight neurofilament protein	2111	—	—	1635
Gallus domesticus nicotinic acetylcholine receptor α-5 subunit	—	—	—	1365
G. domesticus nicotinic acetylcholine receptor α-3 subunit	—	—	—	1491

Table 1.3. (*continued*)

Entry	Transcript[a]	5' UTR[b]	3' UTR[c]	ORF[d]
R. norvegicus neuronal protein (NP25)	1007	68	279	660
Rat neuronal nicotinic acetylcholine receptor α-2 subunit	1931	—	—	1535
R. norvegicus neurocan	5191	—	—	3926
Rat neuronal nicotinic acetylcholine receptor β-3 subunit	2188	—	—	1395
Rat cholinergic neuronal differentiation factor	—	—	—	609
Rat delayed rectifier potassium channel (K-V-4)	3977	1161	1058	1758
Drosophila hairy gene homolog	1609	—	—	846
Rat neuronal growth protein 43 (GAP-43)	1153	—	—	701
Rat β-alanine-sensitive GABA transporter	2062	—	—	1884
R. rattus GABA-A receptor γ-2 subunit	1838	—	—	1401
R. rattus GABA-A receptor δ-subunit gene	1794	—	414	1350
Rat (clone nclk) cdc2-related protein kinase	1161	—	189	879
Rat calcium channel β-subunit-III	2525	—	—	1455
Mouse neuronal proto-oncogene *c-src* mRNA encoding tyrosine-specific protein kinase	—	—	—	1626
M. musculus SNAP-25	2040	—	—	621
Mouse TAFG-1-like neuronal glycoprotein	3448	—	—	3087
Mouse neuronal dihydropyridine-sensitive L-type calcium channel α-1 subunit	9014	1166	1428	6420
Mouse AE3	4060	—	—	3684
Human protein phosphatase 2A β-subunit	3441	525	1584	1332
Human protein phosphatase 2A α-subunit	2131	105	682	1344
Human α-3 nicotinic acetylcholine receptor subunit	1880	—	299	1512
Human neurofibromatosis protein type I (NF1)	—	—	—	1197
Human neuronal growth protein 43 (GAP-43)	1231	—	—	717
Human DHP-sensitive, voltage-dependent, calcium channel α-1D subunit	7635	—	—	6486
Human DHP-sensitive, voltage-dependent, calcium channel α-2b subunit	3600	—	—	3276
Human DHP-sensitive, voltage-dependent, calcium channel β-2 subunit	1546	—	—	1437
H. sapiens nicotinic acetylcholine receptor α-5 subunit	1679	—	—	1407
H. sapiens nicotinic acetylcholine receptor α-3 subunit	1584	—	—	1509
Rabbit protein phosphatase 2A β-subunit	1506	—	264	1242
Grasshopper fasciclin I	3137	—	—	1989
D. melanogaster Pros protein (prospero)	6404	—	1093	4224
D. melanogaster G nucleotide binding protein α subunit	1340	—	—	1065
D. melanogaster fasciclin I	2993	—	—	1959
D. melanogaster fasciclin II (Fas2B)	3070	—	—	2622
D. melanogaster fasciclin II (Fas2A)	2818	—	—	2436
D. melanogaster DNA-binding prot. (erect wing)	4812	1962	—	2202

[a] Length in nucleotides. Dashes indicate entries which only contained the protein coding region of the mRNA.

[b] Length in nucleotides. Dashes indicate entries with no or partial 5' UTR.

[c] Length in nucleotides. Dashes indicate entries with no or partial 3' UTR.

[d] Length in nucleotides.

Note: the set of mRNA sequences listed here comprise those database entries accessed by using the terms 'neuronal' and 'complete' in Entrez, with some exclusions (see Section 1.4.2). Despite the text terms used to search, these mRNAs are not all complete sequences and are not necessarily neuron-specific.

correlated. *Figure 1.2* shows a plot of transcript length against 3' UTR length for the subset of human mRNAs in the databases which have a complete 3' UTR. As can be seen there is no strong correlation between the length of the transcript and the length of the 3' UTR. There is a suggestion of a clustering of 3' UTR lengths below 1000 bp.

1.4.4 Conclusions of the analysis of brain-expressed mRNA structure

Using the Entrez software via the World Wide Web, we have analyzed the available sequence information for 799 brain-expressed mRNAs. Comparing our data with those of Sutcliffe (1988), we conclude that in general brain mRNAs are indeed larger than nonbrain mRNAs and that rarer transcripts are larger still. Brain transcripts have longer ORFs, 3' and 5' UTRs than liver transcripts. Less highly expressed brain transcripts have longer 5' UTRs and ORFs than average brain transcripts, but the 3' UTRs are of similar lengths. However, the average brain mRNA lengths in this larger study are less than in the 1988 study. This is accounted for almost entirely by the observed shorter average length of the 3' UTR. Indeed, in the case of transcripts defined as neuronal rather than brain, the average 3' UTR length is less than half that found by Sutcliffe in rarer transcripts. We also found no correlation between transcript length and the length of the 3' UTR. The differences between these data and the previous set are that 5' UTRs are longer and 3' UTRs shorter, although still long.

The occurrence of longer ORFs in the mRNAs of brain and neuronal genes reflects a higher frequency of large proteins in the brain; this is perhaps not surprising in view of the large array of adhesion molecules, receptors and channels expressed in the brain, and the likelihood that the 'neuronal' database is somewhat biased towards such proteins. There is growing evidence, largely from work in yeast, for important roles of both 3' and 5' UTR sequences in determining susceptibility to specific mRNA degradation systems (Beelman *et al.*, 1996) and thus intrinsic mRNA turnover rates. The 5' UTR in particular is involved in determining translation efficiency also, and may interact with the 3' UTR in this function; moreover, interaction of 3' and 5' UTR RNA–protein complexes has been implicated in control of localization of maternal

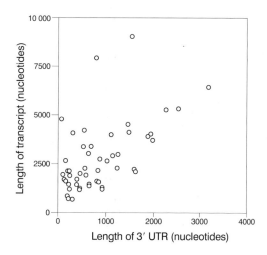

Figure 1.2. Human brain mRNA against 3' UTR.

mRNAs. The fact that the 3' and 5' UTRs of brain and neuronal genes are particularly long presumably reflects a particularly important and complex role for mRNA secondary structure in regulating neuronal mRNA translation efficiency and stability, and also such widespread neuronal phenomena as RNA editing, alternative RNA splicing and mRNA localization to cellular compartments.

References

Adams MD, Dubnick M, Kerlavage AR, Moreno R, Kelley JM, Utterback TR, Nagle JW, Fields C, Venter JC. (1992) Sequence identification of 2375 human brain genes. *Nature* 355: 632–634.

Adams MD, Kerlavage AR, Fields C Venter JC. (1993) 3400 new expressed sequence tags identify diversity of transcripts in human brain. *Nature Genetics* 4: 256–257.

Altschul SF, Gish W, Miller W, Myers EW, Lipman DJ. (1990) Basic local alignment search tool. *J. Mol. Biol.* 215: 403–410.

Ashworth LK, Batzer MA, Brandriff B *et al.* (1995) A metric physical map of human chromosome 19. *Nature Genetics* 11: 422–427.

Bauer D, Warthue P, Rohde L, Struss M. (1994) In: *PCR Methods and Applications.* Cold Spring Harbor Laboratory Press, Cold Spring Harbor, NY, pp. S97–S108.

Beelman CA, Stevens A, Caponigro G, LaGrandeur TE, Hatfield L, Fortner DM, Parker R. (1996) An essential component of the decapping enzyme required for normal rates of mRNA turnover. *Nature* 382: 643–647.

Bertioli DJ, Schlichter UHA, Adams MJ, Burrows PR, Steinbiss H-H, Antoniw JF. (1995) An analysis of differential display shows a strong bias towards high copy number messenger RNAs. *Nucleic Acids Res.* 23: 4520–4523.

Cooley L, Berg C, Spradling A. (1988) Controlling P-element insertional mutagenesis. *Trends Genet* 4: 254–258.

Dalal SS, Welsh J, Tkachenko A, Ralph D, Dicicco-Bloom E, Bordas L, McClelland M, Chada K. (1994) Rapid isolation of tissue-specific and developmentally regulated brain cDNAs using RNA arbitrarily primed PCR (RAP-PCR). *J. Mol. Neurosci.* 5: 93–104.

Davies RW, Roberts AB, Morris AJ, Griffith GW, Jerecic J, Ghandi S, Kaiser K, Savioz A. (1994) Enhanced access to rare brain cDNAs by prescreening libraries: 207 new mouse brain ESTs. *Genomics* 24: 456–463.

Diatchenko L, Lau Y-F C, Campbell AP *et al.* (1996) Suppression subtractive hybridization: a method for generating differentially regulated or tissue-specific cDNA probes and libraries. *Proc. Natl Acad. Sci. USA* 93: 6025–6030.

Drescher U, Kremoser C, Handwerker C, Löschinger J, Noda M, Bonhoeffer F. (1995) *In vitro* guidance of retinal ganglion cell axons by RAGS, a 25 kDa tectal protein related to ligands for Eph-receptor tyrosine kinases. *Cell* 82: 359–370.

Duguid JR, Rohwer RG, Seed B. (1988) Isolation of cDNAs of scrapie-modulated RNAs by subtractive hybridization of a cDNA library. *Proc. Natl Acad. Sci. USA* 85: 5738–5742.

Fickett JW. (1996) Finding genes by computer: the state of the art. *Trends Genet.* 12: 316–320.

Guo Y, Gillan A, Török T, Kiss I, Dow JAT, Kaiser K. (1996) Site-selected mutagenesis of the *Drosophila* second chromosome via plasmid rescue of lethal P-element insertions. *Genome Res.*, in press.

Hubank M, Schatz DG (1994) Identifying differences in messenger RNA expression by representational difference analysis of cDNA. *Nucleic Acids Res.* 22: 5640–5648.

Human Genome News (1995) 7, no.3/4: 4–9.

Human Genome News (1996) 7, no.5: 10–12.

Jockusch H, Nave K-A, Grenningloh G, Schmitt-John T. (1996) Molecular genetics of nervous and neuromuscular systems. In: *Molecular Biology of the Neuron* (eds RW Davies, B Morris). BIOS Scientific Publishers, Oxford, pp. 21–66.

Kato K. (1992) Finding new genes in the nervous system by cDNA analysis. *Trends Neurosci.* 15: 319–323.

Khan AS, Wilcox AS, Polymeropoulos MH, Hopkins JA, Stevens TJ, Robinson M, Orpana AK, Sikela JM. (1992) Single-pass sequencing and physical and genetic mapping of human brain cDNAs. *Nature Genetics* 2: 180–185.

Klein RD, Gu Q, Goddard A, Rosenthal A. (1996) Selection for genes encoding secreted proteins and receptors. *Proc. Natl Acad. Sci. USA* 93: 7108–7113.

Kuwada J. (1995) Development of the zebrafish nervous system: genetic analysis and manipulation. *Curr. Opin. Neurobiol.* **5**: 50–54.

Liang P, Pardee A. (1992) Differential display of eukaryotic messenger RNA by means of the polymerase chain reaction. *Science* **257**: 967–970.

Lisitsyn N, Lisitsyn N, Wigler M. (1993) Cloning the differences between two complex genomes. *Science* **259**: 946–951.

Milosavljevic A, Zeremski M, Strezoska Z et al. (1996) Discovering distinct genes represented in 29,750 clones from infant brain cDNA libraries by applying sequencing by hybridization methodology. *Genome Res.* **6**: 132–141.

Porteus MH, Brice EJ, Bulfone A, Usdin TB, Ciaranello RD, Rubenstein JLR. (1992) Isolation and characterization of a library of cDNA clones that are preferentially expressed in the embryonic telencephalon. *Mol. Brain Res.* **12**: 7–22.

Rhyner TA, Fauco Biguet N, Berrard S, Borbely AA, Mallet J. (1986) An efficient approach for the selective isolation of specific transcripts from complex brain mRNA populations. *J. Neurosci. Res.* **16**: 167.

Rubenstein JLR, Brice AEJ, Ciaranello RD, Denney D, Porteus MH, Usdin TB. (1990) Subtractive hybridization system using single-stranded phagemids with directional inserts. *Nucleic Acids Res.* **18**: 4833–4842.

Savioz A, Davies RW. (1995) Discovering genes with localised expression in the mouse brain: cDNAs specific to the substantia nigra. *Gene* **154**: 225–230.

Schuler GD, Epstein JA, Ohkawa H, Kans JA. (1996) Entrez: molecular biology database and retrieval system. *Meth. Enzymol* **266**: 141–62.

Seeger M, Tear G, Ferres-Marco D, Goodman CS. (1993) Mutations affecting growth cone guidance in *Drosophila*: genes necessary for guidance toward or away from the midline. *Neuron* **10**: 409–426.

Sentry JW, Goodwin SF, Milligan CD, Duncanson A, Yang M, Kaiser K. (1994) Reverse genetics of *Drosophila* brain structure and function. *Prog. Neurobiol.* **42**: 299–308.

Siebert PD, Chenchik A, Kellogg DE, Lukyanov KL, Lukyanov SA. (1995) An improved PCR method for walking in uncloned DNA. *Nucleic Acids Res.* **23**: 1087–1088.

Skarnes WC, Auerbach BA, Joyner AL. (1992) A gene trap approach in mouse embryonic stem cells: the lacZ reporter is activated by splicing, reflects endogenous gene expression, and is mutagenic in mice. *Genes Dev.* **6**: 903–918.

Skarnes WC, Moss JE, Hurtley SM, Beddington RSP. (1995) Capturing genes encoding membrane and secreted proteins important for mouse development. *Proc. Natl Acad. Sci. USA* **92**: 6592–6596.

Sompayrac L, Jane S, Burn TC, Tenen DG, Danna KJ. (1995) Overcoming limitations of the messenger RNA differential display technique. *Nucleic Acids Res.* **23**: 4738–4739.

Stewart GA, Savioz A, Davies RW. (1996) Sequence analysis of 497 mouse brain ESTs expressed in the substantia nigra. *Genomics*, in press.

Stahl B, Müller B, von Boxberg Y, Cox EC, Bonhoeffer F. (1990) Biochemical characterization of a putative axonal guidance molecule of the chick visual system. *Neuron* **5**: 733–743.

Sutcliffe GJ. (1988) mRNA in the mammalian central nervous system. *Annu. Rev. Neurosci.* **11**: 157–98.

Swaroop A, Xu J, Agarwal N, Weissman SM. (1991) A simple and efficient cDNA library subtraction procedure: isolation of human retina-specific cDNA clones. *Nucleic Acids Res.* **19**: 1954.

Tashiro K, Tada H, Heilker R, Shirozu M, Nakano T, Honjo T. (1993) Signal sequence trap – a cloning stategy for secreted proteins and type-1 membrane proteins. *Science* **261**: 6000–6003.

Török T, Tick G, Alvarado M, Kiss I. (1993) P-lacW insertional mutagenesis on the second chromosome of *Drosophila melanogaster*: isolation of lethals with different overgrowth phenotypes. *Genetics* **133**: 347–359.

Welsh J, Chada K, Dalal SS, Ralph D, Cheng L, McClelland M. (1992) Arbitrarily primed PCR fingerprinting of RNA. *Nucleic Acids Res.* **20**: 4965–4970.

Molecular genetics of nervous and neuromuscular systems

Harald Jockusch, Klaus-Armin Nave, Gabriele Grenningloh and Thomas Schmitt-John

2.1. Introduction

2.1.1 'Physiological genetics' as applied to the nervous system

The study of genetics is fundamental to all biology because it deals with the material basis of continuity of life from viruses to man. By the exploitation of natural and induced mutations, genetics can be a powerful tool to elucidate the control mechanisms that allow complicated biological structures to emerge. This principle has been used for many decades to unravel metabolic pathways and was first applied to the analysis of morphogenesis in the case of a virus, bacteriophage T4. It is less obvious how genetics would contribute to the understanding of the emergence of a nervous system from the very beginning of the fertilized egg, or to the understanding of its function and maintenance, of neuronal plasticity, learning and behavior.

In classical neurobiology, the analysis of cellular and molecular mechanisms of function was usually based on surgical and pharmacological experiments. Several natural toxins, of both plant and animal origin, bind with high specificity to certain receptors as well as to chemosensitive and voltage-gated ion channels of the nervous system. Thus, it was possible to apply these molecules as research tools to dissect functional cascades in the central nervous and neuromuscular systems and to allow for a biochemical approach to neurobiology despite the extremely low concentrations of receptor and channel proteins involved. However, there are no toxins that would be particularly helpful in studying development in general and neurogenesis in particular. In classical neuroembryology, surgical experiments (ablation, reconstitution) and experiments using organ cultures were of great importance. Yet, the more recent genetic approach has led to remarkable insights, and its importance for basic neurobiology is ever growing.

2.1.2 Neurogenetics and disease

With spina bifida (Epstein *et al.*, 1991) and epilepsy (Steinlein *et al.*, 1995) as examples, it is obvious that both developmental and functional aspects of the nervous

Molecular Biology of the Neuron, edited by R.W. Davies and B.J. Morris.
© 1997 BIOS Scientific Publishers Ltd, Oxford.

system are susceptible to pathological aberrations, and hence may be targets of genetic mutations. Thus, there is growing interest in understanding neurological conditions in genetic terms. In contrast with the physiological and pharmacological approaches to neurological diseases, the genetic approach can be successful without any physiological or biochemical concept or prejudice with regard to the affected function. In human and mouse genetics, this approach, called 'positional cloning', starts with the chromosomal localization of the 'disease gene' under investigation and ends, if successful, with the molecular description of disease-causing mutations. Examples of this type of analysis will be given in this chapter: quite often the results obtained with this method have been rather surprising. Another application of the genetic approach to human neurological diseases is their analysis and simulation by transgenic animal models.

Mutations are the essence of genetics – they reveal themselves as a phenotypic difference, called a 'mutant phenotype' with reference to a standard or 'wild-type' phenotype. Initially genetics relied on spontaneous mutations, such as 'albino' mutations in vertebrates. Their lack of pigmentation turned out to be due to a simple enzyme defect, inactive or absent tyrosinase, which incidentally has interesting side effects on the wiring of optic nerves (Guillery, 1974). Experimentally induced mutations, among these the gene locus targeted 'knockouts', are at present essential research tools in the recursive method of correlating gene structure and genomic organization with gene function and phenotype. An important feature of present-day genetics is the cyclic nature of analysis, as exemplified by the study of human neurological disease genes. Depending on one's expertise, one may step on to the 'carousel of experimental genetics' at any place, using gene mapping, physiological and protein biochemical analysis, expression studies, or sequence homology screens. If the gene is known but no mutation available, a functional analysis requires the specific elimination of this gene function. For vertebrates, the experimental approach is the targeted 'knockout' of a gene, introduced by Capecchi and co-workers (Thomas and Capecchi, 1987) for the mouse. This method is applicable to any gene function, essential or nonessential, yet requires the genomic structure of the gene to be known (Brandon *et al.*, 1995a,b,c).

Despite advanced methodology, experimental geneticists still rely on what Nature presents: some organisms are amenable to genetic analysis, and others are simply not. Marine organisms that play such an important role in neurophysiology (e.g. *Limulus*, crustaceans, *Aplysia*, *Loligo*, and *Torpedo*) cannot at present be analyzed by the methods of experimental genetics, mostly because their life cycles are too elaborate and/or take too much time. The clawfrog *Xenopus*, chickens and cats are favorite experimental animals of neuroembryologists and neurophysiologists, mostly used in conjunction with surgical approaches. Again, experimental genetics has so far not been feasible with these animals. This is the reason why the following chapter will deal with only a few species of animals ('model organisms'; *Table 2.1*), like the fruitfly and the house mouse, and man himself, the only organism that can report his ailments, and therefore has an extremely low threshold for discovering mutations with marginal effects.

2.2 Developmental neurogenetics: emergence and compartmentalization of the nervous system

In current developmental biology three players dominate the stage: transcription factors, nuclear proteins that regulate gene expression by binding to specific DNA

Table 2.1. Favored organisms used in neurogenetics

Species	Duration of life cycle (days)	Number of chromosomes	Genome size	Number of neurons	Special features
Nematode *Caenorhabditis elegans*[a]	3	2×5 XX, X0	8×10^7 bp	3×10^2	Self fertile hermaphrodite. Can be stored frozen and grown in fermenters
Fruitfly *Drosophila melanogaster*	11	2×3 XX, X0	1.6×10^8 bp	10^5	Genetic control of embryonic morphogenesis well known
Zebrafish *Danio rerio*	90	2×29	1.7×10^9 bp	10^8	Parthenogenetic development possible
Mouse *Mus musculus*	90	2×19 XX, XY	2.7×10^9 bp	10^9	Gene knockouts possible
Man[b] *Homo sapiens*	10 000	2×22 XX, XY	3.3×10^9 bp	10^{12}	Many alleles available for most disease genes

[a] Sequencing of the entire genome will be completed in 1998.
[b] This species designation refers to both sexes.

sequences; signaling molecules, secreted or cell-surface bound polypeptides which transmit messages from one cell to another; and their receptors, allosteric transmembrane proteins which, upon the binding of the corresponding signaling molecule, transduce the message to the interior of the cell, often by activating their own intracellular catalytic (kinase) domain and by phosphorylating other proteins. This signal cascade in turn influences the activity of transcription factors.

2.2.1 Neurons vs. epidermal cells

The divergence between the presumptive nervous system and cells destined for other tissues is among the earliest events in metazoan development. Considering that unicellular organisms like protozoa combine, within one cell, properties typical of the nervous system, such as light sensitivity and an excitable plasma membrane, with the 'vegetative physiology' of ingesting and digesting food particles, and the potential to divide, one might expect that the fate of becoming a neuron is less in need of specification than is the suppression of excitability and other neuronal properties that are absent from nonneural cells. This view is indeed supported by observations on *Drosophila* mutants that cause an imbalance between neuronal and nonneuronal cells.

The mutation *Notch*, discovered in *Drosophila* many decades ago (1916) by Morgan, has taught us fascinating lessons on the initiation of the nervous system, both in insects and in vertebrates. The gene *Notch* codes for a receptor, and the corresponding ligand is coded for by the gene *Delta*. These genes are expressed in the same ectodermal cells in the *Drosophila* embryo. Defective mutations (the ones after which the genes have been named, as is the usage in *Drosophila* genetics) cause an overproduction of neurons. Hence, the neuronal development of ectodermal cells is the default pathway, the suppression of which favors epidermal determination. Thus, the *Notch–Delta* system, in its functional wild-type state, has a negative cell-fate-determining function which is exerted by lateral inhibition: cells that, within the ectodermal layer, happen to have a slight head start towards neurogenesis, secrete the Delta protein which acts on the Notch receptor of their neighbors. The signal received, in turn inhibits the initial stages of neurogenesis. With this simplified description, it may not be evident that this interpretation was the result of ingenious and extensive genetic analyses on *Drosophila*. After the identification of the genes at the DNA level and with nucleic acid (or 'molecular') methods at hand, it took much less time to demonstrate the relevance of the homologs of *Notch* and *Delta* in vertebrate systems. The principle is obviously similar in the amphibian to that realized in the *Drosophila* embryo: the *Notch–Delta* signaling pathway serves to suppress the default determination of neurons in favor of that of epidermal cells. Interestingly, the Notch transmembrane protein carries, in a 36-fold repetition, a sequence motif related to the epidermal growth factor. The same motif, though with much lower repeat numbers, is found in *Caenorhabditis* homologs of *Notch*. In *Drosophila* and in *Caenorhabditis*, the *Notch–Delta* system is also used in germ layers other than ectoderm to promote the decision between two cell types (review: Nye and Kopan, 1995).

As *Drosophila* geneticists found out, among the targets of the *Notch–Delta* signal are neuron-determining transcription factors. In *Drosophila* wild-type, the *Notch–Delta* system suppresses neurogenesis by suppressing the activity of *achaete-scute* transcription factors. In the claw frog *Xenopus*, gene transplantation studies have shown that the homolog of *achaete-scute* 'Xash' (for '*Xenopus achaete scute homolog*') is able to induce supernumerary neurons in the dorsal ectoderm. Are the *achaete-scute* homologs required for the formation of the central nervous system (CNS) in vertebrates (i.e. what is the consequence of loss-of-function mutations?). Here knockout mice provided an answer: loss of the mammalian gene '*Mash1*' eliminates parts of the nervous system, olfactory sensory neurons and the peripheral autonomic system (Guillemot *et al.*, 1993).

As in myogenesis, determination in neurogenesis is followed by the first steps of cell type-specific differentiation, again governed by transcription factors. A screen was conducted for new transcription factors of the basic–helix–loop–helix (bHLH) type, using a yeast expression system and interaction with the partner proteins, E proteins, that form bHLH-E heterodimers. The expectation was that transcription factors of the bHLH family would play a role in neurogenesis analogous to that of myogenic bHLH transcription factors in muscle formation. A factor termed NeuroD was discovered which, in the mouse, shows an expression pattern compatible with a role in postmitotic neuronal differentiation. Furthermore, the corresponding gene, when injected into *Xenopus* embryos, could override the inhibitory dermal influences on the ectoderm and convert it into neural ectoderm (Lee *et al.*, 1995). There is as yet no direct evidence for the role of this gene family in mammalian development.

2.2.2 Subdivision of the neural tube

The molecular mechanisms for the principal decision making in development are similar in mammals and flies, despite the fundamental differences in their anatomy, such as a dorsally located spinal cord in vertebrates vs. a ventral nerve cord in arthropods. The usefulness of *Drosophila* genetics for the understanding of vertebrate neuroembryology is witnessed not only by the *Notch–Delta* system but also by another gene, *hedgehog* (*hh*). This gene was discovered in *Drosophila*, cloned and its vertebrate homolog identified and dubbed *sonic hedgehog* (*shh*, after a 'hero' in a cartoon; Echelard *et al.*, 1993). *Drosophila hh* and vertebrate *shh* both provide important signals for patterning, but in different contexts. *Drosophila hh* was discovered as a segmentation gene of the segment polarity-determining type (i.e. the wild-type allele functions in the last steps of the subdivision of the arthropod body along the anterior–posterior axis) and loss-of-function mutant larvae are abnormally segmented and therefore reminiscent of a hedgehog (i.e. with a higher density of bristles). The *Drosophila* gene product was recognized as a secreted protein that autoproteolyzes to yield peptides which act as diffusible signaling factors. In the vertebrate embryo, the source of the homologous sonic hedgehog SHH signal is the notochord, the axial skeletal structure which induces ventral specializations in the neural tube, the floor plate and the motoneurons (*Figure 2.1*). With progressing development, the neural tube itself expresses SHH with a temporal pattern dependent on anterior–posterior position, and the *shh* gene may thus contribute to the axial compartmentalization of both the spinal cord and the brain (for review see: Lumsden and Graham, 1995). Furthermore, SHH secretion by the forebrain is important for the proximal differentiation of the eye, as exemplified by the *cyclops* mutation in zebrafish, in which SHH secreting cells are lacking in the forebrain (Ekker *et al.*, 1995). No spontaneous mutations in the *shh* gene(s) of vertebrates or a disease associated with its function are known at present. Obviously, a knockout of the *shh* gene would be of great interest.

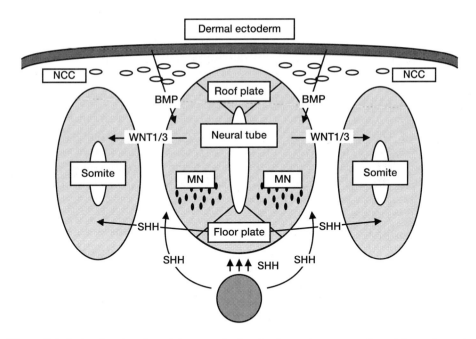

Figure 2.1. Inductive signals and the neural tube. A schematic cross-section of the embryonic neural tube and the notochord is shown. The dorsoventral specificity of the neural tube is induced by antagonistic external signals. The dermal ectoderm induces dorsal specificity by secreting peptides of the bone morphogenic protein (BMP) type. These inductive influences are suppressed by the sonic hedgehog peptide (SHH) secreted by the notochord. SHH independently induces the floor plate and motoneurons, the characteristic neurons of the ventral spinal cord and brain stem. The neural tube in turn by secretion of Wnt type signaling molecules (WNT; dorsal) and of SHH (ventral) induces neighboring somites to differentiate (see Liem *et al.*, 1995; Munsterberg *et al.*, 1995; Tanabe *et al.*, 1995). NCC, neural crest cells; MN, motoneurons.

The signaling pathways in vertebrates have been elucidated mainly by ablation, transplantation and organ culture experiments, but the identity of the molecules involved (i.e. diffusible factors and their receptors and that of the markers of region-alization) were based on *Drosophila* genetics. Such markers are *paired box* (*pax*) and *homeobox* (*hox*) genes. The *hox* genes were discovered in *Drosophila* as their loss-of-function and gain-of-function mutant alleles lead to bizarre transformations of one organ into another. Some of these mutations, like *antennapedia* or *bithorax* are compat-ible with the life of an adult fly, the 'imago' on the phenotype of which classical *Drosophila* genetics was based. The *paired* type genes were identified in mutant screens for segmentation abnormalities, as scored on larvae. They function in the second stage of axial subdivision from a tripartite stage to seven double segments, which is followed by the division into 14 proper segments, and their subdivision into anterior and posterior compartments, by the segment polarity genes mentioned above. The study of homeotic genes of *Drosophila* paved the way for a whole new area of molecu-lar developmental biology. They are characterized by a typical sequence stretch of 60 amino acid residues, the homeobox (HOX), which was found to be highly conserved among a wide variety of organisms. A gene complex of at least nine homeobox genes was defined in *Drosophila*, and the expression of these genes along the body axis turned out to be correlated with their chromosomal position.

After characterizing *Hox* genes in vertebrates on the basis of molecular homology it was found that in mouse and man, there are four *Hox* gene complexes, instead of one as in *Drosophila* and that there is a correlation between the position of single genes within a complex and their expression along the anterior–posterior axis. Thus not only is the homeobox conserved, but also the organization of *Hox* gene clusters (*Figure 2.2*; McGinnis and Krumlauf, 1992).

In both cases, the regional pattern of expression reflects that these genes respond to positional signals. What is the function of *Hox* genes in the development of verte-brates, specifically of their CNS? Knockouts (KO) of single *Hox* genes in most cases did not have very dramatic effects in the mouse. Some defects were observed in the *Hox* A1-KO mouse in the formation of the axial skeleton and the CNS, but these were relatively mild. More pronounced homeotic transformations were found in another mouse mutant which lacked HOX C8 function (Le Mouellic *et al.*, 1992): certain skeletal segments had assumed a more anterior phenotype so that segment identity was transformed. However, the neurological symptoms of surviving HOX C8-KO mice showed no clear relationship to homeotic segment transformation. In verte-brates, genuine neural segmentation is confined to the brain and is particularly appar-ent in the rhombomere organization of the hindbrain. *Hox* gene expression follows rather than produces this pattern. The anatomical segmentation of the spinal cord is obviously not of neural origin but is imposed by the primary segmentation of the adjacent mesoderm into somites. Therefore, a direct and general genetic mechanism for segmentation of the vertebrate CNS might not exist.

The *Pax* genes, the other example of genes borrowed from *Drosophila*, have been more useful in elucidating the basis of hereditary diseases in man and mouse. The eye is a specialized evagination of the brain. The mutation '*small eye*' (*sey*) of the mouse and a human disease mutation '*aniridia*' (lack of iris) are genetically homologous, and both turned out to be due to defects in the gene *Pax6*, one member of the *Pax* gene family of transcription factors. Although the mutant effects in humans mainly con-cern the iris, the *Pax6* /aniridia gene is expressed in the neural retina and other parts

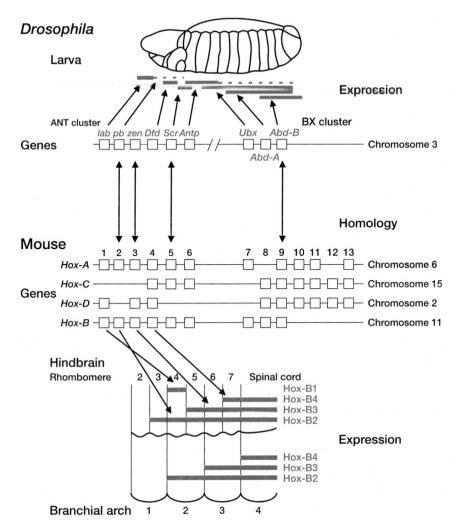

Figure 2.2. Axial expression patterns of homeobox (*Hox*) genes in *Drosophila* and mouse. Homeotic genes determine segment identity in *Drosophila* (upper part). They are grouped on chromosome 3 in gene complexes *Antennapedia* and *Bithorax*. The chromosomal order of the genes within the complexes is correlated with their axial expression pattern. In the mouse (lower part), four homeobox (HOX) gene complexes are located on four different chromosomes. Mouse *Hox* genes show a segmental expression pattern related to the axial subdivision of the brain, especially the segmentation into rhombomeres of the hindbrain. The spinal cord is secondarily segmented by interaction with the segmented somites. Modified after McGinnis and Krumlauf (1992).

of the neural ectoderm. Most likely *Pax6* is involved in inductive pathways between the eyecup and the overlying epidermis so that several different tissues can be affected by loss-of-function mutations of *Pax6* (Grindley *et al.*, 1995; Ton *et al.*, 1991). On the other hand, ectopic expression of *Pax6* in *Drosophila* has a gain-of-function effect and induces extra eyes (Halder *et al.*, 1995). This supports the hypothesis that *Pax6* is the master gene in eye development.

The counterparts of transcription factors are signaling molecules. A striking example of regional importance of a gene coding for a putative signaling molecule (a secreted peptide) for the nervous system is *Wnt1*. The *Wnt1* gene is exclusively expressed in the CNS and in testis. Originally *Wnt1* was discovered in the mouse as a proto-oncogene, an integration site for a retrovirus, and therefore designated *int1*. The wild-type allele *int1* was found to share amino acid sequence homology with the *Drosophila* segment polarity gene *wingless* (*wg*) and was therefore renamed *Wnt1*. *Wnt1* was knocked out in mice, and this led to highly defined ablations in the CNS: most of the midbrain and part of the rostral metencephalon were missing in affected (i.e. homozygous KO) mouse midgestation embryos. In neonates, midbrain and cerebellum were missing, and the mice died within 24 h (McMahon and Bradley, 1990; Thomas and Capecchi, 1990).

Similar regional effects have been found in mice in which a zinc finger-type transcription factor gene, termed *Krox20* (the name is derived, by fusion, from *Krüppel*, a *Drosophila* homeobox gene and *Hox*), had been knocked out. This gene is specifically transcribed in two alternate segments (rhombomeres r3 and r5) of the developing hindbrain. Affected mice die during the first 2 weeks after birth. Rhombomeres r3 and r5 are either reduced in size or missing. Thus, *Krox20* activity is specifically required for further development of two particular rhombomeres, whereas another regulatory pathway is responsible for the delimitation of rhombomeres and the assignment of their identity (Schneider-Manoury *et al.*, 1993).

The following overall picture emerges as to the genetic control of origin and compartmentalization of the nervous system: the initial decision within the ectoderm of 'neural vs. nonneural' is brought about by intercellular signaling. The response (i.e. fate determination) to these signals involves transcription factors as the main players. Intercellular signaling controls the number and distribution of neurons in the context of the developing embryo. The following regionalization is again due to an interplay between cell-to-cell signaling and specific patterns of gene activity in response to these signals, mediated by another set of transcription factors responsible for cell determination and early differentiation. Quite often, the signaling pathways important for neural development are used elsewhere in the embryo for analogous tasks of determination and differentiation.

Two generalizations may be allowed: first, in contrast to the situation in the *Drosophila* embryo, the regionalization of the CNS in the vertebrate embryo seems to be governed more by inductive interactions than by primary compartmentalization events. Second, whereas the subdivision of the brain is due to an axial segmentation process of the neural ectoderm itself, the segmental pattern of the spinal cord probably reflects the primary segmentation events in mesodermal structures, the somites from which the axial skeleton with its primary segmentation is derived. Fundamental genes responsible for the axial subdivision of the vertebrate nervous system may still have to be discovered. Zebrafish developmental genetics is promising in this respect as the developing larva can easily be observed under the microscope. In the mouse, 'gene trapping' by insertional mutagenesis with reporter gene constructs is currently used to discover new genes relevant to the early development of the nervous system (Joyner, 1991; Skarnes *et al.*, 1992).

2.3 Pathfinding and guidance of axons

One of the fundamental questions of developmental neurobiology is how neurons find their targets to establish the stereotypical patterns of connections characteristic of the adult nervous system. A specialized structure at the tip of a growing axon, the growth cone, accomplishes the pathfinding, often over long distances. In cell culture, the behavior of growth cones can be influenced by differential adhesion, chemo-attraction and repulsion. *In situ*, it is likely that the growth cone receives signals simultaneously from molecules on the surface of other cells, molecules in the extra-cellular matrix, and diffusible factors. To understand at the molecular level the nature and function of these signals and how they are coordinated to guide the growth cone to the target cell, much work has aimed at searching for axon guidance molecules.

A successful approach is the genetic analysis in the nematode *Caenorhabditis elegans* and in particular in the fruitfly *Drosophila melanogaster*. These large-scale mutant screens which covered the entire genome and focused on a variety of systems, includ-ing the *Drosophila* central nervous, neuromuscular, and visual systems, identified many candidate genes for guidance molecules and may reveal their regulatory path-ways. Mutations in the *commissureless* (*comm*) and *roundabout* (*robo*) genes affect growth cone guidance at the midline (see *Figure 2.3*) (Seeger *et al.*, 1993). Several other genes have been identified that are necessary for axons of motoneurons to navigate past particular choice points in the pathfinding process and for the ability of motoneurons to recognize their appropriate muscle targets (Van Vactor *et al.*, 1993). As a vertebrate model, the zebrafish has recently been established for systematic screens and is already yielding a number of interesting phenotypes affecting pathfinding in the retinotectal system (Kuwada, 1995). These mutants support a model in which the reti-nal growth cones are guided by sequential cues as they navigate from the eye to the tectum.

A number of genes recently identified in *Drosophila* that are thought to play impor-tant roles in growth cone guidance, such as those coding for the fasciclins, connectin and receptor-like tyrosine phosphatases (RTP) were not identified through mutant phenotypes; instead, their relevance was discovered by their expression pattern within the nervous system or on the basis of sequence homology to other character-ized gene families. The specific function of a number of these genes in axon guidance was further investigated using 'reverse' genetics by controlling the presence or absence of the gene product at a specific time and place.

Another route that has been successfully followed for the molecular cloning of guidance molecules is the use of culture bioassays for biochemical purification. By this approach, the first chemoattractants, called netrins, were identified by their func-tion (Kennedy *et al.*, 1994; Serafini *et al.*, 1994). In vertebrates, commissural axons pioneer a circumferential pathway to the floor plate at the ventral midline of the embryonic spinal cord. Floor plate cells secrete a diffusible factor that promotes the outgrowth of commissural axons *in vitro*. Because of the small size of the floor plate, embryonic chick brain was used to purify two novel proteins, netrin-1 and netrin-2, which possess outgrowth-promoting activity for commissural axons. They are secreted proteins that are related to each other and exist in both membrane-associated and in soluble forms. The amino acid sequences of the two netrins are 50% homolo-gous to that of UNC-6, a protein identified in *C. elegans* by mutational analysis (the designation 'unc' in *C. elegans* genetics stands for 'uncoordinated movement', due to the original screening criterion; genes with different functions bear this designation). In UNC-6 null mutants, the guidance of axons that normally travel circumferentially around the worm is disrupted. Both UNC-6 and the netrins are in part further homol-ogous to certain domains of laminin, a giant, heterotrimeric glycoprotein of the ver-tebrate extracellular matrix.

Organ culture assays have demonstrated that in the developing chick tectum, the regional expression of repulsive guidance molecules plays an important role in the formation of the retinotectal map. Two candidate proteins of molecular masses 33 kDa and 25 kDa which show repulsive activities have been purified (Drescher *et al.*, 1995; Stahl *et al.*, 1990). The cDNA corresponding to the 25 kDa protein, named RAGS (for repulsive axonal guidance signal), has been cloned, and its sequence shows significant homology to ligands of the Eph-subclass of receptor tyrosine kinases (RTKs). Another member of the Eph-receptor ligand family, AL-1, appears to be involved in axon fasciculation in co-cultures of cortical neurons and astrocytes (Winslow *et al.*, 1995). Both, RAGS and AL-1 are linked to the membrane via a phosphatidylinositol anchor (GPI-link). Many members of the receptors for these molecules, the Eph-related RTKs, are expressed in the developing avian nervous system in a pattern that is consistent with a role in map formation.

Another family of proteins with a potential role in receptor-mediated signaling in

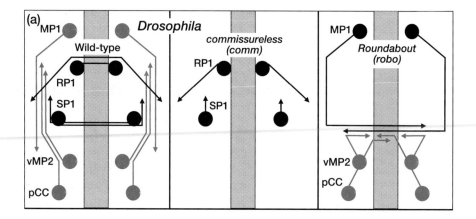

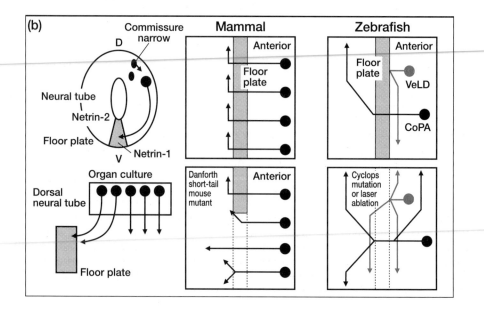

axon guidance are the RTPs. Three RTPs are expressed on developing axons in the embryonic *Drosophila* CNS (Tian *et al.*, 1991; Yang *et al.*, 1991). This class of proteins shares motifs with recognition/adhesion proteins in their extracellular domains: immunoglobulin-like domains and fibronectin type III repeats.

Various cell adhesion molecules (CAMs) have been implicated as axon guidance molecules, usually on the basis of suggestive expression patterns or cell culture studies. However, targeted disruption of mouse genes encoding CAMs has failed to yield obvious abnormalities of axon pathfinding. The potential of genetic analysis of CAM function was demonstrated by studies of fasciclin II in *Drosophila*. Fasciclin II belongs to the immunoglobulin superfamily of cell-surface receptors, related to the neural cell adhesion molecule (N-CAM), and mediates homophilic cell adhesion in culture (Grenningloh *et al.*, 1991). In the embryo, fasciclin II is expressed in a subset of developing CNS axons that selectively fasciculate with one another to form several longitudinal fascicles. The phenotypes of the various mutants point to a role of fasciclin II in mediating selective fasciculation. Ectopic expression increases axon fasciculation and leads to subsequent errors in pathfinding. The loss-of-function mutation results in defasciculation of the longitudinal CNS axon pathways that selectively express the protein. Remarkably, 'follower' growth cones are able to project in the appropriate direction in the absence of contact with their pioneer axons, implying that other guidance cues are present (Lin and Goodman, 1994; Lin *et al.*, 1994).

In several species a variety of experimental approaches have indicated that members of the semaphorin/collapsin gene family play a repulsive role in axon guidance, target recognition, or both. The insect molecule fasciclin IV (later called semaphorin I) and the growth cone collapse-inducing chick protein collapsin were the first members of

---

Figure 2.3. Pathfinding mutations affecting guidance at the midline of insects and vertebrates. (a) In the *Drosophila* embryonic nerve cord, the growth cones of a number of identified neurons project across the midline (black), whereas others project on only their own side (gray). In *commissureless* mutant embryos, growth cones fail to cross the midline and thus commissural axon pathways do not form. The *comm* gene product might be involved in the attractive signal that guides commissural growth cones toward the midline. In embryos mutant in the *roundabout* gene, growth cones that normally project on their own side instead abnormally cross the midline. The *robo* gene product might therefore be involved in a repulsive signal that keeps growth cones away from the midline. (b) Left: cross-section of vertebrate neural tube showing the floor plate at the ventral midline and of the commissural neurons at the dorsal side. The growth cones of the commissural neurons follow a circumferential path down toward the floor plate where they cross the midline and extend toward the brain. Produced in the floor plate and lower two-thirds of the developing spinal cord, the netrins may attract commissural axons. Shown below is the organ culture bioassay in which commissural neurons and pieces of floor plate are co-cultured at a distance from one another. The growth cones of commissural neurons closest to the floor plate turn and extend toward it, suggesting chemotropic guidance. Middle and right: fillets of neural tubes viewed as if sliced down the dorsal midline and opened up. Middle: in mice carrying the Danforth short-tail mutation, which eliminates variable portions of the floor plate (dashed lines), the growth cones of commissural neurons still extend toward the ventral midline but, once reaching this region, take abnormal pathways. Right: in zebrafish, some growth cones project toward the ventral midline and then across the floor plate (CoPA, black), whereas others extend toward the midline but remain on the same side (VeLD, gray). When the floor plate is removed by either mutation (cyclops) or laser ablation, these growth cones still extend toward the ventral midline, but once reaching this region, take aberrant pathways. Adapted from Goodman and Shatz (1993) with permission from Cell Press.

this family. Based on sequence homologies, many more related genes were identified in insects and vertebrates (human, mouse, chick), encoding both secreted and transmembrane proteins. This protein family is characterized by the presence of a conserved semaphorin domain of 500 amino acids and 16 conserved cysteine residues (Kolodkin et al., 1993). Whether the semaphorins act locally, being anchored on a cell surface, or also exert more distant effects on pathfinding by diffusing freely through the embryo is not yet clear.

The *Drosophila* cell surface protein connectin plays a role in motoneuron growth cone guidance and the formation of specific synaptic connections. This GPI-linked protein of the leucine-rich repeat family is expressed on a subset of muscles and on the axons and growth cones of motoneurons that innervate these muscles. Connectin mediates homophilic adhesion in cell transfection experiments which suggests that it may function as an attractive cue for motor axon guidance and during neuromuscular innervation (Nose et al., 1992). However, ectopic expression of connectin on the surface of neighboring muscles which do not normally express this protein causes abnormal behavior of connectin-negative motoneurons that normally innervate these muscles. Their growth cones take detours, grow past the muscles or stall and fail to form synapses, consistent with a repulsive function for connectin during motoneuron pathfinding and synapse formation (Nose et al., 1994). Therefore, it is likely that connectin is a bifunctional molecule, mediating attractive interactions between some growth cones and muscles and repulsive interactions between others. Connectin's two-faced role may be shared by many other guidance cues. There is evidence that netrin-1 is another bifunctional guidance molecule with the ability to attract some axons while repelling others (Colamarino and Tessier-Lavigne, 1995). Different axons may therefore respond differently to the same molecule, and how a growth cone reacts to any specific guidance cue may depend on the types of receptors present on its surface.

2.4 Genetics of cell migration

The preceding section described how elongating cell processes find their way to their target cells, being guided by molecular cues through the jungle of surrounding cells and extracellular matrix, to provide the basis of sensory perception and coordinated motor output in metazoa. However, even at the lowest level of multicellularity (e.g. during the formation of the fruiting body of the cellular slime mold *Dictyostelium*), another principle is evident: the movement of whole cell populations relative to each other, called 'migration' with regard to the minority population. Cell migration is particularly important during the formation of the CNS and peripheral nervous systems (PNS) of vertebrates, and the principles of guidance of migrating cells are very similar to those of the guidance of growth cones, involving both positive 'attractive' and negative 'repulsive' signals carried by cell surfaces, extracellular matrix compounds or diffusible 'factors'.

Two types of cell migration can be distinguished in vertebrates: radial migration (with respect to the neural tube topology) within the CNS, and long distance migration of cells derived from the neural crest, to form peripheral sympathetic and parasympathetic ganglia which innervate internal organs. In both cases, mutations may interfere with the migratory activity. In the case of the PNS, the effect is often not specific for neurons but affects other migratory cell types as well.

Radial migration is essential in the development of the vertebrate CNS, as glial and neuronal precursor cells originate from a germinal epithelium lining the lumen of the neuronal tube and differentiate at the periphery, forming a mantle zone of neuronal cell bodies (to become 'gray matter') and peripheral to that a zone of neuronal cell processes which later are myelinated by glial cells (to become 'white matter'). In the cerebellum, neuronal migration is not only centrifugal but also centripetal. A subclass of neurons, the granule cells, forms an external germinal layer from which they migrate back, apparently guided by radially oriented glia cells (the 'Bergmann glia'), to form the internal granular layer. The resulting architecture of the cerebellum is rather stereotypical with four morphologically distinct classes of neurons: the small and numerous granule cells, the basket cells, the stellate cells, and the large Purkinje cells. The function of the cerebellum is the coordination of the motor activities by means of the inhibitory output of the Purkinje cells which themselves integrate a highly complex input. About 30 mutations in the mouse affect the structure of the cerebellum and lead to easily recognizable defects in motor coordination like tremor and ataxias. The affected (homozygous mutant) mice were given descriptive names like *weaver*, *reeler* or *staggerer*. Because the cerebellum develops postnatally, and motor coordination is not so critical for mice raised under laboratory conditions, it was possible to thoroughly analyze a number of these mutations. Typically, such mutants have a cerebellum of greatly reduced size and a disrupted internal organization. There is cell loss by degeneration of neurons which may also be found in other parts of the brain. In the case of *weaver* and *reeler* mutants, more detailed neurohistological and cell culture studies indicated a severe disturbance of granule cell migration. Thus the primary defect would be a faulty interaction between the neuronal precursor cells, and the Bergmann glia and the degeneration of the granule cells and other neurons a secondary consequence of their improper positioning and failure to establish normal contacts. Cell adhesion or extracellular matrix components would thus appear to be candidate molecules for the *reeler* or *weaver* defects. Alternatively, either granule cells or Bergmann glia cells could be blocked at some step of differentiation. Both genes have recently been identified, and the sequence of the *reeler* gene does in fact indicate that it codes for an extracellular matrix protein, 'reelin', probably secreted by granule cells (D'Arcangelo *et al.*, 1995). Surprisingly the *weaver* mutant turned out to be affected in an ion channel (see Section 2.11). Reelin is a large polypeptide of 3461 amino acids, with repeated epidermal growth factor domains homologous to those found in other extracellular matrix and signaling proteins, among these the delta protein of *Drosophila*. The amino terminus of reelin bears some homology to F-spondin, a protein secreted from the floor plate of the spinal cord which is thought to be involved in regulation of adhesion and extension of commissural neurons (Klar *et al.*, 1992). Reelin is not only expressed in the cerebellum but also in the cerebral cortex, hippocampus and the olfactory bulb.

An example of a human hereditary disease due to a defect in cell migration is Kallmann's syndrome. The patients have a greatly reduced ability to perceive odors and show hypogonadism due to gonadotropin deficiency. These symptoms point to defects in the olfactory lobe, a rostral extrusion of the telencephalon, and of the hypophysis, the neuroendocrine posterior lobe of which is derived from the mesencephalon, and responsible for the release of gonadotropins by the nonneural anterior lobe. The gene *KAL1* mutated in Kallmann's syndrome is located on the X and Y chromosomes. The *KAL1* gene product predicted from the gene structure (Franco *et al.*, 1991) shares homology with neuronal cell adhesion molecules and tyrosine kinases. It probably mediates signals for the migration of olfactory neurons and precursors of the hypothalamic gonadotropin-releasing hormone producing neurons.

The most prominent guiding signal for neural crest cells is the c-Kit-receptor (*W*)-Kit-Ligand (*Sl*) system (Fleischman, 1993). The receptor is produced by a subset of migrating neural crest cells and the ligand is expressed by the cells in the target region. The Kit-ligand is synthesized as a diffusible as well as a membrane-bound protein, and may therefore act as a chemoattractant and/or a homing signal. Mouse mutants have contributed to the understanding of this case of migration signaling which affects pigment cells, blood cell precursors and germ cells: White spotting (*W*) mice lack the Kit receptor (Geissler *et al.*, 1988) and Steel (*Sl*) mice lack the ligand (Huang *et al.*, 1990). In both cases the most obvious effect is the regional lack of melanocytes. Little is known about the genetic control of migratory signals guiding neuronal precursors from the neural crest to the periphery. Hirschsprung's disease and the mouse mutations piebald (*s*), piebald lethal (*s'*) as well as lethal spotting (*ls*), all of which lead to hypopigmentation and megacolon, provide some insights. The megacolon is due to a lack of neural crest-derived intestinal neurons. The knockout of the mouse endothelin-B-receptor gene (*Ednrb*) leads to a phenotype similar to that of the piebald lethal (*s'*) mutation, and it transpired that *s'* is a null-allele of this gene, whereas the milder phenotype of piebald (*s*) mice is due to a reduced level of structurally intact endothelin-B-receptor mRNA in *s/s* mice (Hosoda *et al.*, 1994). Mutations within the human endothelin receptor gene were shown to be responsible for some forms of Hirschsprung's disease (Baynash *et al.*, 1994), a syndrome characterized by hypopigmentation and megacolon, whereas the loss of the ligand endothelin-3 (*EDN3*) was shown to be affected in other Hirschsprung patients (Edery *et al.*, 1996; Hofstra *et al.*, 1996). The mouse homolog to the latter form is probably 'lethal spotting' because the gene maps close to the locus coding for endothelin-3 (Pavan *et al.*, 1995).

Mutations affecting the migration of neural crest cells, be they precursors of pigment, blood, germ cells or those destined to become neurons of the PNS, thus illustrate that similar phenotypes may result from genes coding for a receptor and those coding for the corresponding ligand.

2.5 Neurotrophic factors and their receptors

One of the most successful fields in modern neurobiology is based on serendipity. In 1948, Bueker observed that a certain tumor transplanted into a chick embryo caused excessive sprouting of nerve fibers. This observation was followed up by Victor Hamburger and Rita Levi-Montalcini and was the beginning of the identification and characterization of nerve growth factor (NGF), a polypeptide which not only stimulates neurite outgrowth but also, when injected into neonatal mice, can reorient the direction of nerve fiber growth. Furthermore, NGF supports the survival of certain classes of neurons, sympathetic neurons and a subpopulation of sensory neurons, both in culture and *in situ*. For this to occur, a receptor and a signal transduction pathway were postulated to be present in responsive neurons. Further growth of this field (for review see Davies, 1994; Snider, 1994, and Chapter 13) and the characterization of additional factor–receptor systems were not based on genetics but rather on model experiments using embryo or organ extracts on cultured cells. The analysis of neurotrophic factors thus led from biological effects to purified proteins, from there to cDNA sequences, and finally to the identification of gene loci. Because neurotrophic factors support neuronal differentiation and survival, the genes that code for these factors or their receptors must be considered as candidate genes for neurodegenerative diseases. *Figure 2.4* shows a chromosome map of the mouse, with known locations of some of the genes coding for neurotrophic factors and their receptors as well as of disease genes.

Any hypothesis on the biological function of a molecule derived from a cell culture system needs to be verified in the context of the whole organism, and here genetics

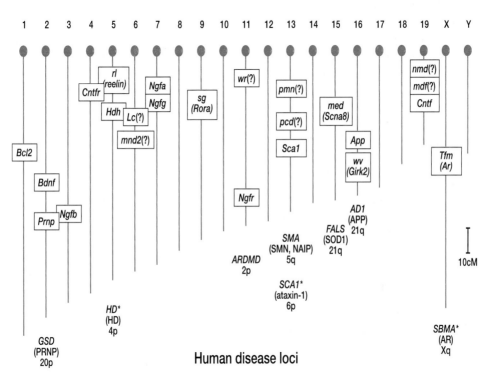

Figure 2.4. Chromosome map of the mouse, model organism for human neurological diseases. The 19 autosomes (in order of decreasing length, as given in recombination units, cM) and sex chromosomes of the mouse are shown with loci for neurotrophic factors (*Bdnf* coding for BDNF; *Ngfa, Ngfb, Ngfg*, coding for α-, β- and γ-subunits of NGF; *Cntf*, CNTF) and their receptors (*Cntfr*, CNTF-R; *Ngfr*, NGF-R), neurodegenerative diseases of the mouse (cerebellar: *lc, sg, pcd, wv, rl*; brainstem/spinal cord: *mnd2, wr, pmn, med, nmd, mdf*; see Section 2.7) and loci homologous to human disease loci. The mouse gene locus *Bcl2* (B-cell leukemia 2) codes for an anti-apoptotic protein discovered in the immune system but active also in other cells including neurons. Human disease genes (symbols in capitals) with their chromosomal location are given below the mouse chromosomes on which their mouse homologs map. Asterisk, trinucleotide repeat. Designations in brackets refer to identified genes or known products/proteins. '(?)' indicates that the gene product is not yet known. Mutations in the androgen receptor (locus *Tfm/Ar*) cause testicular feminization (loss of function in male mice and spinobulbar muscular atrophy (trinucleotide repeat) in man (see also Sections 2.7 and 2.11).

comes into play by targeted mutagenesis. In the case where there is a one-to-one relation between neurotrophic factor/ligand and receptor, genetic knockout of either one should lead to a similar phenotype. Such an observation has been made on natural mutations affecting certain ligand–receptor pairs [e.g. in the case of the pair 'White spotting' (W) and 'Steel' (Sl), as mentioned above]. In the case of the knockout of the genes for NGF and an NGF receptor, the defects were not identical. Genetic elimination of NGF leads to an extensive loss of sensory and sympathetic neurons, as expected from cell culture experiments and manipulations of neonatal mice (e.g. injection of anti-NGF antibody), and perinatal death (Crowley et al., 1994). The elimination of one of the known NGF receptors had much milder effects, implying that another NGF receptor is more important for development (Lee et al., 1992).

A result opposite to that found for the NGF system has been obtained with the ciliary neurotrophic factor (CNTF), and its receptor. The peptide CNTF was discovered in cell culture experiments, as a diffusible molecule that would support the survival of parasympathetic motoneurons, obtained from the ciliary ganglia of chick embryos. Subsequently it was found to act also on other embryonic neurons, such as ganglionic and preganglionic sympathetic neurons, peripheral sensory neurons and cranial and spinal motoneurons. Furthermore, when CNTF was applied to the chick embryo or to newborn mice previously subjected to axotomy it suppressed neuronal death that occurs as a consequence of the surgical disconnection from the periphery. CNTF was also found to slow down the progression of motoneuron degeneration in mouse models of neuromuscular disease (Sendtner et al., 1992). These findings implied that CNTF was the neurotrophic factor long searched for, by which muscles regulate the size of motoneuron pools and suppress programmed neuronal death in the limb girdle regions during embryogenesis. Very recently a novel potent neurotrophic factor, cardiotrophin-1 (CT-1), has been discovered, which like CNTF belongs to the family of interleukin-6 cytokines. CT-1 like CNTF protects motoneurons in culture and, after axotomy, in the organism (Pennica et al., 1996).

One might have suspected that already known neurodegenerative diseases of the mouse were due to mutations in the Cntf gene or the gene(s) for subunits of the CNTF receptor. Disappointingly, CNTF knockout mice turned out to be indistinguishable from wild-type mice, and required quantitative analysis to detect subtle and late effects of the loss of this gene on muscle performance (Masu et al., 1993). Furthermore, none of the known mouse mutations causing neurodegeneration (cf. Section 2.7) mapped to the Cntf locus on chromosome 19 (disease gene hunters would have called the Cntf gene a 'candidate gene by function' and the procedure to refute it 'exclusion mapping'). On the other hand, the knockout of the gene for the α-subunit of the CNTF receptor which maps to chromosome 4, had dramatic effects: these mice died around birth, due to severe defects in motoneurons (DeChiara et al., 1995). This result proves the fundamental importance of this receptor, the physiological ligand of which, however, is obviously not identical with the CNTF peptide.

The last factor to be discussed is brain-derived neurotrophic factor, BDNF. BDNF had first been described as an 'activity' present in brain extracts that would support the survival of cultured neurons. This was a lucky discovery as BDNF seems to be essential for development in situ. In contrast to CNTF knockout mice, BDNF knockout mice are severely affected: their sensory ganglia are deficient, and they die around birth (Ernfors et al., 1994; Jones et al., 1994).

A combined treatment with CNTF and BDNF has been reported to alleviate the motoneuron degeneration of a mutant mouse termed '*wobbler*' (Mitsumoto *et al.*, 1994, cf. Section 2.7) although, from exclusion mapping, it became clear that the gene affected in *wobbler* is not identical with either the *Cntf* or the *Bdnf* gene (*Figure 2.4*). So far, no defect in a neurotrophic factor gene or in a gene for a neurotrophic factor receptor has turned out to be responsible for the phenotype in any of the known spontaneous neurological mutations of the mouse.

2.6 Genetic control of cell death

The concept of programmed cell death applies to all processes of organogenesis in which the final number of cells, the creation of gaps or holes in tissues, or the adjustment to functional requirements is achieved by the elimination of cells during normal development or during cyclic processes (e.g. those related to reproductive cycles). Well-known examples in vertebrates are the cyclic cell death in the mammary gland, the elimination of interdigital cells in the development of toes, and the adjustment of the number of spinal motoneurons to the size of the periphery (i.e. presence or absence of limbs). During the last decade, cell biologists and pathologists have learnt to distinguish two types of cell death: 'necrosis', which may be described as 'giving up' under adverse circumstances, and 'apoptosis', a more active, suicide-like response of the cell. These types of cell death are associated with characteristic ultrastructural and biochemical events, especially in the cell nucleus.

One of the most thoroughly studied systems for the genetic control of programmed cell death is the nematode *C. elegans*. Nematodes are cell-constant animals: depending on species, sex and larval stage, their body is made up of a relatively small (about 1000), exactly defined number of cells. Furthermore, the cell-lineage is reproducible, and the program of apoptotic events is accurate to the level of single cells. For this reason and because about a third (302) of the *C. elegans* cells are neurons, this organism has provided valuable insights into the genetic control of cell death and its possible relationship to neurodegenerative diseases.

The technical advantages of *C. elegans* (small genome, small body size, rapid development, cell constancy and translucency) allowed for an accurate observation of programmed cell death during development: about 130 cells undergo apoptosis, an active and cell-autonomous process of (self-)elimination. Obviously this process must be genetically controlled and mutants were isolated that were defective in programmed cell death ('*ced*' mutations). In brief, the essential genetic components of apoptosis in *C. elegans* can be described as follows (*Figure 2.5*) (Hengartner, 1994; Osborne and Schwartz, 1994): two genes, *ced-3* and *ced-4* are necessary for all programmed cell death events in development. While the gene product CED3 (i.e. the protein inferred from the gene structure) bears no similarity to any previously known protein, the structure of CED4 turned out to be homologous to vertebrate cysteine proteases, especially to a protease termed 'interleukin-1β converting enzyme' (ICE) which has been implicated in mammalian apoptosis. The decision to undergo apoptosis, of course, requires specific signals, depending on species, cell type and environmental stresses (e.g. UV irradiation). It also requires a self-protective, anti-apoptotic principle, and in *C. elegans*, this is determined by the gene *ced-9*. Interestingly, its product, CED9, has a mammalian counterpart, termed BCL-2, which is coded for by the gene *Bcl2* (for review see Davies, 1995). These findings indicate that the balance between survival and programmed cell death must have developed early in metazoan evolution. This view was experimentally corroborated: the mammalian gene *Bcl2* was able to prevent programmed cell death in transgenic *C. elegans*, that is to replace the function of *ced-9*. Conversely, CED4, the cysteine protease coded for by the *C. elegans* gene, can induce cell death in mammalian cells, that is replace ICE in cell culture (see Hengartner, 1994). The significance of this regulatory system is not confined to the nervous system, and genetic defects interfering with apoptosis are thought to be the cause of a variety of tumors, including those of the hematopoietic and immune systems.

In vertebrates, the topic of neuronal programmed cell death is interwoven with the role of neurotrophic factors. Thus, a classical method of inducing neuronal apoptosis in cell culture is the withdrawal of NGF from NGF-dependent cells, for example sensory neurons or PC12 rat phaeochromocytoma tumor cells that previously had been induced by NGF to undergo neuronal differentiation. While the genetic basis of the elimination of neurons is not yet known in vertebrates, a link between programmed cell death and hereditary neuromuscular diseases may exist: it is conceivable that a pathological loss of neurons is due to a dysregulation of apoptosis with regard to its time window and extent. However, from genetic mapping studies in mouse and man there is so far no positive support for any specific case of that kind. Saturation mutagenesis for neurological defects, now possible in zebrafish (Mullins *et al.*, 1994) might reveal such connections in the near future.

The genetics of *C. elegans* has made a second contribution to the field of neurodegeneration, due to the discovery of dominant mutations leading to neurodegeneration ('*mec*' genes for 'mechanosensory' and '*deg*' genes for 'degeneration'). When these genes were cloned, a homology to a specific class of mammalian epithelial sodium channels, the amiloride-sensitive Na^+-channel was evident. The conclusion was that ion channels (in this case a complex of ion channels) involved in mechanoreception, may turn into 'gain-of-function killers' by certain mutations. One can imagine that unscheduled ion fluxes have deleterious effects on neuronal cells, in this case the sensory neurons. Such a mechanism may be related to the phenomenon of excitotoxicity in vertebrate neurons. Excitotoxic events are usually thought to involve the influx of calcium ions which may trigger destructive protease activities.

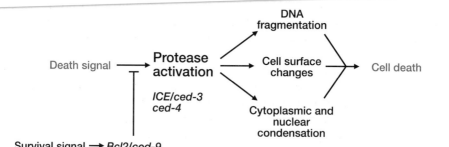
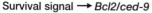

Figure 2.5. Genes involved in apoptosis. Cellular and biochemical steps involved in programmed cell death (apoptosis) and genes involved (mammalian genes, *Bcl-2* and *ICE*; *ced-*, nematode genes). There is structural and functional homology between the apoptosis protease genes *ICE* and *ced-3* and between the anti-apoptotic genes *Bcl-2* and *ced-9*. See text for further explanation. Adapted from Hengartner (1994).

2.7 Hereditary neurodegenerative diseases: natural and transgenic models

Typically, apoptosis is associated with defined developmental processes as described above. What about genetic defects that lead to unscheduled cell death in the nervous system? As it turns out, such diseases are not at all mechanistically understood, despite the fact that a number of relevant genes have been identified. Neurodegeneration can often be diagnosed under the light microscope by a swelling of the affected neurons, fading of the cell contents, and finally the disappearance of the neuron, typically accompanied by extensive hyperplasia and hypertrophy of surrounding astrocytes (astrogliosis). In the age- and infection-related neurodegenerative diseases as described at the end of this chapter, accumulation of insoluble protein deposits within or around dying neurons is pronounced. In hereditary neurodegenerative diseases of the mouse, typical apoptotic processes seem to be the exception rather than the rule. One such case is the semidominant mutation *Lurcher* which causes Purkinje cells to undergo apoptosis (Norman *et al.*, 1995).

Which are the most thoroughly investigated hereditary diseases, in man and in animal models? Which genes have been identified as being responsible? Examples of human neurodegenerative diseases that are due to single gene mutations are given by Bailey *et al.* in Chapter 14.

It is evident that there is no common denominator as to their genetic basis: diseases may be dominant or recessive, may affect ubiquitously expressed genes, and these may code for enzymes, ion channels or hitherto unknown proteins. Formally, a dominant mutation could be explained by a 'gain of function' (e.g. prolonged opening of an ion channel, or the exertion of a 'toxic' effect by some product of the mutant allele), and in these cases, the presence of a functional wild-type allele would be irrelevant for the disease, or there could be a haploinsufficiency, that is insufficiency of a single gene dosage (of an autosomal gene) in connection with a standard loss-of-function mutation (i.e. a case of 'pseudodominance').

A prominent group of dominant neurodegenerative diseases is due to a particular type of genetic abnormality, the expansion of a trinucleotide repeat. A generalized neurological condition, myotonic dystrophy (dystrophia muscularis, DM) belongs to this class of mutations and has recently served to clarify the issue of dominance. The gene affected in DM is called DM kinase whose function is unknown. It carries a CTG repeat in the 3'-untranslated region of the gene and mRNA, and a late onset disease is observed when the CTG repeat is expanded beyond a 40-fold repetition. The toxic product in dominant hereditary diseases could either be the transcript itself or a protein translated from it or a metabolite produced by the mutant protein but not by the wild-type version. For the transcript to be toxic, the mutated site need not be located in the translated sequence, it may even be intronic. In fact, a noncoding trinucleotide expansion seems to be responsible in DM, possibly by causing the transcript to remain in the nucleus. As the DM kinase is expressed in a variety of tissues, the relative severity of the disease symptoms in the neuromuscular system may be due to the nuclei being postmitotic and unable to clear themselves from the harmful deposits (Taneja *et al.*, 1995).

In a number of neurodegenerative diseases, for example Huntington's disease, spinocerebellar ataxia type I (SCA1), and spinobulbar muscular atrophy, CAG triplet repeat expansions are found within the coding region where they translate into polyglutamine tracts (Brooks and Fishbeck, 1995). The complete sequence of the *Sca1* gene product of 'ataxin-1' is known and antibodies directed against it are available. Although ataxin-1 does not resemble known proteins and its cellular function remains elusive, recent experiments have contributed to the understanding of the etiology of SCA. Transgenic mice have been produced for different alleles (differing in the lengths of their CAG repeats) of the *Sca1* gene, and these experiments have conclusively shown that the severity of the neurological symptoms in the transgenic mouse, as in patients correlates with the length *n* of the trinucleotide repeat. In the mouse *Sca1* gene, there are only two CAGs, $n = 2$. Yet, the repeat length found in normal humans, $n = 30$, is still not pathogenic in mice, but an allele with $n = 82$ that is harmful in humans also causes neurodegeneration in the mouse. Nonneural cells express ataxin-1 in their cytoplasm, and neurons express it in the nucleus. Only Purkinje cells express ataxin-1 both in their cytoplasm and nuclei, and their specific susceptibility to toxic influences of overlength polyglutamine tracts may be related to the localization of ataxin-1. Although this issue is not quite clarified yet, the arguments for SCA-1 seem to be in favor of the protein rather than the mRNA being the toxic agent (Burright *et al.*, 1995).

Neurodegenerative mutations in the mouse are shown in *Figure 2.4*. In order to search for a possible genetic homology between murine and human diseases, one makes use of an evolutionary argument, the conservation of synteny: not only has (nearly) each human gene a homologous equivalent in the mouse (and probably all other mammals as well), but in addition genes that map closely together on a human chromosome tend to be close together in the mouse genome. In the case of the X-linked genes, the whole gene content (but not the mapping positions) seems to be conserved among mammals. Based on these observations, one can assign to any chromosomal segment in the mouse genome a region of conserved synteny in the human genome, or vice versa (DeBry and Sedlin, 1996). If a newly mapped gene falls between two marker genes in a conserved synteny group in one species, one can predict its location with considerable confidence and accuracy in the other species. The genetic map in *Figure 2.4* shows mouse chromosomes with the gene loci relevant for neurodegeneration and human disease loci below the mouse chromosomes on which their homologs are expected to map.

Obviously, genes for neurodegenerative diseases are scattered all over the genome. The most important human neurodegenerative disease, Werdnig–Hoffmann spinal muscular atrophy (SMA) does not have a homologous counterpart in the mouse. The human *SMA* gene is located on the short arm of chromosome 5 (5q), and after extensive positional cloning efforts two candidate genes have been molecularly identified. The genes were termed '*SMN*' for 'survival motor neuron (gene)' (Lefebvre *et al.*, 1995) and '*NAIP*' for 'neuronal apoptosis inhibitory protein' (Roy *et al.*, 1995). The murine counterpart of the 5q *SMA* gene should be located on mouse chromosome 13. The mouse disease 'peripheral motor neuronopathy', a spontaneously arisen neurodegenerative disease seemed to map in the right region to be a homolog of human SMAs but finally turned out *not* to be homologous to Werdnig–Hoffmann disease (Brunialti *et al.*, 1995). Thus one will have to wait for SMN and NAIP knockout mice.

For another human neurodegenerative disease, familial amyotrophic lateral sclerosis (FALS), the affected gene locus has been shown to code for the well known enzyme cytosolic superoxide dismutase, SOD-1, an ubiquitously expressed enzyme thought to protect cells against oxidative stress. However, the etiology was not clear, as in some affected persons the catalytic activity of SOD-1 was not affected, and, again no homologous mouse mutants were available to clarify the issue. Recently, a SOD-1 knockout mouse has been produced and found to display no neurological symptoms under standard conditions. However, when the animals were challenged by axotomy, neurons degenerated rather than extending new axons as in control mice (Reaume *et al.*, 1996). This surgically induced stress situation in the mouse may simulate the cumulative long-term effects of oxidative stress during the lifetime of man.

More relevant to the human disease may be a transgenic mouse bearing a FALS allele of the human *SOD1* gene (i.e. a situation analogous to the SCA1 transgenic mouse). Here the innocent looking amino acid replacement glycine to alanine at position 93 does not impair enzyme activity but, in a gain-of-function mechanism, causes neurodegeneration. The same symptom was observed in mice made transgenic for this allele but not in mice transgenic for wild-type SOD (Gurney *et al.*, 1994). A gain-of-function mechanism of mutant SOD1 is supported by experiments on isolated mutant protein (Yim *et al.*, 1996).

Neurodegenerative diseases in mouse models have been found to affect neurons in the brain, for example Purkinje cells and granule cells in the cerebellum, motoneurons in the brain stem and ventral spinal cord, and sensory neurons. In addition to spontaneous mutations which have been intensely studied for 30 years, there are a growing number of mutations induced by gene manipulation. In lucky cases, random insertional mutagenesis, which introduces a known sequence of DNA into an undetermined gene, has led to the creation of new alleles of known disease genes and facilitated their molecular identification because cumbersome positional cloning could be circumvented. In contrast to myelin and excitability diseases, neurodegenerative diseases are often very difficult to approach, because there is usually no useful hint as to the biochemical nature of the affected gene product. Furthermore, as exemplified by the *SOD1* gene and the candidate genes for human SMA on 5q, the affected gene may be expressed ubiquitously, so that the expression pattern is not helpful for its identification either.

Two diseases affecting central neuronal differentiation and peripheral neuronal function in the mouse turned out to be ion channel diseases. These were the cerebellar mutation '*weaver*' (*wv*) in which granule cells fail to properly migrate and degenerate, and *motor endplate disease* (*med*) which appeared as a presynaptic defect in motor endplates of skeletal muscles, and hence a disease of the spinal cord, but in addition causes neuronal degeneration in the cerebellum. The former is a mutation in a GTP-binding protein-regulated potassium channel, GIRK-2, the human gene for which, *GIRK2*, was already known (Goldowitz and Smeyne, 1995; Patil *et al.*, 1995). This is a case where conserved synteny between mouse and human genomes was helpful in identifying the disease gene, in this case in the mouse. The *GIRK2* gene is expressed rather specifically, in the cerebellum and in testis, and indeed '*weaver*' mice not only show ataxia, but also have a defect in spermiogenesis. The concomitant effect of genes on the nervous system and on testis without the common denominator of a humoral defect is observed in a number of neurological mouse mutants (e.g. *wobbler* and *quaking*).

In the case of motor endplate disease (MED), serendipity was helpful in that an insertional mutation produced the same symptoms, mapped to the same chromosome (15) and did not complement the authentic *med* mutation. In addition, the expression pattern of the candidate gene, coding for a new sodium channel and therefore termed *Scna8* (for 'sodium channel α-subunit 8'), was helpful: its mRNA was found in brain and spinal cord but not in other organs including skeletal muscle. Muscle was thought to be secondarily affected in the paralyzed MED animals (Burgess *et al.*, 1995).

Another cerebellar neurodegenerative mutation of the mouse, the gene for which has recently been identified, is *staggerer* (*sg*). In this mutation, the gene locus for a nuclear receptor, Ror-α, is affected. The ligand of this 'orphan receptor' is not known but might be thyroxin (Hamilton *et al.*, 1996). This would make sense in the light of the known dependence on thyroid hormone of cerebellar maturation.

Many of the mouse disease genes that affect motoneurons such as '*motoneuron degeneration 2*' (*mnd2*, chromosome 6), '*wobbler*' (*wr*, chromosome 11), '*peripheral motor neuronopathy*' (*pmn*, chromosome 13) and '*muscle deficient*' (*mdf*, chromosome 19) have only recently been mapped (see *Figure 2.4*) and are presently investigated by positional cloning approaches as there is no idea as to the nature of the gene products.

If apoptosis is an important factor in a neurodegenerative disease, one might think of an anti-apoptotic gene being mutated to loss-of-function. One of the candidate genes for 5q SMA in man, *NAIP* (Roy *et al.*, 1995), would explain the disease by the loss of an anti-apoptotic function – as some hereditary tumor susceptibilities are explained by the loss of anti-tumor transcription factors. This idea is based on the sequence homology of *NAIP* to a gene coding for baculovirus anti-apoptosis protein. However, at present, the correlation between SMA and mutations in the alternative candidate gene, *SMN*, favors the latter as the relevant *SMA* gene, especially because deletions are seen with a high frequency in patients. As the *SMA* region seems to be complicated by gene repetitions, pseudogenes and a structural instability (i.e. high mutability) in humans, the whole question of the genetic basis of SMA is not yet resolved. To further complicate matters, the disease phenotype of SMA may be absent despite homozygosity for seemingly deleterious mutations in the *SMN* candidate gene. Hence, either a hitherto undetected gene in that region is the true SMA gene, or unlinked modifying genes are involved in the etiology of SMA.

In order to test the concept of pathological apoptosis experimentally, a known anti-apoptotic gene, *Bcl2*, was artificially introduced (by transgene construction and appropriate crosses) into various mouse mutants with neurodegenerative diseases. So far, the results have been modest, probably for two reasons: first, curing of a hereditary neurodegenerative disease by an anti-apoptotic transgene requires the mechanism of neuron loss to be indeed due to apoptosis and not to necrosis. Second, for a functional restoration, it would seem necessary that apoptosis is the *only* defect. Function and programmed cell death may be interwoven in that nonfunctional cells may be eliminated by apoptosis. In such a case, saving their lives would not help. In the *wobbler* mouse, neuron loss seems to be of necrotic rather than apoptotic type. Accordingly, the *Bcl2* transgene failed to rescue the mutant (Ait-Ikhlef *et al.*, 1995). However, in mice homozygous for the *pmn* mutation a partial restoration of neuronal function by the *Bcl2* transgene was observed (Sagot *et al.*, 1995).

2.8 Myelin genetics

A good example of how genetics can be applied to analyze the development of the vertebrate nervous system is provided by mouse mutants with genetic defects of myelination. Myelin, the structural prerequisite for rapid saltatory impulse conduction in vertebrates, is elaborated by glial cells, oligodendrocytes in the CNS and Schwann cells in the PNS. Both glial cell types spirally enwrap segments of neuronal axons with a multi-layered sheath of cell membrane which subsequently forms a compact structure (for review see Bunge and Fernandez-Valle, 1995; Szuchet, 1995). The myelin membrane insulates a neuronal axon, sparing only the 'nodes of Ranvier' which are equally spaced along its length and to which action potentials are restricted. In most species, including humans and rodents, myelination takes place postnatally.

The lack of normal myelin in neurological mouse mutants is associated with striking behavioral symptoms, such as ataxia and tremor, which reflect the loss of motor control. This late-onset phenotype has allowed the identification of a number of spontaneous mutations with both CNS and PNS dysmyelinations (Nave, 1995; Sidman et al., 1964). Most of these developmental mutants have now been molecularly defined as mutations in genes coding for myelin-associated proteins. More recently, gene targeting techniques have been used to generate additional mouse mutants using cloned genes. Some of the myelin-deficient mice serve as genetic animal models or 'genocopies' for equivalent human neurological diseases. Myelin membranes contain only 20% protein (dry mass), but some of the myelin proteins are highly abundant. They are assumed to serve a structural function in the myelin architecture.

Myelin proteins of the CNS and PNS are encoded by an overlapping albeit not identical set of genes, the expression of which is largely restricted to oligodendrocytes and Schwann cells (for review see Campagnoni, 1995; Mikoshiba et al., 1991; Nave, 1995). Structural proteins are most likely required for glial process outgrowth and axonal recognition at early time points, and later for the spiral ensheathment and membrane interactions that underlie myelin compaction. Most identified myelin proteins are integral membrane components and some belong, by structural homology, to known protein families.

Many ultrastructural features of the myelin architecture are directly related to myelin structural proteins. Thus, one would expect genetic defects to allow visualization of a structure–function relationship of these proteins. Specific interest has focused on the genes that are candidates for specification of the 'major dense line' of myelin (MDL; an electron-dense zone which marks the intracellular adhesion of the compacted myelin), the 'intraperiod line' (IPL; the extracellular apposition zone), and the axonal–glial junction.

The myelin basic protein (MBP) gene encodes a group of small positively charged proteins derived by alternative mRNA splicing (Campagnoni, 1995). MBPs range in size from 14 to 21 kDa and are abundant in myelin (30–40% by mass in the CNS, 10–20% in the PNS). The *MBP* gene is by itself contained within a much larger unit, termed *'Golli-mbp'* (the *Golli-mbp* gene, expressed in glial and a nonglial cells, includes additional exons and generates, by alternative splicing, MBP-related proteins of unknown function). The *shiverer* mutation of the mouse is defined by a large deletion within the *MBP* gene (Molineaux et al., 1986; Roach et al., 1985). Homozygous *shiverer* mice illustrate how the nervous system develops in the complete absence of this protein: at the cellular level, CNS myelin is very thin and largely uncompacted. The MDL is missing, suggesting that MBP participates in membrane adhesion, possibly as the major MDL component itself. The *shiverer* defect has been rescued by complementation with a wild-type *MBP* transgene, an experiment which demonstrated that the amount of MBP available to oligodendrocytes is a rate-limiting condition of myelination (Popko et al., 1987; Readhead et al., 1987).

In contrast to the dysmyelinated CNS, peripheral myelin of *shiverer* mice is ultra-structurally normal because its major protein component, protein zero (P0), shares functions with MBP (Kirschner and Ganser, 1980; Privat *et al.*, 1979). Experimental proof of this theoretical concept has come from 'double mutant' mice (Martini *et al.*, 1995a). P0 is a highly abundant, glycosylated membrane protein of 30 kDa with two major domains: an extracellular immunoglobulin-like domain and an intracellular basic region (Lemke *et al.*, 1988). The abundance of P0 and its bipartite domain structure suggest an involvement in both intracellular and extracellular myelin compaction. This has been visualized in mutant mice with a targeted disruption of the P0 gene (Giese *et al.*, 1992; Martini *et al.*, 1995a). In the absence of P0, the PNS is severely dysmyelinated. Whereas most axons are engulfed by the P0-deficient Schwann cells in the normal 1:1 ratio, nearly all myelin structures remain thin and lack a normally compacted IPL. The cellular phenotype is not uniform, although this has been attributed to an overlapping function with other membrane proteins, some of which are not found in normal peripheral myelin [for example proteolipid protein (PLP) and N-CAM]. These proteins appear to compensate and mask, at least in part, the full effect of P0 deficiency (Giese *et al.*, 1992). Such compensatory effects have also been observed in several other systems and are complications that may be encountered in any knockout mouse. Heterozygous P0-deficient mice (P0/+) are behaviorally normal but long-term observation has revealed that their myelin is unstable (Martini *et al.*, 1995b). Loss of one P0 allele in mice leads to ultrastructural abnormalities reminiscent of myelin in Charcot–Marie–Tooth (CMT) disease type 1B, previously associated with point mutations in the human P0 gene (Hayasaka *et al.*, 1993).

Mutations should illustrate how development proceeds in the absence of a gene function, but some mouse mutants have a more complex phenotype, due to the presence of an abnormal gene product. Thus, the assignment of a gene's functions, based on one mutant phenotype alone, can be difficult. This is demonstrated by the naturally occurring mutations of the PLP and peripheral myelin protein-22 (PMP-22) genes, which display a combination of gain of function and loss-of-function effects.

PLP is the major integral membrane protein of CNS myelin, constituting about 50% of total protein (Nave and Milner, 1989). PLP and its smaller isoform DM-20 (derived by alternative RNA splicing) are highly conserved in evolution and belong to a diverse group of 'four helix bundle' proteins (Weimbs and Stoffel, 1992). The *PLP* gene is X chromosome-linked in mouse and man and several allelic mutants have been described. The *jimpy* mouse (*jp*), discovered more than 40 years ago, was the first known mutant affected in the *PLP* gene, and *jp* is a point mutation leading to a fatal error of mRNA splicing (Hudson *et al.*, 1987; Nave *et al.*, 1986). All other murine alleles are point mutations causing single amino acid substitutions. *PLP* gene mutations have also been found in other mammalian species, including over 30 different mutations in human patients with Pelizaeus–Merzbacher disease (Hodes *et al.*, 1994). *Jimpy* mice display a CNS-specific dysmyelination with behavioral consequences much more severe than in *shi* (the disorder is lethal at 3–4 weeks of age). Histologically most striking is the apoptotic death of the majority of oligodendrocytes which accounts for a nearly complete lack of CNS myelin (Knapp *et al.*, 1986). Only a small percentage of *jimpy* oligodendrocytes differentiate to the stage of myelin formation. Such residual myelin has a unique ultrastructural defect: it is compacted but the IPL is fused to a single electron dense structure that can not be distinguished from the MDL. This suggests that PLP serves as a 'strut' in myelin and not as a 'glue'-type molecule

(Duncan *et al.*, 1989; Schneider *et al.*, 1995). One allele of *jimpy*, termed *rumpshaker*, differs from *jimpy* and most PLP mutations in that dysmyelination is associated with little cell death and a normal number of mature oligodendrocytes (Schneider *et al.*, 1992). *Rumpshaker* mice demonstrated for the first time that the role of PLP in oligodendrocyte cell death and in dysmyelination can be genetically uncoupled. Is PLP required for oligodendrocyte survival? PLP-dependent cell death is always associated with point mutations and the expression of misfolded polypeptides. Most striking is the allele *jimpy*^{msd}, defined by the conservative substitution A242V in a putative transmembrane domain of PLP (Gencic and Hudson, 1990). Recent experiments, using transgenic complementation with a wild-type *PLP* gene and a targeted complete inactivation of the *PLP* gene have revealed that oligodendrocyte death is not the consequence of the loss of PLP function but rather a specific 'gain-of-function' effect of the misfolded protein (Boison and Stoffel, 1994; Schneider *et al.*, 1995). The latter may relate to another surprising finding: oligodendrocytes are very sensitive to an increase of the PLP gene dosage. Already a two-fold overexpression of a wild-type *PLP* gene leads to a lethal dysmyelination in mice, and this is the most frequent cause of Pelizaeus–Merzbacher disease in humans (Kagawa *et al.*, 1994; Readhead *et al.* 1994).

The problems in establishing protein function from mutant phenotypes are exemplified by PMP-22, an integral membrane protein of peripheral myelin (Spreyer *et al.*, 1991; Welcher *et al.*, 1991). PMP22 has been independently cloned as a growth arrest-specific protein from fibroblasts and is thus not myelin-specific (Schneider *et al.*, 1988). Mutations of this small glycoprotein were first identified in the autosomal-dominant *Trembler* mouse (Falconer, 1951; Suter *et al.*, 1992a,b) and later in human patients with one form of CMT, type 1A (Snipes *et al.*, 1993; Valentijn *et al.*, 1992, for review). Following the normal association of Schwann cells with axons, myelin sheaths remain disproportionately thin or unmyelinated. Is the primary defect architectural or a failure of Schwann cell growth control? Continued Schwann cell proliferation leads to hypertrophy and 'onion bulb' formation in the nerve. Homozygous *Trembler* mice have virtually no peripheral myelin (nevertheless, the mutants are fully viable; Henry and Sidman, 1988). In contrast, in the complete absence of PMP-22 expression PMP-22 KO mice have another neuropathy with local hypermyelination and myelin instability (Adlkofer *et al.*, 1995). In humans, the frequent peripheral neuropathy CMT1A, a progressive demyelinating disorder, is associated with a duplication of the *PMP-22* gene. This gene dosage effect has been modeled in a transgenic rat (Sereda *et al.*, 1996). Thus, very different genetic disorders (overexpression, point mutations, and loss of function) result in similar peripheral neuropathies. Whereas these genetic observations demonstrate that PMP-22 plays a critical role in Schwann cell growth, myelin assembly and myelin maintenance, the 'real' cellular function of this protein remains obscure.

Most spontaneous myelin mutants have been 'preselected' by an obvious behavioral phenotype, but the outcome of engineered mutations cannot be predicted. The myelin-associated glycoprotein (MAG), an integral membrane protein and member of the immunoglobulin superfamily, is specific to myelinating glial cells. MAG has raised considerable interest because of its unique distribution along the glial–neuronal interface, and has been suggested to mediate axonal recognition and ensheathment (Martini and Schachner, 1986; Trapp, 1988). Surprisingly, the targeted disruption of MAG expression did not cause dysmyelination or obvious alteration of the myelin architecture (Li *et al.*, 1994; Montag *et al.*, 1994). MAG-deficient mice are, by first approximation, behaviorally and histologically normal, demonstrating that MAG is not essential for axon recognition and myelin ensheathment (for a discussion see Meyer-Franke and Barres, 1994). There is some evidence that other cell-surface proteins may compensate for MAG, but no candidate has been experimentally identified. Subtle abnormalities of MAG-deficient myelin, such as the occasional collapse of the periaxonal 'cytoplasmic collar' (the innermost lamella of myelin is normally uncompacted) point to a rather minor role of MAG in the myelin architecture. It is possible that MAG serves a quite different role than initially thought. A widely expressed serine-threonine protein kinase, Fyn, associates with and phosphorylates the intracellular carboxyl terminus of MAG. Targeted disruption of the Fyn gene causes a significant hypomyelination in mice (Umemori *et al.*, 1994). This suggests that MAG is part of an as yet poorly understood signal transduction pathway which communicates axonal information to myelin-forming glial cells.

2.9 Genetics of ion channels and of neuromuscular functions

A major weight fraction of the metazoan body is made up of cells with excitable membranes: skeletal muscles, cardiac muscle, in addition to neurons and sensory receptors. In fact, the egg cell from which all these cells derive is excitable as well. The typical excitable membrane is characterized by a set of ion channels that fall into two categories: chemosensitive and voltage-sensitive, and fulfill the functions of reception of external signals (excitatory or inhibitory), production and self-propagation of a wave of depolarization (the spike or action potential), as well as termination and modulation of the excited state. The latter is brought about by inhibitory (hyperpolarizing) and dampening (short-circuiting) anion channels. Ion channels are often oligomers of identical or different protein subunits and may be associated with peripheral membrane proteins and/or components of the cytoskeleton. Therefore, a variety of genes may be involved in functional disturbances of a given channel. An additional complication is the occurrence of developmental and/or tissue-specific isoforms that derive from different genes or by differential splicing from a single gene (or by a combination of the two).

The excitability of muscle and neuromuscular transmission have played a pioneer role in the elucidation of membrane excitability in general, and the molecular mechanisms of synapse formation and function, respectively. These processes are related to the membrane and extracellular matrix (basal lamina) of the muscle fiber, and by mass, these are only minor constituents of skeletal muscle tissue. For preparative biochemistry, a naturally transformed muscle, the electroplax tissue of the electric ray (*Torpedo*) was extremely helpful. In this tissue, the cells are largely devoid of contractile elements and consist mainly of layers of matrix and membranes with extended synaptic contacts. Therefore, it was possible to biochemically isolate the two proteins most important for neuromuscular transmission, the nicotinic acetylcholine receptor (AChR or nAChR, the plant alkaloid nicotine acts as an agonist), a chemosensitive cation channel, and its physiological counterpart, the extracellular matrix enzyme, acetylcholinesterase, from this material.

AChR is a heteropentameric transmembrane glycoprotein of the composition $\alpha 2\beta(\gamma$ or $\epsilon)\delta$ (see Chapter 8 by Glencorse and Davies). Once the structure of the AChR was known, it could be studied in less favorable material like developing or adult skeletal muscle of mammals. Thus, a number of observations made by electrophysiologists found their biochemical explanation. It was found that the shorter opening of adult as compared to embryonic AChRs in mammals are due to the replacement of an embryonic (γ) by the adult (ϵ) isoform of one of the subunits. The genes of all five kinds of subunits are well characterized and chromosomally localized in mouse and man. Mutations in different subunits of the nAChR have recently been associated with muscle diseases the symptoms of which resemble classical myasthenia gravis, an autosomal disease with auto-antibodies directed against muscular AChR, and are therefore called congenital myasthenias. In these, muscle weakness is caused by a decreased channel efficiency, abnormal opening times, or abnormal affinity to the ligand, acetylcholine, due to point mutations (amino acid replacements) in either the α or the ϵ subunit (Ohno *et al.*, 1996 and references therein). A mutation in the α subunit (isoform α 4) of brain AChR has been implicated in a form of epilepsy (Steinlein *et al.*, 1995).

The developmental changes regarding AChR distribution and formation of the neuromuscular synapse can be summarized as follows: as immature muscle fibers (or 'myotubes') develop by fusion from mononuclear precursor cells, the expression of AChR increases, and the receptor is distributed all over the surface of the myotube, first uniformly then in patches called 'hot spots'. Upon nerve contact, the fiber matures, and the receptor becomes extremely concentrated at the subsynaptic membrane and nearly disappears elsewhere from the sarcolemma. Upon denervation, the receptor spreads again over the whole surface which leads to what electrophysiologists call 'denervation supersensitivity'. Some other proteins, like the cell adhesion molecule N-CAM, follow the same pattern. Obviously, there is a cross-talk between two types of excitable cells, the motoneuron and the muscle fiber, amounting to some kind of 'negotiation' whether and where to form a synapse. Neuromuscular transmission and excitation may be components of this interaction but other elements are necessary in addition, especially for the early phases of neuromuscular contacts. Therefore, the neuromuscular synapse or 'endplate' provides a good model for cell interaction during synaptogenesis, a process more difficult to study in the CNS. Recently the molecular syntax of this cross-talk has become partially understood. The motor nerve terminal secretes a specific isoform of agrin, a proteoglycan, into the extracellular matrix of the synaptic cleft, and this is recognized by the subsynaptic muscle membrane. This recognition in turn leads to the local aggregation of AChRs on the myotube surface. Originally, agrin had been isolated from *Torpedo* electroplax (Godfrey *et al.*, 1984). The muscular agrin receptor has recently been identified as a muscle-specific tyrosine kinase, a transmembrane protein termed muscle-specific kinase (MuSK) (*Figure 2.6*). The recognition of agrin by MuSK is obviously the key event in neuromuscular synaptogenesis (Glass *et al.*, 1996): genetic elimination of either the agrin (Gautam *et al.*, 1996) or the MuSK (DeChiara *et al.*, 1996) gene in mice has dramatic effects that lead to death due to a blockade of endplate formation. Interestingly, not only is the subsynaptic specialization in muscle absent or reduced in these knockout mice, but in addition nerve endings sprout 'desperately' on muscle, in their futile attempt to establish localized stable relations with their target tissue.

So far, no hereditary disease in man or spontaneously occurring mutations in the mouse have been identified as being due to defects in the development of neuromuscular contacts. However, a host of mutations affect ion channel function in muscles, and, in order to understand these, a brief description of signaling in normal muscle will be given.

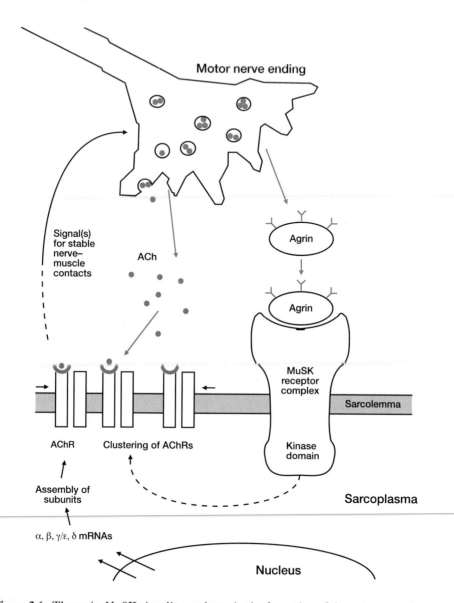

Figure 2.6. The agrin-MuSK signaling pathway in the formation of the neuromuscular synapse. This schematic drawing shows the signaling between the motor nerve ending (above) and the skeletal muscle (below, only a small peripheral segment is shown). The nerve ending releases the transmitter acetylcholine (ACh) and macromolecules influencing the differentiation of the target muscle fiber. One of these is the proteoglycan agrin, which is the ligand for a muscle specific receptor kinase, MuSK. Its activation is the key event to induce subsynaptic specializations in the muscle membrane (sarcolemma), notably the clustering of acetylcholine receptors (AChR), a hetero-oligomeric cation channel made of subunits α-, β-, γ- or ε-, and δ. Adapted from DeChiara *et al.* (1996).

Once the chemical signal of the nerve has been received by the subsynaptic AChR and translated into a local depolarization ('generator potential'), the voltage-sensitive channels of the sarcolemma transmit the excitation along the muscle fiber, usually in the form of an all or none signal, the action potential. This depolarization wave is finally translated into an intracellular calcium release which in turn triggers contraction of the actomyosin complex. The channels involved in this process, Na^+, K^+, Ca^{2+}, and Cl^- channels (see Chapter 6, by Edwards and Weston) can be the target of mutations which may lead to hyperexcitability or paralysis.

An important route into the genetics and molecular biology of ion channels led through the analysis of mutants of *Drosophila* which showed a legshaking phenotype under ether anesthesia (Isacoff *et al.*, 1990). In these flies a so-called A type potassium channel is affected which is expressed in central neurons and in muscle fibers. There is one *shaker* locus coding for a large variety of K^+ channels by elaborate differential splicing. The channel subunit itself is relatively simple and corresponds to a quarter of the large Na^+ and Ca^{2+} channel polypeptides (Isacoff *et al.*, 1990; Pongs *et al.*, 1988; *Figure 2.7*). In vertebrates, there is a multiplicity of homologous genes, comprising four subfamilies of the *shaker* family, the genes of which are scattered but also partially clustered in the mouse genome (Klocke *et al.*, 1993). A typical channel of this class is termed Kv.1.1 in mammals, and point mutations in Kv1.1 were found to change the excitability of Purkinje cells and the cerebellum and thereby to cause episodic ataxia with myokymia (Browne *et al.*, 1995). Another class of K^+ channels is gated not by voltage changes but by second messengers. In general, K^+ channel proteins share features of the cation conducting pore and are small compared to Na^+ and Ca^{2+} channel polypeptides (*Figure 2.7*).

As the neuromuscular synapse has served as a model to elucidate the biochemistry and molecular biology of synapses in general, the skeletal muscle fiber may serve to exemplify the genetic control of excitability. Channel proteins that are possible targets of mutations are: (i) the voltage-gated cation channels like the skeletal muscle Na^+ channel and a variety of K^+ channels, and (ii) a voltage-gated Cl^- channel, ClC-1. Whereas the sarcolemmal K^+ channels have a variety of physiological functions in the excitation–inactivation process, the α-subunit of the Na^+ channels (in vertebrates) comes in two isoforms, a tetrodotoxin (TTX)-resistant embryonic form and a TTX-sensitive adult form, but the two, though pharmacologically different, are functionally equivalent: Their voltage-dependent rapid opening is the basis of the self-propagating depolarization wave, the essence of excitability. The molecular structure of these channel subunits, which are large proteins of 1800 amino acid residues, is given in *Figure 2.7* (for review see Cannon, 1996).

Loss-of-function mutations in any of the two Na^+ channels would be expected to be a recessive lethality unless the juvenile form could replace the adult form. What has been found in humans instead are dominant mutations with a defect in channel inactivation rather than activation, leading to a class of relatively mild diseases called, depending on the clinical symptoms, paramyotonia, hyperkalemic periodic paralysis (hyperYPP) or potassium-aggravated myotonia. These names indicate whether the aspect of muscle stiffness (myotonia) or paralysis is more important, and what ionic conditions accompany or influence the episodes of muscle dysfunction. Obviously these are a highly selected and therefore biased subclass of all possible mutations that lead to only a marginal dysfunction at the single channel level. Such mutations have also been found in a specific breed of horse, the American quarterhorse, specifically

A type K⁺ channel (*shaker, Drosophila; episodic ataxia,* human)

K⁺ channel, Girk2 (*weaver,* mouse)

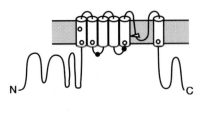
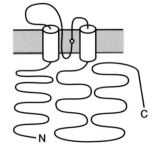

Muscular Na⁺ channel (paramyotonia, and related diseases, human, horse)

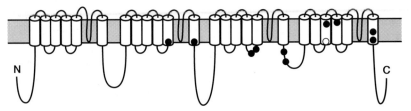

Muscular L-Ca²⁺ channel (*muscular dysgenesis,* mouse; hypokalemic periodic paralysis, human)

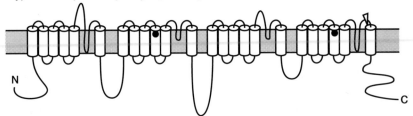

Muscular chloride channel ClC-1 (*myotonia,* mouse, human)

Glycine receptor α-subunit (*spasmodic,* mouse; hyperekplexia, human)

Glycine binding

Figure 2.7. Molecular structure of ion channel subunits and mutations causing disease. Schematic drawing of channel subunits in the cell membrane (outside up, inside down) helical transmembrane domains (cylinders), and intra- and extracellular connecting loops have been inferred from the primary sequences and ligand binding studies. The functional channel is made up either of homo-oligomers or of hetero-oligomers involving additional subunits not shown here (like β-subunits of the Na⁺ and K⁺ channels and the glycine receptor). The upper four channels are cation channels, the lower two anion (Cl⁻) channels. Girk2 is G-protein regulated, the glycine receptor is chemosensitive, all others are voltage gated. Shown are mutations that cause hereditary diseases in animals (empty symbols) or man (filled symbols). Circles, amino acid replacements; wedges, mutations leading to a premature termination of the polypeptide (stop codons, frame shift mutations, splice defects). Hyperekplexia is a startle disease.

bred for quarter mile races and selected for the prominent looks of its musculature (which is due to myotonia-induced hypertrophy). Not a single mutant of that type has been found in mice, the mammalian species that has been most extensively screened for abnormalities. The spontaneous point mutations in human patients are related to functional domains of the α-subunit polypeptide, with a number of amino acid replacements localizing to those polypeptide stretches that are responsible for the inactivation or voltage-dependent closing of the ion gate (see Hoffman *et al.*, 1995).

True myotonias have made essential contributions to our understanding of the physiological role of Cl⁻ channels in skeletal muscle. Myotonias like paramyotonias are diseases that lead to muscle stiffness due to a hyperexcitability of the muscle membrane. They have been observed in humans (dominant 'congenital' or Thomsen, and recessive, 'generalized' or Becker forms), in the goat (dominant, Bryant, 1979) and in several mouse mutants (recessive only). In the organism, these hereditary diseases can be simulated (or 'phenocopied') by drugs (like anthracene-9-carboxylic acid) that block chloride conductance, and in isolated muscle preparations the same effect is achieved by replacing external chloride by an impermeant anion, like methane sulfonate or gluconate. Hence, the structural gene that codes for the major muscular Cl⁻ channel was a favorite (though not the only) candidate gene based on function. Once sequences of this channel had become available, based on the pioneering work on the major Cl⁻ channel ClC-0 of *Torpedo* electroplax (Jentsch *et al.*, 1990), it turned out that both, murine and human myotonias are due to mutations in the structural gene for ClC-1 and were therefore homologous to each other (Gronemeier *et al.*, 1994; Koch *et al.*, 1992; Steinmeyer *et al.*, 1991). Hence, in this case, recessive and dominant myotonia mutations occur at the same gene locus. Whereas the recessive ones indicate that the function of ClC-1 is not absolutely required for the organism to survive, the dominant forms suggest that the channel is composed of several (e.g. two or four) subunits, and that mutated subunits can compromise channel function when associated with normal, wild-type subunits (Steinmeyer *et al.*, 1994).

Finally, mutations have been described in the slow Ca²⁺ channel responsible for excitation contraction coupling in muscle, the α1-subunit of the dihydropyridine receptor (DHP-R). The human disease connected to this channel is called hypokalemic periodic paralysis (hypoPP, see Hoffman *et al.*, 1995). During an episode of paralysis, serum K⁺ levels are low in contrast to the Na⁺ channel disease hyperPP. The physiological function of the DHP receptor is to activate another, juxtaposed, sarcolemmal Ca²⁺ channel, the Ca²⁺ release channel or ryanodine receptor. In hypoPP the mutated DHP-R shows a reduced activity. Obviously a total loss of this activity would interrupt excitation–contraction coupling and hence lead to total paralysis of muscle, despite a normally excitable sarcolemma and a normal contractile apparatus. This is in fact observed in a mutation of the mouse called *muscular dysgenesis, mdg*. This loss-of-function or 'null'-mutation causes perinatal death in the homozygous state (Chaudhari, 1992; see Henderson, 1990). As the mutant designation implies, affected myotubes deteriorate in late embryogenesis, so that the mice are born with only vestigial amounts of skeletal muscle. In cell culture, mutant myotubes do not spontaneously contract, but survive like wild-type myotubes. This indicates that there may be, in excitable cells, a connection between proper function and survival, exerted by a control mechanism which is only active in the context of the organism, not in cell culture.

For neurons, an interesting contribution to the function of anion channels has come from the molecular analysis of chemosensitive Cl⁻ channels, the glycine receptors, GlyR, of vertebrate motoneurons. Glycine is an inhibitory neurotransmitter. When it binds to the GlyR chloride channel, the channel is opened. This counteracts depolarization, by lowering the membrane potential. Hence, blockade of these channels causes de-inhibition or hyperexcitability. In the spinal cord, glycine is produced by inhibitory interneurons, the Renshaw cells, that form synapses with motoneurons, which express GlyRs on their surface. The activity of motoneurons and hence of voluntary muscles is determined by the balance of the excitatory input from descending fibers on the motoneurons and the inhibitory input from Renshaw cells, reflecting sensory signals from muscle spindles. Coordinated limb movement relies on alternating cycles of contraction and relaxation of agonist and antagonistic muscle groups. The alkaloid strychnine causes simultaneous cramps of all groups of voluntary muscles, and thus lethal convulsions, by binding to the GlyR and inactivating it. Thus, mutations interfering with the ligand binding or channel function of the GlyR can be expected to simulate strychnine intoxication. This phenotype is observed as a result of two mutations in the mouse, 'spastic' (spa) and 'spasmodic' (spd) that are located on different chromosomes.

Both mutations affect subunits of the pentameric GlyR. The molecular and genetic basis of spasticity is somewhat complicated by the fact that the GlyR is heteromeric with three α- and two β-subunits forming the channel. It is the α-subunits that bind, at the same sites, glycine and its antagonist strychnine. Furthermore the subunits occur in isoforms with regional and developmental specific expression patterns. The spasmodic mutation in the mouse and the human disease hyperekplexia, a startle disease, are both due to amino acid exchanges in the α1-subunit; the spastic mutation in the mouse is caused by a splicing defect in the transcript coding for the β-subunit (Becker, 1995; Mülhardt et al., 1994; Saul et al., 1994).

Myotonia and spastic/spasmodic are examples of well understood ion channel diseases in which effects previously known from pharmacology are faithfully mimicked by null or dominant-negative mutations. In both cases, the respective ion channel function is not essential for development and early postnatal life, so that these mutants were easily detected in the mouse.

Other ion channel mutations, such as motor endplate disease and weaver of the mouse have already been mentioned in Section 2.7.

2.10 A glimpse of the genetics of behavior and learning

Behavior is the output of the motor system in response to internal cues and sensory input, as translated by the complex machinery of the nervous system. This implies that behavior and its heritable interspecies variations must be dependent on the interaction of a host of gene functions, the unraveling of which might seem a hopeless enterprise. Yet, relatively simple relationships between gene mutations and behavioral variations or defects can be imagined. 'Pseudo-behavioral genes' would act on the effector molecules involved in the motor output rather than the processing within the nervous system. An example of this is the misnomer originally given to the first discovered myotonic mouse mutant, 'arrested development of righting response', adr, which (as described in the previous section) suffers from the absence of Cl⁻ conductance in mature muscle rather than from a defect in the development of a behavioral trait. A block in the first step, the sensory input would also cause mutants to be picked up in screens for abnormal behavior. This has indeed happened in *C. elegans* and *Drosophila*, organisms that lend themselves to mass analysis based on principles borrowed from microbial genetics. In fact, behavioral genetics has even been applied to unicellular organisms like bacteria and ciliates and yielded interesting mutants affected in 'sensory input' by receptors and 'motor output' (of flagellae or cilia) as well as defects in signal transduction.

In vertebrates, one is faced with a system containing about 10^{12} neurons. Yet nontrivial situations of relatively simple genetic controls can still be imagined. Levels of hormones, transmitters, or receptors which determine thresholds of behavioral switches (e.g. from 'peaceful' to 'aggressive' behavior) may be controlled by single genes. In fact, with the behavioral differences between males and females, nature provides a model of how a simple genetic difference (the presence or absence of the testis-determining factor *Tdf* or other genes on the Y chromosome) triggers a cascade of hormonal differences which in turn lead to the anatomical and behavioral divergence between sexes, the degree of which depends on the species.

In the analysis mutants, it makes a conceptual difference whether behavior has been altered by knocking out a gene function (loss-of-function mutation), proving, with luck, that this gene function (e.g. an ion channel or receptor) is *necessary* for normal behavior, or whether an altered or added gene (as in the case of the *Tdf* transgenic female mouse) causes altered behavior (gain-of-function) indicating that the gene is *sufficient* to produce a specific difference in behavior.

Sometimes the genetic control of a particular type of behavior might be revealed by studies in a seemingly unrelated field, such as nutritional physiology. In some parts of the world obesity poses a medical problem, and this has led to an investigation of spontaneous mutations in the mouse that cause obesity, the long-known mutations *obese* (*ob*) and *diabetic* (*db*). The identification, by positional cloning, of the *ob* gene of the mouse was 'satisfying' in a double sense: the gene identified coded for a hitherto unknown secreted protein, which seems to act as the satiety factor long searched for. This finding explained a great deal about the feedback control of body weight and furthermore was in line with classical experiments that had used the technique of parabiosis (i.e. surgical joining of the circulation of two individuals), to analyze the defect in *ob/ob* and *db/db* mice. When an *ob/ob* mouse was joined to a wild-type mouse, its feeding behavior was normalized, and it lost weight. When a *db/db* mouse was joined to a normal mouse, it was *not* normalized but the latter stopped eating and starved.

From these experiments it had been concluded that there is a factor that suppresses food intake which is missing in the 'obese' mouse (which however remains responsive to it), but is overproduced in the 'diabetic' mouse which has lost responsiveness. The factor missing in the *ob/ob* mouse (i.e. the product of the wild-type allele of *ob*), turned out to be a hormone-like polypeptide which was termed 'leptin' (from greek 'leptos', 'thin', 'slim'), and was found to be produced by adipose tissue (Zhang *et al.*, 1994) and to act on the brain. Injection of leptin into the blood or directly into the brain reduced food uptake in wild-type and obese, but not in diabetic mice, that is the same responses were found as in the parabiosis experiments performed decades earlier. Leptin controls feeding behavior by suppressing the release of another peptide from the hypothalamus, neuropeptide Y which by physiological experiments had been found to stimulate eating. As expected, the *db* mutation turned out to inactivate the leptin receptor (Lee *et al.*, 1996) and this, by interruption of a feedback loop, leads to overproduction of leptin, as demonstrated by the response of a wild-type mouse joined to a *db/db* mouse. The leptin receptor belongs to the family of cytokine receptors and is thus related to the CNTF receptor. When activated by their ligand these receptors bind to and activate tyrosine kinases. The leptin receptor is produced in different splice variants and a particularly large isoform is produced by the hypothalamus where presumably feeding behavior is controlled by leptin, acting as an antagonist to the release of neuropeptide Y. These findings are a beautiful illustration of how a relatively simple genetic system controls the threshold of a well-defined behavioral activity, in this case food intake, by levels of antagonistic signaling molecules (for review see Miller and Bell, 1996).

As feeding is controlled by biochemical thresholds so may be aggressive behavior. The notion that aggressiveness may have a simple genetic basis in humans (Brunner *et al.*, 1993), apart from the well known gender differences, has stirred considerable excitement and controversies. This genetic analysis led into the field of neurotransmitters, specifically into the metabolism of serotonin (5-hydroxytryptamine, 5-HT) and CNS serotonin receptors. From pharmacological evidence it was long known that the biogenic amine 5-HT acts both in the CNS and PNS and affects a wide variety of behavioral activities such as sleep, locomotion, aggression and sexual activity. Genetic analysis provides an approach to the metabolism of the transmitter, via mutations affecting synthesizing or degrading enzymes, or receptor mutations. There are two isoenzymes which degrade 5-HT and other biogenic amines, monoamine oxidases A and B (MAOA and MAOB) and in mammals the genes are both located on the X chromosome. The more abundant MAOA acts in mitochondria. Loss-of-function mutations in MAOA go unnoticed in female carriers but display the fatal phenotype in hemizygous males. An analysis of a family in which a number of males had a criminal record of impulsive aggressiveness (including arson and attempted rape) has revealed a stop codon mutation in the MAOA gene (Brunner *et al.*, 1993). Mice in which the MAOA gene had been knocked out showed hyperaggressiveness in addition to other behavioral abnormalities. In both cases, the behavioral effects might be attributed to elevated 5-HT levels in the brain and this was corroborated in mice, by pharmacologically suppressing the mutant symptoms with inhibitors of 5-HT synthesis. The effect of MAOA deficiency by itself is, of course, not quite specific as levels of the other biogenic amines are elevated as well. It seems likely that the genetic lack of MAOA has long-term effects on the development of the nervous system, at least in humans. The link between aggressive behavior and serotonin receptors is complicated by the fact that at least 30 receptors exist in mammals. Unexpectedly in the light of the MAOA deficiency, the knockout of one specific subtype, 5-HT$_{1B}$, causes increased aggressiveness, whereas that of another subtype 5-HT$_{2C}$, causes excessive feeding in addition to other abnormalities (see Heath and Hen, 1995).

The gaseous messenger nitric oxide, NO, plays a regulatory role in blood vessels and skeletal muscle and is a neurotransmitter of the CNS. NO is synthesized by NO synthase, and this comes in tissue-specific isotypes. The gene for the neuronal isoform, nNOS, has been knocked out. Surprisingly, the knockout mice showed normal overall appearance and behavior, but the aggressiveness of males was drastically elevated. This seems to be a rather specific effect as other functions, such as olfaction and fear that might influence aggressiveness were not changed (Nelson *et al.*, 1995).

Learning requires memory, and memory has been studied by training in combination with pharmacological treatment. The distinction of short-term and long-term memory is common knowledge (see Chapter 12 for a detailed discussion). More precise definitions were possible when learning and memory were studied by training *Drosophila* with combinations of odor and electroshocks. Retention times were tested by the time schedule of conditioning and the decay of trained behavior. A short-term memory in the minute range is followed by an anesthetic-sensitive intermediate memory and this by long-term memory (see deZazzo and Tully, 1994). A biochemical distinction between short-term and long-term memory had previously been defined in vertebrates, particularly in the goldfish: long-term memory could be blocked by cycloheximide, an inhibitor of protein synthesis. Because of these biochemical differences it should be possible to find mutations specifically affecting different steps from learning to long-term memory.

Mutations affecting different steps in learning and memory formation have been detected in *Drosophila* and pointed to the importance of cAMP-dependent intracellular signal transduction, as previously found by microbiochemical methods in giant neurons of *Aplysia*. In *Drosophila* there are two types of long-term memory, anesthesia-resistant memory with little sensitivity against cycloheximide, and a long-term memory, comparable to that of vertebrates, which is highly sensitive to inhibitors of protein synthesis (*Figure 2.8*). Mutations in *Drosophila* genes coding for cAMP-phosphodiesterase, Ca^{2+}/calmodulin-dependent adenylate cyclase and a catalytic subunit of the cAMP-dependent protein kinase all disrupt learning and memory. Signaling by cAMP at the gene expression level is mediated by the cAMP response element binding protein, CREB protein, the 'responsive element' being a specific DNA sequence; cAMP-regulated gene expression is expected to require CREB protein. To test its importance for memory and learning, the CREB protein gene has been functionally knocked out: in *Drosophila* by a dominant-negative transgene (Yin *et al*., 1994), and in mouse by homologous recombination leading to a loss of function. In both cases, long-term memory was affected. In a shock-conditioning test, CREB protein knockout mice which were otherwise normal indeed failed to retain memory for longer than about 30 min, whereas wild-type controls did so for at least 24 h (Bourtchuladze *et al*., 1994; Hummler *et al*., 1994).

2.11. Neurodegeneration due to aging and infections: genetic factors

Old age and its ailments are the predominant issue of public health. The most common neurological disease of aged people is the senile dementia called Alzheimer's disease (AD). This comes in sporadic and familial, late-onset (>65 years) and early-onset (30–60 years) forms. The familial forms, sometimes characteristic for certain ethnic groups, especially the early-onset varieties have recently become accessible to genetic analysis. In one instance, the approach has been a biochemical one in the first place, the characterization of protein crystals deposited in the brains of AD patients. As these resemble starch, amylum, in their microscopical appearance, the protein was termed β-amyloid. With its amino acid sequence determined, the corresponding gene was identified and localized to human chromosome 21. This chromosome is present in three instead of two copies in people with Down's syndrome and therefore the amyloid gene was also associated with mental retardation and premature aging observed in Down's patients. In familial AD, an important disease gene locus, termed *AD1*, is indeed the β-amyloid gene *βAPP* itself. The β-amyloid crystals are water insoluble proteolytic cleavage products of the amyloid precursor protein βAPP, a transmembrane protein of unknown function which is coded for by the *AD1/βAPP* gene. Mutations in the *βAPP* gene causing familial AD are amino acid replacements usually localized in the β-amyloid portion of the precursor protein that act in a dominant fashion, implying a gain-of-function type of etiology in which the mutant protein exerts toxic effects.

Two additional AD genes have been discovered on other chromosomes, the *STM2* gene on chromosome 1 (*AD2*), and the *S182* candidate gene on chromosome 14 (*AD3*, for review see: van Broeckhoven, 1995). These two newly discovered genes are

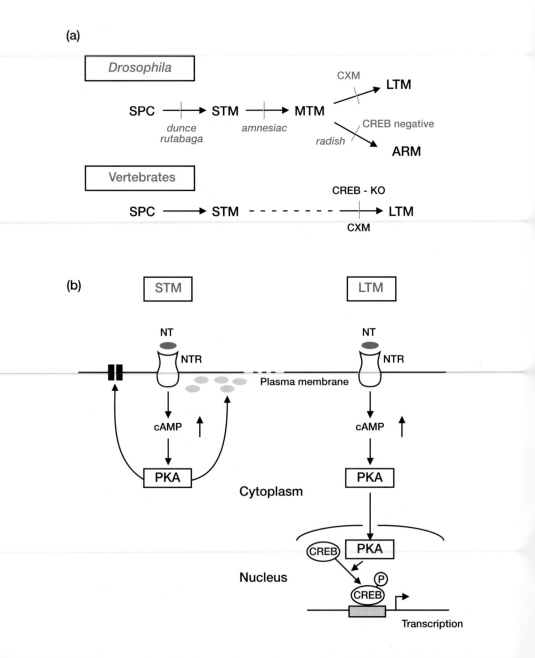

homologous to each other and to a spermatozoal protein of the nematode *C. elegans*. They code for receptor-like transmembrane proteins, now termed presenilins. Some alleles of the polymorphic apolipoprotein E locus on chromosome 19 apart from being involved in cholesterol levels and vascular disease seem to exert a strong modifying influence on AD dementia. The allele ε4 enhances the AD symptoms in a dosage dependent fashion, whereas ε2 seems to suppress them, other alleles being neutral (see Charlesworth, 1996). Thus, AD appears as a typical case of a polygenic etiology which will take several more years to fully unravel, and the support of genetic animal models in which AD-like effects can be observed within short periods of time (months).

A transgenic construct with the neurofilament light chain promoter (to direct over-expression specifically to neurons), and the mouse β-amyloid gene aβ (LaFerla *et al.*, 1995) was used to produce such a mouse model. Although specific cognitive deterioration was not observed in this mouse, neurodegeneration including apoptotic processes, seizures and premature death were reported. It may well be that pathological processes physically similar to those observed in AD patients have very different neurological consequences in the mouse. In another transgenic AD mouse model a pathogenic human *AD1* was used. A construct coding for a mutant (valine to phenylalanine at position 717) form of the human amyloid gene, was introduced into the mouse genome and was found to be expressed at high levels. At age 6–9 months (i.e. a quarter of the normal lifespan) the *AD1* transgenic mice developed regional histopathological changes in the brain similar to those found in AD patients. However, cognitive properties of these mice have not been tested yet.

Another topic of public interest are neurodegenerative diseases of the Creutzfeldt–Jakob/Gerstmann–Sträussler or Kuru type, known in sheep as scrapie and in cattle as bovine spongiform encephalitis. These are infectious diseases in the sense that they can be transmitted accidentally (via feeding) or experimentally (by the intracerebral injection of brain or spinal cord extracts). Originally designated slow virus

---

Figure 2.8. Genetics and biochemistry of short- and long-term memory. (a) Pathways of learning and memory as defined by genetics and pharmacological experiments, in *Drosophila* and vertebrates. SPC, sensory perception of conditioning stimuli; STM, short-term memory; MTM, middle-term memory; LTM, long-term memory; ARM, anesthesia-resistant memory. The last two constitute 'consolidated memory' in *Drosophila*. ARM, in contrast to LTM, is relatively resistant to cycloheximide treatment (CXM) and specifically blocked by the '*radish*' mutation. Other mutations block earlier steps of memory formation by interfering with cAMP metabolism: '*dunce*' is a gene for cAMP phosphodiesterase, '*rutabaga*' for calmodulin-dependent adenylate cyclase. In vertebrates MTM and ARM have not been experimentally defined, but LTM similar to *Drosophila* is blocked by CXM and interference with the function of CREB, the protein binding to the cAMP responsive element. NT, neurotransmitter; NTR, receptor for NT. Modified after Tully *et al.* (1994). (b) Presumed biochemical events underlying STM and LTM in fly and mouse. In both cases, the binding of neurotransmitter (NT) to its receptor (NTR) raises the intracellular cAMP level. This in turn activates protein kinase A (PKA) which may phosphorylate ion channels and peripheral membrane proteins near the synapse, thereby leading to a short-term modulation of its efficiency. During the formation of LTM, sustained elevated levels of cAMP cause the catalytic subunit of PKA to translocate to the nucleus, where it can phosphorylate CREB. This, in turn, activates the transcription of so-called 'immediate early genes' many of which code for transcription factors that activate 'late response genes'. The products of late response genes contribute to lasting structural changes at the synapse. Modified from Frank and Greenberg (1994).

infections, these diseases are now believed to be due not to the transfer of conventional genetic material (nucleic acid) of a pathogen but to an abnormal conformer of a species-intrinsic protein, the prion. This is the famous 'protein only' hypothesis which has recently received strong support from ingenious experiments using transgenic animals. In brief, it was shown that when the prion gene *Prnp* on chromosome 2 of the mouse was knocked out, the mouse became resistant to mouse prion infection. Its susceptibility could be restored by re-introducing the gene. In the same type of experiment, the relative species specificity of prion infection could be reproduced: the mouse is relatively resistant to infection with hamster prion but becomes highly susceptible to it when harboring a hamster prion transgene (see Beyreuther and Masters, 1994; Brandner *et al.*, 1996). Thus the prion protein gene is a classical case of a susceptibility gene. Its presence or absence determines the response to an external disease-causing agent, in these case with a covalent structure identical to that of the susceptibility gene product.

2.12. Conclusions

In recent years, concepts have developed that allow for a mechanistic understanding of metazoan development and morphogenesis. These involve the interpretation of prepatterns of graded morphogen concentrations by cascades of gene regulation, with key roles played by genes coding for transcription factors which control downstream 'realizator' genes (review: St Johnston and Nüsslein-Vollhard, 1992), in conjunction with theoretical concepts of the self-organization of patterns, starting from random fluctuations of morphogen concentration (Gierer and Meinhardt, 1971). Hence, a genetic understanding of a subset of metazoan differentiation and morphogenesis events, namely the emergence of a nervous system with an elaborate wiring pattern, should be possible. The genetic analysis of pathfinding of nerve processes, which has made great progress both in favorable invertebrates (e.g. *C. elegans* and *Drosophila*) and in vertebrate systems (e.g. zebrafish) is a most promising approach.

Neurogenetics as applied to medicine will progress even if a full understanding of the emergence of the nervous system has a long way to go. In terms of scientific advancement this chapter ranges from well-understood, relatively straightforward gene–protein–phenotype relationships, as in some ion channel and myelin diseases, to the complicated field of neurodegeneration, which is just starting to become unraveled.

A generalization that can be made from genetic analysis of the nervous and neuromuscular systems is that aspects of the life of an excitable cell that conceptually may appear separate (such as cell differentiation, cell migration, interaction with accessory cells, electrical activity, and survival of an excitable cell) may in fact be interwoven and share genetic functions, because there are feedback loops from function to the advancement of differentiation, and from both to survival, that govern the career of a cell in the social environment of a multicellular organism.

Examples given in this chapter clearly show that genetics is useful, even indispensable for cellular neurobiology and is making its way into higher levels of integrative functions such as behavior and learning. But what about consciousness, a scientific explanation of which would appear to be the ultimate goal of neurobiology? Will there ever be such a thing as the 'genetics of consciousness'? One currently promising scientific approach to the identification of the neural correlates of consciousness is by the physiology of perception (see Crick, 1996). Is it possible then, in analogy to the genetics of behavior and learning, to imagine a genetic analysis of consciousness? Maybe not: genetics may be of as little relevance to the analysis of consciousness as quantum mechanics is for embryology. No scientist doubts that quantum mechanics is valid during embryonic development, but even the most successful embryologists do not resort to that universal theory. As a basis of explanation it is too many levels below the level of the phenomena to be explained. An analogous relation may exist between genetics and consciousness.

Acknowledgments

We thank R. Klocke for help with typing, J.W. Bartsch for contributions to the bibliography, A. Lengeling, P. Heimann, M. Gronemeier, G. John and B.M. Jockusch for carefully reading the manuscript, and R.W. Davies for his patience.

References

Adlkofer K, Martini R, Aguzzi A, Zielasek J, Toyka KV, Suter U. (1995) Hypermyelination and demyelinating peripheral neuropathy in PMP22-deficient mice. *Nature Genetics* **11**: 274–280.

Ait-Ikhlef A, Murawsky M, Blondet B, Hantaz-Ambroise D, Martinou JC, Rieger F. (1995) The motoneuron degeneration in the wobbler mouse is independent of the overexpression of *Bcl2* transgene in neurons. *Neurosci. Lett.* **199**: 163–166.

Baynash AG, Hosoda K, Giaid A, Richardson JA, Emoto N, Hammer RE, Yanagisawa M. (1994) Interaction of endothelin-3 with endothelin-B receptor is essential for development of epidermal melanocytes and enteric neurons. *Cell* **79**: 1277–1285.

Becker C-M. (1995) Glycine receptors: molecular heterogeneity and implications for disease. *Neuroscience* **1**: 130–141.

Beyreuther K, Masters CL. (1994) Catching the culprit prion. *Nature* **370**: 419–420.

Boison D, Stoffel W. (1994) Disruption of the compacted myelin sheath of axons of the central nervous system in proteolipid protein-deficient mice. *Proc. Natl Acad. Sci. USA* **91**: 11 709–11 713.

Bourtchuladze R, Frenguelli B, Blendy J, Cioffi D, Schütz G, Silva AJ. (1994) Deficient long-term memory in mice with a targeted mutation of the cAMP-responsive element-binding protein. *Cell* **79**: 59–68.

Brandner S, Isenmann S, Raeber A, Fischer M, Sailer A, Kobayashi Y, Marino S, Weissmann C, Aguzzi A. (1996) Normal host prion protein necessary for scrapie-induced neurotoxicity. *Nature* **379**: 339–343.

Brandon EP, Idzerda RL, McKnight GS. (1995a) Targeting the mouse genome: a compendium of knockouts I. *Curr. Biol.* **5**: 625–634.

Brandon EP, Idzerda RL, McKnight GS. (1995b) Targeting the mouse genome: a compendium of knockouts II. *Curr. Biol.* **5**: 758–765.

Brandon EP, Idzerda RL, McKnight GS. (1995c) Targeting the mouse genome: a compendium of knockouts III. *Curr. Biol.* **5**: 873–881.

Brooks BP, Fischbeck KH. (1995): Spinal and bulbar muscular atrophy: a trinucleotide-repeat expansion neurodegenerative disease. *Trends Neurosci.* **18**: 459–461.

Browne DL, Brunt ER, Griggs RC, Nutt JG, Gancher ST, Smith EA, Litt M. (1995) Identification of two new KCNA1 mutations in episodic ataxia/myokimia families. *Hum. Mol. Genet.* **4**: 1671–1672.

Brunialti ALB, Poirier C, Schmalbruch H, Guénet J-L. (1995) The mouse mutation progressive motor neuronopathy (*pmn*) maps to chromosome 13. *Genomics* **29**: 131–135.

Brunner HG, Nelen M, Breakefield XO, Ropers HH, van Oost BA. (1993) Abnormal behavior associated with a point mutation in the structural gene for monoamine oxidase A. *Science* **262**: 578–580.

Bryant SH. (1979) Myotonia in the goat. *Proc. Natl Acad. Sci. USA.* **317**: 314–325.

Bunge RP, Fernandez-Valle C. (1995) Basic biology of the Schwann cell. In: *Neuroglial Cells* (eds H Kettenmann, B Ransom). Oxford University Press, Oxford, pp. 44–57.

Burgess DL, Kohrman DC, Galt J, Plummer NW, Jones JM, Spear B, Meisler H. (1995) Mutation of a new sodium channel gene, *Scn8a*, in the mouse mutant 'motor endplate disease'. *Nature Genetics* **10**: 461–465.

Burright EN, Clark HB, Servadio A, Matilla T, Feddersen RM, Yunis WS, Duvick LA, Zoghbi HY, Orr HT. (1995) *SCA1* transgenic mice: a model for neurodegeneration caused by an expanded CAG trinucleotide repeat. *Cell* 82: 937–948.

Campagnoni A. (1995) Molecular biology of myelination. In: *Neuroglial Cells* (eds H Kettenmann, B Ransom). Oxford University Press, Oxford, pp. 555–570.

Cannon SC. (1996) Ion-channel defects and aberrant excitability in myotonia and periodic paralysis. *Trends Neurosci.* 19: 3–10.

Charlesworth B. (1996) Evolution of senescence: Alzheimer's disease and evolution. *Curr. Biol.* 6: 20–22.

Chaudhari N. (1992) A single nucleotide deletion in the skeletal muscle-specific calcium channel transcript of muscular dysgenesis (mdg) mice. *J. Biol. Chem.* 267: 25 636–25 639.

Colamarino SA, Tessier-Lavigne M. (1995) The axonal chemoattractant netrin-1 is also a chemorepellent for trochlear motor axons. *Cell* 81: 621–629.

Crick F. (1996) Visual perception: rivalry and consciousness. *Nature* 379: 485.

Crowley C, Spencer SD, Nishimura MC, Chen KS, Pitts MS, Armanini MP. (1994) Mice lacking nerve growth factor display perinatal loss of sensory and sympathetic neurons yet develop basal forebrain cholinegic neurons. *Cell* 76: 1001–1011.

D'Arcangelo G, Miao GG, Chen S-C, Soares HD, Morgan JI, Curran T. (1995) A protein related to extracellular matrix proteins deleted in the mouse mutant *reeler*. *Nature* 374: 719–723.

Davies AM. (1994) The role of neurotrophins in the developing nervous system. *J. Neurobiol.* 25: 1334–1348.

Davies AM. (1995) The Bcl-2 family of proteins, and the regulation of neuronal survival. *Trends Neurosci.* 18: 355–358.

DeBry RW, Seldin MF. (1996) Human/mouse homology relationships. *Genomics* 33: 337–351.

DeChiara TM, Vejsada R, Poueymirou WT *et al.* (1995) Mice lacking the CNTF receptor, unlike mice lacking CNTF, exhibit profound motor neuron deficits at birth. *Cell* 83: 313–322.

DeChiara TM, Bowen DC, Valenzuela DM *et al.* (1996) The receptor tyrosine kinase MuSK is required for neuromuscular junction formation *in vivo*. *Cell* 85: 501–512.

DeZazzo J, Tully T. (1995) Dissection of memory formation: from behavioral pharmacology to molecular genetics. *Trends Neurosci.* 18: 212–218.

Drescher U, Kremoser C, Handwerker C, Löschinger J, Noda M, Bonhoeffer F. (1995) *In vitro* guidance of retinal ganglion cell axons by RAGS, a 25 kDa tectal protein related to ligands for Eph-receptor tyrosine kinases. *Cell* 82: 359–370.

Duncan ID, Hammang JP, Goda S, Quarles RH. (1989) Myelination in the jimpy mouse in the absence of proteolipid protein. *Glia* 2: 148–154.

Echelard Y, Epstein DJ, St-Jacques B, Shen L, Mohler J, McMahon JA, McMahon AP. (1993) Sonic hedgehog, a member of a family of putative signalling molecules, is implicated in the regulation of CNS polarity. *Cell* 75: 1417–1430.

Edery P, Attie T, Amiel J *et al.* (1996) Mutation of the endothelin-3 gene in the Waardenburg-Hirschsprung disease (Shah-Waardenburg syndrome). *Nature Genetics* 12: 442–444.

Ekker SC, Ungar AR, Greenstein P, von Kessler DP, Porter JA, Moon RT, Beachy PA. (1995) Patterning activities of vertebrate hedgehog proteins in the developing eye and brain. *Curr. Biol.* 5: 944–955.

Epstein DJ, Vekemans M, Gros P. (1991) Splotch (Sp^{2H}), a mutation affecting development of the mouse neural tube, shows a deletion within the paired homeodomain of Pax-3. *Cell* 67: 767–774.

Ernfors P, Lee KF, Jaenisch R. (1994) Mice lacking brain-derived neurotrophic factor develop with sensory deficits. *Nature* 368: 147–150.

Falconer DS. (1951) Two new mutations, trembler and reeler, with neurological action in the house mouse. *J. Genet.* 50: 192–201.

Fleischman RA. (1993) From white spots to stem cells: the role of the Kit receptor in mammalian development. *Trends Genet.* 9: 285–289.

Franco B, Guioli S, Pragiola A *et al.* (1991) A gene deleted in Kallmann's syndrome shares homology with neural cell adhesion and axonal path-finding molecules. *Nature* 353: 529–536.

Frank DA, Greenberg ME. (1994) CREB: a mediator of long-term memory from mollusks to mammals. *Cell* 79: 5–8.

Gautam M, Noakes PG, Moscoso L, Rupp F, Scheller RH, Merlie JP, Sanes JR. (1996) Defective neuromuscular synaptogenesis in agrin-deficient mutant mice. *Cell* 85: 525–535.

Geissler EN, Ryan MA, Houseman DE. (1988) The dominant-white spotting (*W*) locus of the mouse encodes the *c-kit* proto-oncogene. *Cell* 55: 185–192.

Gencic S, Hudson L. (1990) Conservative amino acid substitution in the myelin proteolipid protein of jimpy^{msd} mice. *J. Neurosci.* **10:** 117–124.

Gierer A, Meinhardt H. (1971) A theory of biological pattern formation. *Kybernetik* **12:** 30–39.

Giese KP, Martini R, Lemke G, Soriano P, Schachner M. (1992) Disruption of the P0 gene in mice leads to abnormal expression of recognition molecules, and degeneration of myelin and axons. *Cell* **71:** 565–576.

Glass DJ, Bowen DC, Stitt TN *et al.* (1996) Agrin acts via a MuSK receptor complex. *Cell* **85:** 513–523.

Godfrey EW, Nitkin RM, Wallace BG, Rubin LL, McMahan UJ. (1984) Components of *Torpedo* electric organ and muscle that cause aggregation of acetylcholine receptors on cultured muscle cells. *J. Cell Biol.* **99:** 615–627.

Goldowitz D, Smeyne RJ. (1995) Tune into the weaver channel. *Nature Genetics* **11:** 107–109.

Goodman CS, Shatz CJ. (1993) Developmental mechanisms that generate precise patterns of neuronal connectivity. *Cell* **72** (Suppl.): 77–98.

Grenningloh G, Rehm EJ, Goodman CS. (1991) Genetic analysis of growth cone guidance in *Drosophila*: fasciclin II functions as a neuronal recognition molecule. *Cell* **67:** 45–57.

Grindley JC, Davidson DR, Hill RE. (1995) The role of *Pax-6* in eye and nasal development. *Development* **121:** 1433–1442.

Gronemeier M, Condie A, Prosser J, Steinmeyer K, Jentsch TJ, Jockusch H. (1994) Nonsense and missense mutations in the muscular chloride channel gene *Clc-1* of myotonic mice. *J. Biol. Chem.* **269:** 5963–5967.

Guillemot F, Lo LC, Johnson JE, Auerbach A, Anderson DJ, Joyner AL. (1993) Mammalian achaete-scute homolog 1 is required for the early development of olfactory and autonomic neurons. *Cell* **74:** 463–476.

Guillery RW. (1974) Visual pathways in albinos. *Sci. Am.* **230:** 44–54.

Gurney ME, Pu H, Chiu AY *et al.* (1994) Motor neuron degeneration in mice that express a human Cu, Zn superoxide dismutase mutation. *Science* **264:** 1772–1775.

Halder G, Callaerts P, Gehring WJ. (1995) Induction of ectopic eyes by targeted expression of the *eyeless* gene in *Drosophila*. *Science* **267:** 1788–1792.

Hamilton BA, Frankel WN, Kerrebrock *et al.* (1996) Disruption of the nuclear hormone receptor RORα in *staggerer* mice. *Nature* **379:** 736–739.

Hayasaka K, Himoro M, Sato W, Takada G, Uyemura K, Shimizu N, Bird TD, Conneally PM, Chance PF. (1993) Charcot-Marie-Tooth neuropathy type 1B is associated with mutations of myelin P0 gene. *Nature Genetics* **5:** 31–34.

Heath MJS, Hen R. (1995) Genetic insights into serotonin function. *Curr. Biol.* **5:** 997–999.

Henderson C. (1990) Making mouse muscle move. *Trends Neurosci.* **13:** 39–41.

Hengartner MO. (1994) A rich harvest. *Curr. Biol.* **4:** 950–952.

Henry EW, Sidman RL. (1988) Long lives for homozygous trembler mutant mice despite virtual absence of peripheral nerve myelin. *Science* **241:** 344–346.

Hodes ME, Pratt VM, Dlouhy SR. (1994) Genetics of Pelizaeus-Merzbacher disease. *Devel. Neurosci.* **15:** 383–394.

Hoffman EP, Lehmann-Horn F, Rüdel R. (1995) Overexited or inactive: ion channel in muscle disease. *Cell* **80:** 681–686.

Hofstra RM, Osinga J, Tan-Sindhunata G *et al.* (1996) A homozygous mutation in the endothelin-3 gene associated with a combined Waardenburg type 2 and Hirschsprung phenotype (Shah-Waardenburg syndrome). *Nature Genetics* **12:** 445–447.

Hosoda K, Hammer RE, Richardson JA, Bayanash AG, Cheung JC, Giaid A, Yanagisawa M. (1994) Targeted and natural (piebald-lethal) mutations of endothelin-B receptor gene produce megacolon associated with spotted coat color in mice. *Cell* **79:** 1267–1276.

Huang E, Nocka K, Beier DR, Chu T-Y, Buck J, Lahm H-W, Wellner D, Leder P, Besmer P. (1990) The hematopoetic growth factor KL is encoded by the *Sl* locus and is the ligand of the *c-kit* receptor, the gene product of the W locus. *Cell* **63:** 225–233.

Hudson LD, Berndt JA, Puckett C, Kozak CA, Lazzarini RA. (1987) Aberrant splicing of proteolipid protein mRNA in the dysmyelinating jimpy mutant mouse. *Proc. Natl Acad. Sci. USA* **84:** 1454–1458.

Hummler E, Cole, Blendy JA, Ganss R, Aguzzi A, Schmid W, Beermann F, Schütz G. (1994) Targeted mutation of the CREB gene: compensation within the CREB/ATF family of transcription factors. *Proc. Natl Acad. Sci. USA* **91:** 5647–5651.

Isacoff E, Papazian D, Timpe L, Jan Y-N, Jan L-Y. (1990) Molecular studies of voltage-gated potassium channels. *CSH Symposia Quantitative Biology*, Vol. **LV**. Cold Spring Harbor Laboratory Press, Cold Spring Harbor, NY.

Jentsch TJ, Steimeyer K, Schwarz G. (1990) Primary structure of *Torpedo marmorata* chloride channel isolated by expression cloning in *Xenopus* oocytes. *Nature* **348**: 510–514.

Jones KR, Farinas I, Backus C, Reichardt LF. (1994) Targeted disruption of the BDNF gene perturbs brain and sensory neuron development but not motor neuron development. *Cell* **76**: 989–999.

Joyner AL. (1991) Gene targeting and gene trap screens using embryonic stem cells: new approaches to mammalian development. *Bioessays* **13**: 649–656.

Kagawa T, Ikenaka K, Inoue Y *et al.* (1994) Glial cell degeneration and hypomyelination caused by overexpression of the myelin proteolipid protein gene. *Neuron* **13**: 427–442.

Kennedy TE, Serafini T, de la Torre JR, Tessier-Lavigne M. (1994) Netrins are diffusible chemotropic factors for commissural axons in the embryonic spinal cord. *Cell* **78**: 425–435.

Kirschner DA, Ganser AL. (1980) Compact myelin exists in the absence of basic protein in the shiverer mutant mouse. *Nature* **283**: 207–210.

Klar A, Badassare M, Jessell TM. (1992) F-spondin: a gene expressed at high levels in the floor plate encodes a secreted protein that promotes neural cell adhesion and neurite extension. *Cell* **69**: 95–110.

Klocke R, Roberds SL, Tamkun MM, Gronemeier M, Augustin A, Albrecht B, Pongs O, Jockusch H. (1993) Chromosomal mapping in the mouse of eight K$^+$ channel genes representing the four *Shaker*-like subfamilies *Shaker*, *Shab*, *Shaw* and *Shal*. *Genomics* **18**: 568–574.

Knapp PE, Skoff RP, Redstone DW. (1986) Oligodendroglial cell death in jimpy mice: an explanation for the myelin deficit. *J. Neurosci.* **6**: 2813–2822.

Koch MC, Steinmeyer K, Lorenzc *et al.* (1992) The skeletal muscle chloride channel in dominant and recessive human myotonia. *Science* **257**: 797–800.

Kolodkin AL, Matthes DJ, Goodman CS. (1993) The semaphorin genes encode a family of transmembrane and secreted growth cone guidance molecules. *Cell* **75**: 1389–1399.

Kuwada J. (1995) Development of the zebrafish nervous system: genetic analysis and manipulation. *Curr. Opin. Neurobiol.* **5**: 50–54.

LaFerla FM, Tinkle BT, Bieberich CJ, Haudenschild CC, Jay G. (1995) The Alzheimer's Aβ peptide induces neurodegeneration and apoptotic cell death in transgenic mice. *Nature Genetics* **9**: 21–30.

Lee KF, Li E, Huber LJ, Landis SC, Sharpe AH, Chao MV, Jaenisch R. (1992) Targeted mutation of the gene encoding the low affinity NGF receptor p75 leads to deficits in the peripheral sensory nervous system. *Cell* **69**: 737–749.

Lee JE, Hollenberg SM, Snider L, Turner DL, Lipnick N, Weintraub H. (1995) Conversion of *Xenopus* ectoderm into neurons by NeuroD, a basic helix–loop–helix protein. *Science* **268**: 836–844.

Lee G-H, Provenca R, Montez JM, Carroll KM, Darvishzadeh JG, Lee JI, Friedman JM. (1996) Abnormal splicing of leptin receptor in *diabetic* mice. *Nature* **379**: 632–635.

Lefebvre S, Bürglen L, Reboullet S *et al.* (1995) Identification and characterization of a spinal muscular atrophy-determining gene. *Cell* **80**: 155–165.

Lemke G, Lamar E, Patterson J. (1988) Isolation and analysis of the gene encoding peripheral myelin protein zero. *Neuron* **1**: 73–83.

Le Mouellic H, Lallemand Y, Brulet P. (1992) Homeosis in the mouse induced by a null mutation in the *Hox-3.1* gene. *Cell* **69**: 251–264.

Li C, Tropak MB, Gerial R, Clapoff S, Abramov-Newerly W, Trapp B, Peterson A, Roder J. (1994) Myelination in the absence of myelin-associated glycoprotein. *Nature* **369**: 747–750.

Lichinghagen R, Stocker M, Wittka R, Boheim G, Stuhmer W, Ferrus A, Pongs O. (1990) Molecular basis of altered excitability in *Shaker* mutants of *Drosophila melanogaster*. *EMBO J.* **9**: 4399–4407.

Liem KF, Tremmel G, Roelink H, Jessell TM. (1995) Dorsal differentiation of neural plate cells induced by BMP-mediated signals from epidermal ectoderm. *Cell* **82**: 969–979.

Lin DM, Goodman CS. (1994) Ectopic and increased expression of fasciclin II alters motoneuron growth cone guidance. *Neuron* **13**: 507–523.

Lin DM, Fetter RD, Kopczynski C, Grenningloh G, Goodman CS. (1994) Genetic analysis of fasciclin II in *Drosophila*: defasciculation, refasciculation, and altered fasciculation. *Neuron* **13**: 1055–1069.

Lumsden A, Graham A. (1995) A forward role for Hedgehog. *Curr. Biol.* **5**: 1347–1350.

Martini R, Schachner M. (1986) Immunoelectron microscopic localization of neural cell adhesion molecules (L1, N-CAM, and MAG) and their shared carbohydrate epitope and myelin basic protein in developing sciatic nerve. *J. Cell Biol.* **103**: 2439–2448.

Martini R, Mohajeri MH, Kasper S, Giese KP, Schachner M. (1995a) Mice doubly deficient in the genes for P0 and myelin basic protein show that both proteins contribute to the formation of the major dense line in peripheral nerve myelin. *J. Neurosci.* **15**: 4488–4495.

Martini R, Zielasek J, Toyka KV, Giese KP, Schachner M. (1995b) Protein zero (P0)-deficient mice show myelin degeneration in peripheral nerves characteristic of inherited human neuropathies. *Nature Genetics* **11**: 281–286.

Masu Y, Wolf E, Holtmann B, Sendtner M, Brem G, Thoenen H. (1993) Disruption of the CNTF gene results in motor neuron degeneration. *Nature* **365**: 27–32.

McGinnis W, Krumlauf R. (1992) Homeobox genes and axial patterning. *Cell* **68**: 283–302.

McMahon AP, Bradley A. (1990) The Wnt-1 (int-1) proto-oncogene is required for development of large region of the mouse brain. *Cell* **62**: 1073–1085.

Meyer-Franke A, Barres B. (1994) Myelination without myelin-associated glycoprotein. *Curr. Biol.* **4**: 847–850.

Mikoshiba K, Okano H, Tamura T, Ikenaka K. (1991) Structure and function of myelin protein genes. *Annu. Rev. Neurosci.* **14**: 201–217.

Miller RJ, Bell GI. (1996) JAK/STAT eats fat. *Trends Neurosci.* **19**: 159–161.

Mitsumoto H, Ikeda K, Klinkosz B, Cedarbaum JM, Wong V, Lindsay RM. (1994) Arrest of motor neuron disease in wobbler mice cotreated with CNTF and BDNF. *Science* **265**: 1107–1110.

Molineaux SM, Engh H, deFerra F, Hudson L, Lazzarini RA. (1986) Recombination within the myelin basic protein gene created the dysmyelinating shiverer mouse mutation. *Proc. Natl Acad. Sci. USA* **83**: 7542–7546.

Montag D, Giese K-P, Martini R et al. (1994) Mice deficient for the myelin-associated glycoprotein show subtle abnormalities of myelin. *Neuron* **13**: 229–246.

Mülhardt C, Fischer M, Gass P, Simon-Chazottes D, Guénet J-L, Kuhse J, Betz H, Becker C-M. (1994) The spastic mouse: aberrant splicing of glycine receptor β subunit mRNA caused by intronic insertion of L1 element. *Neuron* **13**: 1003–1015.

Mullins MC, Hammerschmidt M, Haffter P, Nüsslein-Vollhard C. (1994) Large-scale mutagenesis in zebrafish: in search of genes controlling development in a vertebrate. *Curr. Biol.* **4**: 189–202.

Munsterberg AE, Kitajewski J, Bumcrot DA, McMahon AP, Lassar AB. (1995) Combinatorial signalling by Sonic hedgehog and Wnt family members induces myogenic cHLH gene expression in somite. *Genes Dev.* **9**: 2911–2922.

Nave K-A. (1995) Myelin-specific genes and their mutations in the mouse. In: *Glial Cell Development* (eds. KR Jessen, WD Richardson). BIOS Scientific Publishers, Oxford, pp.141–164.

Nave K-A, Milner RJ. (1989) Proteolipid proteins: Structure and genetic expression in normal and myelin-deficient mutant mice. *CRC Crit. Rev. Neurobiol.* **5**: 65–91.

Nave K-A, Lai C, Bloom FE, Milner RJ. (1986) Jimpy mutant mouse: a 74-base deletion in the mRNA for myelin proteolipid protein and evidence for a primary defect in RNA splicing. *Proc. Natl Acad. Sci. USA* **83**: 9264–9268.

Nelson RJ, Demas GE, Huang PL, Fishman MC, Dawson VL, Dawson TM, Snyder SH. (1995) Behavioural abnormalities in male mice lacking neuronal nitric oxide synthase. *Nature* **378**: 383–386.

Norman DJ, Feng L, Cheng SS, Gubbay J, Chan E, Heintz N. (1995) The lurcher gene induces apoptotic death in cerebellar Purkinje cells. *Development* **121**: 1183–1193.

Nose A, Mahajan VB, Goodman CS. (1992) Connectin: a homophilic cell adhesion molecule expressed on a subset of muscles and the motoneurons that innervate them in *Drosophila*. *Cell* **70**: 553–567.

Nose A, Takeichi M, Goodman CS. (1994) Ectopic expression of connectin reveals a repulsive function during growth cone guidance and synapse formation. *Neuron* **13**: 525–539.

Nye JS, Kopan R. (1995) Vertebrate ligands for Notch. *Curr. Biol.* **5**: 966–969.

Ohno K, Wang H-L, Milone M et al. (1996) Congenital myasthenic syndrome caused by decreased agonist binding affinity due to a mutation in the acetylcholine receptor ε subunit. *Neuron* **17**: 157–170.

Osborne BA, Schwartz LM. (1994) Essential genes that regulate apoptosis. *Trends Cell Biol.* **4**: 394–399.

Patil N, Cox DR, Bhat D, Faham M, Myers RM, Peterson AS. (1995) A potassium channel mutation in weaver mice implicates membrane excitability in granule cell differentiation. *Nature Genetics* **11**: 126–129.

Pavan WJ, Liddell RA, Wright A, Thibaudeau G, Matteson PG, McHugh KM, Siracusa LD. (1995) A high-resolution linkage map of the lethal spotting locus: a mouse model for Hirschsprung disease. *Mamm. Gen.* **6**: 1–7.

Pennica D, Arce V, Swanson TA et al. (1996) Cardiotrophin-1, a cytokine present in embryonic muscle, supports long-term survival of spinal motorneurons. *Neuron* **17**: 63–74.

Pongs O, Kecskemethy N, Müller R, Krah-Jentgens I, Baumann A, Kiltz HH, Canal I, Llamazares S, Ferrus A. (1988) *Shaker* encodes a family of putative potassium channel proteins in the nervous system of *Drosophila*. *EMBO J.* **7**: 1087–1096.

Popko B, Puckett C, Lai E, Shine HD, Readhead C, Takahashi N, Hunt SW III, Sidman RL, Hood L. (1987) Myelin deficient mice: expression of myelin basic protein and generation of mice with varying levels of myelin. *Cell* **48**: 713–721.

Privat A, Jaque C, Bourre JM, Dupouye P, Baumann N. (1979) Absence of the major dense line in myelin of the mutant mouse 'shiverer'. *Neurosci. Lett.* **12**: 107–112.

Readhead C, Popko B, Takahashi N, Shine HD, Saavedra RA, Sidman RL, Hood L. (1987) Expression of a myelin basic protein gene in transgenic shiverer mice: correction of the dysmyelinating phenotype. *Cell* **48**: 703–712.

Readhead C, Schneider A, Griffiths I, Nave K-A. (1994) Premature arrest of myelination in transgenic mice with increased proteolipid protein gene dosage. *Neuron* **12**: 583–595.

Reaume AG, Elliott JL, Hoffman EK *et al.* (1996) Motor neurons in Cu/Zn superoxide dismutase-deficient mice develop normally but exhibit enhanced cell death after axonal injury. *Nature Genetics* **13**: 43–47.

Roach A, Takahashi N, Pravtcheva D, Ruddle F, Hood L. (1985) Chromosomal mapping of mouse myelin basic protein gene and structure and transcription of the partially deleted gene in shiverer mutant mice. *Cell* **42**: 149–155.

Roy N, Mahadevan MS, McLeal M *et al.* (1995) The gene for neuronal apoptosis inhibitory protein is partially deleted in individuals with spinal muscular atrophy. *Cell* **80**: 167–178.

Sagot Y, Dubois-Dauphin M, Tan SA, de Bilbao F, Aebischer P, Martinou J-C, Kato AC. (1995) Bcl-2 overexpression prevents motoneuron cell body loss but not axonal degeneration in a mouse model of a neurodegenerative disease. *J. Neurosci.* **15**: 7727–7733.

Saul B, Schmieden V, Kling C, Mülhardt C, Gass P, Kuhse J, Becker C-M. (1994) Point mutation of glycine receptor α1 subunit in the *spasmodic* mouse affects agonist responses. *FEBS Lett.* **350**: 71–76.

Schneider C, King RM, Philipson L. (1988) Genes specifically expressed at growth arrest of mammalian cells. *Cell* **54**: 787–793.

Schneider A, Montague P, Griffiths IR, Fanarraga M, Kennedy P, Brophy P, Nave K-A. (1992) Uncoupling of hypomyelination and glial cell death by a mutation in the proteolipid protein gene. *Nature* **358**: 758–761.

Schneider A, Griffiths IR, Readhead C, Nave K-A. (1995) Dominant-negative action of the *jimpy* mutation in mice complemented with an autosomal transgene for myelin proteolipid protein. *Proc. Natl Acad. Sci. USA* **92**: 4447–4451.

Schneider-Maunoury S, Topilko P, Seitandou T, Levi G, Cohen-Tannoudji M, Pournin S, Babinet C, Charnay P. (1993) Disruption of *Krox-20* results in alteration of rhombomeres 3 and 5 in the developing hindbrain. *Cell* **75**: 1199–1214.

Seeger M, Tear G, Ferres-Marco D, Goodman CS. (1993) Mutations affecting growth cone guidance in *Drosophila*: genes necessary for guidance toward or away from the midline. *Neuron* **10**: 409–426.

Sendtner M, Schmalbruch H, Stöckli KA, Carroll P, Kreutzberg GW, Thoenen H. (1992) Ciliary neurotrophic factor prevents degeneration of motor neurons in mouse mutant progressive motor neuronopathy. *Nature* **358**: 502–504.

Serafini T, Kennedy TE, Galko MJ, Mirzayan C, Jessel TM, Tessier-Lavigne M. (1994) The netrins define a family of axon outgrowth-promoting proteins homologous to *C. elegans* UNC-6. *Cell* **78**: 409–424.

Sereda M, Griffiths I, Magiar J *et al.* (1996) Slowed nerve conduction and demyelination in a PMP-22 transgenic rat model of Charcot-Marie-Tooth disease type 1A. *Neuron* **16**: 1049–1060.

Sidman RL, Dickie M, Apple SH. (1964) Mutant mice (quaking and jimpy) with deficient myelination in the central nervous system. *Science* **144**: 309–311.

Skarnes WC, Auerbach BA, Joyner AL. (1992) A gene trap approach in mouse embryonic stem cells: the lacZ reporter is activated by splicing, reflects endogenous gene expression, and is mutagenic in mice. *Genes Dev.* **6**: 903–918.

Snider WD. (1994) Functions of the neurotrophins during nervous system development: what the knockouts are teaching us. *Cell* **77**: 627–638.

Snipes GJ, Suter U, Shooter E. (1993) The genetics of myelin. *Curr. Opin. Neurobiol.* **3**: 694–702.

Spreyer P, Kuhn G, Hanemann CO, Gillen C, Schaal H, Kuhn R, Lemke G, Müller HW. (1991) Axon-regulated expression of a Schwann cell transcript that is homologous to a growth arrest-specific gene. *EMBO J.* **10**: 3661–3668.

Stahl B, Müller B, von Boxberg Y, Cox EC, Bonhoeffer F. (1990) Biochemical characterization of a putative axonal guidance molecule of the chick visual system. *Neuron* 5: 733–743.

Steinlein OK, Mulley JC, Propping P, Wallace RH, Phillips HA, Sutherland GR, Scheffer IE, Berkovic SF. (1995) A missense mutation in the neuronal nicotinic acetylcholine receptor α4 subunit is associated with autosomal dominant nocturnal frontal lobe epilepsy. *Nature Genetics* 11: 201–203.

Steinmeyer K, Klocke R, Ortland C, Gronemeier M, Jockusch H, Gründer S, Jentsch TJ. (1991) Inactivation of muscle chloride channel by transposon insertion in myotonic mice. *Nature* 354: 304–308.

Steinmeyer K, Lorenz C, Pusch M, Koch MC, Jentsch TJ. (1994) Multimeric structure of ClC-1 chloride channel revealed by mutations in dominant myotonia congenita (Thomson). *EMBO J.* 13: 737–743.

St Johnston D, Nüsslein-Vollhard C. (1992) The origin of pattern and polarity in the *Drosophila* embryo. *Cell* 68: 201–219.

Suter U, Welcher AA, Ozcelik T, Snipes GJ, Kosaras B, Francke U, Billings-Gagliardi S, Sidman RL, Shooter EM. (1992a) *Trembler* mouse carries a point mutation in a myelin gene. *Nature* 356: 241–244.

Suter U, Moskow JJ, Welcher AA, Snipes GJ, Kosaras B, Sidman RL, Buchberg AM, Shooter EM. (1992b) A leucine-to-proline mutation in the putative first transmembrane domain of the 22-kDa peripheral myelin protein in the trembler-J mouse. *Proc. Natl Acad. Sci. USA* 89: 4382–4386.

Szuchet S. (1995) The morphology and ultrastructure of oligodendrocytes and their functional implications. In: *Neuroglial Cells* (eds H Kettenmann and B Ransom). Oxford University Press, Oxford, pp. 23–43.

Tanabe Y, Roelink H, Jessell TM. (1995) Induction of motor neurons by Sonic hedgehog is independent of floor plate differentiation. *Curr. Biol.* 5: 651–658.

Taneja KL, McCurrach M, Schalling M, Houseman D, Singer RH. (1995) Foci of trinucleotide repeat transcripts in nuclei of myotonic dystrophy cells and tissues. *J. Cell Biol.* 128: 995–1002.

Thomas KR, Capecchi MR. (1990) Targeted disruption of the murine int-1 proto-oncogene resulting in severe abnormalities in midbrain and cerebellar development. *Nature* 346: 847–850.

Tian S-S, Tsoulfas P, Zinn K. (1991) Three receptor-like tyrosine phosphatases are selectively expressed on central nervous system axons in the *Drosophila* embryo. *Cell* 67: 675–685.

Ton CCT, Hirvonen H, Miwa H et al. (1991) Positional cloning and characterization of a paired box- and homeobox containing gene from the aniridia region. *Cell* 67: 1059–1074.

Trapp BD. (1988) Distribution of the myelin-associated glycoprotein and P_0 protein during myelin compaction in *quaking* mouse peripheral nerve. *J. Cell Biol.* 107: 675–685.

Tully T, Preat T, Boynton SC, Del Vecchio M. (1994) Genetic dissection of consolidated memory in *Drosophila*. *Cell* 79: 35–47.

Umemori H, Sato S, Yagi T, Aizawa S, Yamamoto T. (1994) The initial events of myelination involve Fyn tyrosine kinase signalling. *Nature* 367: 572–576.

Valentijn LJ, Baas F, Wolterman RA, Hoogendijk JE, van den Bosch N, Zorn I, Gabreels-Festen A, de Visser M, Bolhuis PA. (1992) Identical point mutation of PMP-22 in trembler-J mouse and Charcot-Marie-Tooth disease type 1A. *Nature Genetics* 2: 288–291.

Van Broeckhoven CL. (1995) Molecular genetics of Alzheimer disease: identification of genes and gene mutations. *Eur. Neurol.* 35: 8–19.

Van Vactor D, Sink H, Fambrough D, Tsoo R, Goodman CS. (1993) Genes that control neuromuscular specificity in *Drosophila*. *Cell* 73: 1137–1153.

Weimbs T, Stoffel,W. (1992) Proteolipid protein (PLP) of CNS myelin: positions of free, disulfide-bonded, and fatty acid thioester-linked cysteine residues and implications for the membrane topology of PLP. *Biochemistry* 31: 12 289–12 296.

Welcher AA, Suter U, De Leon M, Snipes GJ, Shooter EM. (1991) A myelin protein is encoded by the homologue of a growth arrest-specific gene. *Proc. Natl Acad. Sci. USA* 88: 7195–7199.

Winslow JW, Moran P, Valverde J et al. (1995) Cloning of AL-1, a ligand for an Eph-related tyrosine kinase receptor involved in axon bundle formation. *Neuron* 14: 973–981.

Yang X, Seow KT, Bahri SM, Oon SH, Chia W. (1991) Two *Drosophila* receptor-like tyrosine phosphatase genes are expressed in a subset of developing axons and pioneer neurons in the embryonic CNS. *Cell* 67: 675–685.

Yim MB, Kang J-H, Yim H-S, Kwak H-S, Chock PB, Stadtman ER. (1996) A gain-of-function of an amyotrophic lateral sclerosis-associated Cu,Zn-superoxide dismutase mutant: an enhancement of free radical formation due to a decrease in K_m for hydrogen peroxide. *Proc. Natl Acad. Sci. USA* 93: 5709–5714.

Yin JCP, Wallach JS, Del Vecchio M, Wilder EL, Zhou H, Quinn WG, Tully T. (1994) Induction of a dominant negative CREB transgene specifically blocks long-term memory in *Drosophila*. *Cell* **79**: 49–58.
Zhang Y, Proenca R, Maffei M, Barone M, Leopold L, Friedman JM. (1994) Positional cloning of the mouse *obese* gene and its human homologue. *Nature* **372**: 425–432.

Further reading

Brown MC, Hopkins WG, Keynes RJ. (1991) *Essentials of Neuronal Development.* Cambridge University Press, Cambridge.
Gilbert SF. (1994) *Developmental Biology.* Sinauer Associates, Sunderland, MA.
Hall ZW. (1992) *Molecular Neurobiology.* Sinauer Associates, Sunderland, MA.
Jockusch H. (1996) Genetic control of muscle function and molecular basis of diseases. In: *Comprehensive Human Physiology* Vol. 1. Springer-Verlag, Berlin, pp. 959–967.
Kandel ER, Schwartz JH, Jessell TM. (1991) *Principles of Neural Science*, 3rd Edn, Elsevier, New York.
Kandel ER, Schwartz JH, Jessell TM. (1995) *Essentials of Neural Science and Behaviour.* Appleton & Lange, Norwalk, CT.
Lehmann-Horn F, Rüdel R. (1996) Molecular pathophysiology of voltage-gated ion channels. *Rev. Physiol. Biochem. Pharmacol.* **128**: 195–268.
Shepherd GM. (1994) *Neurobiology*, 3rd Edn. Oxford University Press, New York.

Neuron-specific gene expression

Andrea L. Grant and William Wisden

3.1 Introduction

The key to understanding biological regulation lies – to the delight of some and the dismay of others – 'all in the details'.

[McKnight and Schibler, 1993].

The nervous system is the most complex of tissues. Many different types of neuron are present in the brain but there is little understanding of how this diversity is controlled at the genetic level. It is clearly a central tenet that selective gene expression is important in determining neuronal and glial cell type (He and Rosenfeld, 1991; Lewin, 1994; Mandel and McKinnon, 1993; McKay, 1989; Sutcliffe, 1988; Twyman and Jones, 1995), and some investigators estimate that about one-third of the expressed mammalian genome is exclusively dedicated to brain function (Sutcliffe, 1988). However, no all-encompassing model has so far emerged to explain how such differential gene expression is governed.

Transcription of protein-encoding eukaryotic genes requires the assembly of a multiprotein 'core transcription complex' composed of RNA polymerase II (RNA pol II) and numerous auxiliary factors (Gill, 1994). In many genes this complex binds at a sequence-specific site called the TATA box which lies approximately 30 bp upstream of the start site of transcription in a region known as the 'promoter' (Conaway and Conaway, 1993). However, many genes do not have TATA boxes and the RNA polymerase complex binds to, and initiates transcription from, these promoters using less well defined initiator elements (Gill, 1994). *In vivo*, the formation of the core initiation complex on the TATA box or initiator element is usually insufficient to attain physiological levels of gene transcription. Additional *cis*-regulatory DNA elements, known as enhancers (elements which mediate transcriptional activation) and silencers (elements which mediate transcriptional repression) are also required. These elements bind transcription factor proteins (TFs) in a sequence-specific manner. It is through this binding and the combinatorial interactions of the TFs with each other, and with the core transcription complex, that constitutive, inducible and tissue-specific regulation of gene expression can be achieved (Struhl, 1991; Tjian and Maniatis, 1994) (*Figure 3.1*). Other mechanisms such as chromatin structure and differential methylation of CpG sites are also important in regulating differential gene

---

Molecular Biology of the Neuron, edited by R.W. Davies and B.J. Morris.
© 1997 BIOS Scientific Publishers Ltd, Oxford.

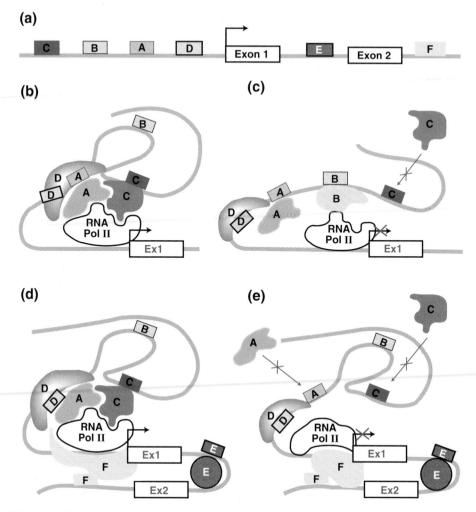

Figure 3.1. A schematic view of some possible mechanisms of transcriptional regulation through protein binding enhancers and silencers in eukaryotic genes. (a) Organization of regulatory elements in genomic regions of a prototypical gene. Multiple positive and negative regulatory elements can be distributed in the 5′ promoter, intronic and 3′ regions. (b) Gene activation via 5′ DNA elements. The binding of TFs A, C and D to their respective DNA sequences, and their intermolecular interactions with each other and the RNA pol II–protein complex, ensures co-ordinate assembly of a functional transcriptional complex at the promoter and gene transcription is activated. (c) Gene repression through 5′ DNA elements. The presence of TF B binding to its DNA element sterically blocks the binding of TF C to its binding site. Additionally, the occupancy of element B disrupts the TF A:RNA pol II–core complex associations. Thus, the D:A:C protein complex seen in panel (a) is not formed and gene transcription is repressed. (d) Gene activation via 5′, intronic and 3′ DNA element interaction. The binding of TF E to its corresponding DNA element effects a conformational change that brings the positive activating TF F, which is bound to its 3′ DNA element, into contact with the promoter, and this further activates transcription. (e) Similar to (d), but TF F may also be negatively regulating. In this case, F acts by distorting the proximal promoter region and the RNA pol II complex, with the consequence that TFs A and C are sterically inhibited from binding their DNA elements, and thus the D:A:C complex is not formed and transcription is repressed.

expression (Bird and Tweedie, 1995; Grosschedl, 1995; McKnight and Schibler, 1993; Paranjape *et al.*, 1994), but the extent to which these mechanisms are important in specifically determining neuron-specific gene expression is unknown.

When considering neuron-specific gene expression there are two broad themes:

(i)   What mechanisms are used to enable precursor cells to differentiate into neurons rather than say liver cells (i.e. how do neurons differ from nonneurons?). One way of specifying at least some types of neuronal identity is to utilize master activating TFs that act at the top of regulatory hierarchies. Such networks lead to the restricted expression of target genes. Examples of putative master 'neuronal' regulators are the eyeless/pax-6 and NeuroD transcription factors (Anderson, 1995; Halder *et al.*, 1995a,b; Lee *et al.*, 1995). Another mechanism of specifying neurons uses the neuronal phenotype as the default state (Lewin, 1994; Simpson, 1995). In these cases, certain neuronal-specific genes are actively repressed in nonneural tissues (Mandel and McKinnon, 1993; Simpson, 1995).

(ii) The activation of 'housekeeping' genes such as those encoding neurotransmitter synthesizing enzymes, neurotransmitter receptors or various cytoskeletal elements represents the endpoint of cell differentiation, and such genes are stably expressed in specific cell types. Thus, once the commitment to differentiate into the neuronal class has been made, how are different types of neurons specified? Many genes tend to be expressed in complex and distributed patterns in the central nervous system (CNS). *Figure 3.2* illustrates this phenomenon for the kainate receptor subunit genes – part of a large gene superfamily encoding ligand-gated ion channel receptor subunits for the neurotransmitter glutamate (Wisden and Seeburg, 1993). As assayed by *in situ* hybridization to localize gene transcripts, the *KA-1* subunit gene expression pattern is largely confined to CA3 pyramidal cells and dentate granule cells of the hippocampus (*Figure 3.2h*), whereas the *KA-2* subunit gene is expressed in many types of neuron throughout the brain (*Figure 3.2i* and *j*). Other genes, such as *GluR-5*, are expressed mainly in septal and thalamic nuclei (*Figure 3.2a* and *b*). For each subunit gene there are likely to be unique combinations of DNA regulatory elements that determine these complex cell type-specific expression patterns.

3.1.1 The diversity of gene regulatory mechanisms used in the brain

Although there are basic similarities in the regulation of all genes, with the underlying aim being the regulation of RNA pol II binding and subsequent transcriptional activation, the regulatory architecture of neuron-specific genes can vary considerably. This probably reflects the fact that regulatory circuits are not necessarily based on economical design principles, but often on the ease by which these circuits can and have been reconfigured during evolution (Johnson, 1995). For example, some genes such as those encoding the neurotrophins and choline acetyl transferase (ChAT), have multiple promoters which are preferentially utilized in different neuronal types and which may serve to increase regulatory flexibility (Berse and Blusztajn, 1995; Timmusk *et al.*, 1993, 1995; *Figure 3.3*). Other genes such as those for dystrophin and aromatic L-amino acid decarboxylase have two promoters, one of which is neural-specific while the other directs transcription in other tissues (Albert *et al.*, 1992; Chelly *et al.*, 1990). In many other cases, regulatory enhancer/silencer regions do not necessarily lie exclusively 5' to the promoter, but are found in intragenic/intronic regions including exon sequences, or are found 3′ to the polyadenylation site of the gene (e.g. Echelard *et al.*, 1994; Marshall *et al.*, 1994; Sakimura *et al.*, 1995; Vidal *et al.*, 1990; Yao and White, 1994; Zimmerman *et al.*, 1994). In these cases, the TFs binding to the downstream regions are believed to physically contact the basal transcriptional machinery via looping of DNA (see *Figure 3.1d* and *e*). Clusters of genes may also share a common regulatory region known as a locus control region (LCR) which enables efficient co-ordinate reg-

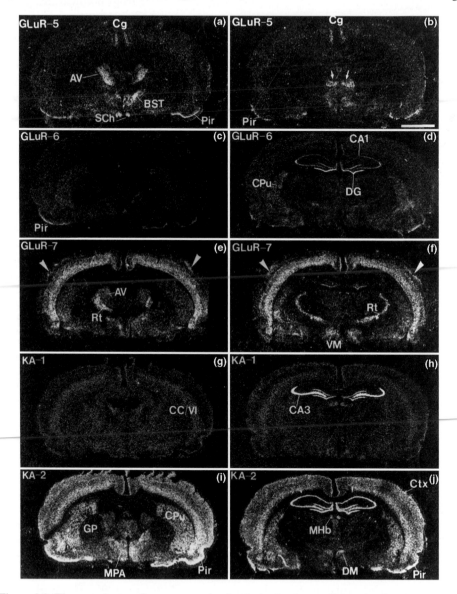

Figure 3.2. The complexity of gene expression in the brain. Autoradiographs showing the distribution of kainate receptor subunit mRNAs (GluR-5, -6, -7, KA-1, -2) in the adult rat brain. It can be seen that each gene has a completely different transcription pattern. Coronal sections were hybridized with antisense ^{35}S-labeled oligonucleotide probes. White areas correspond to the expression of mRNA. Reproduced from Wisden and Seeburg (1993) with permission from the Society for Neuroscience.

ulation (Orkin, 1995; see Section 3.6). The co-ordinate regulation of β-globin gene expression in blood cells provides the most rigorously studied system for LCRs (Orkin, 1995), but it has been proposed that similar mechanisms may be involved in the co-ordinate regulation of, for example, GABA$_A$ receptor subunit genes (McLean *et al.*, 1995). Evolution has neatly solved one particular problem of co-ordinate regulation using a nested gene strategy. In the rat and mouse genomes the vesicular acetylcholine transporter (VAChT) gene lies within the first intron of the *ChAT* gene and has the same transcriptional orientation (Benjanin *et al.*, 1994; Erickson *et al.*, 1994) (*Figure 3.3*). Both proteins are required for cholinergic synaptic transmission and the nested structure may facilitate co-regulation through shared regulatory sequences (Berrard *et al.*, 1995; Berse and Blusztajn, 1995). Thus, it is clear that a large variety of strategies are used in the regulation of gene expression in neurons.

3.2 Gene silencing

Models of eukaryotic gene expression usually emphasize transcriptional activation. Specific gene regulatory proteins are viewed as activators, serving to turn on particular genes for transcription within a background of nonexpressed genes. However, the expression of many genes is actively repressed in some tissues (Johnson, 1995), and in particular negative regulation of an otherwise ubiquitously expressed gene plays an important role in regulating neuron-specific gene expression. DNA regions which are involved in specifically repressing expression have been collectively referred to as 'silencers'. When considering neuron-specific gene expression there are two possible levels of silencing; first, the repression of neuronal genes in nonneuronal cells ('global silencing'). Secondly, within neural tissue, silencing can act at the level of fine tuning, to direct the expression of a neuron-specific gene to only a subset of neurons ('restricted silencing').

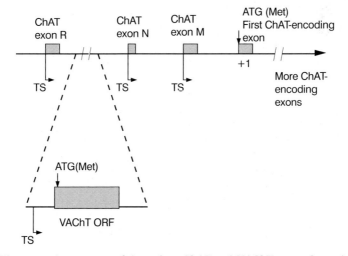

Figure 3.3. The genomic structure of the rodent *ChAT* and *VAChT* genes. Several *ChAT* transcripts which differ at their 5′ untranslated region are synthesized through the differential use of the transcription start site (TSS) of exons R, N and M, and by alternative splicing (Kengaku *et al.*, 1993; Misawa *et al*, 1992). The intronless open reading frame (ORF) of the *VAChT* gene is located in intron 1 of the *ChAT* gene between exons R and N. Adapted from Berse and Blusztajn (1995).

3.2.1 Global silencing

The neural restrictive silencer element (NRSE) is a DNA sequence that has been identified in the promoters of many neuron-specific genes that have disparate patterns of expression, and might reflect a common mechanism used to inhibit neuronal gene expression in nonneuronal tissues.

Table 3.1 lists NRSEs from various genes which have been demonstrated to have some functional role in silencing nonneuronal gene expression. An NRSE sequence has also been described in the promoter region of the brain-derived neurotropic factor (BDNF) gene, although no functional role for this has yet been demonstrated (Timmusk *et al.*, 1993). Furthermore, sequence analysis has identified putative NRSE sequences in other neuron-specific genes including the NR1 subunit of the *N*-methyl-D-aspartate receptor, synaptotagmin, glycine receptor and the β2 neuronal nicotinic receptor subunit genes (Bessis *et al.*, 1995; Schoenherr and Anderson, 1995; Schoenherr *et al.*, 1996).

The NRSEs in the synapsin I, SCG10 and sodium channel subunit (NaII) genes all bind a sequence-specific protein present in nonneuronal cells but not in neuronal cells (Kraner *et al.*, 1992; Li *et al.*, 1993; Mori *et al.*, 1992). Two separate studies have isolated a cDNA encoding a zinc finger TF with homology to the GLI-Krüppel family (Chong *et al.*, 1995; Schoenherr and Anderson, 1995). This protein, called neuron restrictive silencer factor (NRSF) or RE-1-silencing transcription factor, binds NRSE sequences from SCG10, NaII channel, synapsin I and BDNF genes (Schoenherr and Anderson, 1995), and can repress transcription from an NRSE containing reporter plasmid in PC12 cells (Chong *et al.*, 1995; Schoenherr and Anderson, 1995). NRSF is expressed in a wide range of nonneuronal tissues, both during development and in adulthood. It is also found in neuronal progenitor cells but is absent from fully differentiated neurons (Schoenherr and Anderson, 1995). These data support the role of NRSF as a silencer binding protein which mediates the repression of many specific NRSE containing genes in nonneuronal tissues. Furthermore, its presence in neuronal progenitor cells suggests that its own down-regulation may be coupled to neuronal differentiation.

Although the NRSE may prove to be a common mechanism of silencing neuronal genes, many neuron-specific genes possess functionally defined negative regulatory regions which bear no similarity to the NRSE. It is clear that there are other mecha-

Table 3.1. Consensus NRSE sequences for which a functional activity in nonneuronal cells has been demonstrated by deletion analysis and protein binding studies. The NRSE sequences of the SCG10, sodium channel type II (NaII), dopamine β-hydroxylase (DBH), synapsin I and the Na,K-ATPase α3 subunit (α3 NKA) genes are shown

Gene	NRSE sequence
SCG10[a]	TTCAGAACCACGGACAGCACC
NaII[b]	TTCAGAACCACGGACAGCACC
DBH[c]	AGCAGCTCCTCGGACCTCA–G
Synapsin I[d]	TTCAGCACCGCGGACAGTGCC
α3 NKA[e]	CTTAGCTTCTCGGTGG–CGCC

[a]Mori *et al.* (1992), [b]Maue *et.al.* (1990), [c]Ishiguro *et al.* (1993), [d]Li *et al.* (1993), [e]Pathak *et al.* (1994).

nisms of gene repression in nonneuronal cells which are common to many neuron-specific genes. In particular, a role for E boxes [DNA binding sites for the basic helix–loop–helix (bHLH) class of TFs] in silencing nonneuronal expression has been demonstrated for the gene which encodes the tyrosine hydroxylase (TH) enzyme.

A 23 bp segment of the upstream promoter region of the *TH* gene which is important for tissue-specific expression contains an AP-1 motif (the binding site for leucine zipper TFs such as c-fos and c-jun) which overlaps with a dyad symmetry element centered about an E box consensus site (Yoon and Chikaraishi, 1992). Reporter constructs containing the AP-1 site alone are expressed in both neuronal and nonneuronal cells with higher expression levels in the nonneuronal cell type. However, on inclusion of the dyad symmetry element into the reporter gene, nonneuronal expression is abolished whilst expression levels in neuronal cells increases 25-fold. This implies a dual role of both activation and repression for the AP-1 site with the decisive factor being the interaction that occurs at the dyad symmetry element. The mechanism of this interaction however is unclear. Gel shift assays indicate similar protein binding complexes at this site in both neuronal and nonneuronal cells (Yoon and Chikaraishi, 1992). Also, two novel E-box binding factors, termed rITF2 and CDP2, which are expressed in both TH expressing and nonexpressing tissues have been shown to bind the TH-dyad (Yoon and Chikaraishi, 1994). Thus, the contrasting effects of the AP-1/dyad symmetry element in neuronal and nonneuronal cells does not appear to be simply mediated by the differential expression of a 'dyad binding TF'. The different functions may arise from more subtle differences between the proteins involved in neuronal and nonneuronal cells, or through differential interactions with other proteins at further sites on the promoter which are mediated only when the dyad symmetry element is occupied.

3.2.2 Restricted silencing

The phenotypic diversity of the cells of the nervous system relies largely on the fact that many neuron-specific genes are only expressed in a small subset of neurons. For example, the ChAT protein is restricted to the cholinergic neurons of the nervous system. In the rodent, multiple ChAT mRNAs are expressed from three alternative promoters coupled with the use of differential RNA splicing (Kengaku *et al.*, 1993; Misawa *et al.*, 1992, *Figure 3.3*). Therefore, the regulation of cell-specific ChAT expression in the nervous system is likely to be quite complex. The existence of similar multiple promoters in the human *ChAT* gene is unreported. However, a silencer which can act to fine tune *ChAT* gene expression such that it is only expressed in a subset of neurons has been identified (Li *et al.*, 1993).

The promoter of the human gene encoding ChAT has been characterized using transient transfection assays and contains two major silencing regions which work co-operatively to repress ChAT expression in noncholinergic cells (Li *et al.*, 1993). The proximal silencer element contains two E-box sequences both of which must be present to repress transcription in noncholinergic cells (Li *et al.*, 1995). Gel shift experiments indicate protein binding activity to both boxes in the nonexpressing adrenergic cell line. However, binding activity to one of the boxes is absent in the expressing cholinergic cell line. This lack of binding activity in cholinergic cells may explain the lack of silencing activity in cholinergic cells. Either the E box binding factor is absent in the cholinergic cell line, or a dominant negative bHLH protein may be expressed in these cells which is incapable of binding the E-box site, for example due to the lack of a functional DNA binding domain. A dominant negative bHLH could also work by forming a heterodimer with the TF that normally binds the E-box site thus rendering the latter incapable of binding. A similar example of a TF operating in this way is seen in muscle-specific gene expression. Muscle-specific genes are activated by the binding of the MyoD class of TFs binding to multiple E-box motifs in their promoter regions (Buckingham, 1994). In nonmuscle cells these genes are repressed by the expression of the Id TF which forms a heterodimer with the MyoD, which is then incapable of activating transcription (Benezra *et al.*, 1990).

Global and restricted silencing are not mutually exclusive. The gene encoding glial fibrillary acidic protein (GFAP), an intermediate filament protein expressed in astrocytes and Schwann glial cells of the nervous system, provides an example of both mechanisms of silencing at work. Two negative elements named GDR1 and GDR2 reside between the first intron to fifth exon and 3' to the poly-adenylation site of the gene respectively. Both elements are necessary to suppress *GFAP* expression in neuronal cell lines (i.e. in nonglial cell lines) and GDR1 alone is sufficient to suppress expression in nonneuronal and nonglial cell lines (Kaneko and Sueoka, 1993). Thus, GDR1 is acting as a global silencer and is responsible for brain-specific expression, and the interaction of GDR1 and GDR2 provides a more restricted silencing mechanism responsible for glial-specific expression.

3.3 Gene activation via single positive enhancers

Some neuron-specific genes are only expressed in one or two cell types. One way of ensuring co-ordinate expression of different genes in a single cell type would be to give the regulatory regions of the genes the same transcriptional 'address'. For example, they might all share a common enhancer element which then binds a TF that is only expressed in that cell type. Many of the proteins involved in olfactory transduction (e.g. olfactory marker protein) are expressed exclusively or predominantly in the sensory neurons of the olfactory system (Wang *et al.*, 1993). Analysis of the regulatory regions (upstream and introns) of six of these olfactory-specific genes, using footprinting and the electrophoresis mobility shift assay (EMSA), identified a common nucleotide sequence as a putative TF binding site (Kudrycki *et al.*, 1993; Wang *et al.*, 1993). This motif alone, derived from the *OMP* gene, is sufficient to direct reporter gene expression exclusively to the olfactory epithelium (Kudrycki *et al.*, 1993). The TF which binds this motif was isolated using a yeast one-hybrid system and named Olf-1 (Wang and Reed, 1993). The Olf-1 binding protein is a TF possessing a novel structural domain, similar to the domain found in the family of bHLH proteins such as MyoD, called the repeat helix–loop–helix (Wang and Reed, 1993).

Thus, the binding of the Olf-1 TF, which itself is found only in the nuclei of olfactory neurons, to an Olf-1 motif seems sufficient and indeed critical to mediate olfactory neuron-specific expression of many genes. A similar example is provided by the nematode *Caenorhabditis elegans* UNC-30 homeodomain TF. This is a transcriptional activator of the gene encoding glutamic acid decarboxylase, an enzyme required for the synthesis of the inhibitory amino acid neurotransmitter γ-aminobutyric acid (GABA) (Jin *et al.*, 1994). UNC-30 protein is usually only found in GABA-positive neurons of the worm nervous system. Ectopic expression of UNC-30 in other neuronal types using transgenic methods induces the transcription of glutamic acid decarboxylase in these cells which results in their assuming a GABA-positive phenotype (Jin *et al.*, 1994). Thus, just as Olf-1 regulates the differentiation of olfactory neurons by switching on olfactory-specific genes, UNC-30 activates a gene which is critical for GABA synthesis and thereby regulates terminal differentiation of GABA neurons.

Perhaps the ultimate in cell specificity is a TF that controls the phenotype of a *single* neuron (Lewin, 1994). The putative TF ODR-7, a member of the steroid receptor superfamily, is only found in a single pair of *C. elegans* olfactory receptor neurons – the AWA cell (Sengupta *et al.*, 1994). Physiological studies of ODR-7 mutants suggest that the ODR-7 protein specifically regulates olfactory receptor gene expression, and is responsible for the unique array of receptors expressed by the AWA neuron (Sengupta *et al.*, 1994).

This conceptually simple method of ensuring expression of different genes in only one cell type can be extended further. Many neuronal genes are expressed in more than one, but still a limited number of cell types. Such expression can be manifested by the presence of several cell-specific positive enhancers, which bind cell-specific TFs for each cell type in which the gene is expressed. For example, the promoter region of the fruit fly *Drosophila FMRFamide* neuropeptide gene is composed of multiple discrete enhancer regions which are required for expression in different neuronal cell types in the fly brain (Schneider *et al.*, 1993).

3.4 Multiple positive and negative elements direct cell type-specific expression within the nervous system

So far, the incidence of gene activation and gene repression in the nervous system has been considered in isolation. However, more typically, many neuron-specific genes are regulated via both multiple positive and negative regulatory regions. Specific examples of genes regulated in this way are *synapsin I, dopamine-β-hydroxylase (DBH)* and *L7/pcp-2* genes. These are discussed in detail below.

3.4.1 The synapsin I gene

The *synapsin I* gene encodes a neuron-specific phosphoprotein involved in neurotransmitter release which is expressed in many neuronal cell types. Transient transfection studies showed that the expression of *synapsin I* is regulated by multiple positive and negative regions in the 5′ upstream promoter region (Sauerwald *et al.*, 1990; Thiel *et al.*, 1991). One of these regions operates through an NRSE (Li *et al.*, 1993) (see Section 3.2.1). Also, adjacent to the NRSE, two conserved sequences have been identified called SNN (acronym for synapsin I, neurofilament, NGF). The SNNs are also found in the neuron-specific 68 kDa neurofilament and the nerve growth factor genes (Lewis and Cowan, 1986; Sehgal *et al.*, 1988), but no clear functional role has been demonstrated for them (Sauerwald *et al.*, 1990). In isolation, the SNNs are insufficient to enhance reporter gene expression in neuronal cell lines, and thus they may not act as positive enhancers of transcription (Thiel *et al.*, 1991).

Figure 3.4 illustrates the possible interactions that can occur to result in the neuron-specific regulation of the *synapsin I* gene. The core promoter is active in both neuronal and nonneuronal cells. The NRSF is found in nonneuronal cells and, when bound to the promoter region at the NRSE, prevents activation of transcription and acts to globally silence transcription in nonneuronal cells (Schoenherr and Anderson, 1995). Site 'E' represses transcription in both neuronal and nonneuronal cell lines, indicat-

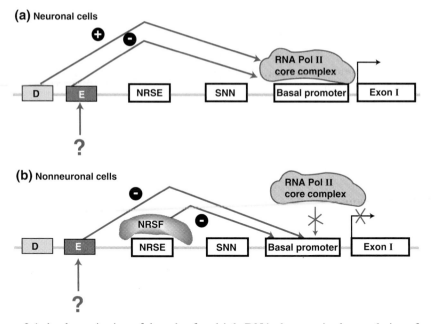

Figure 3.4. A schematic view of the role of multiple DNA elements in the regulation of *synapsin I* gene expression. (a) In neuronal cells transcription arises through a highly active basal promoter which is also positively activated by a more upstream region D. In addition, region E negatively regulates neuronal transcription. However, the question mark symbol indicates that it is unclear how important this negative effect is or, how it may be regulated *in vivo*. (b) *Synapsin I* gene expression is repressed in nonneuronal cells mostly by the presence of the NRSF protein which binds the NRSE site and globally represses transcription. In addition the positively enhancing effect of region D is absent. Region E also inhibits *synapsin I* gene transcription in nonneuronal cells. The function of the SNN sequences identified by functional homology to sequence elements found in other neuron-specific genes is undefined.

ing a possible silencing role for this region, and that some component that gives site 'E' a differential activity in neuronal and nonneuronal cells is missing (e.g. a TF that binds a site further upstream and that interacts with TF 'E'). TF 'D' is only present or active in neurons and is positively enhancing.

3.4.2 The dopamine-β-hydroxylase *gene*

Figure 3.5 illustrates those sites, as identified by transgenic analysis, found to be important in regulating the human *DBH* gene whose expression is limited to adrenergic and noradrenergic cells of the nervous system (Hoyle *et al.*, 1994). Two positive activator regions, 'A' and 'C', were identified. Region 'A' directs expression to noradrenergic cells and other regions, particularly the olfactory bulb, septum and hypothalamus. A negatively regulating region ('B') which suppresses this ectopic expression was also identified. Region 'C' has widespread activity in many areas of the brain. This activity must presumably be repressed *in vivo* by a silencing region 'D' located either further 5', intronically, or 3' to the gene (Hoyle *et al.*, 1994). As is the case for the *synapsin I* gene, the actual TFs acting on these regions are not yet identified.

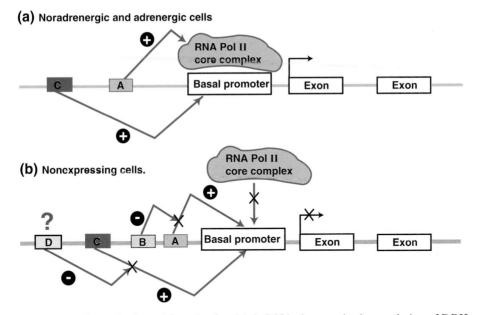

Figure 3.5. A schematic view of the role of multiple DNA elements in the regulation of *DBH* gene expression. (a) *DBH* expression is positively enhanced in both expressing and many nonexpressing cells by the presence of regions C and A. (b) In order to repress this transcription in non-DBH-expressing cells, two sites D (the exact location of which is unclear, as indicated by the question mark symbol) and B are required to inhibit the positive enhancing effects of C and A respectively.

3.4.3 The L7/pcp-2 gene

The *L7/pcp2* gene, encoding a protein of unknown function, is expressed specifically in cerebellar Purkinje cells and retinal bipolar cells (Nordquist *et al.*, 1988; Oberdick *et al.*, 1988). Despite such a simple expression pattern, the regulation of the gene cannot be explained simply by the presence of one positive enhancer (cf. Olf-1, Section 3.3), but involves multiple regulatory elements in the 5′, intronic and 3′ regions of the gene as illustrated in *Figure 3.6*.

The proximal promoter of the *L7/pcp-2* gene contains a positive enhancer 'P' (Oberdick *et al.*, 1993; Vandaele *et al.*, 1991), which directs expression predominantly to the Purkinje cells of the cerebellum and also to some ectopic sites in the CNS. This ectopic expression is only abolished on the inclusion of intronic and 3′ sequences into the construct which implies the presence of a suppressor of expression, 'B', somewhere in these regions (Oberdick *et al.*, 1993). Additionally, sequences between 4 kb and 0.4 kb upstream of the transcription start site (TSS) also act to restrict expression to the Purkinje cells (Vandaele *et al.*, 1991). Since retinal bipolar cell expression was only observed when the transgenic construct contained intronic sequences downstream of exon 2 and 2 kb of the 3′ region (Oberdick *et al.*, 1990), there must be a retinal-specific positive enhancer somewhere in this region. Interestingly, elements involved in regulating the compartmentalized expression of the *L7/pcp-2* gene during development have also been identified in the 5′ promoter region (Oberdick *et al.*, 1993).

Since only 250 bp of *L7/pcp-2* proximal promoter is required for Purkinje cell-

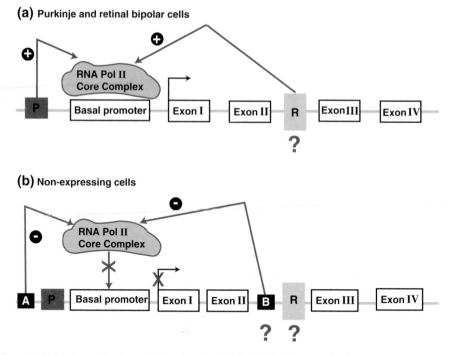

Figure 3.6. A schematic view of the role of multiple DNA elements in the regulation of *L7/pcp-2* gene expression. (a) The proximal promoter contains a positive element(s) P, which directs expression mainly to the Purkinje cells of the cerebellum but also to other sites in the brain. Retinal bipolar cell-specific expression requires an additional positive element R, of unknown location, as indicated by the question mark symbol, but which resides somewhere in the intronic or 3′ regions. (b) Non-Purkinje and nonretinal bipolar cell expression is repressed by a negative element A, which lies upstream to the proximal promoter. Also, an additional element(s) B, with an unknown location(s) in the intronic or 3′ regions of the gene are important to repress *L7/pcp-2* expression in other cell types.

specific expression with some expression in ectopic sites, there are likely to be Purkinje cell-specific positive enhancer elements in this region. Footprint analysis of the 0.25 kb proximal promoter detected an AT-rich region which was protected by recombinant Pit-1, a pituitary-specific member of the POU family of transcription factors (Oberdick *et al.*, 1993). This suggests that a similar factor to Pit-1 may play a role in regulating *L7/pcp-2* expression *in vivo*. In a separate study, the yeast one-hybrid system was used to screen other regions of the *L7/pcp-2* promoter for transcription factor binding activities. The c-Maf transcription factor, a member of the basic-zipper superfamily, has been shown to bind regions –200 to –210 and –209 to –318 of the *L7/pcp-2* proximal promoter and thereby activate transcription (Kurschner and Morgan, 1995). The nrl protein, a c-Maf family member that is expressed exclusively in the retina and fetal brain (Swaroop *et al.*, 1992), can substitute for c-maf in this system and possesses the same sequence binding specificity. Other basic-zipper proteins such as c-fos and c-jun do not substitute in this manner. Thus, the largely ubiquitous c-Maf and the nrl, which is more restricted in its expression, may also interact to regulate *L7-pcp2* expression.

The *synapsin I*, *DBH* and *L7/pcp-2* genes illustrate the complex interplay of positive and negative regulation that is involved in determining neuron-specific gene expression. When considering one particular gene in isolation, it appears that more factors than necessary are required to achieve the correct expression pattern. For example, often a positive enhancer may be present in a gene that needs a complementary silencer to bring about the required expression pattern. However, a different gene with the same positive regulatory element but different silencer elements can generate a different or overlapping expression pattern. Thus a network of factors that exert different effects depending on their combinatorial interactions may be one mechanism that has evolved for regulating cell-specific expression (Hoyle *et al.*, 1994).

3.5 Intronic and downstream (3′) regulatory elements in neuronal genes

Not all regulatory elements reside in the 5′ regions of genes. As illustrated in *Figure 3.1*, transcriptional elements can also reside in intronic and 3′ regions of genes. The proteins which bind these elements may mediate their effects, which can be either enhancing or repressive, by interacting with the RNA pol II transcription complex directly (*Figure 3.1d*), or through protein:protein interactions with other TF components of the transcriptional complex. In both these cases, it is clear that some structural rearrangement of the gene (e.g. looping of DNA) must be achieved for these interactions to occur. In addition, some intronic and 3′ enhancers and the proteins that they bind sometimes mediate this structural rearrangement. In such cases these regulatory elements do not themselves interact directly with the transcriptional complex but have a secondary effect on regulating transcription by bringing other positive or negative enhancing TFs into the transcriptional complex (*Figure 3.1e*).

3.5.1 The nestin gene

Nestin is an intermediate filament protein whose expression is observed in multipotential neuroepithelial cells which give rise to terminally differentiated neurons and astrocytes. This differentiation into the mature neuronal phenotype is marked by a down-regulation of nestin expression. Similarly, nestin expression is observed transiently in the presomitic mesoderm and striated cells of the myotome layer in the somites during muscle development. On differentiation into mature muscle, nestin is also down-regulated (Zimmerman *et al.*, 1994).

The 5′ region of the nestin gene alone is insufficient to direct expression of a β-galactosidase (*lacZ*) reporter gene to the neural tube or somites of embryonic day 10.5–11.5 mice (Zimmerman *et al.*, 1994). However, on inclusion of intronic regions, significant reporter gene expression is observed in a pattern similar to that of endogenous nestin (Zimmerman *et al.*, 1994). Deletion of the 5′ upstream region from this construct has no effect on expression. Thus the regulatory elements that govern the cell-specific and transitory expression of the *nestin* gene are located exclusively in the intronic regions of the *nestin* gene. The upstream region of the gene apparently only serves as a basal promoter and binding site for RNA polymerase.

A positive enhancer which drives expression to somites resides in intron 1 of the *nestin* gene, and in the second intron a CNS-specific regulatory region is present. This CNS control region is active regardless of orientation or distance from the transcription start site and thus fits the classic definition of an enhancer (Zimmerman *et al.*, 1994). The gene encoding the cell-surface glycoprotein Thy-1 is similar to the *nestin* gene in that it has a brain-specific enhancer in the first intron and a thymus-specific element in the third intron (Vidal *et al.*, 1990). Other neuron-specific or glial-specific genes are similarly regulated by multiple positive and negative elements that lie in the intronic and 3' regions. Examples include the *GAP-43* (Vanselow *et al.*, 1994), *peripherin* (Belecky-Adams *et al.*, 1993), *neurofilament light* (Hsu *et al.*, 1995) and *GFAP* genes (Kaneko and Sueoka, 1993) (see Section 3.2.2).

3.6 Locus control regions

The red and green photoreceptor pigments involved in color vision are expressed exclusively in the red/green cones of the retina and multiple genes encoding variant isoforms of the red/green pigment receptor proteins lie in a head-to-tail array on the X chromosome (Neitz and Neitz, 1995). In most mammals a single gene from the array is expressed per cone cell (Rölich *et al.*, 1994). The selection of which gene to express from this tandem array could occur by one or a combination of the two mechanisms shown in *Figure 3.7*. Each gene may possess a unique binding site for a specific positively enhancing TF(s). These TFs are themselves expressed in different and nonoverlapping cells in the retina and thus only the gene with the binding site for the particular TF found in any one cell will be transcribed (*Figure 3.7a*). This mechanism is similar to that proposed for the selection of sensory olfactory neuron-specific genes from a background of nonolfactory expressed genes by the positive olfactory-specific TF Olf-1 (see Section 3.3).

Alternatively, there may be one single regulatory region which is uniquely accessible to the transcriptional apparatus, and which mediates transcriptional activation of all the genes from the cluster. The gene whose promoter is most proximal to this single active locus is expressed, and the proximity of any given gene is possibly determined by differentially regulated DNA looping (*Figure 3.7b*). Such single active loci, known as locus control regions (LCRs), have been demonstrated to be important in regulating the selection of globin genes from the human β-globin tandem array (Orkin, 1995).

In the retina, there is evidence that an 'LCR-like' element is involved in regulating red/green pigment gene expression. Deletion of a 0.6 kb region, found 5' to the cluster of red/green pigment receptor genes, from transgenic reporter constructs which otherwise direct retina-specific expression, completely abolishes transgene expression. The presence of this region in reporter constructs alone can confer retinal-specific expression in transgenic mice (Wang *et al.*, 1992). This region is also found to be a common deletion in nearly half of a group of individuals known as 'blue cone monochromats'. These patients are unable to detect light at long and middle wavelengths due to their complete inability to express red and green pigment genes (Nathans *et al.*, 1989). Thus this region of DNA might act as an LCR, in that it is essential for the expression of one photoreceptor gene from a cluster.

An intriguing possibility would be that control of odorant receptor gene expression also utilizes an 'LCR-like' mechanism. The mammalian olfactory system uses some 1000 or so individual seven-transmembrane-domain receptors encoded by genes which are expressed in unique patterns in specific sensory cells of the olfactory epithelium (Buck and Axel, 1991; Chess *et al.*, 1992). The receptor genes are organized into clusters, comprising 10–100 genes, scattered throughout the genome (Ben-Arie *et al.*, 1994). The selection of a single gene to be expressed from the cluster

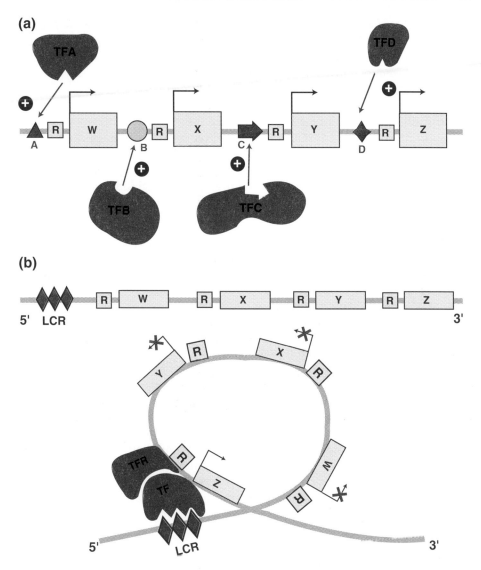

Figure 3.7. A schematic view of two possible methods of selection of a single gene from a multiple gene cluster arranged in tandem array along one chromosome. (a) Each gene is transcriptionally activated by its own unique cell-specific TF. W, X, Y and Z are genes arranged in a tandem array from which only one gene is expressed at any one time. The region-specific positive enhancer element R ensures all these genes are expressed in a single cell type (e.g. retinal neurons). However, gene W will only be expressed in the sub-class of retinal neurons which express TF A, as this is the only gene of the array with the positive DNA element A upon which TF A binds. Similarly, gene X will only be expressed in the subset of retinal neurons expressing TF B and so on. (b) An LCR-based strategy. The genes W, X, Y and Z are under the co-ordinate regulation of an LCR located 5′ to the cluster. The LCR is a site at which specific positively activating TFs bind. Looping of the DNA can juxtapose one of the proximal promoter elements of either W, X, Y or Z to the LCR where the TFs at the LCR and the region-specific TF R can interact to activate transcription of that gene from the cluster.

may be mediated through an LCR. In addition, studies investigating the timing of replication of the two alleles of specific olfactory receptors demonstrated that the alleles are replicated asynchronously (Chess *et al.*, 1994). Asynchronous replication of maternal and paternal alleles is similarly observed in female X-inactivation (Rastan, 1994) and male imprinting (Kitsberg *et al.*, 1993.) Therefore, by analogy, one allelic form of any given odorant receptor gene cluster may also be inactivated. Consequently, selection of genes to be expressed via an LCR might only occur at one gene locus, thus refining the selection process even further. Although chemosensory receptor genes of the nematode *C. elegans* are also grouped in clusters of two to nine genes like their vertebrate counterparts (Troemel *et al.*, 1995), genes within these clusters can have very different expression patterns, suggesting that they do not share identical regulatory elements, and that clustering is not necessarily related to gene regulation (Troemel *et al.*, 1995).

3.7 Summary

The specification of neuronal phenotype is predominately determined at the level of gene expression. Regulatory regions containing multiple *cis*-acting sequence elements control both the level of gene expression and its restriction to appropriate cell types. The regulatory regions of a small minority of neuronal genes have been identified, but the TFs and the associated proteins which act with them remain largely unknown. It has been estimated that there are 100 000 or so mammalian genes, and that 30–50% of these are expressed in brain tissue (Sutcliffe, 1988). Many of these have unique patterns of transcription (see *Figure 3.2*). Even with the use of combinatorial mechanisms, there are likely to be thousands of TFs needed for regulating gene expression in the brain (He and Rosenfeld, 1991; Twyman and Jones, 1995). In the simplest cases, cell-specific gene expression is achieved through DNA binding of a TF restricted to a particular cell type (e.g. Olf-1, UNC-30, ODR-7). More often, expression of neuronal genes (e.g. *synapsin I* and *DBH*) is restricted to certain cell types by unique combinations of sequence elements binding more broadly expressed proteins. It will be a considerable challenge to further elucidate these regulatory circuits.

Acknowledgments

We thank Hilmar Bading, Sabine Bahn, Stephen Hunt, Alison Jones and Richard Twyman for critical comments and suggestions, Mary-Anne Starkey for her help in the preparation of the manuscript, and Shirley Wheeler (MRC Visual Aids) for assistance in producing the figures. ALG holds an MRC Research Studentship. The writing of this review was supported by the Medical Research Council (WW).

References

Albert VR, Lee MR, Bolden AH, Wurzburger RJ, Aguanno A. (1992) Distinct promoters direct neuronal and nonneuronal expression of rat aromatic L-amino acid decarboxylase. *Proc. Natl Acad. Sci. USA* **89**: 12053–12057.

Anderson, D.J. (1995) Spinning skin into neurons. *Curr. Biol.* **5**: 1235–1238.

Andrews PW. (1984) Retinoic acid induces neuronal differentiation of a cloned human embryonal carcinoma cell-line *in vitro*. *Devel. Biol.* **103**: 285–293.

Arnold D, Feng L, Kim J, Heintz N. (1994) A strategy for the analysis of gene expression during neural development. *Proc. Natl Acad. Sci. USA* **91:** 9970–9974.

Bading H, Ginty DD, Greenberg ME. (1993) Regulation of gene expression in hippocampal neurons by distinct calcium signaling pathways. *Science* **260:** 181–186.

Banerjee SA, Hoppe P, Brilliant M, Chikaraishi DM. (1992) 5′ flanking sequences of the rat tyrosine hydroxylase gene target accurate tissue-specific, developmental, and transsynaptic expression in transgenic mice. *J. Neurosci.* **12:** 4460–4467.

Barthel F, Loeffler JP. (1995) β₂-adrenoreceptors stimulate *c-fos* transcription through multiple cyclic AMP- and Ca²⁺-responsive elements in cerebellar granular neurons. *J. Neurochem.* **64:** 41–51.

Bejanin S, Cervini R, Mallet J, Berrard S. (1994) A unique gene organization for two cholinergic markers, choline acetyltransferase and a putative vesicular transporter of acetylcholine. *J. Biol. Chem.* **269:** 21944–21947.

Belecky-Adams T, Wight DC, Kopchick JJ. (1993) Intregenic sequences are required for cell type-specific and injury-induced expression of the rat peripherin gene. *J. Neurosci.* **13:** 5056–5065.

Ben-Arie N, Lancet D, Taylor C *et al.* (1994) Olfactory receptor gene-cluster on human-chromosome-17 – possible duplication of an ancestral receptor repertoire. *Hum. Mol. Genet.*, **3:** 229–235.

Benezra R, Davis RL, Lassar A, Tapscott S, Thayer M, Lockshon D, Weintraub H. (1990) A negative regulator of helix-loop-helix DNA-binding proteins: control of terminal myogenic differentiation. *Ann. NY Acad. Sci.* **599:** 1–11.

Berrard S, Varoqui H, Cervini R, Israël M, Mallet J, Diebler M-F. (1995) Coregulation of two embedded gene products, choline acetyltransferase and the vesicular acetylcholine transporter. *J. Neurochem.* **65:** 939–942.

Berse B, Blusztajn JK. (1995) Coordinated up-regulation of choline acetyltransferase and vesicular acetylcholine transporter gene expression by the retinoic acid receptor α, cAMP, and leukemia inhibitory factor/ciliary neurotrophic factor signaling pathways in a murine septal cell line. *J. Biol. Chem.* **270:** 22 101–22 104.

Bessis A, Salmon A-M, Zoli M, Le Novere N, Picciotto M, Changeux J-P. (1995) Promoter elements conferring neuron-specific expression of the β2-subunit of the neuronal nicotinic acetylcholine receptor studied *in vitro* and in transgenic mice. *Neuroscience.* **69:** 807–819.

Bird A, Tweedie S. (1995) Transcriptional noise and the evolution of gene number. *Phil. Trans. R. Soc. Lond. B* **349:** 249–253.

Buck L, Axel R. (1991) A novel multigene family may encode odorant receptors: a molecular basis for odor recognition. *Cell* **65:** 175–187.

Buckingham ME. (1994) Muscle: the regulation of myogenesis. *Curr. Opin. Genet. Dev.* **4:** 745–751.

Carter DA. (1993) Transgenic rodents and the study of the central nervous system. In: *Methods in Molecular Biology,* Vol. 18, *Transgenesis Techniques: Principles and Protocols* (eds D Murphy, DA Carter). Humana Press, Totowa, NJ, pp. 7–22.

Chelly J, Hamard G, Koulakoff A, Kaplan J-C, Kahn A, Berwald-Netter Y. (1990) Dystrophin gene transcribed from different promoters in neuronal and glial cells. *Nature* **344:** 64–65.

Chess A, Buck L, Dowling MM, Axel R, Ngai J. (1992) Molecular biology of smell: expression of the multigene family encoding putative odorant receptors. *Cold Spring Harb. Symp. Quant. Biol.* **57:** 505–516.

Chess A, Simon I, Cedar H, Axel R. (1994) Allelic inactivation regulates olfactory receptor gene expression. *Cell* **78:** 823–834.

Chong JA, Tapia-Ramirez J, Kim S *et al.*, (1995) REST: a mammalian silencer protein that restricts sodium channel gene expression to neurons. *Cell* **80:** 949–957.

Conaway RC, Conaway JW. (1993) General initiation factors for RNA polymerase. *Annu. Rev. Biochem.* **62:** 161–190.

Crystal RG. (1995) Transfer of genes to humans: early lessons and obstacles to success. *Science* **270:** 404–409.

Davidson BL, Allen ED, Kozarsky KF, Wilson JM, Roessler BJ. (1993) A model system for *in vivo* gene transfer into the central nervous system using an adenoviral vector. *Nature Genetics* **3:** 219–223.

Dawson SJ, Yoon SO, Chikaraishi DM, Lillycrop KA, Latchman DS. (1994) The Oct-2 transcription factor represses tyrosine hydroxylase expression via a heptamer TAATGARAT-like motif in the gene promoter. *Nucleic Acids Res.* **22:** 1023–1028.

Dent CL, Latchman DS. (1993) The DNA mobility shift assay. In: *Transcription Factors: a Practical Approach* (ed. DS Latchman). IRL Press, Oxford, pp. 1–26.

Echelard Y, Vassileva G, McMahon AP. (1994) *Cis*-acting regulatory sequences governing *Wnt-1* expression in the developing mouse CNS. *Development* **120**: 2213–2224.

Erickson JD, Varoqui H, Schäfer MK-H *et al.* (1994) Functional identification of a vesicular acetylcholine transporter and its expression from a 'cholinergic' gene locus. *J. Biol. Chem.* **269**: 21 929–21 932.

Gao W-Q, Hatten ME. (1994) Immortalizing oncogenes subvert the establishment of granule cell identity in developing cerebellum. *Development* **120**: 1059–1070.

Gill G. (1994) Taking the initiative. *Curr. Biol.* **4**: 374–376.

Grant AL, Jones A, Thomas KL, Wisden W. (1996) Characterization of the rat hippocalcin gene: the 5′ flanking region directs expression to the hippocampus. *Neuroscience*, in press.

Grosschedl R. (1995) Higher-order nucleoprotein complexes in transcription: analogies with site-specific recombination. *Curr. Opin. Cell Biol.* **7**: 362–370.

Halder G, Callaerts P, Gehring WJ. (1995a) Induction of ectopic eyes by targeted expression of the *eyeless* gene in *Drosophila*. *Science* **267**: 1788–1792.

Halder G, Callaerts P, Gehring WJ. (1995b) New perspectives on eye evolution. *Curr. Opin. Genet. Dev.* **5**: 602–609.

He X, Rosenfeld MG. (1991) Mechanisms of complex transcriptional regulation: implications for brain development. *Neuron* **7**: 183–196.

Hogan B, Beddington R, Costantini F, Lacy E. (1994) *Manipulating the Mouse Embryo: a Laboratory Manual*, 2nd Edn. Cold Spring Harbor Laboratory Press, Cold Spring Harbor, NY.

Holt CE, Garlick N, Cornel E. (1990) Lipofection of cDNAs in the embryonic vertebrate central nervous system. *Neuron* **4**: 203–214.

Hoyle GW, Mercer EH, Palmiter RD, Brinster RL. (1993) Cell-specific expression from the human dopamine β-hydroxylase promoter in transgenic mice is controlled via a combination of positive and negative regulatory elements. *J. Neurosci.* **14**: 2455–2463.

Hsu C, Janicki S, Monteiro MJ. (1990) The first intron of the mouse neurofilament light gene (NF-L) increases gene expression. *Mol. Brain Res.* **32**: 241–251.

Jin Y, Hoskins R, Horvitz HR. (1994) Control of type-D GABAergic neuron differentiation by *C. elegans* UNC-30 homeodomain protein. *Nature* **372**: 780–783.

Johnson AD. (1995) The price of repression. *Cell* **81**: 655–658.

Jones-Villeneuve EMV, McBurney MW, Rogers KA, Kalnins V. (1982) Retinoic acid induces embryonal carcinoma cells to differentiate into neurons and glial cells. *J. Cell Biol.* **94**: 253–262.

Kaneko R, Sueoka N. (1993) Tissue-specific versus cell type-specific expression of the glial fibrillary acidic protein. *Proc. Natl Acad. Sci. USA* **90**: 4698–4702.

Kengaku M, Misawa H, Deguchi T. (1993) Multiple messenger-RNA species of choline-acetyltransferase from rat spinal-cord. *Mol. Brain Res.* **18**: 71–76.

Kaplitt MG, Kwong AD, Kleopoulos SP, Mobbs CV, Rabkin SD, Pfaff DW. (1994) Preproenkaphalin promoter yields region-specific and long-term expression in adult brain after direct *in vivo* gene transfer via a defective herpes simplex viral vector. *Proc. Natl Acad. Sci. USA* **91**: 8979–8983.

Kitsberg D, Selig S, Brandeis M, Simon I, Keshet I, Driscoll DJ, Nicholls RD, Cedar H. (1993) Allele-specific replication timing of imprinted gene regions. *Nature* **364**: 459–463.

Kobayashi M, Takamatsu K, Saitoh S, Miura M, Noguchi T. (1992) Molecular cloning of hippocalcin, a novel calcium-binding protein of the recoverin family exclusively expressed in hippocampus. *Biochem. Biophys. Res. Commun.* **189**: 511–517.

Konradi C, Cole RL, Green D, Senatus P, Leveque J-C, Pollack AE, Grossbard SJ, Hyman SE. (1995) Analysis of the proenkephalin second messenger-inducible enhancer in rat striatal cultures. *J. Neurochem.* **65**: 1007–1015.

Kraner SD, Chong JA, Tsay H-J, Mandel G. (1992) Silencing the type II sodium channel gene: a model for neural-specific gene regulation. *Neuron* **9**: 37–44.

Kudrycki K, Stein-Izsak C, Behn C, Grillo M, Akeson R, Margolis FL. (1993) Olf-1-binding site: characterization of an olfactory neuron-specific promoter motif. *Mol. Cell. Biol.* **13**: 3002–3014.

Kurschner C, Morgan JI. (1995) The *maf* proto-oncogene stimulates transcription from multiple sites in a promoter that directs *Purkinje* neuron-specific gene expression. *Mol. Cell. Biol.* **15**: 246–254.

Lakin ND. (1993) Determination of DNA sequences that bind transcription factors by DNA footprinting. In: *Transcription factors: a Practical Approach* (ed. DS Latchman). IRL Press, Oxford, pp. 27–47.

Le Gal La Salle G, Robert JJ, Berrard S, Ridoux V, Stratford-Perricaudet LD, Perricaudet M, Mallet J. (1993) An adenovirus vector for gene transfer into neurons and glia in the brain. *Science* **259**: 988–990.

Lee JE, Hollenberg SM, Snider L, Turner DL, Lipnick N, Weintraub H. (1995) Conversion of *Xenopus* ectoderm into neurons by NeuroD, a basic helix–loop–helix protein. *Science* **268**: 836–844.

Lee V, Andrews P. (1986) Differentiation of NTera-2 clonal human embryonal carcinoma cells into neurons involves the induction of all three neurofilament proteins. *J. Neurosci.* **6**: 514–521.

Lewin B. (1994) On neuronal specificity and the molecular basis of perception. *Cell* **79**: 935–943.

Lewis SA, Cowan NJ. (1986) Anomalous placement of introns in a member of the intermediate filament multigene family: an evolutionary conundrum. *Mol. Cell. Biol.* **6**: 1529–1534.

Li L, Suzuki T, Mori N, Greengard P. (1993) Identification of a functional silencer element involved in neuron-specific expression of the synapsin I gene. *Proc. Natl Acad. Sci. USA* **90**: 1460–1464.

Li Y-P, Baskin F, Davis R, Wu D, Hersh LB. (1995) A cell type-specific silencer in the human choline acetyltransferase gene requiring two distinct and interactive E boxes. *Mol. Brain Res.* **30**: 106–114.

Lo DC, McAllister K, Katz LC. (1994) Neuronal transfection in brain slices using particle-mediated gene transfer. *Neuron* **13**: 1263–1268.

Loeffler J-P, Behr J-P. (1993) Gene transfer into primary and established mammalian cell lines with lipopolyamine-coated DNA. *Methods Enzymol.* **217**: 599–618.

Loeffler JP, Barthel F, Feltz P, Behr JP, Sassone-Corsi P, Feltz A. (1990) Lipopolyamine-mediated transfection allows gene expression studies in primary neuronal cells. *J. Neurochem.* **54**: 1812–1815.

Mandel G, McKinnon D. (1993) Molecular basis of neural-specific gene expression. *Annu. Rev. Neurosci.* **16**: 323–345.

Marshall H, Studer M, Pöpperl H, Aparicio S, Kuroiwa A, Brenner S. (1994) A conserved retinoic acid response element required for early expression of the homeobox gene *Hoxb-1*. *Nature* **370**: 567–571.

Matter J-M, Matter-Sadzinski L, Ballivet M. (1995) Activity of the β3 nicotinic receptor promoter is a marker of neuron fate determination during retina development. *J. Neurosci.* **15**: 5919–5928.

Matter-Sadzinski L, Hernandez M-C, Roztocil T, Balliver M, Matter J-M. (1992) Neuronal specificity of the α7 nicotinic acetylcholine receptor promoter develops during morphogenesis of the central nervous system. *EMBO J.* **11**: 4529–4538.

Maue RA, Kraner SD, Goodman RH, Mandel G. (1990) Neuron-specific expression of the rat brain type II sodium channel gene is directed by upstream regulatory elements. *Neuron* **4**: 223–231.

McKay RDG. (1989) The origins of cellular diversity in the mammalian central nervous system. *Cell* **58**: 815–821.

McKnight SL, Schibler U. (1993) Gene expression and differentiation. *Curr. Opin. Genet. Dev.* **3**: 201–202.

McLean PJ, Farb DH, Russek SJ. (1995) Mapping of the α4 subunit gene (GABRA4) to human chromosome 4 defines an α_2-α_4-β_1-γ_1 gene cluster: further evidence that modern GABA$_A$ receptor gene clusters are derived from an ancestral cluster. *Genomics* **26**: 580–586.

Mellon PL, Windle JJ, Goldsmith PC, Padula CA, Roberts JL, Weiner RI. (1990) Immortalization of hypothalamic GnRH neurons by genetically targeted tumorigenesis. *Neuron* **5**: 1–10.

Mercer EH, Hoyle GW, Kapur RP, Brinster RL, Palmiter RD. (1991) The dopamine β-hydroxylase gene promoter directs expression of *E. coli lacZ* to sympathetic and other neurons in adult transgenic mice. *Neuron* **7**: 703–716.

Min N, Joh TH, Kim KS, Peng C, Son JH. (1994) 5′ upstream DNA sequence of the rat tyrosine hydroxylase gene directs high-level and tissue-specific expression to catecholaminergic neurons in the central nervous system of transgenic mice. *Mol. Brain Res.* **27**: 281–289.

Misawa H, Ishii K, Deguchi T. (1992) Gene expression of mouse choline acetyltransferase. *J. Biol. Chem.* **267**: 20 392–20 399.

Mori N, Schoenherr C, Vandenbergh DJ, Anderson DJ. (1992) A common silencer element in the SCG10 and type II Na$^+$ channel genes binds a factor present in non-neuronal cells but not in neuronal cells. *Neuron* **9**: 45–54.

Nathans J, Davenport CM, Maumenee IH *et al.* (1989) Molecular genetics of human blue cone monochromacy. *Science* **245**: 831–838.

Neitz M, Neitz J. (1995) Number and ratios of visual pigment genes for normal red–green color vision. *Science* **267**: 1013–1016.

Nordquist DT, Kozak CA, Orr HT. (1988) cDNA cloning and characterization of three genes uniquely expressed in cerebellum by Purkinje neurons. *J. Neurosci.* **8**: 4780–4789.

Oberdick J, Levinthal F, Levinthal C (1988) A Purkinje cell differentiation marker shows a partial DNA sequence homology to the cellular sis/PDGF2 gene. *Neuron* **1**: 367–376.

Oberdick J, Smeyne RJ, Mann JR, Zackson S, Morgan JI. (1990) A promoter that drives transgene expression in cerebellar Purkinje and retinal bipolar neurons. *Science* **248**: 223–226.

Oberdick J, Schilling K, Smeyne RJ, Corbin JG, Bocchiaro C, Morgan JI. (1993) Control of segment-like patterns of gene expression in the mouse cerebellum. *Neuron* **10:** 1007–1018.

Orkin SH. (1995) Regulation of globin gene expression in erythroid cells. *Eur. J. Biochem.* **231:** 271–281.

Palmiter RD, Brinster RL. (1986). Germ-line transformation of mice. *Annu. Rev. Genet.* **20:** 465–499.

Paranjape SM, Kamakaka RT, Kadonaga JT. (1994) Role of chromatin structure in the regulation of transcription by RNA polymerase II. *Annu. Rev. Biochem.* **63:** 265–297.

Pathak BG, Neumann JC, Croyle ML, Lingrel JB. (1994) The presence of both negative and positive elements in the 5′-flanking sequence of the rat Na,K-ATPase α3 subunit gene are required for brain expression in transgenic mice. *Nucleic Acids Res.* **22:** 4748–4755.

Pleasure SJ, Page C, Lee VMY. (1992) Pure, postmitotic, polarized human neurons derived from NTera 2 cells provide a system for expressing exogenous proteins in terminally differentiated neurons. *J. Neurosci.* **12:** 1802–1815.

Rastan S. (1994) X-chromosome inactivation and the Xist gene. *Curr. Opin. Gen. Dev.* **4:** 292–297.

Roemer K, Johnson P, Friedmann T. (1995) Transduction of foreign regulatory sequences by a replication-defective herpes simplex virus type-1: the rat neuron-specific enolase promoter. *Virus Res.* **35:** 81–89.

Roessler BJ, Davidson BL. (1994) Direct plasmid mediated transfection of adult murine brain cells *in vivo* using cationic liposomes. *Neurosci. Lett.* **167:** 5–10.

Röhlich R, Veen Tv, Szél A. (1994) Two different visual pigments in one retinal cone cell. *Neuron* **13:** 1159–1166.

Sakimura K, Kushiya E, Ogura A, Kudo Y, Katagiri T, Takahashi Y. (1995) Upstream and intron regulatory regions for expression of the rat neuron-specific enolase gene. *Mol. Brain Res.* **28:** 19–28.

Sauerwald A, Hoesche C, Oschwald R, Kilimann MW. (1990) The 5′-flanking region of the synapsin I gene. *J. Biol. Chem.* **265:** 14 932–14 937.

Schneider LE, Roberts MS, Taghert PH. (1993) Cell type-specific transcriptional regulation of the Drosophila *FMRFamide* neuropeptide gene. *Neuron* **10:** 279–291.

Schoenherr CJ, Anderson DJ. (1995) The neuron-restrictive silencer factor (NRSF): a coordinate repressor of multiple neuron-specific genes. *Science* **267:** 1360–1363.

Schoenherr CJ, Paquette AJ, Anderson DJ. (1996) Identification of potential target genes for the neuron-restrictive silencer factor. *Proc. Natl Acad. Sci. USA* **93:** 9881–9886.

Sehgal A, Patil N, Chao M. (1988) A constitutive promoter directs expression of the nerve growth-factor receptor gene. *Mol. Cell. Biol.* **8:** 3160–3167.

Sengupta P, Colbert HA, Bargmann CI. (1994) The *C. elegans* gene *odr-7* encodes an olfactory-specific member of the nuclear receptor superfamily. *Cell* **79:** 971–980.

Simpson P. (1995) Positive and negative regulators of neural fate. *Neuron* **15:** 739–742.

Stocker KM, Brown AMC, Ciment G. (1993) Gene transfer of *LacZ* into avian neural tube and neural crest cells by retroviral infection of grafted embryonic tissues. *J. Neurosci. Res.* **34:** 135–145.

Struhl K. (1991) Mechanisms for diversity in gene expression patterns. *Neuron* **7:** 177–181.

Sutcliffe JG. (1988) mRNA in the mammalian central nervous system. *Annu. Rev. Neurosci.* **11:** 157–198.

Swaroop A, Xu JZ, Pawar H, Jackson A, Skolnick C, Agarwal N. (1992) A conserved retina-specific gene encodes a basic motif leucine zipper domain. *Proc. Natl Acad. Sci. USA* **89:** 266–270.

Thiel G, Greengard P, Südhof TC. (1991) Characterization of tissue-specific transcription by the human synapsin I gene promoter. *Proc. Natl Acad. Sci. USA* **88:** 3431–3435.

Timmusk T, Palm K, Metsis M, Reintam T, Paalme V, Saarma M, Persson H. (1993) Multiple promoters direct tissue-specific expression of the rat BDNF gene. *Neuron* **10:** 475–489.

Timmusk T, Lendahl U, Funakoshi H, Arenas E, Persson H, Metsis M. (1995) Identification of brain-derived neurotrophic factor promoter regions mediating tissue-specific, axotomy-, and neuronal activity-induced expression in transgenic mice. *J. Cell Biol.* **128:** 185–199.

Tjian R, Maniatis T. (1994) Transcriptional activation: a complex puzzle with few easy pieces. *Cell* **77:** 5–8.

Troemel ER, Chou JH, Dwyer ND, Colbert HA, Bargmann CI. (1995) Divergent seven transmembrane receptors are candidate chemosensory receptors in *C. elegans. Cell* **83:** 207–218.

Twyman RM, Jones EA. (1995) The regulation of neuron-specific gene expression in the mammalian nervous system. *J. Neurogenet.* **10:** 67–101.

Vandaele S, Nordquist DT, Feddersen RM, Tretjakoff I, Peterson AC, Orr HT. (1991) *Purkinje cell protein-2* regulatory regions and transgene expression in cerebellar compartments. *Genes Dev.* **5:** 1136–1148.

Vanselow J, Grabczyk E, Ping J, Baetscher M, Teng S, Fishman MC. (1994) GAP-43 transgenic mice: dispersed genomic sequences confer a GAP-43-like expression pattern during development and regeneration. *J. Neurosci.* **14**: 499–510.

Vidal M, Morris R, Grosveld F, Spanopaulou E. (1990) Tissue-specific control elements of the *Thy-1* gene. *EMBO J.* **9**: 833–840.

Wang MM, Reed RR. (1993) Molecular cloning of the olfactory neuronal transcription factor Olf-1 by genetic selection in yeast. *Nature* **364**: 121–126.

Wang Y, Macke JP, Merbs SL, Zack DJ, Klaunberg B, Bennett J, Gearhart J, Nathans J. (1992) A locus control region adjacent to the human red and green visual pigment genes. *Neuron* **9**: 429–440.

Wang MM, Tsai RYL, Schrader KA, Reed RR. (1993) Genes encoding components of the olfactory signal transduction cascade contain a DNA binding site that may direct neuronal expression. *Mol. Cell. Biol.* **13**: 5805–5813.

Watson JD, Gilman M, Witkowski J, Zoller M. (1992) *Recombinant DNA.* Scientific American Books, W.H. Freeman, New York.

Wisden W, Seeburg PH. (1993) A complex mosaic of high-affinity kainate receptors in the rat brain. *J. Neurosci.* **13**: 3582–3597.

Wolfe JH, Deshmane SL, Fraser NW. (1992) Herpesvirus vector gene transfer and expression of β-glucuronidase in the central nervous system of MPS VII mice. *Nature Genetics.* **1**: 379–384.

Wong SC, Moffat MA, O'Malley KL. (1994) Sequences distal to the AP1/E box motif are involved in the cell type-specific expression of the rat tyrosine hydroxylase gene. *J. Neurochem.* **62**: 1691–1697.

Yao K-M, White K. (1994) Neural specificity of *elav* expression: defining a *Drosophila* promoter for directing expression to the nervous system. *J. Neurochem.* **63**: 41–51.

Yoon SO, Chikaraishi DM. (1992) Tissue-specific transcription of the rat tyrosine hydroxylase gene requires synergy between an AP-1 motif and an overlapping E box-containing dyad. *Neuron* **9**: 55–67.

Yoon SO, Chikaraishi DM. (1994) Isolation of two E-box binding factors that interact with the rat tyrosine hydroxylase enhancer. *J. Biol. Chem.* **269**: 18 453–18 462.

Zimmerman L, Lendahl U, Cunningham M, McKay R, Parr B, Gavin B, Mann J, Vassileva G, McMahon A. (1994) Independent regulatory elements in the nestin gene direct transgene expression to neural stem cells or muscle precursors. *Neuron* **12**: 11–24.

Appendix. A description of methods for studying promoters and enhancers of neuronal genes

A region of DNA can be said to be functionally involved in the regulation of tissue-specific expression of a particular gene if the presence or absence of the region has any effect on mRNA synthesis *in vivo*. *Figure 3.8* illustrates the basic strategy used to study cell type-specific gene expression. All methods rely on 'reporter constructs' or 'transgenes'. These contain the putative DNA regulatory regions under investigation linked to a promoterless or enhancerless reporter gene cassette. Commonly used reporters are β-galactosidase (*LacZ*), chloramphenicol acetyl transferase or luciferase. These proteins are not endogenously expressed, and so the activation of the reporter gene can be clearly distinguished from the promoter activity of the endogenous gene. The reporter constructs are introduced into cell cultures, tissue slices or whole organisms. If the reporter construct can support the neuron-specific pattern of expression that is observed for the endogenous gene, then in the ideal case, specific DNA sequences are deleted or mutated to pinpoint which regions of the DNA are important in controlling this expression. This, together with assays such as EMSA and footprinting (Dent and Latchman, 1993; Lakin, 1993), results in the characterization of specific regulatory sequences. Further studies, using techniques such as the yeast one-hybrid selection system (Wang and Reed, 1993), can characterize the TFs which bind these elements. However, most studies on brain-specific gene expression have not so far reached this point.

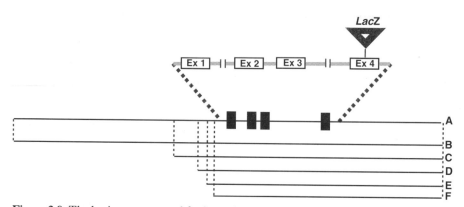

Figure 3.8. The basic strategy used for investigating cell type-specific gene expression using reporter genes (A). In this example, taken from the Purkinje cell-specific *L7* gene, the whole native gene is used as a construct for preliminary analysis in transgenic mice, with the *LacZ* coding region inserted into exon 4. (B–F), The entire gene (B) directs the correct pattern of expression in transgenic mice. Sequential deletions of specific DNA regions, in this example all from the 5′ end (C–F), are made to isolate smaller elements that are involved in specifying the correct expression pattern. Adapted from Oberdick *et al.* (1993) with permission from Cell Press.

A major consideration is whether to assay reporter gene expression *in vitro* (e.g. in primary neurons or neuronal cell lines) or *in vivo* (e.g. transgenic mice). A second consideration is how to get the reporter gene into the cells or neurons (e.g. transfection, microinjection, ballistics or viral vectors). Studying neural gene expression with reporter genes is difficult but not impossible. Neurons are very delicate cells and many methods routinely used on other cell types to introduce foreign DNA (e.g. calcium phosphate precipitation, electroporation) kill neurons.

Analyzing cell-specific gene expression in vitro: transient transfection of cell cultures and primary neurons

Transfection of primary neuronal cultures. Tissue-specific gene expression can be studied by comparing the expression of a plasmid reporter construct in cell cultures derived from the tissue in which the gene is normally expressed with those from a nonexpressing tissue. This *in vitro* method has been particularly successful in the study of muscle-specific and liver-specific gene expression. Primary cultured muscle and liver cells are extremely characteristic of those found *in vivo* and are very receptive to transfection of foreign DNA. Primary neuronal cultures (cells derived directly from dissociated nervous tissue), however, are extremely difficult to transfect using procedures such as calcium phosphate precipitation and electroporation. The development of specific DNA delivery agents however, has greatly improved prospects for transfecting primary neuronal cultures. These lipopolyamine agents are comprised of cationic lipids that form positively charged liposomes which complex spontaneously with polynucleotides. The positively charged complexes then interact with the negatively charged cell surface, fusing and releasing their DNA into the cytoplasm (Loeffler and Behr, 1993; Loeffler *et al.*, 1990).

Lipopolyamine-mediated transfer of DNA into primary neuronal cultures has been useful, for example, in analyzing c-*fos* gene expression in cerebellar neurons and hippocampal neurons (Bading *et al.*, 1993; Barthel and Loeffler, 1995), proenkephalin gene expression in striatal neurons (Konradi *et al.*, 1995), and $\alpha7$ and $\beta3$ nicotinic acetylcholine receptor subunit gene expression in dissociated retinal cells (Matter *et al.*, 1995; Matter-Sadzinski *et al.*, 1992). Cationic liposome:DNA complexes have also proved a useful means of transfecting neuronal tissues *in vivo*, either through injection directly into the brain (Roessler and Davidson, 1994) or by direct incubation of embryonal tissue with a liposome:DNA mixture (Holt *et al.*, 1990). However, although the techniques for transfection of primary neurons are improving, the efficiency of transfection is still very low and this makes the technique difficult to work with.

Transfection of neuronal cell lines. Neuronal cell lines, derived from central or peripheral neurons, ideally retain an established neuronal phenotype, but are by definition transformed due to their ability to divide and grow indefinitely *in vitro*. The effects of this deregulated growth on the control of gene expression, although poorly understood, are obviously of paramount importance when using the system to identify DNA elements normally involved in phenotypic cell type-specific gene expression in nonmitotic cells. It is possible that the molecular milieu of TFs and accessory factors in the nuclei of cell lines is different from that found in nontransformed neurons. Furthermore, reporter plasmids introduced into primary cells or cell lines do not integrate into the genome and remain episomal. Gene expression from episomal plasmids is not necessarily reflective of expression of a gene contained in a chromosome, primarily because chromosomal structures are believed to have some effect on, and in some cases may even regulate, transcription initiation (Paranjape *et al.*, 1994).

Nevertheless, the advantages of studying cell-specific gene expression in cell lines are ease of application, reproducibility and speed of analysis. It is possible to analyze a large number of deletion constructs to define putative silencers and enhancers in a relatively short time. In addition, some pluripotent embryonal carcinoma cell lines can be induced by certain treatments to differentiate into mature 'neuron-like' cells, a process which resembles commitment to the neuronal phenotype *in vivo* (Andrews, 1984; Jones-Villeneuve *et al.*, 1982; Lee and Andrews, 1986). The undifferentiated stem cells can be stably transfected with reporter constructs which are subsequently maintained in both undifferentiated cells and post-mitotic neurons upon differentiation (Pleasure *et al.*, 1992). Thus, such cell lines are potentially useful for studying neuron-specific gene regulation both in development and in the mature neuron.

Nearly all 'neuronal-like' cell lines have peripheral origins (e.g. PC12 cells). There are only a few neuronal cell lines which are derived from the CNS, although targeted tumorigenesis using transgenic mice or viral infection may be a way of making more of them (e.g. Gao and Hatten, 1994; Mellon *et al.*, 1990). Most CNS neuronal cell types are not represented by a cell line. This can lead to conflicting results between different cell line transfection analyses and transgenic analyses which are difficult to interpret. This point is well illustrated by studies on *TH* gene regulation. The AP1/dyad element shown to be sufficient to regulate *TH* expression in the PC8b cell line (Yoon and Chikaraishi, 1992) (see Section 3.2.1) appears to play no role in *TH* expression in the PC12 cell line (Wong *et al.*, 1994). Another study conducted in entirely different cell lines demonstrated a previously unreported regulatory role for an Oct-2 binding motif in the proximal promoter of the *TH* gene (Dawson *et al.*, 1994). In contrast, short transgene constructs containing 150 bp of rat *TH* gene upstream region, which includes this Oct-2 motif, were unable to drive any *LacZ* expression in transgenic mice, and sequences between –9 kb and –2.4 kb of the start site were necessary to confer high-level and tissue-specific expression to cate-cholaminergic neurons in mice (Min *et al.*, 1994). An additional transgenic analysis also demonstrated that at least 4.8 kb of 5′ flanking region of the *TH* gene is needed to direct appropriate cell type-specific expression (Banerjee *et al.*, 1992). Possibly these disparate results between *in vitro* and *in vivo* systems may reflect genuine differences in the mechanisms used to regulate *TH* expression in the wide variety of neurons in which it is expressed *in vivo*. None the less, it is clear that results can differ between different experimental systems and the use of both *in vitro* and *in vivo* approaches is often necessary in order to fully understand the intricate complexities of gene regulation.

Studying cell-specific expression in vivo

The best way to look at biological regulation is in cells which most clearly resemble the natural situation. In studying neuron-specific gene expression the major obstacle to this is getting the reporter gene into neuronal cells. The following sections illustrate methods that have been used to introduce foreign DNA into primary nervous tissue.

Transfection of brain slices. The brain slice has an advantage over primary neuronal cultures in that it preserves all the neuronal and glial cell types as well as the 3-D architecture and synaptic connections found in the tissue *in vivo*. However, conventional methods of transfecting neuronal tissue slices have poor efficiency (see Section 3.8.1). A recent study successfully introduced plasmid DNA into neuronal cells and glia of brain slices using particle-mediated-transfer, the firing of micro-sized gold particles coated with DNA at high velocities at the tissue (Lo *et al.*, 1994). This technique, originally developed as a method to introduce DNA into plant cells, has been used to demonstrate cell-specific regulation of the brain lipid-binding protein gene in Bergmann glia, astrocytes and migrating granule cells of cerebellar slices (Arnold *et al.*, 1994). This methodology has many advantages; it is quick, the vectors being plasmid based are easy to construct, and it is possible to co-transfect multiple vectors into the same cell thus allowing for cell marking and internal controls. Not all the cells in the slice are bombarded, but as the study by Arnold *et al.* demonstrates, it is still useful for studying cell type-specific gene expression provided sufficient numbers of each cell type are transfected. Because of the accessibility of the system, the nature of the tissue's structure, its speed and simplicity relative to transgenic methods, this technique may well prove popular for looking at cell-specific expression both in the adult and during development.

Viral infection of neural tissue. Gene transfer *in vivo* by means of viral vectors (retroviruses and replication defective or latency-prone neurotropic viruses [e.g. herpes simplex virus (HSV) and adenovirus vectors] is proving to be a promising technique in gene therapy studies (Crystal, 1995). However, the use of these vectors in studying gene regulation may be limited. Problems arise from the fact that the vectors are technically difficult to construct and package in large numbers compared with the routine construction of simple plasmid vectors. This makes the analysis of large numbers of constructs difficult. Additionally, the size of insert that can be cloned into a viral vector is limited and there is also evidence that the site of insertion of the test DNA into the viral genome can affect expression levels (Roemer *et al.*, 1995). Furthermore, retroviruses require the cell to be in a replicative state in order to integrate into the genome, and most mature neurons do not replicate. However, neuronal precursors from developing embryos can be infected with a retro-viral vector containing the reporter gene of interest and then grafted back into a host organism. The resultant graft gives rise to neuronal cells expressing the reporter gene (Stocker *et al.*, 1993). Stereotaxic injection of HSV (Wolfe *et al.*, 1992) and adenovirus vectors (Davidson *et al.*, 1993; Le Gal La Salle, 1993) have also successfully introduced DNA into specific regions of the nervous system, and this technique has been used to study the pre-proenkephalin gene promoter regions (Kaplitt *et al.*, 1994).

Transgenic mice. Transgenic mouse technology, whereby the reporter gene is introduced directly into the nucleus of a mouse oocyte, bypasses many of the problems faced by other techniques of analyzing cell type-specific expression (Carter, 1993; Hogan *et al.*, 1994; Palmiter and Brinster, 1986; *Figure 3.9*). The transgene is normally incorporated into the genome before the first division of the fertilized oocyte, and thus is present in every cell of a living organism, and so is in principle ideal for studying cell type-specific gene expression. Lines of mice can be generated from the founder mice, enabling extensive characterization of transgene expression.

A current complication of transgenic mice is that the random site of integration of the transgene cannot be controlled; in some cases this can influence the expression of reporter genes. For example, if the transgene integrates downstream of say a powerful muscle-specific enhancer of a nearby gene, or in a region of generally highly transcriptionally active chromatin, this may lead to ectopic expression which is not actually regulated by sequences in the reporter gene construct. Thus, ideally a large number of mice transgenic for any one particular reporter gene must be analyzed, with the premise that it is extremely unlikely that the gene will integrate in the same site more than once, and so influences of site integration can be detected. Additionally, transgenes integrate into a head-to-tail array of multiple copies which might also effect expression in undefined ways.

Figure 3.10 illustrates typical results obtained from transgenic mice, in this case studying the expression of a *LacZ* reporter gene under the control of 4 kb of the 5' region of the brain-specific *hippocalcin* gene (Kobayashi *et al.*, 1992; Grant *et al.*, 1996). The sequence is sufficient to direct β-galactosidase expression to some hippocampal CA1 pyramidal cells which express endogenous hippocalcin (*Figure 3.10*). The β-galactosidase protein is linked to a nuclear localization signal which prevents diffusion and diluting of the signal in neuronal dendrites and axons, and so enables more sensitive detection of the reporter protein in neurons by concentrating the signal in the cell nucleus (Mercer *et al.*, 1991).

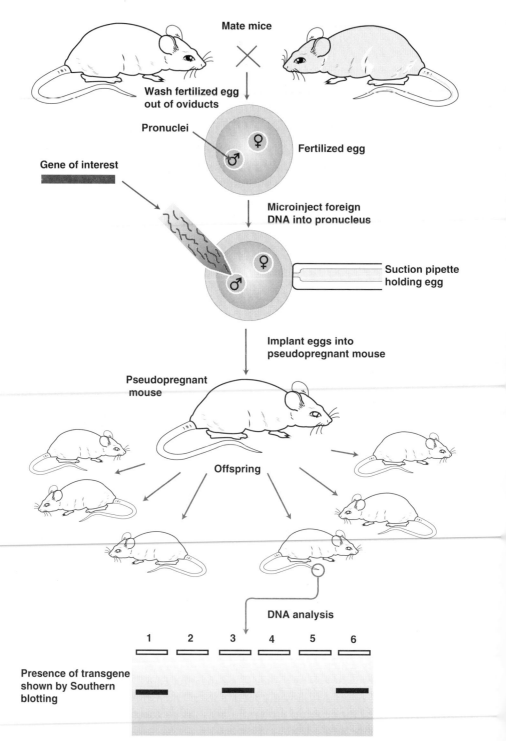

Figure 3.9. The procedure for producing transgenic mice. Adapted from *Recombinant DNA* 2/E by Watson, Gilman, Witkowski and Zoller. Copyright © 1992 by James D. Watson, Michael Gilman, Jan Witkowski and Mark Zoller. Used with permission of W.H. Freeman and Company.

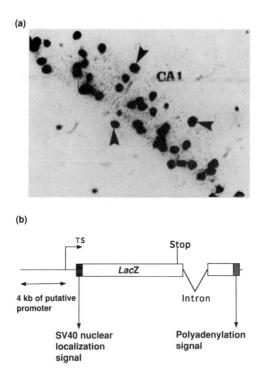

Figure 3.10. (a) A hippocampal tissue section stained for *LacZ*, taken from the brain of a transgenic mouse containing a *LacZ* reporter cassette under the control of 4 kb of the 5′ upstream region of the *hippocalcin* gene. Pyramidal cells in the CA1 region (arrowheads), which express the endogenous *hippocalcin* gene, are shown to be expressing nuclear *LacZ*. (b) Schematic diagram of the structure of the transgene used in (a) (Grant *et al.*, 1996).

The cytoskeleton

Javier Díaz-Nido and Jesús Avila

4.1 Introduction

The intricate circuitry of the nervous system is built of billions of neurons, each of which has a complex morphology with numerous long processes that branch and interconnect through synaptic junctions. In this way, the highly asymmetrical shape of nerve cells is crucial for the functioning of the brain.

At the beginning of the 20th century, neuroanatomists interested in the generation and maintenance of neuronal morphologies observed a 'neurofibril network' which arose in the cell body and extended into the axon and dendrites (Ramón y Cajal, 1904). Electron microscopy later showed that 'neurofibrils' corresponded to bundles of cytoskeletal fibers similar to those found in all eukaryotic cells (Peters *et al.*, 1976). Within the last 20 years, research has progressed impressively in the analysis of cytoskeletal components through the application of immunochemical, biochemical and molecular genetic techniques. This has dramatically improved our knowledge of the cytoskeleton (Bershadsky and Vasiliev, 1988; Burgoyne, 1991; Kreis and Vale, 1993).

The cytoskeleton consists of three types of filament structures: microfilaments, intermediate filaments and microtubules. These fibrous structures are assembled from the polymerization of certain protein subunits. A larger number of additional proteins associate with these filaments, modulating their structural stability and mediating their interaction with other cellular components. The dynamics of the assembly and disassembly of these protein polymers as well as their interactions with other cellular organelles and molecules provide the basis for the understanding of the physiological roles played by the cytoskeleton.

As the word 'cytoskeleton' implies, the skeleton of the cell is firstly required to sustain cell shape. The extraordinary morphologies of neurons consequently demand a highly developed cytoskeleton. Indeed, most cytoskeletal components are more abundant in neurons than in any other cell type. Furthermore, some proteins associated with the cytoskeleton appear to be specific for neurons.

Neuronal morphogenesis may thus be viewed as a process in which the relatively simple cytoskeleton of an undifferentiated neuroblast is progressively converted through a series of rearrangements into the complex cytoskeleton of a mature neuron. In this process, both changes in gene expression and post-translational modifications of cytoskeletal proteins take place.

Interestingly, the very sophisticated shapes of neurons are not unalterable during the entire life of an organism but they exhibit a noteworthy plasticity. Thus, neurons

Molecular Biology of the Neuron, edited by R.W. Davies and B.J. Morris.
© 1997 BIOS Scientific Publishers Ltd, Oxford.

may undergo morphologic changes in response to their synaptic input, providing the nervous system with a flexibility of neuronal connectivity which might contribute to learning and memory mechanisms. Other neuron shape variations arise as the consequence of injury or denervation. Obviously, all these modifications in neuronal morphology are carried out through changes in the cytoskeleton. The regulation of proteins associated with the cytoskeleton by protein kinases and phosphatases activated in response to certain extracellular signals is particularly relevant in this respect.

In addition to its role in the development, maintenance and modification of neuronal morphology, the cytoskeleton is essential in the intracellular organization of the neuron. Thus, the sorting, distribution, transport and anchoring of most cellular organelles depends on their interactions with cytoskeletal components.

Finally, the significance of the cytoskeleton in neuronal physiology is highlighted by the neuropathological effects of agents that disturb the cytoskeleton. This may be the cause of several toxic neuropathies. Moreover, cytoskeletal abnormalities are also found in several naturally occurring neurodegenerative disorders.

This chapter summarizes the main features of the three major cytoskeletal polymers and reviews some aspects of their contribution to neuronal morphogenesis and plasticity, intraneuronal transport and neuropathology.

4.2 Components of the neuronal cytoskeleton

4.2.1 Microfilaments

Microfilaments are produced by the polymerization of a 43 kDa globular protein called actin. Two actin isoforms, β and γ actin, have been identified in neurons (Choo and Bray, 1978). Actin is referred to as G-actin in its soluble form and once polymerized into microfilaments it is named F-actin. Actin monomers are arranged like two intertwined strings of beads giving a double helical filament of about 6 nm in diameter (see *Figure 4.1*). Actin monomers are asymmetric and associate in a particular orientation. This results in the formation of polar microfilaments in which the two ends (the 'barbed' or 'plus' end and the 'pointed' or 'minus' end) are different. Actin is an ATP-binding protein that requires ATP in order to polymerize. Polymerized actin hydrolyzes ATP rather slowly. One end of the microfilament contains ATP-actin and can incorporate new ATP-actin subunits. The other end contains ADP-actin which can dissociate from the polymer. Thus, polymerization of ATP-actin occurs preferentially in one end of the microfilaments whereas depolymerization of ADP-actin takes place in the other. This dynamics of actin microfilaments is usually referred to as 'treadmilling' (Wegner, 1985).

Actin microfilaments are found throughout the neuronal cytoplasm. Oligomers of actin are quite abundant immediately beneath the plasma membrane where they constitute the membrane skeleton (Luna and Hitt, 1992). Actin polymers are mainly enriched in presynaptic terminals and in dendritic spines and postsynaptic densities (Fifková and Morales, 1992; Hirokawa *et al.*, 1989; Ratner and Mahler, 1983). Within axons, short filaments are associated with microtubules (Fath and Lasek, 1988) and are also concentrated in the cortical region under the axonal plasma membrane (Tsukita *et al.*, 1986). In developing neurons, long microfilaments are present within filopodia of nerve growth cones (Gordon-Weeks, 1987; Lewis and Bridgman, 1992; Smith, 1988).

The variety of actin arrangements in different cellular locations as well as their dynamics are controlled by a number of actin-binding proteins (ABPs)

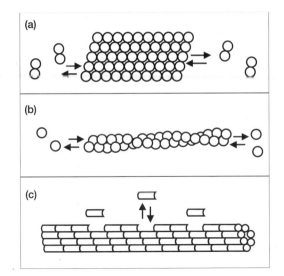

Figure 4.1 Dynamics of cytoskeletal polymers. Microtubule (a) dynamics occur through the incorporation and release of tubulin heterodimers at the ends of the polymer. Microfilament (b) dynamics are also associated with the exchange of actin monomers at the polymer ends. Intermediate filament (c) dynamics mainly involve the lateral replacement of subunits. Reproduced from Atkinson *et al.* (1992) with permission from Current Biology Ltd.

(Vandekerckhove, 1990). *Table 4.1* summarizes the major classes of ABPs.

A class of ABPs regulates the assembly of actin by distinct mechanisms including the catalysis of actin ATP/ADP exchange, the sequestering of G-actin and the severing or capping of F-actin. Interestingly, the activities of some of these ABPs may be modulated by Ca^{2+} or phosphatidylinositol-4, 5-bisphosphate. Thus, actin dynamics and organization may be modified in response to extracellular signals that induce changes in intracellular Ca^{2+} concentration or stimulate phosphatidylinositol bisphosphate hydrolysis. As a case in point, receptors with tyrosine kinase activity phosphorylate phospholipase C-γ which is stimulated to hydrolyze phosphatidylinositol bisphosphate tightly bound to profilin. As a consequence of phosphoinositide hydrolysis, profilin is released to the cytoplasm where it promotes actin polymerization (Aderem, 1992).

The F-actin stabilizing proteins bind along actin filaments, blocking their interaction with other ABPs. For instance, F-actin bound to tropomyosin is resistant to the severing action of ADF (actin depolymerizing factor).

Other classes of ABPs are able to bundle and crosslink F-actin. For instance, fimbrin can make F-actin form bundles of uniform polarity such as those found within filopodia of growth cones.

The best characterized F-actin crosslinking proteins are spectrins (Viel and Branton, 1996). These proteins crosslink actin oligomers, forming a network which is attached to the plasma membrane through the interaction of spectrin with ankyrin molecules. Spectrin can also bind directly to certain membrane proteins. Spectrin–actin complexes are the predominant form of the cytoskeleton immediately underneath the plasma membrane. Spectrin binding to actin can be modulated by Ca^{2+}/calmodulin. There are two major forms of spectrin in neurons: $\alpha\beta$ heterodimers,

Table 4.1. Major actin-binding proteins

Protein	Mass (kDa)	Properties
Assembly-regulating proteins		
ADF	19	Sequesters G-actin. Severs F-actin. Abundant in growth cones and presynaptic terminals
Gelsolin	90	Severs and caps F-actin. Modulated by Ca^{2+} and P1P2. Present in growth cones
Profilin	12–15	Sequesters G-actin. Catalyzes actin nucleotide exchange. Modulated by PIP_2. Abundant in growth cones
F-actin stabilizing proteins		
Tropomyosin	35	Dimer. Present both in dendrites and axons (including growth cones)
F-actin bundling and crosslinking proteins		
α-Actinin	100	Dimer. Modulated by Ca^{2+}. Binds vinculin, integrin and catenin. Present in growth cones
Amelin	80	Bundles F-actin and enhances spectrin binding. Abundant in soma and dendrites of mature neurons
Dystrophin	427	Dimer. Similar to spectrin
Filamin	270	Dimer. Crosslinks F-actin into networks. Present in growth cones.
Fimbrin	68	Bundles F-actin. Present in growth cones
MARCKS	87	Crosslinks F-actin. Modulated by calmodulin binding and PKC phosphorylation
Spectrin (αβ)	240/235	Heterodimer and tetramer. Crosslinks F-actin into networks. Modulated by Ca^{2+}/calmodulin. Abundant in soma and dendrites of mature neurons. Enriched in dendritic spines
Spectrin (αγ)	240/235	Homologous to spectrin. Present in growth cones. Abundant in axons
Synapsin I	76	Bundles F-actin and enhances spectrin binding. Associated with synaptic vesicles. Abundant in presynaptic terminals
Utrophin	400	Dimer. Similar to spectrin
Proteins anchoring F-actin to membranes		
Ankyrin (B-early)	440	Present in unmyelinated axons in the developing brain
Ankyrin (B-late)	220	Present in soma and dendrites of mature neurons
Ankyrin (N)	?	Present in nodes of Ranvier
Ankyrin (R)	206 and 186	Anchors spectrin to membrane proteins. Present in soma and dendrites of mature neurons
Catenin	100	Binds actin, α-actinin and cadherin
Talin	215	Binds vinculin and integrin. Present in growth cones
Vinculin	130	Binds actin, talin and α-actinin. Present in growth cones
Actin-activated ATPases		
Myosin I	110	
Myosin II	540	
Myosin V	190	

ADF, Actin depolymerizing factor; MARCKS, myristoylated alanine-rich C kinase substrate; PIP2, phosphatidylinositol-4, 5-bisphosphate; PKC, protein kinase C.

which are mainly localized in dendrites (including dendritic spines) and αγ heterodimers, which are referred to as fodrin, and are predominantly localized in axons (Riederer *et al.*, 1986). Fodrin appears first in developing neurons whereas αβ spectrin is mainly expressed in mature neurons (Riederer *et al.*, 1987). Other proteins somewhat similar to spectrins include filamin, dystrophin and utrophin.

MARCKS (myristoylated alanine-rich C kinase substrate) is an F-actin crosslinking protein which is localized to the plasma membrane by its myristoylated amino-terminal domain. The actin crosslinking activity of MARCKS is inhibited by either protein kinase C (PKC)-catalyzed phosphorylation or Ca^{2+}/calmodulin binding. MARCKS is therefore a Ca^{2+}/calmodulin- and PKC-sensitive bridge between actin microfilaments and the plasma membrane (Aderem, 1992).

Synapsin I is a multifunctional protein very abundant in presynaptic terminals, which bundles actin filaments, enhances the interaction of spectrin with actin and binds to synaptic vesicles. These activities are inhibited after synapsin phosphorylation by Ca^{2+}/calmodulin-dependent kinase. Synapsin I seems to favor the association of synaptic vesicles with the actin-rich cytoskeleton of the presynaptic terminal. After nerve terminal depolarization, synapsin I becomes phosphorylated and synaptic vesicles are released from actin filaments. These synaptic vesicles are then free to move to the plasma membrane where they can undergo exocytosis to release their neurotransmitter content (Llinás et al., 1985).

An important group of ABPs consists of proteins which anchor F-actin to membranes. These include ankyrins, vinculin, talin and catenin. Spectrins, MARCKS and α-actinin have been mentioned as F-actin crosslinking proteins but could also be included in this group.

Several ankyrin isoforms arise from the expression of three different genes and from the alternative splicing of the primary transcripts. There are two ankyrin (R) isoforms that are generated by alternative splicing of the transcript of the *ANK-1* gene. These proteins are present in the plasma membrane of cell bodies and dendrites of mature neurons. Two ankyrin (B) isoforms arise from alternative splicing of the transcript of the *ANK-2* gene. One 440 kDa isoform appears early during brain development and is present in unmyelinated axons. The other 220 kDa isoform is mainly localized to neuronal cell bodies and dendrites in the adult brain. A less well characterized ankyrin (N) isoform is the product of the *ANK-3* gene and is highly enriched at the nodes of Ranvier (Lambert and Bennett, 1993). Ankyrins mediate the binding of spectrin to the cytoplasmic portion of several integral membrane proteins such as the voltage-dependent Na^+ channel, the Na^+/K^+ ATPase and certain neuronal cell-adhesion proteins (Davis et al., 1993). Phosphorylation of ankyrins by casein kinase 2, PKC and cAMP-dependent protein kinase can affect the association of ankyrins with spectrin and membrane proteins.

Vinculin, talin and α-actinin form a complex that anchors F-actin to integrins. Integrins are transmembrane proteins that function as receptors for extracellular matrix proteins. It has been suggested that these actin-binding protein complexes also bind signaling proteins that are implicated in the signal transduction pathways responsible for integrin-induced changes in cell behavior (Clark and Brugge, 1995). Furthermore, vinculin binding to talin and actin is promoted by phosphatidylinositol-4, 5-biphosphate (Gilmore and Burridge, 1996).

Catenins are involved in the association of F-actin with the cytoplasmic domains of the Ca^{2+}-dependent cell adhesion molecules referred to as cadherins.

Finally, some ABPs are actin-activated ATPases that transduce the chemical energy of ATP into mechanical energy. These actin-dependent motor proteins are involved in growth cone motility (see Section 4.3.1) and in transport of organelles along actin filaments (see Section 4.5.4).

Summarizing, a large variety of ABPs may modulate actin assembly and organization. Moreover, ABPs are regulated by second messengers, phospholipids, protein kinases and other signaling proteins responding to specific extracellular signals. Thus, the actin cytoskeleton is connected to signal transduction pathways.

4.2.2 Intermediate filaments

Intermediate filament proteins (IFP) are a multigene family of polypeptides able to polymerize into filaments about 10 nm in diameter. These proteins share a similar three-domain molecular structure: a variable amino-terminal 'head' domain, a relatively conserved central 'rod' domain, and a variable carboxyl-terminal 'tail' domain. The 'rod' domain contains heptades of hydrophobic amino acids with a tendency to adopt a two chain coiled-coil α-helical configuration. Based on their amino acid sequence homologies, IFP are cataloged into six classes as shown in *Table 4.2* (Steinert and Roop, 1988).

Interestingly, these proteins show a cell type-specific expression. At different stages of differentiation, neuronal cells express distinct IFP. Central nervous system stem cells express nestin (a class VI IFP) at the time of neuroblast migration. Before differentiation, neurons also express vimentin (a class III IFP), which is gradually replaced by neurofilaments.

Neurofilament triplet proteins (NF-L, NF-M and NF-H, class IV IFP) are expressed by differentiating and mature neurons. Most neurons express relatively low levels of NF-L and NF-M at the time of neurite outgrowth. After neuronal maturation, NF-H is expressed and a parallel up-regulation of NF-L and NF-M occurs. Neurofilaments are much more abundant in axons than in dendrites. In fact, neurofilaments are the most prominent cytoskeletal elements within large myelinated axons. Often the number of neurofilaments is an order of magnitude higher than the number of microtubules. Neurofilament numbers may determine the diameter of large myelinated axons and, consequently, the speed of nervous impulse conduction. Ultrastructurally, neurofilaments consist of a core filament assembled form NF-L, with NF-M and NF-H co-assembling on to the core backbone. The 'tail' domains of

Table 4.2. Intermediate filament proteins

Class	Proteins	Mass (kDa)	Distribution
I	Acidic cytokeratins	40–64	Epithelial cells
II	Basic cytokeratins	52–68	Epithelial cells
III	Vimentin	55	Mesenchymal cells
			Immature neuronal and glial cells
	Desmin	53	Muscle cells
	GFAP	51	Astroglial cells
	Peripherin	57	PNS neurons
IV	NF-L	68	Neurons
	NF-M	145	Neurons
	NF-H	200	Neurons
	α-internexin (NF-/66)	66	CNS neurons
V	Lamins	62–72	All cells
VI	Nestin	240	CNS stem cells

CNS, central nervous system; GFAP, glial fibrillary acidic protein; NF-L, neurofilament, low molecular weight; NF-M, neurofilament, middle molecular weight; NF-H, neurofilament, heavy molecular weight; PNS, peripheral nervous system.

NF-M and NF-H extend away from the filament surface (Nixon and Shea, 1992; Nixon and Sihag, 1991).

Some developing neurons in the central nervous system also express α-internexin (NF-66, a class IV IFP), which persists within small caliber axons in the adult brain. α-Internexin is also present within dendrites and dendritic spines within hippocampal neurons. Peripherin (a class III IFP) is expressed by some developing neurons of the peripheral nervous system and is down-regulated during maturation, although it is maintained at low levels in certain neurons (Nixon and Shea, 1992).

Intermediate filaments are far more stable than microfilaments or microtubules. However, they exhibit a certain degree of dynamics which generally involves lateral exchange of subunits (see *Figure 4.1*). Class III intermediate filaments are more dynamic than class IV intermediate filament proteins. The transition from class III IFP to class IV IFP during neuronal development therefore implies a stabilization of the cytoskeleton. The persistence of class III IFP in certain neurons may be correlated with their higher plasticity. For instance, axons from olfactory sensory neurons which are able to regenerate express vimentin as their major IF.

Dynamics of class III intermediate filaments are controlled by phosphorylation. Cyclic AMP-dependent protein kinase and PKC phosphorylate sites on the head domain of class III IFP impeding the polymerization of phosphorylated subunits and inducing the depolymerization of assembled filaments (Inagaki *et al.*, 1989).

Several results indicate that neurofilaments are not entirely stable at least in immature growing axons. Thus, a slow lateral subunit exchange of NF-L has been observed in growing axons. This dynamic behavior declines after axonal maturation (Okabe *et al.*, 1993).

Isolated NF-L proteins are able to polymerize *in vitro*. Subunit exchange is observed in these homopolymers. As for class III IFP, phosphorylation of the 'head' domain by cAMP-dependent protein kinase favors NF-L disassembly. However, homopolymerization of NF-L may not occur *in vivo*. Thus, NF-L is unable to form polymers in transfected cells lacking other intermediate filaments. NF-L can only polymerize if the cells express vimentin, NF-M or NF-H (Lee *et al.*, 1993). In contrast, α-internexin (NF-66) is the only class IV IFP able to assemble in the absence of other intermediate filament proteins (Ching and Liem, 1993). Accordingly, neurofilament triplet proteins are obligate heteropolymers *in vivo*. Perhaps NF-L/NF-M copolymers such as those found in growing axons still retain some dynamic behavior whereas NF-L/NF-M/NF-H polymers such as those found in mature axons are completely stable.

Neurofilaments are extensively phosphorylated at sites on the 'tail' domains of NF-M and NF-H. Most of these sites correspond to repetitive Lys–Ser–Pro motifs and their phosphorylation may be catalyzed by proline-directed protein kinases such as cyclin-dependent kinase 5, glycogen synthase kinase 3 or specific neurofilament protein kinases. Phosphorylation occurs when neurofilaments have entered the axon and continues throughout axonal transport. This gradual phosphorylation is associated with the slowing of neurofilament transport and with the integration of the neurofilaments into a stationary structure (see Section 4.5.2). The large number of phosphorylated residues on the tail domains of NF-M and NF-H possibly increases the electrostatic repulsion between filaments as a consequence of the huge number of negative charges. This extended conformation may be responsible for the increase in interfilament spacing and axonal caliber induced by myelination (see Section 4.3.2). Furthermore, phosphorylation protects neurofilaments against proteolysis by calcium-activated proteases like calpain. Thus, this type of neurofilament phosphory-lation favors the stabilization of the axonal cytoskeleton.

4.2.3 Microtubules

Microtubules are hollow fibers with a diameter of 24 nm. They are formed by 13 lon-gitudinal strands arranged in a helical configuration. Each strand is composed of aligned globular heterodimers consisting of an α-tubulin and β-tubulin subunit. This leads to a polarized polymer with one end having exposed mainly α-subunits and the other end mainly β-subunits. As described for actin microfilaments, one end of the microtubule (the 'plus' end) polymerizes faster than the other (the 'minus' end).

There are different genes coding for distinct isoforms of α- and β-tubulin. In mam-mals six genes for α- and six genes for β-subunits have been found. Some of these gene products are specific for neurons (Sullivan, 1988). A γ-tubulin encoded by a different gene has also been described. This tubulin subunit is not found within microtubules but appears to be localized at the centrosome where it presumably functions as a seed for the initiation of microtubule polymerization (Oakley, 1992).

Further tubulin isoforms are generated on assembled microtubules as the conse-quence of post-translational modifications. There is acetylation of α-tubulin, phos-phorylation of a neuronal-specific β-tubulin and polyglutamination of both α- and β-tubulin. These chemical modifications seem to occur preferentially on stable microtubules.

Tubulin is a GTP-binding protein. Soluble GTP-tubulin has the ability to poly-merize into microtubules. Once tubulin is incorporated into the polymer, the GTP bound to β-tubulin is hydrolyzed to GDP. Possibly α-tubulin facilitates GTP hydrol-ysis. When the proportion of GTP-tubulin at a microtubule end decreases below a threshold level, the microtubule starts to rapidly depolymerize. After this, there is the possibility that the microtubule may again incorporate GTP-tubulin and stop depoly-merizing. This behavior of microtubules has been referred to as 'dynamic instability' and describes well the properties of polymers assembled from purified tubulin *in vitro* (Kirschner and Mitchison, 1986). However, microtubules are less dynamic *in vivo* than they are *in vitro*. There are also differences in the behavior of microtubules in dis-tinct cell types and at different stages of development. For instance, a progressive microtubule stabilization is attained during the maturation of axons and dendrites (Baas *et al.*, 1991).

Microtubules are distributed as bundles throughout the neuronal cytoplasm, although their organization differs in axons and dendrites (see Section 4.3.3). Microtubules are crucial elements in the generation and maintenance of neuronal morphology. Thus, both axons and dendrites shrink back to the cell body after treat-ment of cultured neurons with microtubule-depolymerizing drugs. Microtubules serve also as tracks for bidirectional transport of various organelles and macromole-cules between cell bodies and neurite tips (see Section 4.5.1).

The dynamics of microtubules as well as their interactions with other cellular com-ponents are regulated by microtubule-binding proteins. *Table 4.3* shows the main types of microtubule-binding proteins.

Some microtubule-binding proteins promote the assembly of tubulin into micro-tubules and remain bound to the microtubule surface, resulting in microtubule stabi-lization. These proteins are quite abundant and were the first microtubule-binding

Table 4.3. Major microtubule-binding proteins

Protein	Mass (kDa)	Properties
Assembly-promoting and microtubule-stabilizing proteins		
HMW-Tau	100–120	Present in the peripheral nervous system.
LMW-Tau	50–65	Abundant in axons of the central nervous system. Contributes to microtubule stabilization.
MAP-1A	350	Abundant in dendrites of mature neurons.
MAP-1B (MAP5)	324	Present both in axons and dendrites. Contributes to initial neurite outgrowth.
MAP-2A, B	270	Present in cell bodies and dendrites (including dendritic spines).
MAP-2C, D	70	Present in axon, dendrites and glial cells.
MAP-4	180–220	Present in glial cells and in immature neurons.
Microtubule-destabilizing proteins		
Op18/stathmin	17	Highly abundant. Favors microtubule destabilization.
Microtubule-activated ATPases		
Dynein (MAP1C) (heavy chain)	300	Move organelles from 'plus' to 'minus' ends of microtubules.
Kinesin (heavy chain)	120	Move organelles from 'minus' to 'plus' ends of microtubules.
Kinesin-related proteins		
Proteins linking microtubules and organelles		
CLIP-170	170	Binds endosomes.
Proteins anchoring microtubules to membrane		
Gephyrin	93	Binds glycine receptors.

proteins identified, being named microtubule-associated proteins (MAPs). MAPs bind to the carboxyl-terminal domain of tubulin, a domain implicated in the regulation of tubulin polymerization possibly through its interaction with the GTP-binding domain of the tubulin molecule (Padilla *et al.*, 1993). MAPs are a heterogeneous group of proteins that show developmental stage specific expression as well as subcellular-specific compartmentalization. Interestingly, MAP functionality can be regulated by phosphorylation and dephosphorylation (Avila *et al.*, 1994; Tucker, 1990).

MAP1A and MAP1B are encoded by different genes, but show extensive amino acid sequence homology. These proteins are much more abundant in neurons than in other cell types. MAP1B (also called MAP5) is the first MAP expressed by neurons during differentiation and is particularly abundant in growing axons. Mutant mice lacking MAP1B exhibit gross neuronal abnormalities, thus underlying the essential role of MAP1B in neuronal morphogenesis (Edelmann *et al.*, 1996). The expression of MAP1B diminishes after neuronal maturation, and the remaining protein is localized both in axons and dendrites of adult neurons. MAP1B is highly phosphorylated *in vivo*. There are at least two modes of MAP1B phosphorylation. One is catalyzed by proline-directed protein kinases, mainly takes place in growing axons, and practically disappears after axonal maturation (Mansfield *et al.*, 1992). Interestingly axons from neurons with a high regenerative potential retain this phosphorylated MAP1B. The other mode of MAP1B phosphorylation is catalyzed by casein kinase 2 and is maintained both in axons and dendrites of mature neurons (Ulloa *et al.*, 1994). As for MAP1A, its expression is up-regulated during neuronal maturation, and it is abundant in dendrites and is also *in vivo* phosphorylated.

MAP2, MAP4 and tau proteins share a homologous tubulin-binding domain which is different from that present in MAP1A or MAP1B. MAP2, MAP4 and tau are each encoded by a single gene, but considerable heterogeneity arises from alternative splicing of primary transcripts.

MAP2 isoforms include high molecular weight proteins MAP2A and MAP2B and low molecular weight proteins MAP2C and MAP2D. MAP2C is expressed in the embryonic brain and it is down-regulated during brain maturation. In contrast, MAP2A appears only after brain maturation. MAP2C is present in neuronal cell bodies, dendrites and axons as well as in glial cells, whereas high molecular weight MAP2 is a neuronal-specific protein selectively localized in dendrites and neuronal cell bodies (Tucker, 1990). The compartmentalization of high molecular weight MAP2 into dendrites may be due to the selective transport of the corresponding mRNA into dendrites (Garner *et al.*, 1988). In addition to its association with microtubules, MAP2 is associated with actin in dendritic spines (Fifková and Morales, 1992). Binding of MAP2 to tubulin and actin is regulated by phosphorylation. MAP2 can be modified by cAMP-dependent protein kinase, Ca^{2+}/calmodulin-dependent protein kinase, PKC and proline-directed protein kinases.

MAP4 proteins are mainly expressed in nonneuronal tissues. In the brain, MAP4 is present in glial cells and very immature neurons.

Low molecular weight tau proteins are found in the central nervous system whereas additional high molecular weight tau proteins are present in the peripheral nervous system. In brain, tau proteins are particularly abundant within axons, although some tau is also present in neuronal cell bodies and dendrites. The association of tau with tubulin may also be regulated through phosphorylation by several protein kinases such as cAMP-dependent protein kinase, Ca^{2+}/calmodulin-dependent protein kinase, PKC, casein kinase 1, casein kinase 2 and proline-directed protein kinases. *In vivo*, tau phosphorylation by proline-directed protein kinases is especially prominent in embryonic tau as compared with adult tau. It is plausible that tau dephosphorylation at these sites favors binding of tau to tubulin and therefore contributes to microtubule stabilization during axonal maturation (Ferreira *et al.*, 1993).

A different type of microtubule-binding protein is Op18/stathmin. This 17 kDa protein was initially discovered as a protein which becomes up-phosphorylated in response to a variety of extracellular signals. It is now clear that Op18/stathmin has the ability to bind tubulin and favor rapid microtubule depolymerization (Belmont and Mitchison, 1996).

Other microtubule-binding proteins are microtubule-activated ATPases, also called motor proteins. Kinesin, kinesin-related proteins and cytoplasmic dynein are involved in the transport of organelles along microtubules (see Section 4.5.4).

Whereas motor proteins are essential for the movement of cytoplasmic organelles, other microtubule-binding proteins may link specific organelles to microtubules in order to regulate subsequent translocation by motors and define stable subcellular locations for organelles. This class of proteins has received the name of cytoplasmic linker proteins (CLIPs). The best characterized member of this protein type is CLIP-170, which mediates the binding of endosomes to microtubules. There is some evidence suggesting the existence of other CLIPs linking other organelles such as trans-golgi network-derived exocytic vesicles and phagosomes to microtubules (Rickard and Kreis, 1996).

Microtubules are important not only for the organization of organelles within the cytoplasm but also for the clustering of protein complexes within membranes. Proteins anchoring membrane proteins to microtubules play an essential role in this respect. As a case in point, gephyrin links glycine receptors of postsynaptic membranes to microtubules and microfilaments (Kirsch and Betz, 1996).

A new type of microtubule-binding protein with microtubule severing activity has recently been described. It is not known whether these proteins are present in neurons (Shiina *et al.*, 1995).

4.2.4 Interactions of cytoskeletal components

Microfilaments, intermediate filaments and microtubules are not isolated from each other in the neuronal cytoplasm. Indeed, there are a large number of connections between the three types of cytoskeletal structures. Many proteins are involved in these interactions. For instance, spectrin not only binds actin but also ankyrin, membrane proteins, microtubules and neurofilaments. Certain microtubule-associated proteins have also been reported to bind microfilaments and neurofilaments. Additionally, many membrane organelles and soluble proteins are anchored to the cytoskeleton. The clearest example is the plasma membrane, where the cytoplasmic 'tails' of many membrane proteins are bound to cytoskeletal proteins (Kirsch and Betz, 1996).

Development of the quick-freeze, deep-etch techniques has allowed the observation of the three-dimensional architecture of the unfixed neuronal cytoskeleton. These images have provided evidence that there is a cytoskeletal network that should be considered as an integrated functional entity (Hirokawa, 1982). *Figure 4.2* is a schematic drawing of the cytoskeleton beneath the plasma membrane of the squid giant axon as visualized by the quick-freeze, deep-etch technique (Tsukita *et al.*, 1986).

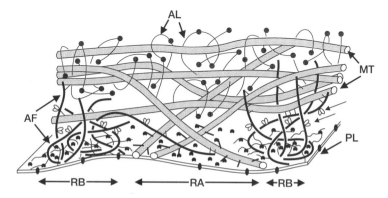

Figure 4.2. Diagram showing the architecture of the cytoskeleton underneath the plasma membrane of a squid giant axon. The plasma membrane (PL) consists of actin microfilament-associated (RB) and microtubule-associated (MT) domains. The cross-linkers between microtubules (MT) and actin filaments (AF), between MT and PL, and between AF and PL are apparent. Microtubules are surrounded by axolinin (AL) molecules. Axolinin is a squid giant axon MAP. Reproduced from *The Journal of Cell Biology* (1986), vol. 102, pp. 1710–1725 by copyright permission of The Rockefeller University Press.

The existence of connections between microtubules and microfilaments and between these cytoskeletal polymers and the plasma membrane is apparent.

4.3 The cytoskeleton in neuronal morphogenesis

4.3.1 Neurite growth

An essential event for neuronal morphogenesis is the extension of the neurites that are the hallmark of neuronal cell shape. All neurites, both axon and dendrites, grow at specialized terminal appendages called growth cones, which were first observed by Ramón y Cajal in the embryonic chick spinal cord. Growth cones are primarily involved in the extension of the neurite and in the guidance of the developing neurite to reach its target. Accordingly, growth cones function as sensory devices that decode extracellular signals in order to direct neurite growth through the regulation of intracellular cytoskeletal dynamics.

Typical growth cones appear as fan-shaped or leaf-shaped expansions of neurite tips. Growth cones are characterized by the presence of long thin projections called filopodia which are embedded within broad expansions named lamellipodia. Microtubules are mostly located in the central portion of the growth cone. Bundled unipolar actin microfilaments constitute the cytoskeleton of filopodia and a network of crosslinked actin predominates within lamellipodia (Lewis and Bridgman, 1992).

Neurite outgrowth occurs through the protrusion of filopodia and lamellipodia and the subsequent invasion of the expanded bases of filopodia and lamellipodia by microtubules. The bundling of the invading microtubules constitutes the consolidation of the growth of the neurite. The protrusive activity of lamellipodia and filopodia of cultured neurons is inhibited by F-actin depolymerizing drugs like cytochalasin B, while it persists in the presence of microtubule-depolymerizing drugs like nocodazole or colchicine. In contrast, neurite elongation is blocked in the presence of microtubule-depolymerizing drugs and continues in the presence of F-actin depolymerizing drugs. This indicates the existence of two linked processes during neurite outgrowth that can be uncoupled by different drugs. One is the growth cone motility, which is presumably involved in neurite guidance and depends on actin dynamics. The other process is neurite elongation which depends on microtubules. Under physiological conditions, both processes are connected.

The molecular mechanisms responsible for the protrusive activity of filopodia and lamellipodia are not entirely understood. However, a hypothetical description has been proposed (Lin et al., 1994, 1996; Mitchison and Kirschner, 1988; Smith, 1988; Stossel, 1993). Figure 4.3 shows a schematic drawing that explains how forward movement of filopodia and lamellipodia might occur. It is well known that there is a retrograde flow of F-actin in filopodia and lamellipodia. This retrograde flow is particularly robust in immotile growth cones and it is easily observed when neurons are plated on a poly-L-lysine substrate lacking certain extracellular matrix proteins. When a growth cone is on a more permissive substrate, the retrograde F-actin flow slows down and the growth cone advances. This suggests that the advance of the growth cone depends on the coupling of the cytoskeleton to the substrate. Figure 4.3a depicts a growth cone in which the cytoskeleton is not linked with the extracellular substrate. In this situation, motor proteins (presumably myosin molecules anchored to the rigid membrane skeleton) can produce the retrograde movement of actin microfilaments that are undergoing 'treadmilling' (see Section 4.2.1). Figure 4.3b depicts the situation in

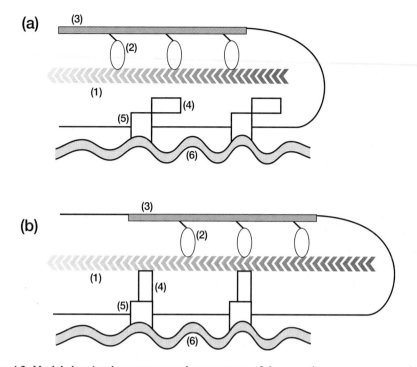

Figure 4.3. Model showing how anterograde movement of the growth cone may occur when the retrograde flow of actin microfilaments ceases as the consequence of anchoring to the extracellular substrate. In (a), actin microfilaments (1) are subjected to 'treadmilling': assembling at the 'barbed' end (shaded chevrons) and disassembling at the 'pointed' end (faded chevrons). There is a retrograde flow of actin microfilaments (1) driven by myosin molecules (2) anchored on to the membrane skeleton (3). In (b), actin filaments become stationary because of their association with anchoring proteins (4) bound to transmembrane proteins (5) which are linked to extracellular matrix molecules (6). Addition of new actin monomers to the 'barbed' end also occurs. Myosin (3) and the membrane skeleton (3) crawl to the leading edge of the growth cone. Reproduced from Mitchison and Kirschner (1988) with permission from Cell Press.

which the cytoskeleton of the growth cone is firmly attached to the extracellular substrate. When this occurs, the actin microfilaments are stationary and the motor protein myosin and the membrane skeleton crawl to the edge of the growth cone. Actin polymerization at the 'plus' ends of microfilaments also occurs in parallel, thus leading to growth cone advance.

Extracellular signal molecules may modulate growth cone motility through the regulation of actin dynamics and motor protein activity by second messengers and protein kinases acting on ABPs. Many ABPs are present in growth cones (see *Table 4.1*) but their precise implication in the control of growth cone motility is not yet known.

In particular, proteins of the Rho subfamily of Ras-related GTPases (CDC42, Rac and Rho) are involved in the signal transduction pathways leading to the remodeling of the actin cytoskeleton within growth cones in response to certain extracellular signals. CDC42 primarily stimulates filopodia formation, Rac stimulates the formation of lamellipodia and Rho could participate in growth cone retraction (MacKay *et al.*, 1995). It is not yet clear how actin dynamics and organization are modified after the activation of CDC42, Rac and Rho. These GTPases regulate some membrane enzymes such as phosphoinositide-3-kinase, phosphoinositide-5-kinase and phospholipase D which may generate phospholipid-derived molecules that in turn can modify actin-binding proteins (Gilmore and Burridge, 1996; Symons, 1996). Furthermore, CDC42, Rac and Rho can also trigger protein kinase cascades that could lead to the phosphorylation of cytoskeletal proteins (Symons, 1996).

The forward movement of the growth cone is accompanied by neurite extension. This presumably occurs through the translocation and polymerization of microtubules from the central part of the growth cone to the expanded initial portions of the protrusive filopodia and lamellipodia. This microtubule extension may simply be favored by the fact that actin filament density is decreasing at the base of filopodia and lamellipodia when these are advancing. Alternatively, there might be molecules crosslinking actin microfilaments and microtubules that could pull microtubules to the base of filopodia and lamellipodia. Some evidence favors the first possibility, namely, that microtubules tend to extend when not restrained by the retrograde flow of actin microfilaments. Thus, treatment of growth cones with microfilament-depolymerizing drugs stimulates the extension of microtubules (Forscher and Smith, 1988).

As mentioned above, neurite elongation is completely dependent on microtubules. Both the transport of microtubules from the cell body and the elongation of microtubules contribute to neurite growth (Joshi and Baas, 1993). *Figure 4.4* shows that short microtubules destined for the neurites are initiated at the centrosome within the cell body, after which they are released from the centrosome and transported into the neurite. Nothing is known about the motor proteins responsible for catalyzing microtubule transport within growing neurites. During their transit down the neurite, these short microtubules are elongated. The central region of the growth cone is particularly enriched in microtubule 'plus' ends that are actively polymerizing by incorporation of tubulin subunits.

In addition to microtubule transport and elongation, the consolidation of the growing neurite is produced by the bundling of microtubules. Microtubule-associated proteins are possibly involved in the bundling of microtubules. In particular, an essential role for MAP1B in the initiation of neurite growth is supported by experiments using

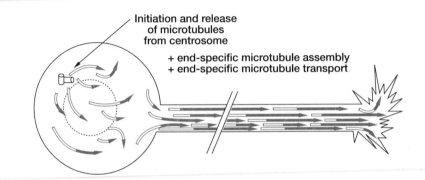

Figure 4.4. Model describing the origin of axonal microtubules. Microtubules are nucleated at the centrosome, then released and transported into the axon where microtubule polymerization takes place at the 'plus' ends. The growth cone is a major site of microtubule assembly. Reproduced from *The Journal of Cell Biology* (1993), vol. 121, pp. 1191–1196, by copyright permission of The Rockefeller University Press.

antisense oligonucleotides which inhibit MAP1B expression in cultured neuronal-like cells (Brugg *et al.*, 1993). Furthermore, MAP1B must be phosphorylated by casein kinase 2 to perform its function in neurite growth (Ulloa *et al.*, 1993).

Microtubules in distal neurite regions are more dynamic than those in the proximal domain, which suggests a progressive stabilization of microtubules during neurite extension. Different MAPs may stabilize microtubules in axons and dendrites. Thus, tau proteins are possibly implicated in a partial microtubule stabilization within growing axons (Harada *et al.*, 1994) and high molecular weight MAP2 protein may perform a similar role in growing dendrites. Microtubules are not completely stable in extending neurites because these need a flexible cytoskeleton to allow growth. In mature neurites, the cytoskeleton becomes less plastic since the maintenance of morphology and the transport of organelles are its major functions. Thus, microtubule stabilization is increased with axonal and dendritic maturation (Baas *et al.*, 1991). Dephosphorylation of certain sites on MAP1B and tau molecules can contribute to axonal microtubule stabilization (Ferreira *et al.*, 1993; Ulloa *et al.*, 1994) whereas the appearance of new MAPs like MAP1A may favor dendritic microtubule stabilization.

4.3.2 Axonal maturation

When axons reach their targets, the cytoskeleton of the growth cone is remodeled and converted into the cytoskeleton of a presynaptic terminal. Motility and extension cease, and an accumulation of synapsin, which crosslinks synaptic vesicles to actin microfilaments, is observed.

Myelination signals a new phase of axonal maturation, characterized by the radial growth of the axon. It is now clear that this increase in axonal diameter is due to the augmented expression and phosphorylation of neurofilaments. Thus, no radial growth of axons is observed in a mutant quail called *quiver* that lacks neurofilaments as a consequence of a spontaneous mutation in the NF-L gene. The diminished axonal diameter in this mutant is accompanied by a significant decrease in the speed of nervous impulse conduction (Ohara *et al.*, 1993; Sakaguchi *et al.*, 1993). A reduced axonal caliber is also observed in a mutant mouse caller *trembler* in which myelination does not occur as the result of a mutation in the gene encoding myelin basic protein. *Trembler* axons have an increased density of neurofilaments that are closely spaced and underphosphorylated. This suggests that NF-M and NF-H tail domain phosphorylation augments interfilament spacing, contributing to radial growth (see Section 4.2.2). Underphosphorylation results in narrow spacing, increased density and reduced axonal caliber. Interestingly, this is not only observed in *trembler* axons but also in normal axons at the nodes of Ranvier. Thus, myelination seems to control NF-M and NF-H tail domain phosphorylation (see *Figure 4.5*). This indicates that Schwann cell–axon interactions may trigger a signaling pathway that controls a neurofilament kinase or phosphatase (De Waegh *et al.*, 1992).

4.3.3 Neuronal polarity

Axons and dendrites differ in their morphology, rate of growth, organelle content and cytoskeletal composition and organization (see *Table 4.4*). It is plausible that the differences between the cytoskeleton of axons and dendrites are responsible for the differences in their morphology, rate of growth and organelle content (Craig and Banker, 1994).

The formation of axons and dendrites follows a stereotyped pattern in cultured embryonic hippocampal neurons (Dotti *et al.*, 1988). After plating, the cells extend

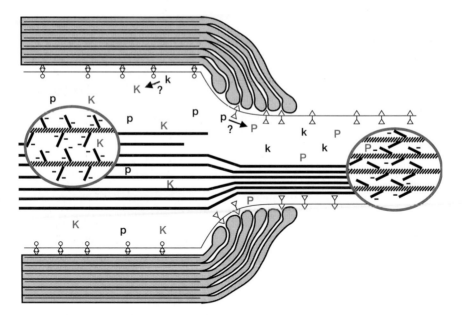

Figure 4.5. Diagram showing the stimulation of axonal neurofilament phosphorylation by myelinating Schwann cells. Putative interactions between Schwann cell membrane and axonal membrane molecules trigger either the activation of a neurofilament kinase (K) or the inhibition of a phosphatase (P), thus leading to an enhanced phosphorylation of the 'tail' domains of NF-H and NF-M. These constitute the lateral projections of the neurofilament polymers and their high degree of phosphorylation may lead to electrostatic repulsion, resulting in a wide interfilament spacing and increased axonal caliber. In nonmyelinated axonal segments, the activity of the phosphatase is higher than the kinase activity, neurofilaments are therefore less phosphorylated, and a narrower interfilament spacing and a reduced axonal diameter are observed. Reproduced from De Waegh *et al.* (1992) with permission from Cell Press.

Table 4.4. Major differences between axons and dendrites

Axons	Dendrites
Uniform caliber	Tapered morphology
Few branches	Highly branched
Lack of polyribosomes	Presence of polyribosomes
Fast growth	Slow growth
Abundance of neurofilaments	Abundance of microtubules
Uniform polarity of microtubules	Mixed polarity of microtubules
Narrow spacing between microtubules	Wide spacing between microtubules
Abundance of tau protein	Presence of MAP2A, B
Presence of $\alpha\gamma$ spectrin	Presence of $\alpha\beta$ spectrin
Highly phosphorylated NF-M and NF-H	Nonphosphorylated NF-M and NF-H

lamellipodia (stage 1). Several short neurites arise from these lamellipodia (stage 2). One of them elongates very rapidly, becoming the axon (stage 3). After a few days, the remaining short neurites begin to grow slowly to become dendrites (stage 4). Finally both axons and dendrites mature (stage 5).

The initiation of fast axonal growth (stage 3) marks the generation of neuronal polarity. A segregation of certain proteins into the nascent axon at this stage has been observed. One of these proteins is neuromodulin, which may have a regulatory function on axonal growth cone motility. Differential protein phosphorylation may also contribute to the development of neuronal polarity. For example, MAP1B phosphorylated by proline-directed protein kinases is mainly localized to growing axons, as shown in *Figure 4.6* (Mansfield *et al.*, 1992; Ulloa *et al.*, 1994). Interestingly, laminin, an extracellular matrix protein that stimulates axonal growth, also promotes MAP1B phosphorylation (Di Tella *et al.*, 1996).

An important event in the establishment of neuronal polarity is the appearance of microtubules with mixed polarity (see *Figure 4.7*). Within the axon, all the microtubules have a uniform polar orientation with their 'plus' ends pointing toward the axon terminal. In contrast, dendritic microtubules are oriented with their 'plus' ends toward the dendrite tip or the cell body (Baas *et al.*, 1989). All microtubules destined for axons or dendrites are probably initiated at the centrosome, released, and then transported into axons and dendrites. Thus, the uniform polarity of axonal micro-

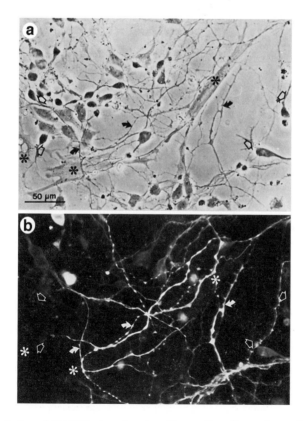

Figure 4.6. Association of MAP1B phosphorylated by proline-directed protein kinases with developing axons. (a) Phase contrast micrograph of cortical neurons and glial cells in culture. (b) Immunofluorescence micrograph with an antibody that recognizes only MAP1B phosphorylated by proline-directed protein kinases. Axons (curved arrows) are intensely stained whereas glial cells (asterisks) and neuronal cell bodies and dendrites (open arrows) are not stained. Reproduced from Mansfield *et al.* (1992) with permission from Chapman and Hall Ltd.

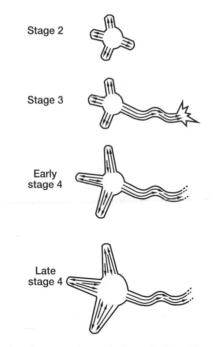

Figure 4.7. Scheme depicting the appearance of microtubules with mixed polarity in developing dendrites of cultured rat hippocampal neurons. Reproduced from *The Journal of Cell Biology* (1989), vol. 109, pp. 3085–3094, by copyright permission of The Rockefeller University Press.

tubules and the mixed polarity of dendritic microtubules must arise from differences in their transport systems (Sharp *et al.*, 1995). However, nothing is known about the molecular mechanism of microtubule transport.

The distinct microtubule patterns within axons and dendrites may constitute a structural basis for organelle distribution in the neuron, as it has been hypothesized that certain organelles, including polyribosomes, are preferentially transported toward the 'minus' ends of the microtubules, which would facilitate their transport into dendrites.

4.4 The cytoskeleton in neuronal plasticity

Both in the developing and adult nervous systems, neurons can undergo structural modifications in response to certain extracellular signals. These modifications may range from the outgrowth of collateral ramifications from neurites, which establish new synapses, to alterations of pre-existing synapses, which include changes in the shape of dendritic spines and more subtle modifications of postsynaptic densities and presynaptic terminals. Some synaptic changes may be associated with learning (Bailey and Kandel, 1993; Greenough and Bailey, 1987; Montague, 1993).

Rearrangements of the neuronal cytoskeleton have been proposed to play a crucial role in these synaptic remodeling events (Fifková and Morales, 1992). Such changes may be triggered by posttranslational modifications of cytoskeletal proteins, mainly through phosphorylation and dephosphorylation. According to this view, certain extracellular signals initiate transduction pathways that modulate cytoskeletal protein phosphorylation, which leads to the structural rearrangements underlying synaptic plasticity. In fact, some preliminary evidence has shown a correlation between MAP2 phosphorylation and certain examples of synaptic plasticity (Aoki and Siekevitz, 1985; Montoro *et al.*, 1993).

Cytoskeletal modifications may not only affect neuronal connectivity through morphological changes but might also control neuronal physiology through the modulation of neurotransmitter receptors and ion channels which are anchored to the membrane skeleton (Johnson and Byerly, 1993; Rosenmund and Westbrook, 1993).

4.5 The cytoskeleton in intraneuronal transport

4.5.1 Axonal and dendritic transport

All neuronal mRNA synthesis and most protein synthesis takes place in the cell body. Specific transport systems allow the delivery of macromolecules from the cell body to axons and dendrites. The fact that axons and dendrites each receive a number of unique proteins (see Section 4.3.3) calls for the existence of molecular sorting mechanisms. Furthermore, certain mRNAs are transported into dendrites where they contribute to local protein synthesis (Steward and Banker, 1992).

Dendritic transport has not been so thoroughly studied as axonal transport. For this reason we will focus on axonal transport. The necessity for an axonal transport mechanism was first appreciated by Ramón y Cajal (1928) who established that the integrity of the axon depends on the neuronal cell body. When a peripheral nerve axon is severed, the segment which is disconnected from the cell body degenerates, while the remaining portion of the axon regenerates. Both axon regeneration in peripheral nerves and axon outgrowth in immature neurons take place as a result of materials continuously supplied from the cell body to the axon.

Axonal transport has been mainly studied by radioisotopic labeling methods. For instance, in the visual system, radiolabeled amino acids injected into the vitreous humor are incorporated into proteins by the retinal ganglion neurons. Labeled proteins are then transported down the axons constituting the optic nerve. The movement of labeled proteins is analyzed by removing the optic nerve, sectioning it into segments and measuring the distribution of radioactivity within these pieces at different times after injection.

The kinetics of axonal transport that emerge from these studies are rather complex, indicating the existence of distinct sets of conveyed proteins according to their rates of transport. These groups of proteins move as coherent waves down the axon at different rates, with no exchange of proteins between them. This has led to the proposal that transported proteins move as parts of cytological structures (Tytell *et al.*, 1981).

Four main components of axonal transport have been identified:

(i) Slow component A. This group of proteins moves at a rate of 0.2–1 mm day^{-1} (0.002–0.01 μm sec^{-1}) and consists primarily of polypeptides associated with microtubules and neurofilaments.

(ii) Slow component B. This is a quite complex group of proteins comprising more than 100 polypeptides moving at 2–8 mm day^{-1} (0.02–0.08 μm sec^{-1}). It seems to correspond to the transport of actin microfilaments and associated proteins. Some of these are metabolic enzymes which bind to actin microfilaments.

(iii) Intermediate component. This corresponds to mitochondria, which are conveyed along microtubules at a rate of 50–100 mm day^{-1} (0.6–1.2 μm sec^{-1}).

(iv) Fast component. This is a rather complex group of membrane-associated proteins moving at a rate of 200–400 mm day^{-1} (2.4–4.8 μm sec^{-1}) and corresponds to the movement of most membrane organelles along microtubules.

4.5.2 Slow axonal transport

The molecular mechanism of slow axonal transport is not yet known. It is generally accepted that cytoskeletal proteins assemble in the cell body and that cytoskeletal polymers are the moving elements in slow axonal transport.

According to the 'structural hypothesis', cytoskeletal polymers enter the axon and there is a continuous movement of the cytoskeletal scaffolding along the axon to the synaptic terminal where microtubules and neurofilaments would be disassembled and proteolyzed. Alternatively to this model, moving cytoskeletal polymers may be transported down the axon and serve as precursors for a stationary axonal cytoskeleton (Nixon, 1991).

The existence of moving and stationary cytoskeletal elements is particularly clear for neurofilaments. Highly phosphorylated NF-H and NF-M isoforms (see Section 4.2.2) are associated with stationary neurofilaments. Thus, it is plausible that non-phosphorylated neurofilaments are assembled in the cell body and enter the axon as moving polymers which become progressively phosphorylated and integrated into a stationary cytoskeleton (Nixon and Sihag, 1991).

Polymer-sliding models have been proposed (Lasek, 1986; Nixon, 1991) as a molecular mechanism for transport. Moving cytoskeletal polymers may slide in relation to stationary polymers or the membrane skeleton. ATPases similar to those mediating fast organelle transport (see Section 4.5.4) might interconnect cytoskeletal polymers and catalyze the sliding between them.

4.5.3 Fast axonal transport

Membrane organelles move along axonal cytoskeletal polymers (mainly microtubules but also actin microfilaments). Fast axonal transport actually comprises an antero-grade (from the cell body to the axon tip) and a retrograde (from the axon tip to the cell body) component (Grafstein and Forman, 1980). For instance, synaptic vesicles move anterogradely, while endocytotic and prelysosomal vesicles move retrogradely. The major function of the fast anterograde axonal transport is the conveying of membrane organelles required for presynaptic events at the axon ending. In developing neurites, anterogradely moving vesicles support the membrane extension which occurs at the growth cone. The retrograde component seems to perform two essential functions. First, it facilitates membrane recycling, since it conveys prelysosomal organelles from the nerve ending to the cell body. Second, it provides a retrograde pathway for the transmission of information through the transport of receptors associated with membrane vesicles. These receptors can convey signaling molecules from the axon tip to the neuronal cell body. For example, the retrograde transport of nerve growth factor and its receptor is well documented (Ehlers *et al.*, 1995).

It now seems clear that axonal microtubules constitute the tracks for organelle transport over long distances whereas actin filaments provide movement to local sites along the axon and within the presynaptic terminal (Atkinson *et al.*, 1992; Langford, 1995). There is a bidirectional movement of organelles on microtubules, whereas transport on actin filaments is unidirectional (toward the 'barbed' end). However, little is known about the coordination of the microtubule-mediated and microfilament-mediated movements of a given organelle.

The video enhancement of images generated by differential interference contrast microscopy, called AVEC-DIC (Allen video enhancement contrast–differential interference contrast microscopy) has allowed the observation of organelles moving on microtubules and microfilaments, which are below the limit of resolution of conventional light microscopy (Allen *et al.*, 1985; Kuznetsov *et al.*, 1992). Using this system, it has been demonstrated that organelle translocation is strictly dependent on ATP hydrolysis.

4.5.4 Molecular motors

Membrane organelle move along microtubules or microfilaments through their association with molecular motors. These motor proteins are microtubule-dependent ATPases (kinesin, kinesin-related proteins and cytoplasmic dynein; see *Figure 4.8*) and actin-dependent ATPases (myosins) (Brady, 1991; Langford, 1995; Walker and Sheetz, 1993).

Conventional kinesin is a tetramer consisting of two heavy chains (110–130 kDa) and two light chains (60–80 kDa). Kinesin has a microtubule-activated ATPase activity and is able to move organelles from the 'minus' to the 'plus' ends of microtubules. The kinesin molecule appears as a long rod with a pair of globular 'head' domains at one end and a 'fan-shaped tail' at the opposite end. Kinesin binds ATP and microtubules through the 'head' domains and presumably interacts with specific proteins on organelle membranes through the 'tail' domain. Recently, kinectin, a 160 kDa transmembrane protein localized to the endoplasmic reticulum, has been shown to serve as a specific attachment protein for kinesin (Kumar *et al.*, 1995). Presumably other kinectin-like proteins may serve as specific receptors for kinesin in other cytoplasmic organelles (Burkhardt, 1996).

The transport of some proteins, including neuromodulin and synapsin I, as well as neurite outgrowth require kinesin, as evidenced from studies in which kinesin heavy chain synthesis was suppressed by treatment of cultured hippocampal neurons with specific antisense oligonucleotides (Ferreira *et al.*, 1992). *In vivo* injection of antisense oligonucleotides for kinesin heavy chain into the eyes inhibits the fast anterograde transport of a large fraction of proteins within the rat optic nerve, thus supporting a role for kinesin in fast axonal transport (Amaratunga *et al.*, 1993).

Molecular genetic techniques have allowed the identification of several kinesin-related proteins in different organisms. Kinesin-related proteins show homology to the 'head' domain of conventional kinesin and are highly divergent in the 'tail'

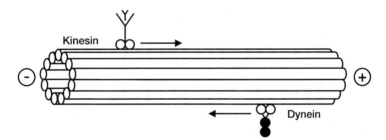

Figure 4.8. Microtubule-dependent motor molecules. Scheme shows kinesin (a 'plus' end-directed motor protein) and dynein (a 'minus' end-directed motor protein).

domains (Goldstein, 1993). It is thus plausible that the different tails may be responsible for the interaction of different motors with distinct membrane organelles (Coy and Howard, 1994). Genetic evidence in the nematode *Caenorhabditis elegans* supports this possibility. Mutations in the *unc-116* gene, which codes for a conventional kinesin heavy chain, yield a lethal phenotype characterized by paralysis. However, synaptic vesicles in this mutant seem to be normally transported. In contrast, mutations in the *unc-104* gene, which codes for a kinesin-related protein, produce a failure in the axonal transport of synaptic vesicles, which become accumulated in the neuronal cell body, without affecting the movement of other membrane organelles. This suggests that the *unc-104* gene product is a specific motor for the anterograde transport of synaptic vesicles along axonal microtubules (Hall and Hedgecock, 1991).

There is evidence suggesting that the phosphorylation of kinesin and certain kinesin-associated proteins may modulate both motor–organelle and motor–microtubule interactions (McIlvain *et al.*, 1994).

Cytoplasmic dynein (which was previously referred to as MAP-1C) contains two 300 kDa heavy chains as well as some associated polypeptides. It has microtubule-activated ATPase activity and can convey organelles from the 'plus' ends to the 'minus' ends of microtubules. Cytoplasmic dynein may participate in fast retrograde axonal as well as in dendritic transport.

Little is known about the possible regulation of cytoplasmic dynein activity. To support retrograde axonal transport without interfering with anterograde movement, dynein may be transported down the axon in an inactivated form and then become activated at the axon tip.

Interestingly, an activator of dynein-catalyzed organelle transport has been identified. This activator is a protein complex referred to as dynactin, and contains ten subunits, p150-Glued, P135-Glued, pG2, p50, Arp-1 (actin-related protein 1), actin, actin-capping protein α-subunit, actin-capping protein β-subunit, p27 and p24. The dynactin complex seems to have a two-domain structure composed of an actin-like filament and a laterally projecting sidearm. The actin-like filament contains Arp-1 and may interact with organelles whereas the sidearm contains p150-Glued and p135-Glued and may interact with dynein and microtubules (Schroer *et al.*, 1996).

The identity of the motor molecules responsible for the movement of organelles along actin microfilaments is not well established. Current evidence indicates that it must be a member of the myosin family (Bearer *et al.*, 1993; Langford *et al.*, 1994). In particular, myosin V is very abundant in brain and has been localized in axons of cultured neurons (Cheney *et al.*, 1993; Espreafico *et al.*, 1992).

4.6 The cytoskeleton in neuropathology

Several neuropathies may arise as the consequence of alterations in the neuronal cytoskeleton. For example, treatment of cultured neurons with colchicine, a microtubule-depolymerizing drug, eventually results in neuronal cell death. Neurodegeneration is also induced in cultured neurons after a treatment with okadaic acid, a potent phosphatase inhibitor that causes cytoskeletal protein hyperphosphorylation and disorganization.

Certain neurotoxins interact with the cytoskeleton. Thus, acrylamide, 2,5-hexanedione and β, β′-iminodipropionitrile interfere with the axonal transport of neurofilaments, giving rise to neurofilament accumulations in central and peripheral axons.

Aluminum intoxication has been implicated in some human encephalopathies. Intracranial injections of aluminum in rabbits cause the accumulation of hyperphosphorylated neurofilaments in neuronal cell bodies and proximal axons. Affected neurons eventually degenerate. Chronic oral administration of aluminum to rats increases the phosphorylation of MAP-2 and NF-H. In addition, *in vitro* studies have shown that aluminum can produce the irreversible aggregation of highly phosphorylated cytoskeletal proteins such as MAPs and neurofilaments. Thus, aluminum may first induce the hyperphosphorylation of cytoskeletal proteins and then cause their aggregation.

Accumulations of cytoskeletal proteins are also found in certain neurodegenerative diseases including amyotrophic lateral sclerosis (ALS) and Alzheimer's disease (AD). Perhaps metabolic disturbances, reductions in neurotropic factor levels, excesses of excitatory neurotransmitters, changes in synaptic interactions or the presence of neurotoxins trigger the cytoskeletal abnormalities observed in these diseases. The resulting disorganization of the cytoskeleton brings about the aberrant accretion of certain cytoskeletal proteins and interferes with intraneuronal transport, thus provoking the death of the affected neurons.

ALS is associated with the specific degeneration of motor neurons. It seems that motor neuron death may be caused in ALS by different mechanisms. A genetic variant of ALS has been associated with the expression of a mutant form of superoxide dismutase. Accumulations of neurofilaments have been described in motor neurons of ALS cases induced by mutations in the superoxide dismutase gene and in transgenic mice expressing the mutant form of human superoxide dismutase. This suggests that oxidative damage induced by the mutant superoxide dismutase may drive neurofilament aggregation in motor neurons. Interestingly, transgenic mice overexpressing the human *NF-H* gene also develop an ALS-like pathology: neurofilaments accumulate in motor neuron cell bodies and proximal axons, axonal transport is defective, and motor neurons eventually degenerate. It thus appears that motor neuron death may be the consequence of the failure in axonal transport produced by neurofilament accumulations (Collard *et al.*, 1995).

AD is associated with the degeneration of neurons in several cortical areas, which gives rise to memory failure and other cognitive deficits. Senile plaques, neurofibrillary tangles, neuropile threads and Hirano bodies are aberrant structures found within the brains of AD patients:

(i)   Senile plaques are constituted by extracellular amyloid deposits made up of a peptide which is a fragment of an integral membrane protein.

(ii) Neurofibrillary tangles (NFTs) are argyrophilic intraneuronal inclusions composed of pairs of approximately 10 nm filaments helically twisted around each other (paired helical filaments or PHFs). PHFs are also found within dystrophic neurites called 'neuropile threads'. Modified tau protein (see Section 4.2.3) is the constituent of PHFs. PHF-tau appears to be highly phosphorylated (Goedert, 1993). Hyperphosphorylated MAP1B may be an accessory component of NFTs through binding to PHFs. Possibly tau and MAP1B are highly phosphorylated by the synergistic action of several protein kinases, which may be enhanced by a deficit in phosphatases (Morishima-Kawashima *et al.*, 1995; Roush, 1995). Tau in AD is probably subjected to other modifications including glycation (Ledesma *et al.*, 1994) and oxidation. AD tau is completely unable to associate with tubulin and may easily self-assemble into PHFs. In fact, purified tau protein can assemble into PHF-like polymers *in vitro* (Montejo de Garcini *et al.*, 1988). In addition, AD tau do not stabilize microtubules. Thus, both NFT formation and microtubule disorganization may lead to a deficit in intraneuronal transport contributing to neuronal cell death in AD.

(iii) Hirano bodies are eosinophilic intraneuronal inclusions composed of actin and several actin-binding protein. MAPs also appear within Hirano bodies.

Other modifications of the cytoskeleton in AD include the proteolysis of fodrin, which is presumably mediated by the activation of a calcium-dependent protease.

Less well characterized intraneuronal fibrillary inclusions also appear in brain from patients affected by other neurodegenerative disorders. These include Lewy bodies which are found in Parkinson's disease and Pick bodies which are characteristic of Pick disease.

The study of the molecular mechanisms responsible for the cytoskeletal abnormalities associated with neurodegenerative diseases is a major research area in contemporary neuroscience, and important progresses are expected in the next few years.

References

Aderem A. (1992) Signal transduction and the actin cytoskeleton: the roles of MARCKS and profilin. *Trends Biochem. Sci.* **17**: 438–443.

Allen RD, Weiss DG, Hayden JH, Brown DT, Fujiwake H, Simpson M. (1985) Gliding movement of and bi-directional organelle transport along single native microtubules from squid axoplasm. Evidence for an active role of microtubules in cytoplasmic transport. *J. Cell Biol.* **100**: 1736–1752.

Amaratunga A, Morin PJ, Kosik KS, Fine RE. (1993) Inhibition of kinesin synthesis and rapid anterograde axonal transport *in vivo* by an antisense oligonucleotide. *J. Biol. Chem.* **268**: 17 427–17 430.

Aoki C, Siekevitz PC. (1985) Ontogenetic changes in the cyclic adenosine 3'–5' monophosphate stimulatable phosphorylation of cat visual cortex proteins, particularly of microtubule-associated protein 2 (MAP2): effects of normal and dark rearing and of the exposure to light. *J. Neurosci.* **5**: 2465–2483.

Atkinson SJ, Doberstein SK, Pollard TD. (1992) Moving off the beaten tracks. *Curr. Biol.* **2**: 326–328.

Avila J, Dominguez J, Díaz-Nido J. (1994) Regulation of microtubule dynamics by microtubule-associated protein expression and phosphorylation during neuronal development. *Int. J. Devel. Biol.* **38**: 13–25.

Baas PW, Black MM, Banker GA. (1989) Changes in microtubule polarity orientation during the development of hippocampal neurons in culture. *J. Cell Biol.* **109**: 3085–3094.

Baas PW, Slaughter T, Brown A, Black MM. (1991) Microtubule dynamics in axons and dendrites. *J. Neurosci. Res.* **30**: 134–153.

Bailey CH, Kandel ER. (1993) Structural changes accompanying memory storage. *Ann. Rev. Physiol.* **53**: 397–426.

Bearer EL, De Giorgis JA, Bodner RA, Kao AW, Reese TS. (1993) Evidence for myosin motors on organelles in squid axoplasm. *Proc. Natl Acad. Sci. USA* **90**: 11 252–11 256.

Belmont LD, Mitchison TJ. (1996) Identification of a protein that interacts with tubulin dimers and increases the catastrophe rate of microtubules. *Cell* **84**: 623–631.

Bershadsky AD, Vasiliev JM. (1988) *Cytoskeleton*. Plenum Press, New York.

Brady ST. (1991) Molecular motors in the nervous system. *Neuron* **7**: 521–533.

Brugg B, Reddy D, Matus A. (1993) Attenuation of microtubule-associated protein 1B expression by antisense oligodeoxynucleotides inhibits initiation of neurite outgrowth. *Neuroscience* **52**: 489–496.

Burgoyne RD. (1991) *The Neuronal Cytoskeleton*. Wiley-Liss, New York.

Burkhardt JK. (1996). In search of membrane receptors for microtubule-based motors. *Trends Cell Biol.* **6**: 127–131.

Cheney RE, Oshea MK, Heuser JE, Coelho MV, Wolenski JS, Espreafico EM, Forscher P, Larson RE, Mooseker MS. (1993) Brain myosin-V is a two-headed unconventional myosin with motor activity. *Cell* **75**: 13–23.

Ching G, Liem R. (1993) Assembly of type IV neuronal intermediate filaments in nonneuronal cells in the absence of preexisting cytoplasmic intermediate filaments. *J. Cell Biol.* **122:** 1323–1335.

Choo Cl, Bray D. (1978) Two forms of neuronal actin. *J. Neurochem.* **31:** 217–224.

Clark EA, Brugge JS. (1995) Integrins and signal transduction pathways: the road taken. *Science* **268:** 233–239.

Collard J.-F, Coté F, Julien J.-P. (1995) Defective axonal transport in a transgenic mouse model of amyotrophic lateral sclerosis. *Nature* **375:** 61–64.

Coy DL, Howard S. (1994) Organelle transport and sorting in axons. *Curr. Opin. Neurobiol.* **4:** 662–667.

Craig AM, Banker G. (1994) Neuronal polarity. *Annu. Rev. Neurosci.* **17:** 267–310.

Davis JQ, McLaughlin T, Bennett V. (1993) Ankyrin-binding proteins related to nervous system cell adhesion molecules: candidates to provide transmembrane and intercellular connections in adult brain. *J. Cell Biol.* **121:** 121–133.

De Waegh SM, Lee VMY, Brady ST. (1992) Local modulation of neurofilament phosphorylation, axonal caliber, and slow axonal transport by myelinating Schwann cells. *Cell* **68:** 451–463.

Di Tella MC, Feiguin F, Carri N, Kosik KS, Cáceres A. (1996) MAP-1B/TAU functional redundancy during laminin-enhanced axonal growth. *J. Cell Sci.* **109:** 467–477.

Dotti CG, Sullivan CA, Banker GA. (1988) The establishment of polarity by hippocampal neurons in culture. *J. Cell Biol.* **108:** 1507–1516.

Edelmann W, Zervas M, Costello P et al. (1996) Neuronal abnormalities in microtubule-associated protein 1B mutant mice. *Proc. Natl Acad. Sci. USA* **93:** 1270–1275.

Ehlers MD, Kaplan DR, Price DL, Koliatsos UE. (1995) NGF-stimulated retrograde transport of trkA in the mammalian nervous system. *J. Cell Biol.* **130:** 149–156.

Espreafico EM, Cheney RE, Matteoli M, Nasimento AC, De Camilli PV, Larson RE, Mooseker MS. (1992) Primary structure and cellular localization of chicken brain myosin-V (p190), an unconventional myosin with calmodulin light chains. *J. Cell Biol.* **119:** 1541–1557.

Fath KR, Lasek RJ. (1988) Two classes of actin microfilaments are associated with the inner cytoskeleton of axons. *J. Cell Biol.* **107:** 613–621.

Ferreira A, Niclas J, Vale RD, Banker G, Kosik K. (1992) Suppression of kinesin expression in cultured hippocampal neurons using antisense oligonucleotides. *J. Cell Biol.* **117:** 595–606.

Ferreira A, Kincaid R, Kosik KS. (1993) Calcineurin is associated with the cytoskeleton of cultured neurons and has a role in the acquisition of polarity. *Mol. Biol. Cell* **4:** 1225–1238.

Fifková, E, Morales M. (1992) Actin matrix of dendritic spines, synaptic plasticity, and long-term potentiation. *Int. Rev. Cytol.* **139:** 267–307.

Forscher P, Smith SJ. (1988) Actions of cytochalasins on the organization of actin filaments and microtubules in a neuronal growth cone. *J. Cell Biol.* **107:** 1505–1516.

Garner CC, Tucker RP, Matus A. (1988) Selective localization of messenger RNA for cytoskeletal protein MAP2 in dendrites. *Nature* **336:** 674–677

Gilmore AP, Burridge K. (1996) Regulation of vinculin binding to talin and actin by phosphatidylinositol-4, 5-biphosphate. *Nature* **381:** 531–535.

Goedert M. (1993) Tau protein and the neurofibrillary pathology of Alzheimer's disease. *Trends Neurosci.* **16:** 460–465.

Goldstein LSB. (1993) With apologies to Scheherazade: tails of 1001 kinesin motors. *Annu. Rev. Genet.* **27:** 319–351.

Gordon-Weeks PR. (1987) The cytoskeleton of isolated growth cones. *Neuroscience.* **21:** 977–989.

Grafstein B, Forman DS. (1980). Intracellular transport in neurons. *Physiol. Rev.* **60:** 1167–1283.

Greenough WT, Bailey CH. (1987) The anatomy of a memory. *Trends Neurosci.* **11:** 142–147.

Hall DH, Hedgecock EM. (1991) Kinesin-related gene *unc-104* is required for axonal transport of synaptic vesicles in *C. elegans. Cell* **65:** 837–847.

Harada A, Oguchi K, Okabe S. et al. (1994) Altered microtubule organization in small-calibre axons of mice lacking tau protein. *Nature* **369:** 488–491.

Hirokawa N. (1982) The crosslinker system between neurofilaments, microtubules and membranous organelles in frog axons revealed by quick freeze, freeze-fracture, deep-etching method. *J. Cell Biol.* **94:** 129–142.

Hirokawa N, Sobue K, Kanda K, Harada A, Yorifuji H. (1989) The cytoskeletal architecture of the presynaptic terminal and molecular structure of synapsin I. *J. Cell Biol.* **108:** 111–126.

Inagaki M, Nishi Y, Nishizawas K, Matsuyama M, Sato C. (1989) Site-specific phosphorylation induces disassembly of vimentin filaments *in vitro. Nature* **328:** 649–652.

Johnson BD, Byerly L. (1993) A cytoskeletal mechanism for Ca^{2+} channel metabolic dependence and inactivation by intracellular Ca^{2+}. *Neuron* **10**: 797–804.

Joshi HC, Baas PW. (1993) A new perspective on microtubules and axon growth. *J. Cell Biol.* **121**: 1191–1196.

Kirsch J, Betz H. (1996) The postsynaptic localization of the glycine receptor-associated protein Gephyrin is regulated by the cytoskeleton. *J. Neurosci.* **15**: 4148–4156.

Kirschner MW, Mitchinson T. (1986) Beyond self assembly: from microtubules to morphogenesis. *Cell* **45**: 329–342.

Kreis T, Vale R. (1993) *Guidebook to Cytoskeletal and Motor Proteins.* Oxford University Press, Oxford.

Kumar J, Yu H, Sheetz MP. (1995) Kinectin, an essential anchor for kinesin-driven vesicle motility. *Science* **267**: 1834–1837.

Kuznetsov SA, Langford GM, Weiss DG. (1992) Actin-dependent organelle movement in squid axoplasm. *Nature* **356**: 722–725.

Lambert S, Bennett V. (1993) From anemia to cerebellar dysfunction. A review of the ankyrin gene family. *Eur. J. Biochem.* **211** 1–6.

Langford GM. (1995) Actin- and microtubule-dependent organelle motors: interrelationships between the two motility systems. *Curr. Opin. Cell Biol.* **7**: 82–88.

Langford GM, Kuznetsov SA, Johnson D, Cohen DL, Weiss DG. (1994) Movement of axoplasmic organelles on actin filaments assembled on acrosomal processes: evidence for a barbed-end-directed organelle motor. *J. Cell Sci.* **107**: 2291–2298.

Lasek RJ. (1986) Polymer sliding in axons. *J. Cell Sci.* **5** (Suppl.): 161–179.

Ledesma MD, Bonay P, Glaxo C, Avila J. (1994) Analysis of microtubule associated tau glycation in paired helical filaments. *J. Biol. Chem.* **269**: 21 614–21 619.

Lee M, Xu Z, Wong P, Cleveland D. (1993) Neurofilaments are obligate heteropolymers *in vivo*. *J. Cell Biol.* **122**: 1337–1350.

Lewis AK, Bridgman PC. (1992) Nerve growth cone lamellipodia contain two populations of actin filaments that differ in organization and polarity. *J. Cell Biol.* **119**: 1219–1243.

Lin C-H, Thompson CA, Forscher P. (1994) Cytoskeletal organization underlying growth cone motility. *Curr. Opin. Neurobiol.* **4**: 640–647.

Lin C-H, Espreafico EM, Mooseker MS, Forscher P. (1996) Myosin drives retrograde F-actin flow in neuronal growth cones. *Cell* **16**: 769–782.

Llinás RT, McGuinness TL, Leonard CS, Sugimori M, Greengard P. (1985) Intraterminal injection of synapsin I or calcium/calmodulin dependent protein kinase II alters neurotransmitter release at the squid giant synapse. *Proc. Natl Acad. Sci. USA* **82**: 3035–3039.

Luna EJ, Hitt AL. (1992) Cytoskeleton–plasma membrane interactions. *Science* **258**: 955–964.

MacKay DJ, Nobes C, Hall A. (1995) The Rho's progress: a potential role during neuritogenesis of the Rho family of GTPases. *Trends Neurosci.* **18**: 496–501.

Mansfield SG, Díaz-Nido J, Gordon-Weeks PR, Avila J. (1992) The distribution and phosphorylation of the microtubule-associated protein MAP1B in growth cones. *J. Neurocytol.* **21**: 1007–1022.

McIlvain JM, Burkhardt JK, Hamm-Alvarez S, Argon Y, Sheetz MP. (1994) Regulation of kinesin activity by phosphorylation of kinesin-associated proteins. *J. Biol. Chem.* **269**: 19 176–19 182.

Mitchison T, Kirschner M. (1988) Cytoskeletal dynamics and nerve growth. *Neuron* **1**: 761–772.

Montague PR. (1993) Transforming sensory experience into structural change. *Proc. Natl Acad. Sci. USA* **90**: 6379–6380.

Montejo de Garcini E, Carrascosa JL, Correas I, Nieto A, Avila J. (1988) Tau factor polymers are similar to paired helical filaments of Alzheimer's disease. *FEBS Lett.* **236**: 150–154.

Montoro, R., Díaz-Nido, J, Avila J, López-Barneo J. (1993) NMDA stimulates the dephosphorylation of the cytoskeletal protein MAP2 and potentiates excitatory synaptic transmission in rat hippocampal slices. *Neuroscience.* **54**: 859–871.

Morishima-Kawashima M, Hasegawas M, Takio K, Suzuki M, Yoshida H, Titani K, Ihara Y. (1995) Proline-directed and nonproline-directed phosphorylation of PHF-tau. *J. Biol. Chem.* **270**: 823–829.

Nixon RA. (1991) Axonal transport of cytoskeletal proteins. In: *The Neuronal Cytoskeleton* (ed. R Burgoyne). Alan R. Liss, New York, pp. 175–200.

Nixon RA, Shea TB. (1992) Dynamics of neuronal intermediate filaments: a developmental perspective. *Cell Motil. Cytoskel.* **22**: 81–91.

Nixon RA, Sihag RK. (1991) Neurofilament phosphorylation: a new look at regulation and function. *Trends Neurosci.* **11**: 501–506.

Oakley BR. (1992) Gamma tubulin: the microtubule organizer? *Trends Cell Biol.* **2**: 1–5.

Ohara O, Gahara Y, Miyake T, Teraoka H, Kitamura T. (1993) Neurofilament deficiency in quail caused by nonsense mutation in neurofilament-L gene. *J. Cell Biol.* **121:** 387–395.

Okabe S, Miyasaka H, Hirokawas N. (1993) Dynamics of the neuronal intermediate filaments. *J. Cell Biol.* **121:** 375–386.

Padilla R, Lopez-Otín C, Serrano L, Avila J. (1993) Role of the carboxy terminal region of beta tubulin on microtubule dynamics through its interaction with the GTP binding region. *FEBS Lett.* **325:** 173–176.

Peters A, Palay SL, De Webster H. (1976) *The Fine Structure of the Nervous System: the Neurons and Supporting Cells.* W B Saunders, Philadelphia, PA.

Ramón y Cajal S. (1904) Variaciones morfológicas normales ó patológicas del reticulo neurofibrilar. *Trab. Lab. Invest. Biol.* **3:** 1–10.

Ramón y Cajal S. (1928) *Degeneration and Regeneration of the Nervous System* (translated by RM May). Oxford University Press, London.

Ratner N, Mahler HR. (1983) Structural organization of filamentous proteins in postsynaptic density. *Biochemistry* **22:** 2446–2453.

Rickard JE, Kreis TE. (1996) CLIPs for organelle–microtubule interactions. *Trends Cell Biol.* **6:** 178–183.

Riederer BM, Zagon IS, Goodman SR. (1986) Brain spectrin (240/235) and brain spectrin (240/235 E): two distinct spectrin subtypes with different locations within mammalian neural cells. *J. Cell Biol.* **102:** 2088–2097.

Riederer BM, Zagon IS, Goodman SR. (1987) Brain spectrin (240/235) and brain spectrin (240/235 E). Differential expression during mouse brain development. *J. Neurosci.* **7:** 864–879.

Rosenmund C, Westbrook GL. (1993) Calcium-induced actin depolymerization reduces NMDA channel activity. *Neuron* **10:** 805–814.

Roush W. (1995) Protein studies try to puzzle out Alzheimer's tangles. *Science* **276:** 793–794.

Sakaguchi T, Okada M, Kitamuru T, Kawasaki K. (1993) Reduced diameter and conduction velocity of myelinated fibers in the sciatic nerve of a neurofilament-deficient mutant quail. *Neurosci. Lett.* **153:** 65–68.

Schroer TA, Bingham JB, Gill SR. (1996) Actin-related protein 1 and cytoplasmic dynein-based motility. *Trends Cell Biol.* **6:** 212–216.

Sharp DJ, Yu W, Baas PE. (1995) Transport of dendritic microtubules establishes their nonuniform polarity orientation. *J. Cell Biol.* **130:** 93–103.

Shiina N, Gotoh, Y, and Nishida E. (1995) Microtubule severing-activity in M phase. *Trends Cell Biol.* **5:** 283–286.

Smith SJ, (1988) Neuronal cytomechanics: the actin-based motility of growth cones. *Science* **242:** 708–715.

Steinert PM, Roop DR (1988) Molecular and cellular biology of intermediate filaments. *Annu. Rev. Biochem.* **57:** 593–625

Steward O, Banker GA. (1992) Getting the message from the gene to the synapse: sorting and intracellular transport of RNA in neurons. *Trends Neurosci.* **15:** 180–186.

Stossel TP, (1993) On the crawling of animal cells. *Science* **260:** 1086–1094.

Sullivan KF. (1988) Structure and utilization of tubulin isotypes. *Annu. Rev. Cell Biol.* **4:** 687–716.

Symons M. (1996) Rho family GTPases: the cytoskeleton and beyond. *Trends Biochem. Sci.* **21:** 178–181.

Tsukita S, Tsukita S, Kobayashi T, Matsumoto G. (1986) Subaxolemmal cytoskeleton in squid giant axon II. Morphological identification of microtubule – and microfilament – associated domains of axolemma. *J. Cell Biol.* **102:** 1710–1725.

Tucker RP. (1990) The roles of microtubule-associated proteins in brain morphogenesis: a review. *Brain Res. Rev.* **15:** 101–120.

Tytell M, Black MM, Gainer J, Lasek RJ, (1981) Axonal transport: each rate component reflects the movement of distinct macromolcular complexes. *Science* **214:** 179–182.

Ulloa L, Díaz-Nido J, Avila J. (1993) Depletion of casein kinase II by antisense oligonucleotide prevents neuritogenesis in neuroblastoma cells. *EMBO J.* **12:** 1633–1640.

Ulloa L, Díez-Guerra FJ, Avila J, Díaz-Nido J. (1994). Localization of differentially phosphorylated isoforms of microtubule-associated protein 1B (MAP1B) in cultured rat hippocampal neurons. *Neuroscience* **61:** 211–223.

Vandekerckhove J. (1990) Actin-binding proteins. *Curr. Opin. Cell Biol.* **2:** 41–50.

Viel A, Branton D. (1996) Spectrin: on the path from structure to function. *Curr. Opin. Cell Biol.* **8:** 49–55.

Walker RA, Sheetz MP. (1993) Cytoplasmic microtubule-associated motors. *Annu. Rev. Biochem.* **62:** 429–451.

Wegner A. (1985) Subtleties of actin assembly. *Nature* **313:** 97–98.

Molecular biology of neurotransmitter release

Julie Staple and Stefan Catsicas

5.1 Introduction

Neurons function to receive, integrate and transmit signals to other neurons or to nonneuronal target cells. While the process of neurotransmission appears relatively simple – neurotransmitter released from one cell binds to a receptor on another cell which results in depolarization or other effects in the target – there are many potentially regulatable components involved in each step. The characteristics of neurotransmission and the opportunities for modification of this process are the subject of intense study since it is these properties and the potential for change with experience that is believed to underlie complex cognitive functions as well as simple forms of adaptation.

5.1.1 Historical perspective on molecular biology at synapses

The neuron. The idea of the synapse necessarily implies a relation between two neurons. Although this statement may seem simplistic, it is interesting to note that it has only been 100 years since neurons were defined as individual cells. Indeed, only 40 years have passed since synapses were first seen and the 'neuron theory' supported by use of the electron microscope (Palade and Palay, 1954; and see Robertson, 1987). As an introduction to the topic of molecular biology of synapses, a brief outline of the history of experiment and observation which led to the definition of neurons and synapses in terms of histology, physiology and biochemistry is presented in this chapter.

The concept of the synapse was essentially dependent on the definition of the neuron in histological terms. A number of debates were waged concerning the relation of axons to cell bodies (it was not clear that these were parts of the same cells) and the relation of one neuron to another (some workers saw all neurons as interconnected, others saw them as individual cells). Steps forward in these arguments were dependent on advances in techniques of fixation and staining (especially on Golgi's silver staining technique) as well as on increased resolution due to better microscopes. More than 150 years later, Robert Remak described for the first time the continuity of a neuronal cell body with an axon in a preparation of sympathetic ganglion.

The relationship of the axon to its own cell body having been established, the controversy which was to interest neurohistologists for 75 years came to the forefront when Joseph von Gerlach published observations of an extensive axonal and dendritic network of neuronal processes. The substance of this argument concerned the direct inter-connection of one nerve cell with another ('reticular theory') as opposed to their exis-tence as individual cells ('nerve cell theory'). Although many others supported this position, Camillo Golgi, became known as the leading proponent of the 'reticular the-ory'. While Golgi denied the existence of the dendritic net proposed by Gerlach, he affirmed an axonal reticular formation based on his observations using his newly devel-oped staining technique. A major contributor to the 'nerve cell theory' was August Forel who believed that nerve cells were separate entities whose individuality was often hard to discern because of the close contacts which they made with each other. Forel based this hypothesis on the pattern of degeneration induced by axonal lesions. He saw that a specific population of cells degenerated in response to axonal injury and that this degen-eration was limited in scope which he believed would not be the case if all cells were connected directly. Santiago Ramon y Cajal, regarded as the main proponent of the 'nerve cell theory' used a modification of the Golgi stain to demonstrate instances of axonal terminations. Wilhelm von Waldeyer introduced the term 'neuron' in 1891 to describe individual nerve cells which were not directly connected to each other. High resolution pictures made possible by the advent of electron microscopy in the 1950s allowed visualization of synapses and showed the membranes that separate the presy-naptic cell from the postsynaptic cell (Palade and Palay, 1954; and see Robertson, 1987).

The synapse. It was in the context of this neuroanatomical debate that Charles Sherrington first used the term 'synapse'.

> '... we are led to think that the tip of a twig of the arborescence is not contiguous with but merely in contact with the substance of the dendrite or cell body on which it impinges. Such a special connection of one nerve cell with another might be called a synapse.' (Foster, 1897, p. 57)

The individual nature of neurons led to questions about how a current propagated along an axon might be transmitted to another cell. Two main theories were proposed in this context, the first being direct transmission of an electrical current and the sec-ond mediation between a neuron and its target by a molecule released from the presy-naptic terminal. Evidence for the possibility that a chemical signal could 'transmit' information was derived especially from work on acetylcholine (ACh) and its actions both at sympathetic ganglia and at the neuromuscular junction. Otto Loewi showed that ACh was the substance which mediated the vagus nerve-induced slowing of car-diac muscle contraction. The 'acetylcholine hypothesis' of neurotransmission was based on a number of observations (detailed in Eccles, 1937) summarized here:

(i) ACh was shown to be released after direct nerve stimulation both from prepara-tions of sympathetic ganglia and from neuromuscular preparations.

(ii) Addition of exogenous ACh or agonists to these preparations mimics the effects on the target of direct nerve stimulation.

(iii) When a nerve is stimulated to exhaustion or when preganglionic fibers degener-ate no more ACh is released.

(iv) Direct stimulation of the target itself in the absence of a motoneuron produces no ACh.

(v) Compounds which block the action of ACh, for example curare, have a similar chemical structure, providing further basis for the idea that it is ACh which is involved in neurotransmission.

The development of intracellular recording techniques allowed detailed analysis of the effects of ACh at neuromuscular junctions and showed that these were inconsistent with direct electrical transmission (Fatt and Katz, 1951).

5.2 Modern concepts in neurotransmitter release

5.2.1 The synaptic vesicle

Intracellular recording techniques also identified discrete units of neurotransmission: small, stereotyped membrane potential changes known as 'quanta'. The smallest events of neurotransmission involve membrane potential changes of single quantum size and larger events always occur as multiples of quanta. Thus, neurotransmission may involve 5 quanta or 200 quanta, but not 2.5 or 154.2 quanta. What is the physical basis for quantal neurotransmission? Soon after the development of intracellular recording, technical advances in electron microscopy made it possible to obtain high resolution images of synapses for the first time. These images showed not only clearly identifiable presynaptic and postsynaptic elements separated by a synaptic cleft, but also a newly discovered synaptic characteristic: vesicles, which were immediately recognized as a possible basis for the release of 'quanta' (*Figure 5.1*). Two main types of vesicles are found at synapses; small, clear vesicles of about 50 nm (SVs) and larger (~100 nm) vesicles characterized by electron-dense cores (LVs) (*Figure 5.2*). These two vesicle types differ functionally as well as morphologically. SVs contain conventional transmitters such as acetylcholine, glutamate, γ-aminobutyric acid (GABA) and glycine whereas LVs contain catecholamines and soluble peptides.

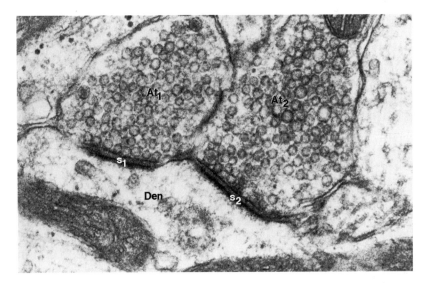

Figure 5.1. Electron micrograph of two synapses (s_1 and s_2) between two axon terminals (At1 and At2) and a dendrite (den). The axon terminals contain many synaptic vesicles and the active zone of the synapses is demarcated by an intercellular cleft and a prominent coating of dense material. Reproduced from *The Fine Structure of the Nervous System: Neurons and Their Supporting Cells*, 3rd Edn, by Alan Peters, Sanford L. Palay and Henry deF. Webster. Copyright © 1990 by Alan Peters. Reprinted by permission of Oxford University Press.

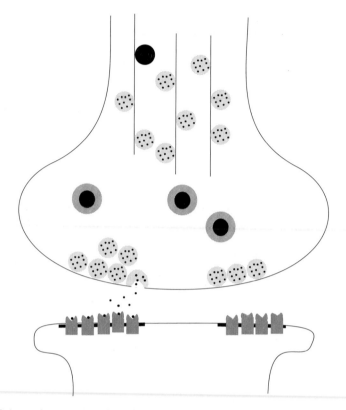

Figure 5.2. Schematic representation of some basic aspects of neurotransmission. Synaptic vesicles (pale orange spheres) filled with neurotransmitter (small black circles) are present in nerve terminals as two functionally different populations. The 'reserve pool' of synaptic vesicles is bound to actin filaments and the releasable pool is present at the presynaptic membrane at the active zone. Following docking of vesicles, fusion of the vesicle with the plasma membrane occurs and neurotransmitter is released into the synaptic cleft. Neurotransmitter molecules then bind to specific receptors present on the postsynaptic cell (shown in solid orange) resulting in signal transmission. Large, dense-core vesicles (pictured as orange spheres with black centers) may be present in the same nerve terminals as small vesicles, though biogenesis and regulation of their fusion is distinct (see text).

5.2.2 Aspects of neurotransmission

When intracellular vesicles fuse with the plasmalemma, the vesicle contents are secreted into the extracellular space and the components of the vesicle membrane become part of the plasmalemma. Thus, vesicle-mediated secretion plays two fundamental roles: intercellular communication and maintenance or renewal of membrane components. There are four main pathways for secretion in all eukaryotic cells. Secretory vesicles can originate from the Golgi apparatus or from endoplasmic reticulum-derived endosomes. Distinct vesicles from both origins contribute to regulated or constitutive secretion. Constitutive fusion is, by definition, independent of extracellular signals and mediates transport and insertion of membrane components. It is thought to play a key role in membrane turn-over as well as membrane insertion underlying changes in cell shape and motility (Catsicas *et al.*, 1994). Regulated secretion occurs upon transient and often fast stimulatory events that induce a cellular response. At the synapse, regulated secretion involves SVs derived from endosomes and LVs derived from the Golgi (see Kelly, 1993). Release of neurotransmitters by SVs requires sequential steps of vesicle trafficking. In the terminal, vesicles can be stored in the so-called reserve pool consisting of vesicles bound to actin filaments (*Figures 5.2* and *5.3*). Vesicles in the reserve pool must be mobilized to progress towards the plasma membrane (Greengard *et al.*, 1993). At the membrane, vesicles are docked to microdomains within the presynaptic active zones and form the 'releasable pool' (Greengard *et al.*, 1993). Docking is an additional storage step as docked vesicles must be primed to become ready to fuse. Membrane fusion and transmitter release are then induced when fast and localized Ca^{2+} gradients are generated by incoming action potentials (see Hu *et al.*, 1993). In contrast, LV progression to the membrane and subsequent fusion seems to involve a single, Ca^{2+}-dependent, cytoskeletal destabilization step (Trifaró and Vitale, 1993). LVs are located at a distance from the presynaptic membrane and their progression is induced by slow and diffuse Ca^{2+} gradients through channels that are distributed more homogeneously in the membrane of the nerve terminal (see Hu *et al.*, 1993). Following fusion, vesicles are retrieved by specific endocytosis mechanisms. SVs remain in the terminal to be filled with transmitters and used again, whereas LVs return to the trans-Golgi network to be packaged with newly synthesized peptides (see Hu *et al.*, 1993). Each of these steps and the main proteins known to be involved are described in the following sections.

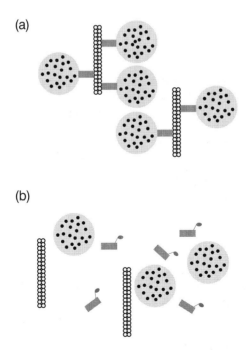

(a)

(b)

Figure 5.3. Schematic representation of a model for regulation of synaptic vesicle mobilization by synapsin. (a) Neurotransmitter-filled synaptic vesicles (pale orange spheres with small black circles) are shown bound via dephosphorylated synapsin (orange bars) to actin filaments (open circles). (b) Depolarization causes Ca^{2+}-dependent phosphorylation of synapsin I (orange-tagged bars) and results in dissociation of synaptic vesicles from actin filaments. The vesicles are now free to move to the active zone to join the releasable pool.

5.2.3 Vesicle storage and mobilization

Synaptic vesicles which contain neurotransmitter are sometimes known as 'mature' synaptic vesicles, a term which suggests their ability to participate in exocytosis. However, since neurotransmission is highly regulated, there are mechanisms which restrain the process of vesicle fusion, and further steps necessary to 'prime' vesicles for exocytosis. A mechanism proposed for restraint of vesicle fusion is the tethering of vesicles to the cytoskeleton in the synaptic terminal. This attachment would prevent vesicles from diffusing to the active zone, but keeping them close to the synapse for recruitment from a 'reserve pool' when needed (*Figures 5.2* and *5.3*).

5.2.4 The synapsin family of phosphoproteins

The synapsins, a family of four phosphoproteins which are associated with synaptic vesicles, have been implicated in reversible binding of vesicles to actin filaments. These abundant proteins, which make up approximately 0.6% of total brain protein and 9% of synaptic vesicle protein (De Camilli *et al.*, 1990; Valtorta *et al.*, 1992), were first characterized as neuronal substrates for cAMP-dependent phosphorylation by Greengard and colleagues (see Greengard *et al.*, 1993). The synapsin family consists of two homologous genes, *synapsin I* and *synapsin II* (reviewed in Südhof *et al.*, 1989). Synapsin I exists in two isoforms, Ia (apparent molecular weight of 86 kDa, 704 a.a. in rat) and Ib (80 kDa, 668 a.a. in rat), which molecular cloning and sequence analysis have shown to be splice products of a single gene. The *synapsin II* gene also encodes two alternatively spliced products, synapsin IIa and IIb, proteins of approximately 74 kDa (586 a.a. in rat) and 55 kDa (479 a.a in rat). Synapsin I isoforms have 70% average sequence identity with synapsin II isoforms over the first 420 amino acids which contain a conserved phosphorylation site and proposed actin binding domains. Comparison of the C-terminal regions of synapsins I and II shows that synapsin II isoforms are missing two Ca^{2+}/calmodulin-dependent kinase phosphorylation sites found in the synapsin I isoforms.

Experiments by Greengard and collaborators suggest that dephosphorylated synapsin I mediates the attachment of SVs to actin filaments, keeping SVs in the 'reserve pool' until needed. Electron microscopic and biochemical techniques have shown that synapsins are peripheral membrane proteins associated with synaptic vesicles (Benfenati *et al.*, 1989; DeCamilli *et al.*, 1983; Thiel *et al.*, 1990; Valtorta *et al.*, 1988) and, additionally, that synapsin I binds actin via specific domains (Bähler and Greengard, 1987; Ceccaldi *et al.*, 1995; Petrucci and Morrow, 1987). The binding of phosphorylated synapsin I both to synaptic vesicles and to actin is reduced compared to the dephosphorylated protein (Huttner *et al.*, 1983; Schiebler *et al.*, 1986; Sihra *et al.*, 1989). Since synapsin I has been shown to be phosphorylated by Ca^{2+}/calmodulin-dependent kinase II in response to various kinds of synaptic stimulation (Forn and Greengard, 1978; Nestler and Greengard, 1982) it has been suggested that activity-dependent phosphorylation regulates the association of SVs with actin, and allows translocation of the vesicles from the stored pool to the releasable pool, near the active zone (*Figure 5.4*). Consistent with this, dephosphorylated synapsin I had an inhibitory effect on neurotransmission at intact synapses (Hackett *et al.*, 1990; Lin *et al.*, 1990; Llinás *et al.*, 1985, 1991) and in synaptosomes (Nichols *et al.*, 1992), whereas phosphorylated synapsin I had no effect on neurotransmission in these studies.

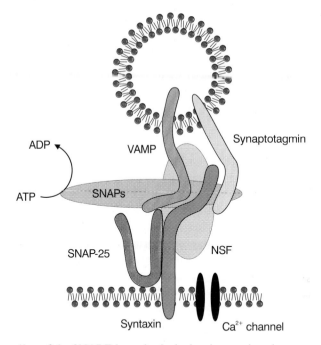

Figure 5.4. An outline of the SNARE hypothesis depicts interactions between vesicles and release sites at the membrane which are mediated by specific proteins. An intrinsic vesicle protein (VAMP, a v-SNARE) binds to plasma membrane proteins (SNAP-25 and syntaxin, both t-SNAREs). The association of these three proteins allows binding of $\alpha/\beta/\gamma$ SNAPs which in turn act as receptors for NSF. The hydrolysis of ATP by NSF results in the dissociation of the complex of proteins and is followed by vesicle fusion. Modified from *Trends Neurosci.*, vol. 17, pp. 368–373, with permission from Elsevier Trends Journals.

Apparently, neither synapsin I nor synapsin II is essential for transmitter release. Recent generation of mice lacking synapsin I, synapsin II or both, results in changes in short-term plasticity but no change has been found in basic neurotransmission or in the ability to induce long-term changes such as those which occur in learning and memory (see Section 5.3; Chin *et al.*, 1995; Li *et al.*, 1995; Rosahl *et al.*, 1995; Spillane *et al.*, 1995). However, altered expression of synapsin I or synapsin II has effects on both the developmental process of synaptogenesis and functional characteristics of mature synapses (Chin *et al.*, 1995; Ferreira *et al.*, 1994, 1995; Han *et al.*, 1991; Lu *et al.*, 1992; Rosahl *et al.*, 1995). These observations are consistent with a role for synapsins in regulation of synaptic vesicle mobilization and further suggest that mobilization is a check point involved in short-term, fast actions on transmitter release, and long-term structural changes.

5.2.5 Vesicle docking

Vesicle fusion occurs in all cells and between many different membrane compartments. Recent evidence indicates that the membrane fusion machinery has been highly conserved during evolution and that different cells use common general protein fusion components (Pevsner and Scheller, 1994). The discovery of the mechanisms that allow correct trafficking of different vesicles as well as recognition between vesicles and their target membranes is a fundamental challenge for cell biologists. During the last few years, a series of novel protein interactions have been demonstrated that have key roles in the docking and fusion of SV to the active zone. The general machinery for intracellular vesicle fusion comprises the N-ethylmaleimide sensitive factor (NSF) and three isoforms of soluble NSF attachment proteins (α, β and γ SNAPs) (Wilson et al., 1992). Biochemical studies by Rothman and his colleagues (Söllner et al., 1993) have shown that the integral SV protein VAMP/synaptobrevin (Trimble et al., 1988), synaptosomal-associated protein 25 (SNAP-25) (Oyler et al., 1989) and syntaxin, an integral protein at the active zone (Bennett et al., 1992), all act as SNAP receptors (SNARES) and thereby can form a complex with the general fusion machinery. Based on these data, Rothman and colleagues have then proposed the so-called SNARE hypothesis, which holds that vesicles select their targets for fusion through specific interactions between vesicle and target SNARES (*Figure 5.4*).

The SNARE hypothesis implies that pairing between proteins specifically expressed on vesicles and their target membranes (v- or t-SNARES) mediates selective vesicle docking and fusion (Rothman and Warren, 1994; Söllner et al., 1993). Recognition between v- and t-SNARES would mediate docking while binding of SNARES to proteins involved in the membrane fusion machinery would mediate vesicle fusion. Thus, VAMP was postulated to be a v-SNARE and SNAP-25 and syntaxin t-SNARES, involved in SV docking and fusion at the presynaptic membrane. Consistent with this, under appropriate conditions, the three proteins form a stable heterotrimeric complex *in vitro* (Chapman et al., 1994; Hayashi et al., 1994). Functional evidence that VAMP, SNAP-25 and syntaxin are involved in transmitter release came from research on the targets of the tetanus and botulinum bacterial neurotoxins (TeNT and BoNT). TeNT and BoNT are metalloproteases that block transmitter release and induce paralysis of skeletal muscles followed by rapid death. Recent studies, pioneered by Montecucco and his colleagues, shortly followed by others (Blasi et al., 1993; Schiavo et al., 1992), showed that blockade of transmitter release by the toxins is due to the proteolytic cleavage of each of the three SNARE proteins identified by Rothman and colleagues. TeNT and BoNT type B, D, F and G cleave VAMP, while BoNT/A and /E cleave SNAP-25 and BoNT/C cleaves syntaxin and SNAP-25 (for review see Ferro-Novick and Jahn, 1994; Montecucco and Schiavo, 1994; see also Osen-Sand et al., 1996, for the role of BoNT/C). Although these data are consistent with the hypothesis that SNARES are involved in vesicle fusion, more recent work suggests that docking can occur in the absence of the SNARES (Osen-Sand et al., 1996; Schweizer et al., 1995; and see Südhof, 1995).

While functionally redundant SNARES could explain this apparent discrepancy (Rothman and Wieland, 1996), these data suggest that docking and fusion may require separate molecular interactions. It is also worth noting that, in addition to their role in release, SNAP-25 and syntaxin may have a structural role in the entire axonal compartment. In differentiated neurons *in vitro*, VAMP or SNAP-25 cleavage with clostridial toxins causes a strong inhibition of spontaneous and evoked release, and does not result in major morphological changes. In contrast, BoNT/C, which cleaves SNAP-25 and syntaxin, induces massive disruption of the axons and neuronal death (Osen-Sand et al., 1996). The fact that cleavage of SNAP-25 by BoNT/A did not induce similar morphological effects suggests that syntaxin plays a major role in axonal maintenance and cell viability. Consistent with this, although knock-out experiments in *Drosophila* indicate that syntaxin 1A is not essential for cell survival at early stages (Schulze *et al.*, 1995), lack of the protein eventually results in massive neurite disruption and degeneration of the nervous system (Schulze and Bellen, personal communication).

The fast toxic effects induced by simultaneous cleavage of SNAP-25 and syntaxin may reflect co-operativity of the two proteins for essential membrane exchanges within the axonal compartment. Consistent with this, syntaxin and SNAP-25 form a heterodimer *in vitro* and this association is believed to exist *in vivo* on the cytosolic face of the axonal membrane (Chapman *et al.*, 1994; Hayashi *et al.*, 1994). In fact, very recent immunochemical studies indicate an extensive co-localization of SNAP-25 and syntaxin on the plasmalemma (Garcia *et al.*, 1995) and a widespread distribution of both proteins throughout the axon (Duc and Catsicas, 1995; Garcia *et al.*, 1995).

These data suggest that both proteins have a more generic role than vesicle fusion and suggest that additional proteins must underlie the specificity required by regulated transmitter release. Since the SNARE proteins described here belong to large families with different tissue, regional or subcellular distribution. This, still expanding, diversity may encompass the specific as well as the general aspects of targeting implied by the SNARE hypothesis (Rothman and Wieland, 1996).

5.2.6 Vesicle fusion

It is clear that SV docking does not necessarily result in fusion (see Kelly, 1993). Electrophysiological evidence from time-resolved capacitance measurements in goldfish bipolar cells suggests that only a fraction of the releasable vesicles fuse in response to the rise of cytosolic Ca^{2+} generated by the action potential (von Gersdorff and Matthews, 1994). These and other data suggest that only a fraction of docked vesicles are ready (primed) to fuse. The molecular basis of priming following docking is not yet understood although recent data implicate the stability of the SNARE complex (Pellegrini *et al.*, 1995). An additional problem that neurons must face is that secretion (fusion) must be highly regulated in time. The rapid arrest of release following the drop of cytosolic Ca^{2+} at the end of the action potential implies the presence of a low affinity Ca^{2+} sensor within the microdomains where fusion occurs (Almers, 1994). Several independent approaches indicate that synaptotagmin, another integral synaptic vesicle protein (Matthew *et al.*, 1981), is a possible Ca^{2+} sensor. Ca^{2+} binds to synaptotagmin and its binding regulates the capacity of the protein to bind phospholipids (Brose *et al.*, 1992). This could in turn affect the possible role of synaptotagmin in fusion. In addition, and most importantly, synaptotagmin can bind to the SNARE complex formed by VAMP, SNAP-25 and syntaxin, and competes with α-SNAP for a common site on the complex (Söllner *et al.*, 1993). Current evidence suggests that α-SNAP can displace synaptotagmin which allows binding of the NSF to the complex and vesicle fusion (Söllner *et al.*, 1993). One possible interpretation of these data is that synaptotagmin acts as a negative regulator, preventing fusion in the absence of appropriate signals. Consistent with this hypothesis, analysis of synaptotagmin mutants of *Caenorhabditis elegans* and *Drosophila* shows that although the protein is not essential for release, it has modulatory functions (DiAntonio *et al.*, 1993; Nonet *et al.*, 1993). There is also additional indirect evidence that Ca^{2+} may regulate protein–protein interactions within the fusion complex, since syntaxin can interact with N-type Ca^{2+} channels within the active zone (Bennet *et al.*, 1992). Taken together, these studies suggest that synaptotagmin is a Ca^{2+}-dependent regulator of release efficiency, acting downstream of SV docking.

5.2.7 Membrane retrieval and neurotransmitter loading

While the cellular mechanisms involved in vesicle docking and fusion are the focus of many studies of neurotransmission, they represent only the initial steps of the exocytotic/endocytotic cycle. Following neurotransmitter release, SVs which fuse with the synaptic membrane do not generally become a permanent part of the plasmalemma (but see Section 5.3). Instead, SV membrane is retrieved to re-form vesicles which are then re-filled with neurotransmitters and take part in further rounds of synaptic activity. The molecules involved in these phases of synapse function are beginning to be characterized: a selection of them are described in the following sections.

Membrane retrieval following fusion. The specific mechanisms of vesicle retrieval remain a matter of debate. The two main hypotheses involve the formation of clathrin coats and subsequent endocytosis, or the rapid opening and closure of a transient exocytotic fusion pore (reviewed by DeCamilli and Takei, 1996). A role for clathrin-coated vesicles in vesicle retrieval seems likely since the number of clathrin-coated vesicles increases after stimulation and these vesicles contain synaptic vesicle proteins (Heuser and Reese, 1973; Maycox *et al.*, 1992). Recently, some of the molecules involved in formation of clathrin-coated pits have been characterized (see DeCamilli and Takei, 1996).

Clathrin coats are formed from heavy (180 kDa) and light (35–40 kDa) clathrin chains, and assembly particles (340 kDa, composed of two copies of three proteins) which form characteristically shaped hetero-oligomers called triskelia. While the components of clathrin coats are found at the plasmalemma as well as in the trans-Golgi network, there are proteins particular to each compartment. A heterotetrameric protein complex, AP2 [comprised of two 100–115 kDa subunits (a and b) and two subunits of 50 and 17 kDa, respectively], functions at the plasmalemma, possibly as an adaptor between clathrin triskelia and membrane proteins (see DeCamilli and Takei, 1996). In addition, synaptotagmin I has been shown to have a role in endocytosis (Fukuda *et al.*, 1995; Jorgensen *et al.*, 1995) and to bind AP2 (Li *et al.*, 1995) suggesting that there are neuron-specific membrane proteins involved in clathrin-mediated vesicle retrieval at synapses.

As indicated above, the initial steps of vesicle endocytosis involve recruitment of clathrin coat components to the synaptic plasma membrane and formation of invaginations. A subsequent step has been identified in which these invaginations break off from the membrane to complete the endocytotic event. A neuron-specific molecule, dynamin I, has been implicated in this process at synapses. Dynamin was first identified as a neuronal microtubule-binding protein which has GTPase activity (Obar *et al.*, 1990; Shpetner and Vallee, 1989). The protein is phosphorylated by protein kinase C (PKC) and it is dephosphorylated in response to neuronal stimulation (Robinson *et al.*, 1993). A number of functional studies, as well as its concentration in nerve terminals (Takei *et al.*, 1995), suggest that dynamin has a major role in endocytosis (for recent review see DeCamilli and Takei, 1996). Dynamin is a mammalian homolog of shibire, a *Drosophila* protein. Mutations of shibire cause arrest of endocytosis after formation of coated pits and subsequent paralysis (Koenig and Ikeda, 1989). Further evidence for the involvement of dynamin in mammalian endocytosis comes from studies of the GTPase activity of this protein. When GTPase-defective mutants of dynamin are transfected into mammalian cells, endocytosis is blocked (Vallee and Okamoto,

1995). Ultrastructural studies of shibire mutants show numerous invaginations with electron dense ring-like structures around a narrow neck (Koenig and Ikeda, 1989). Dynamin has been shown to self-assemble into rings *in vitro* (Hinshaw and Schmid, 1995), and similar structures which are immunopositive for dynamin form when synaptosomes are treated with GTPγS (Takei *et al.*, 1995). Finally, it has been suggested that separation of an endosomal pit from the plasma membrane may be due to a concerted conformational change in the molecules forming the dynamin 'collar', though this remains to be proven (DeCamilli and Takei, 1996; Hinshaw and Schmid, 1995).

Vesicle loading by neurotransmitter transporters. Following exocytosis and membrane retrieval, newly formed vesicles must be reloaded with neurotransmitter. Two classes of neurotransmitter transport activities have been characterized at synapses. These are a family of plasma membrane transporters which move neurotransmitters from the synaptic cleft to the synaptic cytoplasm, and a distinct family of transporters which take up neurotransmitters from the cytoplasm and concentrate them in synaptic vesicles. The plasma membrane transporters were extensively characterized earlier than vesicular transporters (for review see Borowsky and Hoffman, 1995) due to the difficulties involved in obtaining pure synaptic vesicles. Following improvements in isolation techniques, vesicular transport has been demonstrated in synaptic vesicles from various sources for many transmitters, including ACh (Anderson *et al.*, 1982; Parsons and Koenigsberger, 1980; Toll and Howard, 1980), monoamines (Johnson *et al.*, 1978), glutamate (Shioi *et al.*, 1989; Tabb *et al.*, 1992), GABA (Fykse and Fonnum 1988; Hell *et al.*, 1988) and glycine (Kish *et al.*, 1989). Vesicular transport is dependent on ATP and a proton gradient across the vesicle membrane (Maycox *et al.*, 1988; Naito and Ueda, 1983; Tabb *et al.*, 1992). This dependence highlights the fact that two independent proteins are involved in vesicular neurotransmitter transport (*Figure 5.5*)

The first protein needed is a proton pump which generates an electrochemical gradient across the vesicle membrane. The vesicular H^+-ATPase has been characterized and

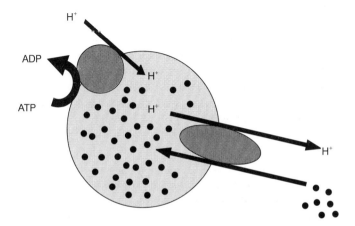

Figure 5.5. Neurotransmitter transport into synaptic vesicles is dependent on two proteins. A H^+-ATPase (orange circle) is essential for creating a H^+ gradient across the vesicle membrane. The neurotransmitter transporter (orange oval) is an H^+ transmitter antiporter.

shown to be similar to the vacuolar H^+-ATPase (see Gluck, 1993). The second protein necessary for vesicular neurotransmitter transport is a neurotransmitter–H^+ antiporter (see Schuldiner et al., 1995; Usdin et al., 1995). Functional reconstitution of purified transport proteins into liposomes has allowed investigators to attribute transport activity of the vesicular monoamine transporter and the vesicular GABA and glutamate transporters to single polypeptides (Carlson et al., 1989; Hell et al., 1990; Maron et al., 1979; Maycox et al., 1988, 1990; Moriyama et al., 1991; Stern-Bach et al., 1990).

Recently, the sequences of three vesicle transporters, two vesicular monoamine transporters (VMATs) and an ACh transporter (AChT) have been isolated. These three proteins share a generally similar structure with a large number of transport proteins, including bacterial drug-resistance genes, sugar transporters, plasma membrane neurotransmitter transporters and the vesicular membrane protein SV2 (for which no function has been identified). A generally similar 12-transmembrane domain functional architecture is proposed for all of these transporters, although sequence homology between these widely differing transporter types is limited. The closer sequence homologies between the three vesicle transporters defines these proteins as a family, more distantly related to other transporters, including those neurotransmitter transporters found at the plasma membrane. cDNAs encoding VMATs have now been cloned in human, bovine and rat (Erickson et al. 1992; Howell et al., 1994; Liu et al., 1992). In addition, two distinct genes have been identified in rat, *VMAT1* and *VMAT2*, which have overall identity of 62% (Schuldiner et al., 1995). Sequence and hydropathy analyses predict 521-amino acid proteins with 12 putative transmembrane segments which differ mostly between the first and second transmembrane domains and at the amino and carboxyl terminals. Functional studies of the two isoforms were performed in stable transfectants of Chinese hamster ovary cells and showed that VMAT2 has a higher affinity for all the monoamines (Peter et al., 1994). VMAT clones from species other than rat are more similar to VMAT2 than VMAT1 based on sequence comparisons (Erickson and Eiden, 1993; Howell et al., 1994; Peter et al., 1993; Vandenburg et al., 1992).

cDNA encoding an AChT have been isolated from *Torpedo marmorata, C. elegans*, rat and human (Alfonso et al., 1993; Erickson et al., 1994). The clone predicts a protein of 532 amino acids with 40% and 38% identity to VMAT1 and VMAT2, respectively (Usdin et al., 1995). Interestingly, the vesicular AChT is encoded within the same gene as an enzyme involved in ACh synthesis, choline acetyltransferase, suggesting that the regulation of transmitter synthesis and transport may be closely related (Usdin et al., 1995). It is not known whether similar mechanisms may be involved for other transmitters.

5.3 Learning and synapses

5.3.1 The neuronal software

The amount of transmitter released at a given synapse may change according to previous 'experience' of the synapse. This parameter is commonly defined as synaptic strength. It is clearly very tempting to relate this adaptive property of the synapse to high order functions of the nervous system. Indeed, learning has now been associated in a variety of systems and animal models with changes in the strength of connections between neurons (Hawkins et al., 1993). Such changes are often referred to as 'synaptic plasticity'. To date, two main types of synaptic plasticity have been identified. Although both types of plasticity can occur at the same synapses, they involve distinct cellular and molecular mechanisms. Short-term changes in synaptic efficiency involve strengthening of existing connections, possibly through modification of the structure and function of preexisting proteins, such as ion channels, protein kinases and receptors (Hawkins et al., 1993). The resulting effects include activation of postsynaptic receptors and modulation of transmitter release itself (Jessel and Kandel, 1993). These adaptations can occur rapidly and usually last for hours but sometimes for days. Long-term changes involve structural modifications of existing synapses or formation of new ones. This type of adaptation has been suggested as one of the possible cellular mechanisms that contributes to the storage of memory. Long-term changes seem to rely on the activation of gene expression and new protein synthesis (see Chapter 12).

Changes in the efficiency, size and number of synapses imply that the adult nervous system is a dynamic network where new terminals can grow and where synapses can be activated, added or removed in response to behavioral experience (Hawkins et al., 1993). Are there common effectors for short- and long-term synaptic plasticity? Are some of the mechanisms involved in synaptic plasticity similar to those that regulate axonal growth and synaptogenesis during development? Both questions are still unanswered, but transmitter release and growth of new connections have at least one mechanism in common: membrane fusion. Indeed, membrane fusion is necessary for vesicle secretion and it is also necessary in order to add new patches of membrane (a prerequisite for growth). The possible relevance of the mechanisms that control membrane fusion events in synaptic plasticity has been clearly demonstrated by the work of Kandel and his collaborators. Figure 5.6 summarizes the different stages that lead

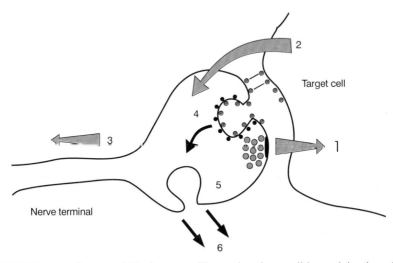

Figure 5.6. Diagram of a 'remodeling' synapse illustrating the possible participation of membrane fusion events during structural changes associated with learning (based on Bailey et al., 1992; Hu et al., 1993). Stimulation of the presynaptic neuron increases the fusion-dependent release of transmitter from SVs (gray circles, 1). When the stimulus is sustained, a target-derived factor (2) induces changes in gene expression in the presynaptic cell (3). In turn, this activates the endosomal pathway (4) and leads to fusion-dependent redistribution of membrane components at the sites of new growth (5,6). Black circles: clathrin. Orange circles: adhesion molecules. Modified from Trends Neurosci., vol. 17, pp. 368–373, with permission from Elsevier Trends Journals.

to a plastic response of a synapse and each stage that can involve membrane fusion is schematically illustrated. According to this model, modulation of transmitter release is the first step of a cascade leading to changes in gene expression and redistribution of membrane components that result in new synapse formation (Bailey *et al.*, 1992; Hu *et al.*, 1993). Each step of vesicle trafficking and fusion described in the previous chapters could contribute to regulated changes of transmitter release.

5.3.2 Functional synaptic plasticity

Changes of efficacy of existing synapses is often referred to as functional synaptic plasticity. One of the most impressive example is long-term potentiation (LTP). Bliss and Lømo, discovered that brief high frequency trains of action potentials produced an increase of synaptic strength in synapses of the hippocampus that use glutamate as a transmitter (Bliss and Lømo, 1973). This was the first demonstration that synaptic strength could change as a function of previous experience. LTP can last for hours or even days and seems to depend on both postsynaptic and presynaptic events. At the level of the postsynaptic cell, high levels of presynaptic stimulation result in the activation of glutamate receptors that are functionally blocked under normal conditions. At the level of the presynaptic cell, LTP involves an increase in transmitter release. This increase is likely to be the result of a retrograde signal originating from the postsynaptic cell. While the precise nature of the diffusible substance remains uncertain, current investigations focus on diffusible membrane-permeant molecules such as nitric oxide (Jessell and Kandel, 1993). While the molecular targets of the retrograde messenger are still unknown, the effects seem to include modifications of the opening time of ion channels in the presynaptic membrane (reviewed in Hawkins *et al.*, 1993). However, the possibility that covalent modifications of the proteins involved in vesicle trafficking and fusion could play a role is also under extensive study. For example, as mentioned in Section 5.2.4, studies on the synapsins indicate that vesicle mobilization may contribute the number of vesicles available for release. Regulating synapsin function may therefore have an indirect effect on synaptic strength. Also, very recent data on the docking and fusion machinery suggest that the function of the proteins involved may be regulated by phosphorylation events occurring during synaptic adaptations (Hirling and Scheller, personal communication). In addition, recent data by Staple and colleagues (Staple *et al.*, 1995) suggest that the relative ratio of proteins involved at different stages of transmitter release can vary in different synaptic boutons of the same neuron and that this variability correlates with synaptic strength.

5.3.3 Morphological synaptic plasticity

Long-term memory has been clearly associated with changes in synaptic structure in a variety of experimental systems (Wallace *et al.*, 1991). Quantitative ultrastructural analysis indicates that four basic morphological parameters of the synapse are strongly correlated. These are total vesicle number, active zone size, presynaptic bouton volume and postsynaptic spine volume (Pierce and Lewin, 1994; Pierce and Mendell, 1993). Interestingly, co-ordinated increases in size of pre- and postsynaptic elements have been reported after LTP in the dentate gyrus. These experiments have shown expansion of the average active zone and apposed surface areas, as well as synaptic bouton volume (see Wallace *et al.*, 1991). These increases imply the fusion and incorporation of new membrane into the synaptic structure. What are the mech-

anisms involved? There are at least two possibilities. Net changes in presynaptic surface could arise from any imbalance between the amount of membrane that is fused
and then retrieved during transmitter release and vesicle recycling. Consistent with
this, ultrastructural analysis of the synapses of the shibire mutant (the *Drosophila*
homolog of dynamin, which has a defect in vesicle endocytosis, see Section 5.2.7)
shows enlarged synapses. To date, there is no evidence that vesicle retrieval is
involved in physiological changes of synaptic size or shape. However, the observation
that membrane retrieval is stimulus dependent (von Gersdorff and Matthews, 1994)
suggests that it may be regulated in response to previous signals received by the neuron. This would provide a mechanism of activity-dependent (or use-dependent or
experience-dependent) control of membrane surface. The data showing that dynamin
(see Section 5.2.7) is phosphorylated by PKC and dephosphorylated by electrical
activity (Robinson *et al.*, 1993; van der Bliek and Meyerowitz, 1991), is also consistent
with this hypothesis.

An alternative way to increase synaptic surface would be the fusion of membrane
vesicles other than SVs. Pfenninger and colleagues have shown that plasmalemmal
expansion involves the fusion of large clear vesicles that were identified as plasmalemmal precursors (PPV) (Pfenninger *et al.*, 1991). These vesicles accumulate in
the growth cones of developing axons (Pfenninger and Friedman, 1993).
Interestingly, data obtained with a cell-free growth cone-expansion assay suggest that
PPV fusion with the plasma membrane is controlled by Ca^{2+} influx (Lockerbie *et al.*,
1991), thereby providing an activity-dependent mechanism of membrane expansion.
If the same mechanism was maintained in adult neurons, growth of new connections,
or morphological changes of existing ones, could be activated by stimulating the
membrane-expansion pathway. If this hypothesis is correct, the cell must be capable
of regulating vesicle fusion for release and vesicle fusion for expansion through distinct mechanisms. Of particular relevance to these observations, is the finding that
SNAP-25 has been shown to be involved in both transmitter release and in axonal
growth. Inhibition of SNAP-25 expression with antisense oligonucleotides prevented
neurite outgrowth in PC12 cells and cortical neurons *in vitro*, and in chick retina neurons *in vivo* (Osen-Sand *et al.*, 1993). These effects could result from inhibition of
transmitter release, but it is also possible that SNAP-25 is involved in the fusion of
PPV. Very recent studies support the latter interpretation. Using clostridial toxins on
primary neurons *in vitro*, Osen-Sand *et al.* (1996) showed that the fusion machineries
for transmitter release and axonal growth involve common but also distinct SNARES.
The v-SNARE VAMP was found to be exclusively involved in transmitter release,
whereas the t-SNARES SNAP-25 and syntaxin have a role in release and growth.
These data suggest that transmitter release (and SV fusion) is not necessary for axonal
growth and that additional v-SNARES must be involved in vesicle fusion for membrane expansion.

In addition to changes in synaptic size, the structural rearrangements that occur
during morphological synaptic plasticity involve the formation of new synapses and
are likely to involve the co-ordinated action of genes that regulate membrane expansion as well as vesicle storage and fusion. Consistent with this, candidate plasticity
genes encoding products involved in the endo- and exocytotic pathways have been
isolated following stimulation of *N*-methyl-D-aspartate receptors in rat hippocampus
(Nedivi *et al.*, 1993), during long-term facilitation in *Aplysia* (Hu *et al.*, 1993) and during synapse formation in the developing chick retina (see Osen-Sand *et al.*, 1993, and

in preparation). These findings demonstrate the importance of the fusion machinery during nerve terminal remodeling in the adult and suggest that the mechanisms involved are also at work during development. Recent work on the regulation of SNAP-25 isoforms expression is in support of this hypothesis. SNAP-25 exists in at least two alternatively spliced variants, differentially regulated during development (Bark, 1993; Bark and Wilson, 1994a; Bark et al., 1995; Boschert et al., 1996). SNAP-25a mRNA is highly and transiently expressed during axonal growth, while SNAP-25b is induced during synapse formation and its levels are maintained throughout adulthood (Bark, 1993; Bark and Wilson 1994b; Bark et al., 1995; Boschert et al., 1996). Further to these observations, Boschert and colleagues (1996) have shown that SNAP-25a (but not b) expression is induced in the adult hippocampus following lesions that are known to induce reactive sprouting. Although indirect, these observations suggest that the two SNAP-25 isoforms may have different roles in transmitter release and membrane expansion. The regulated expression of the two SNAP-25 isoforms, and of additional SNARES, may provide a molecular framework for differential use of the fusion machinery during specific stages of maturation of the terminal. Similarly, heterogeneity of SNARES expression in distinct adult terminals may reflect their capacity to undergo plasticity changes.

5.4 Concluding remarks

Fusion and re-uptake of specialized membrane is involved in a number of processes which affect neuronal morphology and function including, intracellular vesicle trafficking, neurotransmitter release and membrane expansion. We are only beginning to understand the molecular mechanisms of exocytosis/endocytosis which occur at synapses and the role of regulation of these steps on complex cellular behaviors. Our increasingly better understanding of these phenomena will have considerable implications for the molecular basis of synaptic adaptation.

References

Alfonso K, Grundahl K, Duerr JS, Han HP, Rand JB. (1993) The Caenorhabditis elegans unc-17 gene – a putative vesicular acetylcholine transporter. Science 261: 617–619

Almers W. (1994) Synapses. How fast can you get? Nature 367: 682–683.

Anderson DC, King SC, Parsons SM. (1982) Proton gradient linkage to active uptake of [³H]acetylcholine by Torpedo electric organ synaptic vesicles. Biochemistry. 21: 3037–3043.

Bähler M, Greengard P. (1987) Synapsin I bundles F-actin in a phosphorylation-dependent manner. Nature 326: 704–707.

Bailey CH, Chen M, Keller F, Kandel ER. (1992) Serotonin-mediated endocytosis of apCAM: an early step of learning-related synaptic growth in Aplysia. Science 256: 645–9.

Bark IC. (1993) Structure of the chicken gene for SNAP-25 reveals duplicated exon encoding distinct isoforms of the protein. J. Mol. Biol. 233: 67–76.

Bark IC, Wilson-MC. (1994a) Human cDNA clones encoding two different isoforms of the nerve terminal protein SNAP-25. Gene 139: 291–292.

Bark IC, Wilson MC. (1994b) Regulated vesicular fusion in neurons: snapping together the details. Proc. Natl Acad. Sci. USA 91: 4621–4624.

Bark IC, Hahn KM, Ryabinin AE, Wilson MC. (1995) Differential expression of SNAP-25 protein isoforms during divergent vesicle fusion events of neural development. Proc. Natl Acad. Sci. USA 92: 1510–1514.

Benfenati F, Bähler M, Jahn R, Greengard P. (1989) Interaction of synapsin I with small synaptic vesicles: distinct sites in synapsin I bind to vesicle phospholipids and vesicle proteins. J. Cell Biol. 108: 1863–1872.

Bennett MK, Calakos N, Scheller RH. (1992) Syntaxin: a synaptic protein implicated in docking of synaptic vesicles at presynaptic active zones. *Science* **257:** 255–259.

Blasi J, Chapman ER, Link E, Binz T, Yamasaki S, De Camilli P, Südhof TC, Niemann H, Jahn R. (1993) Botulinum neurotoxin A selectively cleaves the synaptic protein SNAP-25. *Nature* **365:** 160–163.

Bliss TV, Lømo T. (1973) Long-lasting potentiation of synaptic transmission in the dentate area of the anaesthetized rabbit following stimulation of the perforant path. *J. Physiol (Lond.)* **232:** 331–356.

Borowsky B, Hoffman BJ. (1995) Neurotransmitter transporters: molecular biology, function, and regulation. *Int. Rev. Neurobiol.* **38:** 139–199.

Boschert U, O'Shaughnessy C, Dickenson R, Tessari M, Bendotti C, Catsicas S, Merlo-Pich E. (1996) Developmental and plasticity-related differential expression of two SNAP-25 isoforms in the rat brain. *J. Comp. Neurol.* **367:** 177–193.

Brose N, Petrenko AG, Südhof TC, Jahn R. (1992) Synaptotagmin: a calcium sensor on the synaptic vesicle surface. *Science* **256:** 1021–1025.

Carlson MD, Kish PE, Ueda T. (1989) Characterization of the solubilized and reconstituted ATP-dependent vesicular glutamate uptake system. *J. Biol. Chem.* **264:** 7369–7376.

Catsicas S, Grenningloh G, Pich EM. (1994) Nerve-terminal proteins; to fuse to learn. *Trends Neurosci.* **17:** 368–373.

Ceccaldi P, Grohovaz F, Benfenati F, Chieregatti E, Greengard P, Valtorta F. (1995) Dephosphorylated synapsin I anchors synaptic vesicles to actin cytoskeleton: an analysis by videomicroscopy. *J. Cell Biol.* **128:** 905–912.

Chapman ER, An S, Barton N, Jahn R. (1994) SNAP-25, a t-SNARE which binds to both syntaxin and synaptobrevin via domains that may form coiled coils. *J. Biol. Chem.* **269:** 27 427–27 432.

Chin LS, Li L, Ferreira A, Kosik KS, Greengard P. (1995) Impairment of axonal development and of synaptogenesis in hippocampal neurons of synapsin I-deficient mice. *Proc. Natl Acad. Sci. USA* **92:** 9230–9234.

De Camilli P, Takei K. (1996) Molecular mechanisms in synaptic vesicle endocytosis and recycling. *Neuron* **16:** 481–486.

De Camilli P, Harris SM, Huttner WB, Greengard P. (1983) Synapsin I (protein I), a nerve terminal-specific phosphoprotein. II. Its specific association with synaptic vesicles demonstrated by immunocytochemistry in agarose-embedded synaptosomes. *J. Cell Biol.* **96:** 1209–1211.

De Camilli P, Benfenati F, Valtorta F, Greengard P. (1990) The synapsins. *Annu. Rev. Cell Biol.* **6:** 433–460.

DiAntonio A, Parfitt KD, Schwarz TL. (1993) Synaptic transmission persists in synaptotagmin mutants of *Drosophila*. *Cell* **73:** 1281–1290.

Duc C, Catsicas S. (1995) Ultrastructural localization of SNAP-25 within the rat spinal cord and peripheral nervous system. *J. Comp. Neurol.* **357:** 1–12.

Eccles, JC. (1937) Synaptic and neuro-muscular transmission. *Physiol. Rev.* **17:** 538–555.

Erickson J, Eiden L, Hoffman B. (1992) Expression cloning of a reserpine-sensitive vesicular monoamine transporter. *Proc. Natl Acad. Sci. USA* **89:** 10 993–10 997.

Erickson J, Eiden L. (1993) Functional identification and molecular cloning of a human brain vesicle monoamine transporter. *J. Neurochem.* **61:** 2314–2317.

Erickson JD, Varoqui H, Schafer MKH, *et al.* (1994) Functional identification of a vesicular acetylcholine transporter and its expression from a 'cholinergic' gene locus. *J. Biol. Chem.* **269:** 21 929–21 932.

Fatt P, Katz B. (1951) An analysis of the end-plate potential recorded with an intracellular electrode. *J. Physiol. (Lond.)* **115:** 320–370.

Ferreira A, Kosik KS, Greengard P, Han H-Q. (1994) Aberrant neurites and synaptic vesicle protein deficiency in synapsin II-depleted neurons. *Science* **264:** 977–979.

Ferreira A, Han H-Q, Greengard P, Kosik KS. (1995) Suppression of synapsin II inhibits the formation and maintenance of synapses in hippocampal culture. *Proc. Natl Acad. Sci. USA* **92:** 9225–9229.

Ferro-Novick S, Jahn R. (1994) Vesicle fusion from yeast to man. *Nature* **370:** 191–193.

Forn J, Greengard P. (1978) Depolarizing agents and cyclic nucleotides regulate the phosphorylation of specific neuronal proteins in rat cerebral cortex slices. *Proc. Natl Acad. Sci. USA* **75:** 5195–5199.

Foster M. (1897) *A Text-book of Physiology.* London, Macmillan.

Fukuda M, Moreira JE, Lewis FMT, Sugimori M, Niinobe M, Mikoshiba K, Llinás R. (1995) Role of the C2B domain of synaptotagmin in vesicular release and recycling as determined by specific antibody injection into the squid giant synapse preterminal. *Proc. Natl Acad. Sci. USA* **92:** 10 708–10 712.

Fykse EM, Fonnum F. (1988) Uptake of gamma-aminobutyric acid by a synaptic vesicle fraction isolated from rat brain. *J. Neurochem.* **50:** 1237–1242.

Garcia EP, McPherson PS, Chilcote TJ, Takei K, DeCamilli P. (1995) rbSec1A and B colocalize with syntaxin 1 and SNAP-25 throughout the axon, but are not in a stable complex with syntaxin. *J. Cell Biol.* **129:** 105–120.

Gluck SL. (1993) The vacuolar H(+)-ATPases: versatile proton pumps participating in constitutive and specialized functions of eukaryotic cells. *Int. Rev. Cytol.* **137:** 105–37.

Greengard P, Valtorta F, Czernik AJ, Benfenati F. (1993) Synaptic vesicle phosphoproteins and regulation of synaptic function. *Science.* **259:** 780–785.

Hackett JT, Cochran SL, Greenfield LJ Jr, Brosius DC, Ueda T. (1990) Synapsin I injected presynaptically into goldfish mauthner axons reduces quantal synaptic transmission. *J. Neurophysiol.* **63:** 701–706.

Han H-Q, Nichols RA, Rubin MR, Bähler M, Greengard P. (1991) Induction of formation of presynaptic terminals in neuroblastoma cells by synapsin IIb. *Nature* **349:** 697–700.

Hawkins RD, Kandel ER, Siegelbaum SA. (1993) Learning to modulate transmitter release: themes and variations in synaptic plasticity. *Annu. Rev. Neurosci.* **16:** 625–665.

Hayashi T, McMahon H, Yamasaki S, Binz T, Hata Y, Südhof TC, Niemann H. (1994) Synaptic vesicles membrane fusion complex: action of clostridial neurotoxins on assembly. *EMBO J.* **13:** 5051–5061.

Hell JW, Maycox PR, Stadler H, Jahn R. (1988) Uptake of GABA by rat brain synaptic vesicles isolated by a new procedure. *EMBO J.* **7:** 3023–3029.

Hell JW, Maycox PR, Jahn R. (1990) Energy dependence and functional reconstitution of the gamma-aminobutyric acid carrier from synaptic vesicles. *J. Biol. Chem.* **265:** 2111–2117.

Heuser JE, Reese TS. (1973) Evidence for recycling of synaptic vesicle membrane during transmitter release at the frog neuromuscular junction. *J. Cell Biol.* **57:** 315–344.

Hinshaw J.E., Schmidt S.L. (1995) Dynamin self-assembles into rings suggesting a mechanism for coated vesicle budding. *Nature* **374:** 190–192.

Howell M, Shirvan A, Stern-Bach Y, Steiner-Mordoch S, Strasser JE, Dean GE, Schuldiner S. (1994) Cloning and functional expression of a tetrabenazine sensitive vesicular monoamine transporter from bovine chromaffin granules. *FEBS Lett.* **338:** 16–22.

Hu Y, Barzulai A, Chen M, Bailey CH, Kandel ER. (1993) 5-HT and cAMP induce the formation of coated pits and vesicles and increase the expression of clathrin light chain in sensory neurons of aplysia. *Neuron* **10:** 921–929.

Huttner WB, Schiebler W, Greengard P, De Camilli P. (1983) Synapsin I (Protein I), a nerve terminal-specific phosphoprotein. III. Its association with synaptic vesicles studied in a highly purified synaptic vesicle preparation. *J. Cell Biol.* **96:** 1374–1388.

Jessell TM, Kandel ER. (1993) Synaptic transmission: a bidirectional and self-modifiable form of cell–cell communication. *Cell* **72:** 1–30.

Johnson RG, Carlson NJ, Scarpa A. (1978) Delta pH and catecholamine distribution in isolated chromaffin granules. *J. Biol. Chem.* **253:** 1512–1521.

Jorgensen EM, Hartwieg E, Schuske K, Nonet ML, Jin Y, Horwitz HR. (1995) Defective recycling of synaptic vesicles in synaptotagmin mutants of *Caenorhabditis elegans. Nature* **378:** 196–199.

Kelly RB. (1993) Storage and release of neurotransmitters. *Cell* **10:** 43–53.

Kish PE, Fischer-Bovenkerk C, Ueda T. (1989) Active transport of gamma-aminobutyric acid and glycine into synaptic vesicles. *Proc. Natl Acad. Sci. USA* **86:** 3877–3881.

Koenig JH, Ikeda K. (1989) Disappearance and reformation of synaptic vesicle membrane upon transmitter release observed under reversible blockage of membrane retrieval. *J. Neurosci.* **9:** 3844–3860.

Li C, Ullrich B, Zhang JZ, Anderson RG, Brose N, Südhof TC. (1995) Ca^{++}-dependent and -independent activities of neural and nonneural synaptotagmins. *Nature* **375:** 594–599.

Lin JW, Sugimori M, Llinás R, McGuinness TL, Greengard P. (1990) Effects of synapsin I and calcium/calmodulin-dependent protein kinase II on spontaneous neurotransmitter release in the squid giant synapse. *Proc. Natl Acad. Sci. USA* **87:** 8257–8261.

Liu Y, Peter D, Roghani S, Schuldiner G, Prive D, Eisenberg N, Brecha N, Edwards R. (1992) A cDNA that suppresses MPP$^+$ toxicity encodes a vesicular amine transporter. *Cell* **70:** 539–551.

Llinás R, McGuiness TL, Leonard CS, Sugimori M, Greengard P. (1985) Intraterminal injection of synapsin I or calcium/calmodulin-dependent kinase II alters neurotransmitter release at the squid giant synapse. *Proc. Natl Acad. Sci. USA* **82:** 3035–3039.

Llinás R, Gruner JA, Sugimori M, McGuinness T, Greengard P. (1991) Regulation of synapsin I and Ca^{++} calmodulin-dependent protein kinase II of the transmitter release in squid giant synapse. *J. Physiol. (London)* **436:** 257–282.

Lockerbie RO, Miller VE, Pfenninger KH. (1991) Regulated plasmalemmal expansion in nerve growth cones. *J. Cell Biol.* **112:** 1215–1227.

Lu B, Greengard P, Poo M-M. (1992) Exogenous synapsin I promotes functional maturation of developing neuromuscular synapses. *Neuron* **8:** 521–529.

Maron R, Fishkes H, Kanner BI, Schuldiner S. (1979) Solubilization and reconstitution of the catecholamine transporter from bovine chromaffin granules. *Biochemistry* **18:** 4781–4785.

Matthew WD, Tsavaler L, Reichardt LF. (1981) Identification of a synaptic vesicle-specific membrane protein with a wide distribution in neuronal and neurosecretory tissue. *J. Cell Biol.* **91:** 257–269.

Maycox PR, Deckwerth T, Hell JW, Jahn R. (1988) Glutamate uptake by brain synaptic vesicles. Energy dependence of transport and functional reconstitution in proteoliposomes. *J. Biol. Chem.* **263:** 15 423–15 428.

Maycox PR, Deckwerth T, Jahn R. (1990) Bacteriorhodopsin drives the glutamate transporter of synaptic vesicles after co-reconstitution. *EMBO J.* **9:** 1465–1469.

Maycox PR, Link E, Reetz A, Morris SA, Jahn R. (1992) Clathrin-coated vesicles in nervous tissues are involved primarily in synaptic vesicle recycling. *J. Cell Biol.* **118:** 1379–1388.

Montecucco C, Schiavo G. (1994) Mechanism of action of tetanus and botulinum neurotoxins. *Mol. Microbiol.* **13:** 1–8.

Moriyama Y, Iwamoto A, Hanada H, Maeda M, Futai M. (1991) One-step purification of *Escherichia coli* H^{+}-ATPase (F0F1) and its reconstitution into liposomes with neurotransmitter transporters. *J. Biol. Chem.* **266:** 22 141–22 146.

Naito S, Ueda T. (1983) Adenosine triphosphate-dependent uptake of glutamate into protein I-associated synaptic vesicles. *J. Biol. Chem.* **258:** 696–699.

Nedivi E, Hevroni D, Naot D, Israeli D, Citri Y. (1993) Numerous candidate plasticity-related genes revealed by differential cDNA cloning. *Nature* **363:** 718–722.

Nestler E, Greengard P. (1982) Distribution of protein I and regulation of its state of phosphorylation in the rabbit superior cervical ganglion. *J. Neurosci.* **2:** 1011–1023.

Nichols RA, Chilcote TJ, Czernik AJ, Greengard P. (1992) Synapsin I regulates glutamate release from rat brain synaptosomes. *J. Neurochem.* **58:** 783–785.

Nonet ML, Grundahl K, Meyer BJ, Rand JB. (1993) Synaptic function is impaired but not eliminated in *C. elegans* mutants lacking synaptotagmin. *Cell* **73:** 1291–1305.

Obar RA, Collins CA, Hammarback JA, Shpetner HS, Vallee RB. (1990) Molecular cloning of the microtubule-associated mechanochemical enzyme dynamin reveals homology with a new family of GTP-binding proteins. *Nature* **347:** 256–261.

Osen-Sand A, Catsicas M, Staple JK, Jones KA, Ayala G, Knowles J, Grenningloh G, Catsicas S. (1993). Inhibition of axonal growth by SNAP-25 antisense oligonucleotides *in vitro* and *in vivo*. *Nature* **364:** 445–448.

Osen-Sand A, Staple JK, Naldi E, Schiavo G, Rossetto O, Petitpierre S, Malgaroli A, Montecucco C, Catsicas S. (1996) Common and distinct fusion proteins in axonal growth and transmitter release. *J. Comp. Neurol.* **367:** 222–234.

Oyler GA, Higgins GA, Hart RA, Battenberg E, Billingsley M, Bloom FE, Wilson MC. (1989) The identification of a novel synaptosomal-associated protein, SNAP-25, differentially expressed by neuronal subpopulations. *J. Cell Biol.* **109:** 3039–3052.

Palade GE, Palay SL. (1954) Electron microscope observations of interneuronal and neuromuscular synapses. *Anat. Rec.* **118:** 335–336.

Parsons SM, Koenigsberger R. (1980) Specific stimulated uptake of acetylcholine by *Torpedo* electric organ synaptic vesicles. *Proc. Natl Acad. Sci. USA* **77:** 6234–6238.

Peter D, Jimenez J, Liu Y, Kim J, Edwards RH. (1994) The chromaffin granule and synaptic vesicle amine transporters differ in substrate recognition and sensitivity to inhibitors. *J. Biol. Chem.* **269:** 7231–7237.

Peter D, Liu Y, Sternini C, de Giorgio R, Brecha N, Edwards RH. (1995) Differential expression of two vesicular monoamine transporters. *J. Neurosci.* **15:** 6179–6188.

Petrucci TC, Morrow JS. (1987) Synapsin I: an actin-bundling protein under phosphorylation control. *J. Cell Biol.* **105:** 1355–1363.

Pellegrini LL, O'Connor V, Lottspeich F, Betz H. (1995) Clostridial neurotoxins compromise the stability of a low energy SNARE complex mediating NSF activation of synaptic vesicle fusion. *EMBO J.* **14**: 4705–4713.

Pevsner J, Scheller RH. (1994) Mechanisms of vesicle docking and fusion: insights from the nervous system. *Curr. Opin. Cell Biol.* **6**: 555–560.

Pfenninger KH, Friedman LB. (1993) Sites of plasmalemmal expansion in growth cones. *Dev. Brain Res.* **71**: 181–192.

Pfednninger KH, de la Houssaye BA, Frame L, Helmke S, Lockerbie RO, Lohse K, Miller V, Negre-Aminou P, Wood MR. (1991) In: *The Growth Cone* (eds PC Letourneau, SB Kater, ER Macagno). Raven Press, New York, pp. 111–123.

Pierce JP, Lewin GR. (1994) An ultrastructural size principle. *Neuroscience* **58**: 441–446.

Pierce JP, Mendell LM. (1993) Quantitative ultrastructure of Ia boutons in the ventral horn: scaling and positional relationships. *J. Neurosci.* **13**: 4748–4763.

Robertson, JD. (1987) The early days of electron microscopy of nerve tissue and membranes. *Int. Rev. Cytol.* **100**: 129–201.

Robinson PJ, Sontag JM, Liu JP, Fykse EM, Slaughter C, McMahon H, Südhof TC. (1993) Dynamin GTPase regulated by protein kinase C phosphorylation in nerve terminals. *Nature* **365**: 163–166.

Rosahl TW, Spillane D, Missler M, Herz J, Selig D, Wolff JR, Hammer RE, Malenka RC, Südhof TC. (1995) Essential function of synapsins I and II in synaptic vesicle regulation. *Nature* **375**: 488–493.

Rothman JE, Warren G. (1994) Implications of the SNARE hypothesis for intracellular membrane topology and dynamics. *Curr. Biol.* **4**: 220–233.

Rothman JE, Wieland FT. (1996) Protein sorting by transport vesicles. *Science* **272**: 227–234.

Schiavo G, Benfenati F, Poulain B, Rossetto O, Polverino de Laureto P, Das Gupta BR, Montecucco C. (1992) Tetanus and botulinum-B neurotoxins block neurotransmitter release by proteolytic cleavage of synaptobrevin. *Nature* **359**: 832–835.

Schuldiner S, Shirvan A, Linial M. (1995) Vesicular neurotransmitter transporters: from bacteria to humans. *Physiol. Rev.* **75**: 369–392.

Schulze KL, Broadie K, Perin MS, Bellen HJ. (1995). Genetic and electrophysiological studies of *Drosophila* syntaxin 1A demonstrate its role in nonneuronal secretion and neurotransmission. *Cell* **80**: 311–320.

Schiebler W, Jahn R, Doucet J-P, Rothlein J, Greengard P. (1986) Characterization of synapsin I binding to small synaptic vesicles. *J. Biol. Chem.* **261**: 8383–8390.

Schweizer FE, Betz H, Augustine GJ. (1995) From vesicle docking to endocytosis: intermediate reactions of exocytosis. *Neuron* **14**: 689–696.

Shpetner HS, Vallee RB. (1989) Identification of dynamin, a novel mechanochemical enzyme that mediates interactions between microtubules. *Cell* **59**: 421–432.

Shioi J, Naito S, Ueda T. (1989) Glutamate uptake into synaptic vesicles of bovine cerebral cortex and electrochemical potential difference of protons across the membrane. *Biochem. J.* **258**: 499–504.

Sihra TS, Wang JKT, Gorelick FS, Greengard P. (1989) Translocation of synapsin I in response to depolarization of isolated nerve terminals. *Proc. Natl Acad. Sci. USA* **86**: 8108–8112.

Söllner T, Bennett MK, Whiteheart SW, Scheller RH, Rothman JE. (1993) A protein assembly–diassembly pathway *in vitro* that may correspond to sequential steps of synaptic vesicle docking, activation, and fusion. *Cell* **75**: 409–418.

Staple JK, Osen-Sand A, Benfenati F, Merlo Pich E, Catsicas S. (1995) Molecular and functional diversity of individual nerve terminals of isolated cortical neurons. *Sci. Neurosci. Abstr.* **21**: 331.

Stern-Bach Y, Greenberg-Ofrath N, Flechner I, Schuldiner S. (1990) Identification and purification of a functional amine transporter from bovine chromaffin granules. *J. Biol. Chem.* **265**: 3961–3966.

Südhof TC. (1995) The synaptic vesicle cycle: a cascade of protein–protein interactions. *Nature* **375**: 645–653.

Südhof TC, Czernik AJ, Kao H-T et al. (1989) Synapsins: mosaics of shared and individual domains in a family of synaptic vesicle phosphoproteins. *Science* **245**: 1474–1480.

Tabb J, Kish P, Vandyke R, Ueda T. (1992) Glutamate transport into synaptic vesicles – roles of membrane potential, pH gradient, and intravesicular pH. *J. Biol. Chem.* **267**: 15 412–15 418.

Takei K, McPherson PS, Schmid SL, DeCamilli P. (1995) Tubular membrane invaginations coated by dynamin rings are induced by GTP-gS in nerve terminals. *Nature* **374**: 186–190.

Thiel G, Südhof TC, Greengard P. (1990) Synapsin II: mapping of a domain in the NH_2-terminal region which binds to small synaptic vesicles. *J. Biol. Chem.* **265**: 16 527–16 533.

Toll L, Howard BD. (1980) Evidence that an ATPase and a protonmotive force function in the transport of acetylcholine into storage vesicles. *J. Biol. Chem.* **255:** 1787–1789.

Trifaró J-M, Vitale ML. (1993) *Trends Neurosci.* **16:** 466–472.

Trimble WS, Cowan DM, Scheller RH. (1988) *Proc. Natl Acad. Sci. USA* **85:** 4538–4542.

Usdin TB, Eiden LE, Bonner TI, Erickson JD. (1995) Molecular biology of the vesicular ACh transporter. *Trends Neurosci.* **18:** 218–224.

Vallee RB, Okamoto PM. (1995) The regulation of endocytosis: identifying dynamin's binding partners. *Trends Cell Biol.* **5:** 43–47.

Valtorta F, Villa A, Jahn R, De Camilli P, Greengard P, Ceccarelli B. (1988) Localization of synapsin I at the frog neuromuscular junction. *Neuroscience* **24:** 593–603.

Valtorta F, Greengard P, Fesce R, Chieregatti E, Benfenati F. (1992) Effects of the neuronal phosphoprotein synapsin I on actin polymerization. I. Evidence for a phosphorylation-dependent nucleating effect. *J. Biol. Chem.* **267:** 11 281–11 288.

Vandenbergh D, Persico A, Uhl G. (1992) A human dopamine transporter cDNA predicts reduced glycosylation, displays a novel repetitive element and provides racially-dimorphic Taqi RFLPs. *Mol. Brain Res.* **15:** 161–166.

Van der Bliek AM, Meyerowitz EM. (1991) Dynamin-like protein encoded by the *Drosophila shibire* gene associated with vesicular traffic. *Nature* **351:** 411–414.

von Gersdorff H, Matthews G. (1994) Dynamics of synaptic vesicle fusion and membrane retrieval in synaptic terminals. *Nature* **367:** 735–739.

Wallace CS, Hawrylak N, Greenough WT. (1991) In: *Long-term Potentiation* (eds M Baudry, JL Davis). MIT Press, Cambridge, MA, pp. 189–232.

Wilson DW, Whiteheart SW, Wiedmann M, Brunner M, Rothman JE. (1992) A multisubunit particle implicated in membrane fusion. *J. Cell Biol.* **117:** 531–538.

Voltage-gated ion channels

Gillian Edwards and Arthur H. Weston

6.1 Introduction

Voltage-gated ion channels are important determinants of cellular excitability. Their functions range from the setting of basal levels of membrane potential to the initiation and termination of both excitatory and inhibitory events. Although chloride channels are important in these processes, we have restricted our comments to voltage-sensitive cation channels individually selective for Na^+, Ca^{2+} and K^+. These not only illustrate many of the general features common to voltage-sensitive ion channels but also their pharmacology is relatively well developed. Indeed, the interaction of these cation-selective channels with drugs has been, and remains, an important factor in understanding the molecular basis of channel diversity and how channel modulation can be exploited in therapeutic applications.

6.2 General principles

Voltage-gated ion channels are membrane-spanning proteins which adopt different structural configurations depending upon the membrane potential. In this way, they flip between a nonconducting, closed state and an open state in which a transmembrane, aqueous pore exists in the center of channel protein(s). This then allows the diffusion of ions across the membrane according to the prevailing transmembrane ionic gradient. Most voltage-sensitive channels are closed when the membrane is normally polarized or hyperpolarized (range typically –60 to –90 mV) and open on depolarization. Most, if not all, native Na^+-, K^+- and Ca^{2+}-channels are complexes of one or more central pore-forming (α-) subunits associated with auxiliary structures (β-, γ- and δ-subunits). However, expression studies have shown that α-subunits alone are capable of forming ion-selective channels.

6.3 General structure of voltage-sensitive K+-channels

K^+-channels possess the simplest α-subunit (see *Figure 6.1*) and on the basis of their structures, voltage-sensitive K^+-channels can be grouped into two main superfamilies. Superfamily 1 includes the delayed-rectifier K^+-channel (K_V), K_A (a rapidly-activating and -inactivating channel which carries the 'A'-current) and the large-conductance calcium-sensitive K^+-channel (BK_{Ca}). The general structure of Superfamily

Molecular Biology of the Neuron, edited by R.W. Davis and B.J. Morris.
© 1997 BIOS Scientific Publishers Ltd, Oxford.

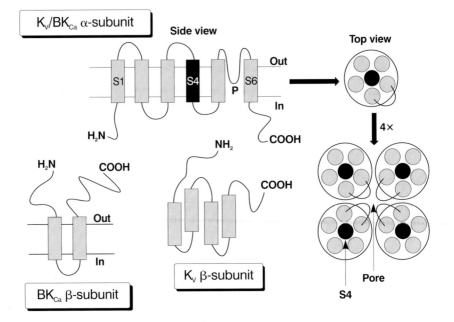

Figure 6.1. Schematic representation of Superfamily 1 K⁺-channel structure. The α-subunit comprises six α-helical membrane-spanning regions (S1–S6). The protein is thought to fold such that the highly charged S4 region is shielded from the membrane by the other transmembrane regions. The inner part of the channel is formed by the association of four α-subunits with the membrane-dipping regions (P) lining the pore. Although the α-subunit carboxyl terminus as depicted is short, that of BK_{Ca} is long (and may traverse the membrane) and probably forms the Ca^{2+} binding site. Four intracellular or transmembrane auxiliary (β-) subunits are thought to associate with the four α-subunits which form K_V or BK_{Ca}, respectively.

1 α-subunits comprises six membrane-spanning α-helical regions (S1–S6), which are connected by alternate extracellular and intracellular linkers, and a membrane-dipping region (P) between S5 and S6; both the carboxyl and amino termini are intracellular (*Figure 6.1*). Approximately every third amino acid of S4 is positively charged (lysine or arginine, separated by hydrophobic residues) and it is thus thought that S4 acts as the voltage sensor of the channel (Catterall, 1995; Dolly and Parcej, 1996; Pongs, 1992).

Superfamily 2 comprises K⁺-selective channels with α-subunits which possess only two membrane-spanning regions (M1 and M2) (*Figure 6.2*; see also Kubo, 1994). The M1 and M2 regions share some homology with the S5 and S6 regions of voltage-sensitive K⁺-channels described above (Kubo *et al.*, 1993). Moreover, M1 and M2 are linked extracellularly by a membrane-dipping region analogous to the pore region of the Superfamily 1 channels (Kubo *et al.*, 1993). The carboxyl and amino termini of the α-subunit protein are located intracellularly and possess multiple consensus phosphorylation sites for several different kinases. Although the activity of several cloned inwardly rectifying K⁺-channel subtypes is modified by protein kinases A and C, other kinases may also be involved in channel regulation (see Doupnik *et al.*, 1995). Recently, it has been proposed (Inagaki *et al.*, 1995) that so-called ATP-sensitive K⁺-

multimers so far widely investigated, Kv1.4, 3.3, 3.4, 4.1 and 4.2 exhibit 'A-channel-like' properties whereas Kv1.1, 1.2, 1.3, 1.5, 1.6, 2.1, 2.2, 3.1, 3.2 homomultimeric channels show little inactivation and appear to be similar to 'delayed rectifiers'. All these channels have been detected in the mammalian central nervous system (Chandy and Gutman, 1995; Weiser et al., 1994).

Mutations of the so-called slowpoke (slo) locus in Drosophila specifically abolish Ca^{2+}-activated K^+-currents in both muscles and neurons (Atkinson et al., 1991). The slo gene, which is present in the mammalian brain, encodes a large-conductance, iberiotoxin-sensitive, K^+-selective channel which is similar to the native BK_{Ca} channel (Butler et al., 1993). The K^+-selective channels which are formed from expression of slo α-subunits are, however, less sensitive to calcium or voltage than the native BK_{Ca}.

Superfamily 1 β-subunits. Five delayed-rectifier K^+-channel β-subunit cDNAs have been identified, three of which arise from the $Kv\beta_1$ gene by alternative splicing (Shi et al., 1996). All seem to be exclusively expressed in the brain (see Pongs, 1995). The $Kv\beta_1$ splice variants are all capable of increasing the rate of inactivation of co-expressed Kv1.x channels and also increase the surface expression and stability of the α-subunits. The increased surface expression of Kv1.x channels when co-expressed with $Kv\beta_2$ suggests that this subunit may play an important chaperone-like role although it does not seem to modify the gating properties of the α-subunit (Isom et al., 1994; Shi et al., 1996). The distribution of $Kv\beta_3$ differs from that of the $Kv\beta_1$ and $Kv\beta_2$ subunits (Heinemann et al., 1995). Channel inactivation by $Kv\beta_{1.1}$ or by $Kv\beta_2$ is sensitive to the intracellular redox potential (Heinemann et al., 1995). To date, only the properties of the channels formed by α-subunits of members of the Kv1 family of channels have been shown directly to be modified by co-expression with the Kvβ-subunits. However, Kv4.2 (but not Kv2.1 or Kv3.1) also strongly associates with co-expressed $Kv\beta_1$ or $Kv\beta_2$, suggesting that these β-subunits may modify the activity of channels in families other than Kv1 (Nakahira et al., 1996).

The Kvβ-subunits are hydrophilic and do not possess sequences typical of membrane-spanning regions. These factors, coupled with the lack of glycosylation sites but with the presence of consensus phosphorylation sites, suggest that the Kvβ-subunits are intracellular (see Pongs, 1995). In this respect, these subunits are more similar to the β-subunits of Ca^{2+}-channels (which are thought to be cytosolic) rather than those of Na^+-channels or of BK_{Ca} (Isom et al., 1994; Pongs, 1995).

In smooth muscle, the α-subunit is tightly associated with a smaller, membrane-spanning β-subunit (Knaus et al., 1994a). If the β-subunit is co-expressed, the cloned channels demonstrate properties similar to those of native channels (Knaus et al., 1994a; McManus et al., 1995). Not only does the β-subunit modify the channel's voltage and calcium sensitivity, it also appears to increase the inhibitory potency of charybdotoxin and is essential for the channel-opening effect of dehydrosoyasaponin-1 (see Section 6.5.3). Although the smooth muscle β-subunit is capable of modifying the properties of a heterologously co-expressed brain slo channel (McManus et al., 1995), any such effects of the recently discovered neuronal BK_{Ca} (Reinhart et al., 1995) remain to be established.

Inwardly rectifying K^+-channels. At least six subfamilies of K_{IR} (Kir1.x–Kir6.x) have been identified (see *Figure 6.5* for proposed lineage) and five of these (Kir2.x–Kir6.x) are strongly expressed in the brain (Doupnik et al., 1995; Inagaki et

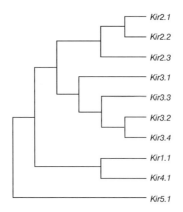

Figure 6.5. Schematic phylogenic tree of Superfamily 2 K$^+$-channel genes based on amino acid sequence similarities. Adapted from Doupnik *et al.* (1995). For an alternative tree which includes Kir6.x see Köhler *et al.* (1996).

al., 1995). Channels of subfamily 2 (Kir2.1, Kir2.2 and Kir2.3), as well as Kir4.1, show strong rectification similar to that of native K_{IR} in neuronal (Constanti and Galvan, 1983) and glial cells (Newman, 1993). Their rectifying properties mean that although these channels will contribute to the resting levels of membrane potential, they almost cease to conduct as the membrane is depolarized during an action potential.

At least four different channels of the Kir3.x family have been cloned from brain cDNA libraries. These channels also show strong inward rectification when expressed alone, but appear to be further activated by co-expression of G protein-coupled receptors (Doupnik *et al.*, 1995). Heterologous expression of one member of this family, Kir 3.3, does not seem to form channels irrespective of whether receptors are co-expressed. Nevertheless, Kir3.3 may combine with other Kir3.x α-subunits to form a heteromultimeric channel and thus could contribute to the diversity of neuronal K$^+$-channels (Doupnik *et al.*, 1995). Similarly, Kir5.1 does not form functional homomultimeric K$^+$-channels after expression in *Xenopus* oocytes but may form part of native heteromultimeric, inwardly rectifying K$^+$-channels (Doupnik *et al.*, 1995).

6.5.3 Modulators of voltage-sensitive K$^+$-channels

Inhibitors. Many of the known toxin K$^+$-channel inhibitors are peptides containing 37–39 residues and derived from scorpion venom. They have been systematically classified as 'α-K$^+$-toxins' (αKTx) and on the basis of sequence similarities they can be divided into four subfamilies (Miller, 1995). They are all neurotoxic, K$^+$-channel-specific and active in the nanomolar range. These toxins have evolved as inhibitors of voltage-sensitive K$^+$-channels and they are known to interact with an αKTx 'receptor' located between the 40 residues which constitute the P-region of the channel pore (*Figure 6.1*). This effectively plugs the channel, an action which prevents or delays neuronal repolarization and induces disruption of the central nervous system.

Toxins in the first subfamily of scorpion toxins, charybdotoxin and iberiotoxin (αKTx1.1 and αKTx1.3), are inhibitors of BK_{Ca}. Early findings that charybdotoxin (isolated from the venom of the scorpion *Leiurus quinquestriatus*) inhibited delayed rectifier K$^+$-channels were essentially due to the presence of impurities such as agitoxins

(Garcia et al., 1994). Thus, in most tissues, inhibition of a K^+-current by charybdotoxin is usually an indication that the underlying channel *is* BK_{Ca}. Nevertheless, even synthetic charybdotoxin is not totally selective for BK_{Ca} since this toxin inhibits Kv1.3 with a K_i value of 0.19 nM (Garcia et al., 1995). Charybdotoxin is thought to bind to the outer vestibule of the channel and thus physically block the movement of K^+ (MacKinnon et al., 1990).

Iberiotoxin is purified from the venom of the scorpion *Bothus tamulus* (Galvez et al., 1990). Although this toxin is of a similar size to charybdotoxin, with which it shares approximately 70% sequence homology, it is a more highly selective inhibitor of BK_{Ca} (Galvez et al., 1990). Thus iberiotoxin is unable to inhibit the binding of charybdotoxin to voltage-sensitive K^+-channels (Kv1.3) in brain or human T-lymphocytes (Garcia et al., 1995). Furthermore, the mechanism by which iberiotoxin inhibits BK_{Ca} (and the *slo* channel) may also differ from that of charybdotoxin and may involve a reduction in the channel mean open time (Galvez et al., 1990).

The second subfamily of scorpion toxins consists of noxiustoxin and margatoxin (αKTx2.1 and αKTx2.2). Noxiustoxin was first described as an inhibitor of delayed rectifier channels in the squid giant axon, although in this tissue its potency is relatively low (K_d approximately 400 nM; Carbone et al., 1982). However, this toxin is a much more potent inhibitor of Kv1.3 heterologously expressed in *Xenopus* oocytes (K_d 0.2 nM). Although it has no effect on BK_{Ca}, noxiustoxin inhibits charybdotoxin binding to Jurkat cells and human T-lymphocytes, suggesting that, like margatoxin, noxiustoxin may be a selective inhibitor of Kv1.3 channels (Garcia et al., 1995).

The primary sequences of margatoxin (from the venom of *Centruroides margaritatus*) and noxiustoxin (from *C. noxius* venom) are highly homologous (79% identity) (Garcia et al., 1995). Margatoxin selectively inhibits Kv1.3 channels (K_d 50 pM) and also inhibits the binding of charybdotoxin to these channels. At concentrations up to 1 μM, margatoxin has no effect on BK_{Ca} (Garcia et al., 1995). The selectivity of margatoxin may aid in the identification of the α-subunit composition of native K^+-channels.

The third subfamily of scorpion toxins consists of kaliotoxin and the agitoxins (αKTx3.1 and αKTx3.2–3.4). As already mentioned, the ability of charybdotoxin to inhibit voltage-sensitive K^+-channels is partly due to impurities co-extracted from the venom of *L. quinquestriatus hebraeus*. These contaminants were subsequently isolated and named agitoxins (Garcia et al., 1994). The agitoxins share a high degree of sequence homology (80–90%) with kaliotoxin (Garcia et al., 1994) and agitoxin$_1$ inhibits Kv1.1, Kv1.3 and Kv1.6 with K_i values of 136 nM, 1.7 nM and 149 nM, respectively. The equivalent values for agitoxin$_2$, the most potent of the agitoxins, are 44 pM, 4 pM and 37 pM, respectively. At concentrations up to 2 μM, the agitoxins do not inhibit Kv2.1 or BK_{Ca} (Garcia et al., 1994).

Despite their similarity to the agitoxins, the kaliotoxins (derived from the venom of the scorpion *Androctonus mauretanicus mauretanicus*) were first described as selective inhibitors of BK_{Ca} in *Helix* neurons and rabbit sympathetic neurons (Crest et al., 1992). Later, the ability of these toxins to inhibit the current carried by cloned Kv1.1 and Kv1.3 channels with half-blocking concentrations of 40 nM and 0.6 nM, respectively, was demonstrated (Grissmer et al., 1994).

The fourth subfamily of scorpion toxins is represented by the tityustoxins (αKTx4.x). These toxins (TsTX-Kα and K^+-β) have been isolated from the venom of the Brazilian scorpion *Tityus serrulatus*. In rat brain synaptosomes, both toxins inhibit a noninactivating voltage-sensitive channel but have no effect on the dendrotoxin-sensitive A-current

(Rogowski *et al.*, 1994). However, TsTX-Kα can completely displace α-dendrotoxin, whereas TsTX-Kβ has no effect (Rogowski *et al.*, 1994). The Kα form of the toxin produces selective blockade of delayed-rectifier K$^+$-channels, and in particular of Kv1.2.

Several dendrotoxins, derived from the venom of green mamba or black mamba snakes have now been isolated and show some selectivity in their inhibition of K$^+$-channels. Thus, whereas α-dendrotoxin (from the green mamba, *Dendroaspis angusticeps*) inhibits I$_A$, dendrotoxin-I (from the black mamba, *D. polylepis*) inhibits a delayed-rectifier K$^+$-channel (see Dreyer, 1990). The dendrotoxin binding site also binds mast cell degranulating peptide (MCDP) (see below), β-bungarotoxin and charybdotoxin (Dreyer, 1990).

Dendrotoxin inhibits A-type K$^+$-channels in both central and peripheral neurons, facilitating transmitter release and producing epileptic-like seizures *in vivo* (Bagetta *et al.*, 1992). In peripheral neurons it also inhibits a delayed rectifier channel (see Bagetta *et al.*, 1992).

Apamin, isolated from the venom of the honey bee, *Apis mellifera*, is a selective inhibitor of the small conductance, calcium-sensitive K$^+$-channel, SK$_{Ca}$, in cultured skeletal muscle cells (Dreyer, 1990) and does not inhibit other K$^+$-channel types in a variety of tissues. Apamin is the only polypeptide neurotoxin which is known to cross the blood–brain barrier. *In vivo* it causes hyperactivity, convulsions and at higher concentrations, death (LD$_{50}$ in mice approximately 4 mg kg^{-1}, i.p.) (see Dreyer, 1990). By extrapolation, it is assumed that the inhibitory effects of apamin on calcium-sensitive afterhyperpolarizations results from its inhibition of SK$_{Ca}$ in autonomic and cortical neurons. Nevertheless, patch-clamp techniques have failed to demonstrate any effect of apamin on neuronal cells. Genes which encode channels with properties resembling those of SK$_{Ca}$ have recently been described (Köhler *et al.*, 1996).

MCDP is also a constituent of the venom of the honey bee, *A. mellifera*. Its name derives from its ability to stimulate degranulation of mast cells and histamine release. In addition, it is a potent inhibitor of Kv1.1 and Kv1.2 delayed-rectifier-type channels, but has essentially no effect on Kv1.3, Kv1.4, Kv1.5 or Kv3.1 (Dolly and Parcej, 1996; Grissmer *et al.*, 1994). Whether other homomultimeric K$^+$-channels are inhibited by MCDP remains to be established. High affinity MCDP binding occurs in all regions of the brain. Intraventricular injection of MCDP produces epileptiform seizures and death (LD$_{50}$ approximately 10 μg kg^{-1} in mice) although its intravenous injection is essentially without effect (see Dreyer, 1990).

Leiurotoxin I (scyllatoxin), isolated from the venom of *L. quinquestriatus hebraeus*, was found to be an inhibitor of SK$_{Ca}$. Although it is structurally unrelated to apamin, it displaces apamin binding from synaptosomes (Dreyer, 1990). Few studies have focused on leiurotoxin I and thus any effect on transmitter release remains to be established.

The finding that a series of indole alkaloids potentiated neurotransmitter release (Norris *et al.*, 1980) prompted their testing in ^{125}I-labeled charybdotoxin binding assays (Knaus *et al.*, 1994b). In these, the alkaloids could be divided into inhibitors and enhancers of binding, typified by penitrem A and paxilline (*Figure 6.6*), respectively. Further studies showed that these effects resulted from a likely interaction of the agents with a single, specific site on the channel β-subunit resulting in a positive or negative allosteric modification of the charybdotoxin binding site itself (Kaczorowski *et al.*, 1996; Knaus *et al.*, 1994b). Paradoxically, however, *both* groups of agent acted as potent inhibitors of BK$_{Ca}$ with IC$_{50}$ values in the range 1–10 nM in both

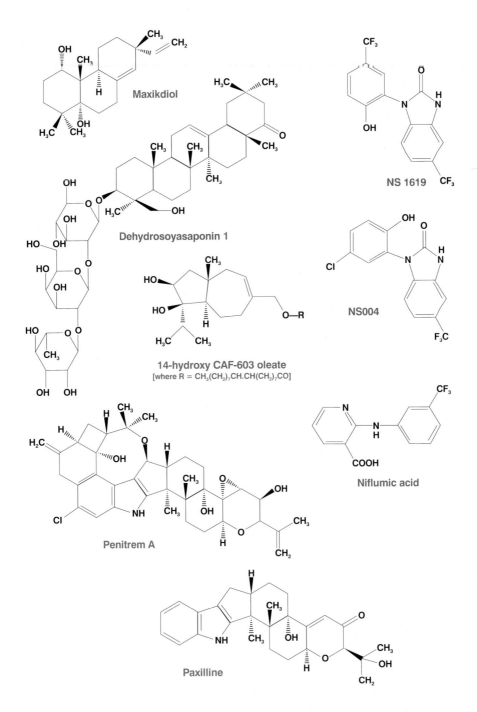

Figure 6.6. Structural formulae of some K$^+$-channel modulators mentioned in the text.

isolated patch and lipid bilayer experiments (Knaus et al., 1994b). In whole-cell studies, at least one of the agents, penitrem A, inhibited current flow through BK_{Ca} induced by the benzimidazolone, NS1619 (Edwards et al., 1994).

Openers. Until recently, the term K^+-channel opener was restricted to agents which could open the voltage-*insensitive* K^+-channel, K_{ATP} (see Edwards and Weston, 1993). Recently, however, openers of voltage-sensitive K^+-channels have been developed but these are currently restricted to agents which interact with BK_{Ca} (*Figure 6.6*). BK_{Ca} is found in virtually all tissues (Edwards and Weston, 1996) and because of its large conductance, the opening of a few such channels would produce significant hyperpolarization. However, the threshold potential at which BK_{Ca} opens seems to vary in different tissues. This channel is thus thought to be mainly involved in action potential repolarization in neurons whereas both this role and the determination of resting membrane potential may be subserved in smooth muscle such as trachealis (Sah, 1996; Small et al., 1996). From the clinical perspective, BK_{Ca} openers may prove useful in the treatment of conditions associated with excessive neuronal discharge such as epilepsy and in the irritable bowel and unstable bladder syndromes in which $[Ca^{2+}]_i$ is likely to be greater than in normally active tissue (Edwards and Weston, 1996).

A series of substituted *benzimidazolones* which open BK_{Ca} has recently been developed. These agents, typified by NS004 and NS1619 (*Figure 6.6*) open native BK_{Ca} in a variety of tissues (Olesen et al., 1994a,b). In addition, the open probability of BK_{Ca} channels derived from rat cortex and incorporated into lipid bilayers is increased over a range of potentials, suggesting that these agents act to shift the voltage sensitivity of the channel (Olesen et al., 1994a) by a direct interaction with its α-subunit (Dworetzky et al., 1994). Both NS004 and NS1619 are membrane permeable. They are capable of activating BK_{Ca} when applied either intra- or extracellularly and their effects are antagonized by various inhibitors including charybdotoxin, iberiotoxin and penitrem A (Olesen et al., 1994a). Although they are an interesting initial development, careful studies have shown that the effects of the benzimidazolones are not selective and that they also inhibit a variety of other voltage-sensitive ion channels including K_V and L-type Ca^{2+}-channels (Edwards et al., 1994).

Derivatives of *fenamic acid* are best known as inhibitors of Ca^{2+}-sensitive chloride channels. However, these agents which include niflumic acid (*Figure 6.6*), are also openers of BK_{Ca} (see Kirkup et al., 1996). Like the benzimidazolones, their site of action is probably the channel α-subunit although the mechanism involved is not understood (Wallner et al., 1995).

A systematic search for naturally occurring openers of BK_{Ca} has been made by Kaczorowski and co-workers (Kaczorowski et al., 1996). Using ^{125}I-labeled charybdotoxin as a marker ligand, several competitive and allosteric inhibitors of binding have been identified. The most potent of these was *dehydrosoyasaponin-1* (*Figure 6.6*), a glycosylated triterpene which acts as an allosteric inhibitor with a K_i value of approximately 120 nM (McManus et al., 1993). Unfortunately, the poor membrane permeability of this compound renders it effective only after intracellular application which precludes any therapeutic potential. Nevertheless, it may be a useful tool with which to provide an insight into the regulation of channel gating. Dehydrosoyasaponin-1 is of additional interest since it is the first compound described which requires the presence of both the α- and the β-subunit of BK_{Ca} before the channel will open (McManus et al., 1995).

Using ^{125}I-labeled charybdotoxin binding, Singh *et al.* (1994) identified a dihydroxy-isoprimane diterpene opener of BK_{Ca} and subsequently named the agent '*maxikdiol*' (*Figure 6.6*). Like dehydrosoyasaponin-1, this agent is an allosteric inhibitor of binding but approximately 10–30 times less potent (Singh *et al.*, 1994). Like the soyasaponin, maxikdiol is active when applied to the cytoplasmic face of BK_{Ca} but in contrast, its action does not require the presence of the channel β-subunit (Kaczorowski *et al.*, 1996).

Several *carotane sesquiterpene* derivatives have been isolated from culture systems of *Trichoderma virens* and found to interfere with ^{125}I-labeled charybdotoxin binding to smooth muscle membranes (Lee *et al.*, 1995). Subsequently, some of these agents were found to exhibit BK_{Ca}-opening properties in isolated patch and lipid bilayer experiments, the most potent compound being 14-hydroxy CAF-603 oleate (*Figure 6.6*; Lee *et al.*, 1995). Like dehydrosoyasaponin-1, this carotane derivative is only active when applied to the inner face of the channel (Lee *et al.*, 1995).

6.6 Ca²⁺ channels

6.6.1 Classification of native Ca²⁺ channels

As was the case with voltage-sensitive K^+-channels (see Section 6.5.1), voltage-sensitive Ca^{2+}-channels are currently classified according to a combination of both electrophysiological and pharmacological properties. The resulting trivial designations (into 'L-type', 'N-type', etc.) are hardly satisfactory but these are likely to remain until the exact subunit composition of the native channels is better understood. The general function of these channels in neurons is to allow Ca^{2+} to influx into the cell with the resultant modulation of a variety of processes, the most important of which are probably the initiation of transmitter release and the modulation of Ca^{2+}-sensitive systems such as ion channels. To date, six classes of voltage-sensitive Ca^{2+}-channels have been described and these can be broadly divided into two groups according to the degree of membrane depolarization which is required to activate them. The majority (L-, N-, P- and Q-types) require substantial membrane depolarization for activation and are sometimes referred to as 'high voltage-activated'. The R-type channel activates after moderate depolarization while the remaining T-type channel opens at relatively negative potentials (Dunlap *et al.*, 1995; Stea *et al.*, 1993; Varadi *et al.*, 1995).

The channels can be further characterized on the basis of their unitary conductance and on their pharmacological properties. In parallel with the approach adopted for voltage-sensitive K^+-channels, the subunit composition of native channels has been inferred by comparing their pharmacological and other properties with those of individual subunits expressed in heterologous systems.

L-type Ca²⁺-channels. These are found not only in neurons and neuroendocrine cells but also in a variety of other tissue types including cardiac, skeletal and smooth muscle. They are involved in neurotransmitter release at some synapses (Perney *et al.*, 1986) and may play a role in long-term potentiation (Johnston *et al.*, 1992). The channels have a unitary conductance of approximately 25 pS and are stimulated to open by depolarization to potentials more positive than approximately –30 mV (high threshold activation). The channel inactivates relatively slowly in most tissues and this property (long-lasting opening) has given rise to the familiar name, 'L'-type. L-type

Ca^{2+}-channels in neurons show little inactivation, apparently due to the absence of a calcium-binding motif which is responsible for calcium-sensitive inactivation in non-neuronal L-type Ca^{2+}-channels (de Leon *et al.*, 1995). L-type Ca^{2+}-channels are distinguished from other calcium channels by the lack of effect of ω-conotoxin GVIA (see Section 6.6.3) and by their sensitivity to inhibition by dihydropyridines, benzothiazepines and phenylalkylamines. Since binding sites for these agents are restricted to the products of the α_{1S}, α_{1C} and α_{1D} genes, it seems likely that these form the core of L-type channels (Section 6.6.2; Dunlap *et al.*, 1995; Varadi *et al.*, 1995).

N-type Ca^{2+}-channels. In contrast to the ubiquitous distribution of L-type Ca^{2+}-channels, N-type Ca^{2+}-channels are restricted to neurons and neuroendocrine cells in which they are involved in neurotransmitter and neurohormone release (Dunlap *et al.*, 1995; Varadi *et al.*, 1995). Like the L-type Ca^{2+}-channel, the N-type requires a substantial depolarizing step for activation and exhibits time-dependent inactivation. Their pore-forming region probably consists of α_{1B} gene products (Dunlap *et al.*, 1995; Varadi *et al.*, 1995).

N-type channels are insensitive to dihydropyridines but are potently and selectively inhibited by ω-conotoxin GVIA and ω-conotoxin MVIIA (Section 6.6.3; Miljanich and Ramachandran., 1995; Olivera *et al.*, 1994). They are also inhibited by several neurotransmitters (e.g. glutamate, γ-aminobutyric acid or adenosine, probably by a mechanism which involves G proteins (Chernevskaya *et al.*, 1991; Cox and Dunlap, 1992; Swartz and Bean, 1992). In addition, they are activated by diadenosine polyphosphates, presumably via purinoceptors (Panchenko *et al.*, 1996).

P-type Ca^{2+}-channels. P-type Ca^{2+}-channels are found in a variety of neurons but are particularly abundant in cerebellar Purkinje neurons, in which they were first identified and from which they derive their name (Llinás *et al.*, 1989). They play a role in neurotransmitter release and are involved in the induction of long-term depression. The channels, which have a unitary conductance of 10–20 pS, have a high-voltage threshold of activation, similar to that of L- and N-types, and inactivate slowly. They are essentially insensitive both to the dihydropyridines and to ω-conotoxin GVIA but are inhibited by ω-agatoxin IVA and a polyamine, FTX, both of which are derived from the venom of the funnel-web spider, *Agelenopsis aperta* (Section 6.6.3; Llinás *et al.*, 1989; Mintz *et al.*, 1992a,b) as well as by ω-conotoxin MVIIC (Section 6.6.3; Hillyard *et al.*, 1992). Like N-type channels, P-type Ca^{2+}-channels appear to be inhibited by a G-protein-coupled mechanism (Mintz and Bean, 1993). Their pore-forming region may comprise the products of the α_{1A} gene (Dunlap *et al.*, 1995; Varadi *et al.*, 1995).

Q-type Ca^{2+}-channels. Q-type Ca^{2+}-channels may be essentially identical to those of the P-type. The innermost part of the latter is believed to be formed from the product of the α_{1A} gene. However, expression of this in *Xenopus* oocytes results in a calcium current with properties which differ from those of the P-channel (Wheeler *et al.*, 1994). Like those of the P-type, Q-type channels are inhibited by neurotransmitters acting via G protein-coupled receptors (Wheeler *et al.*, 1994). These channels are inhibited by high concentrations of ω-conotoxin MVIIC or ω-agatoxin IVA (Hillyard *et al.*, 1992; Randall and Tsien, 1995), toxins which in lower concentrations also inhibit both N-type and P-type Ca^{2+}-channels. They can be distinguished from N-type channels by their insensitivity to ω-conotoxin GVIA.

R-type Ca^{2+}-channels. High-voltage threshold Ca^{2+}-channels which are unaffected by dihydropyridines, phenylalkylamines, and conotoxins have been designated R-type (Randall and Tsien, 1995). These neuronal channels are thought to carry a large proportion of the calcium current which is stimulated by glutamate release in response to ischemia or traumatic brain injury and which results in cell death. Selective inhibitors of this channel remain to be identified. Nonselective inhibitors include amiloride (1 mM) or Ni^{2+} (approximately 50 μM) (see Magee and Johnston, 1995). CNS 2103, a compound derived from spider toxin inhibits both R-type and L-type Ca^{2+}-channels (McBurney *et al.*, 1992) and may prove to be useful in the identification of R-type channels. Furthermore, its nonselectivity may be an asset in inhibiting the toxic effect of glutamate-stimulated calcium influx. Expression experiments tentatively suggest that these channels may be formed from the product of the α_{1E} gene (Dunlap *et al.*, 1995; Varadi *et al.*, 1995).

T-type channels. T-type Ca^{2+}-channels were so named because of their transient opening. These small-conductance channels (unitary conductance approximately 8 pS) are activated by a relatively small depolarization of the membrane (activation threshold approximately –70 mV) and inactivate rapidly. It is thought that they play a major role in repetitive firing in neurons (Coulter *et al.*, 1989). Potent inhibitors of T-type channels remain to be identified and these channels are thus distinguished by their electrophysiological characteristics. T-type channels are relatively unaffected by dihydropyridines, they are insensitive to toxin inhibitors but they are inhibited by nickel, lanthanum ions and amiloride (Bean and Mintz, 1994). The gene product which forms their inner core has not yet been identified (Dunlap *et al.*, 1995; Varadi *et al.*, 1995).

6.6.2 Classification of Ca^{2+}-channel genes and their products

Studies on the L-type Ca^{2+}-channel from skeletal muscle established that it was a complex of five different gene products comprising not only the α_1-subunit, which defines the pore, but also an α_2/δ-, a β- and a γ-subunit (*Figure 6.3*; Dunlap *et al.*, 1995; Perez-Reyes and Schneider, 1994; Varadi *et al.*, 1995). The α_1-, α_2/δ- and γ-subunits which span the membrane or are extracellularly located are associated with the intracellular β-subunit in a 1:1:1:1 ratio. With the exception of the γ-subunit which has not yet been detected in the brain, this complex structure is essentially present in all types of voltage-sensitive Ca^{2+}-channels so far studied.

Ca^{2+}-channel α_1-subunits. In contrast to the innermost part of voltage-sensitive K$^+$-channels belonging to Superfamily 1, this component of voltage-sensitive Ca^{2+}-channels is the product of a single gene. However, because of the repeating nature of domains I–IV, the resulting structure is superficially very similar to that of the K$^+$-channel (*Figures 6.1* and *6.3*). Six α_1-subunit genes have been identified and there are several alternatively spliced variants. There are at least three alternative nomenclature systems in use and we have adopted the α_{1X} system proposed by Snutch *et al.* (1990) from which the genes are designated α_{1A-E} and α_{1S} (*Figure 6.7*; *Table 6.1*).

Each α_1-subunit domain consists of six hydrophobic segments with the S4 component in each domain acting as a voltage sensor. Binding sites for the dihydropyridine, phenyl-

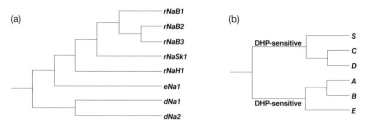

Figure 6.7. Schematic phylogenic trees for genes encoding: (a) Na$^+$-channel α-subunits or (b) Ca^{2+}-channel α_1-subunits. Adapted from Goldin (1995) and Stea *et al.* (1995).

alkylamine and benzothiazepine inhibitors (*Figure 6.8*; see Section 6.6.3) are present only on the α_{1S} (skeletal muscle), α_{1C} (cardiac and smooth muscle, brain) and α_{1D} (brain, endocrine and kidney) gene products which accounts for the selective action of these agents at the sites indicated. Variants which result from alternative splicing at various points in the α_{1S}-subunit are known but the possible functional significance of these is not understood. Ca^{2+}-selective channels can be formed experimentally from the expression of α_1-subunits alone in heterologous systems and co-expression studies have shown that the basic properties of the channel formed by the α_1 polypeptide are modulated by the presence of the β-, α_2/δ- and γ-subunits (Dunlap *et al.*, 1995; Varadi *et al.*, 1995).

Ca^{2+}-channel α_2/δ-subunits. This complex subunit is highly glycosylated and has been isolated from skeletal muscle, brain and heart. It is derived from a single gene, the product of which is cleaved post-translationally to generate the α_2 and δ polypeptides. The latter is probably incorporated into the membrane where it re-combines with the α_2-subunit via disulfide bridges (*Figure 6.3*). Co-expression of α_1 polypeptides with α_2/δ-subunits in *Xenopus* oocytes results in up to a 10-fold increase in current amplitude (Dunlap *et al.*, 1995; Varadi *et al.*, 1995).

Ca^{2+}-channel β-subunits. Four distinct β-subunit genes (β_1–β_4) have been identified following the initial discovery of the gene product in skeletal muscle extracts. Alternatively spliced variants of all forms are known and all four subtypes are present

Table 6.1. Comparison of properties of native calcium channel types

Native Ca^{2+}-channel	α-subunit gene	Unitary conductance	Voltage threshold	Pharmacology
L	α_{1C} α_{1D} α_{1S}	25 pS	High	Dihydopyridines (e.g. nimodipine)
N	α_{1B}	12–20 pS	High	ω-CTX-GVIA, ω-CTX-MVIIC
P	α_{1A}?	10–12 pS	High	ω-Aga-IVA, ω-Aga-IVB, ω-CTX-MVIIC, FTX
Q	α_{1A}	?	High	ω-Ctx-MVIIC, ω-Aga-IVA
R	α_{1E}	15–20 pS	Medium	Ni^{2+}, amiloride; resistant to toxins
T	α_1?	8 pS	Low	Amiloride, flunarizine, ethosuximide, Ni^{2+}; resistant to toxins

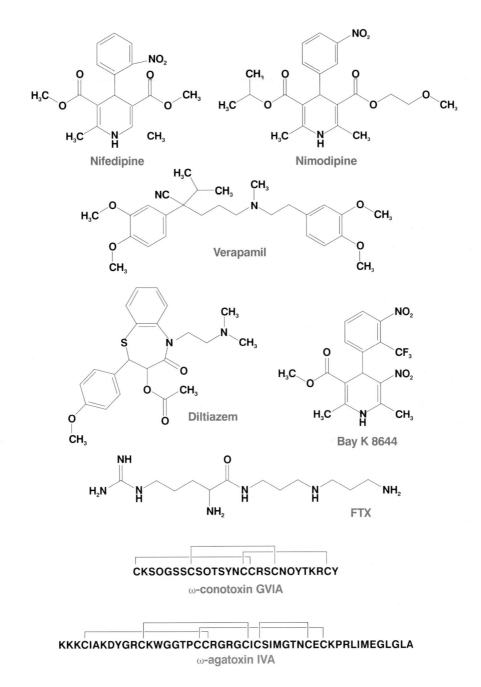

CKSOGSSCSOTSYNCCRSCNOYTKRCY

ω-conotoxin GVIA

KKKCIAKDYGRCKWGGTPCCRGRGCICSIMGTNCECKPRLIMEGLGLA

ω-agatoxin IVA

Figure 6.8. Structural formulae of some Ca²⁺-channel modulators mentioned in the text. The FTX structure shown is a synthetic molecule which mimics the effects of the polyamine found in natural funnel-web spider toxin. The toxins ω-conotoxin GV1A and ω-agatoxin IVA are described by the standard single letter convention for amino acids: disulfide bridges linking cysteine residues are shown.

in brain. They are hydrophilic polypeptides containing 500–600 residues and they are believed to be located intracellularly where they interact with the cytoplasmic linker region between domains I and II of the α_1-subunit. When co-expressed with α-subunits in *Xenopus* oocytes, an increase in current amplitude is observed. Additionally, shifts in voltage-dependence of activation and changes in both activation and inactivation kinetics have been reported depending on the expression system and β-subtype. An increase in the number of dihydropyridine binding sites has also been detected (Dunlap *et al.*, 1995; Perez-Reyes and Schneider, 1994; Varadi *et al.*, 1995).

Ca²⁺-channel γ-subunits. The γ-subunit gene encodes a glycosylated polypeptide containing some 222 amino acid residues with four hydrophobic regions which are putative membrane-spanning components (*Figure 6.3*). Coexpression with α_1-subunits results in an increase in current amplitude and changes in activation kinetics. γ-Subunits have not yet been reported in brain and they may be essentially restricted to skeletal muscle (Perez-Reyes and Schneider, 1994).

6.6.3 *Modulators of voltage-sensitive Ca²⁺-channels*

Inhibitors. The ω-conotoxins are members of a family of peptides (25–29 residues) found in the venom of fish-hunting cone snails, typified by *Conus geographus* and *C. magus*. The designation 'omega' derives from the fact that they inhibit Ca²⁺-channels at nerve *endings* and the prefix 'G' or 'M' indicates the snail species from which the venom is derived. The first one of these to be characterized, ω-conotoxin GVIA, was found to inhibit dihydropyridine-insensitive Ca²⁺-currents in neurons and was instrumental in distinguishing N-type Ca²⁺-currents from the electrophysiologically similar L-type. Two other conotoxins, ω-conotoxin MVIIA and ω-conotoxin MVIIC also inhibit N-type channels. However, ω-conotoxin MVIIC also inhibits P/Q-type channels which are relatively unaffected by ω-conotoxin MVIIA. The site of action of these toxins is assumed to be located in the channel pore but the exact locus is unknown (Olivera *et al.*, 1994).

The venom of the funnel web spider (*A. aperta*) contains several ion channel-active toxins known collectively as agatoxins. Among these, the ω-agatoxins inhibit neuronal Ca²⁺-currents and ω-agatoxins IVA in particular is a potent inhibitor of P/Q-type Ca²⁺-channels (Olivera *et al.*, 1994).

Most of the numerous, so-called 'Ca²⁺-channel antagonists' which are not of toxin origin are drugs selective for L-type Ca²⁺-channels. These agents, typified by the dihydropyridines like nifedipine, the benzothiazepines typified by diltiazem and the phenylalkylamines such as verapamil (*Figure 6.8*; see Triggle, 1994) only inhibit L-type calcium channels. These are formed from α_1-subunits which are the products of the *S, C* and *D* genes (Dunlap *et al.*, 1995; Triggle, 1994; Varadi *et al.*, 1995). Of the inhibitors, nimodipine (*Figure 6.8*) most readily passes the blood–brain barrier and must thus have the greatest therapeutic potential in the regulation of neuronal L-type Ca²⁺-channels.

Although the dihydropyridines, benzothiazepines and phenylalkylamines all interact with the α_1-subunit of the L-type Ca²⁺-channel, they each have distinct binding sites (Spedding and Paoletti, 1992; Varadi *et al.*, 1995). Photo-affinity labeling techniques have located the binding site for the phenylalkylamines to the S6 segment in domain IV and a further sequence in the adjacent carboxylic acid tail. Similar approaches have identified the principal dihydropyridine site to the S6 segment in domain III with a further interaction on S6 in domain IV. Experiments with diltiazem analogs have suggested that the benzothiazepines bind to the extracellular linker between S5 and S6. These experiments are not without their limitations but the broad involvement of regions close to the channel pore is strongly indicated for all three classes of L-type inhibitor. Interestingly, L type Ca^{2+} channels are also inhibited by several anti-epileptic drugs, including benzolamide, ethosuximide, dimethadione, phenobarbital and zonisamide (Gottfried and Chesler, 1995) and this action may thus play a role in their anti-epileptic effects.

L-type channels are widely distributed and are particularly important in the regulation of smooth muscle activity in the vasculature. Since 'Ca^{2+}-antagonists' are hypotensive, their therapeutic usefulness in the modulation of neuronal activity may be limited. In contrast, selective inhibitors of the T-type Ca^{2+}-channel could be effective modifiers of the excessive neuronal activity associated with epilepsy or used to protect against calcium-mediated toxicity. Some anti-convulsants such as phenytoin, ethosuximide and flunarizine are somewhat selective for T-type channels (Bean and Mintz, 1994; Takahashi and Akaike, 1991), the inhibition of which may be clinically relevant. However, selective inhibitors of T-type Ca^{2+}-channels are unknown.

Openers. The dihydropyridines S(–)-Bay-K^+ 8644 (*Figure 6.8*) and S(+)-202791 *prolong* the open time of L-type channels and shift their activation threshold towards a more negative potential (Bean and Mintz, 1994; Triggle *et al.*, 1991). In contrast, the R(+) enantiomer of Bay-K^+ 8644 is a typical inhibitor of this channel. It is assumed that the interaction of S(–)-Bay-K^+ 8644 with sites on the α_1-subunit favors the open state, although this has not been investigated in detail.

6.7 Na+-channels

Voltage-sensitive Na^+ channels are critically important in generating the upstroke of action potentials. In nonneuronal tissues, this is generally the prelude to an excitatory event but in neurons the arrival of the action potential at the nerve terminal can result in the release of either excitatory or inhibitory transmitters.

6.7.1 Classification of native Na+-channels

Electrophysiologically, Na^+-channels in all tissues activate and inactivate rapidly. However, the existence of different subtypes can be inferred from tissue-specific differences in their sensitivity to inhibition by tetrodotoxin and μ-conotoxin (see Section 6.7.3) and by the presence of structurally different α-subunits in different tissues. Tentatively, therefore, evidence for the existence of five subtypes of mammalian Na^+-channel has been obtained but no systematic nomenclature system exists. Types I, II and III are found in the brain, the μ-type is located in skeletal muscle while the variant known as 'H1' is restricted to the heart and to denervated skeletal muscle (Catterall, 1995; Goldin, 1995; Kirsch, 1994).

Structurally, the channels comprise a central pore-forming α-subunit, the membrane-spanning portions of which show homology with the comparable segments of voltage-sensitive Ca^{2+}-channels (*Figure 6.3*). However, the hydrophilic regions which connect the membrane-spanning segments differ from their Ca^{2+}-channel equivalents (Catterall, 1995). In addition to the α-subunit, purification of brain Na^+-channels reveals the presence of both β_1- and β_2-subunits in a stoichiometry of 1:1:1 with the α-polypeptide. The β structures are both probably anchored in the membrane with only the β_2 attached to the α-subunit. In some tissues, no β_1 and/or β_2 peptides seem to be present, resulting in native channels which are monomers or dimers (Catterall, 1995; Goldin, 1995; Isom et al., 1994).

6.7.2 Classification of Na+-channel genes and their products

α-Subunits. Genes have been cloned which encode Na+-channel α-subunits in a variety of mammalian and nonmammalian species. No systematic nomenclature system yet exists but the possible evolutionary relationship between the products of eight of these is shown in *Figure 6.7*. NaB1–3 are expressed in the brain (NaB2 and NaB3 are alternatively spliced products of the same gene) while the skeletal muscle genes, *NaSk1* and *NaSk2*, encode subunits which are tetrodotoxin-sensitive and -insensitive, respectively. NaH1 is predominantly expressed in cardiac muscle, although it also occurs in denervated skeletal muscle.

The α-subunit products of these genes alone are capable of forming Na+-selective channels in heterologous expression systems such as the *Xenopus* oocyte. However, these exhibit two different gating modes, one of which is very rapid and similar to that of native channels while the other is much slower (Isom et al., 1994). In spite of any differences between the behavior of cloned and native channels, it is customary to infer the α-subunit composition of a *native* channel if its properties are only moderately mirrored by those of an expressed α-subunit.

β-Subunits. As is the case with both the K+-channel and Ca2+-channel β-subunits (Sections 6.5.2 and 6.6.2; Isom et al., 1994), Na+-channel β-subunits modify the properties of the associated α-polypeptide. When co-expressed in *Xenopus* oocytes with α-subunits, the β_1-subunit also modifies channel activity by shifting the voltage-threshold in a hyperpolarizing direction and enhancing the rate of channel inactivation to values more typical of native channels (Catterall, 1992). This suggests that the presence of the β_1-subunit favors the rapid gating mode (Catterall, 1992; Isom et al., 1994). Furthermore, the expression of α-subunits is greatly increased when β-subunits are co-expressed, suggesting that their presence might be rate-limiting in the production of mature Na+-channel complexes (Isom et al., 1994).

Relatively little is known about the role played by Na+-channel β-subunits. However, coexpression of β_2- and α-subunits in *Xenopus* oocytes not only increases the functional expression of the α-subunit and modulates channel gating but also increases the cell surface area. This may be related to the presence of a fold similar in structure to that of the cell adhesion molecule, contactin, in the amino-terminal region of the β_2-subunit. This could suggest a role in the expression and localization of the Na+-channel complex in the membrane (Isom et al., 1995).

6.7.3 Modulation of Na+-channel gating

In general, voltage-sensitive Na+-channels are closed at resting membrane potentials and open (activate) when the membrane is stepped to potentials more positive than their activation threshold. Like that of other voltage-sensitive channels, the S4 region of each domain of the Na+-channel protein (see *Figure 6.3*) is thought to act as the channel voltage sensor. The rapid influx of Na+ into the cell when Na+-channels open produces an action potential which is terminated, in part, by the rapid inactivation of the channel (and in part by the opening of voltage-sensitive K^+-channels). Inactivation is associated with the intracellular linker region between domains III and IV. Although there is no sequence homology, this region probably acts in a manner analogous to the inactivating peptide of the K^+-channel (Patton *et al.*, 1993). Indeed, insertion of amino acids corresponding to the peptide which links domain III to domain IV in the Na^+-channel α-subunit into the amino terminus end of a noninactivating K^+-channel α-subunit introduces K^+-channel inactivation (Patton *et al.*, 1993).

Inactivated Na^+-channels are nonconducting and the channels are only reprimed for opening after the membrane is repolarized or hyperpolarized, properties which have been utilized in the evolutionary design of toxins (Hille, 1992). Thus, many of these alter Na^+-channel gating, resulting in paralysis. This can occur as a result of increased channel opening (or inhibition of channel inactivation) which prolongs cellular depolarization and thus increases neurotransmitter release and results in rigid paralysis. Conversely, inhibition of Na^+-channels prevents depolarization and produces a flaccid paralysis.

On the basis of extensive studies, five 'receptor sites' for the action of modulators on the channel α-subunit have been proposed (*Table 6.2*). The best characterized of these is site 1, the locus at which tetrodotoxin and saxitoxin act and which is also involved in the actions of the μ-conotoxins (Catterall, 1992, 1996).

Toxin inhibitors. Tetrodotoxin is responsible for the paralysis (and death) which may occur after ingestion of some puffer fish or other fish of the order Tetraodontiformes. It has also been found in a variety of other species, and it appears likely that it is synthesized in the host by symbiotic bacteria (see Hille, 1992). Saxitoxin is also responsible for potentially fatal food poisoning. This toxin is found in shellfish (including the clam *Saxidomus*) which have fed in water contaminated by dinoflagellates of the genus *Gonyaulax*. Both tetrodotoxin and saxitoxin bind to site 1which is present on a variety of Na^+-channel types to produce a physical blockade of the Na^+-channel pore

Table 6.2. Proposed binding sites of sodium channel modulators and their effects

Site	Modulator	Effect
1	Tetrodotoxin, saxitoxin, μ-conotoxin	Channel inhibition
2	Batrachotoxin, veratridine, aconitine, grayanotoxin	Channel activation
3	α-Scorpion toxins, sea anemone toxins	Channel inactivation slowed or abolished; enhances binding of toxins to site 2
4	β-Scorpion toxins	Voltage threshold of activation more negative
5	Brevetoxin, ciguatoxin	Voltage threshold of activation more negative; channel inactivation abolished
6	Pyrethroid insecticides, tetramethrin	Channel activation and inactivation slowed; enhances binding of toxins to site 2

(Catterall, 1996). The site comprises a critical glutamine residue on the extracellular linker between S5 and S6 in domain I and the three equivalent residues in domains II–IV. These effectively form a ring around the channel mouth and confirm the results of other experiments which indicate that tetrodotoxin plugs the channel pore. Important residues on domains I–IV form an additional binding ring (Catterall, 1996). However, the inability of permeant ions to dislodge the toxin and produce relief from block may be an indication that the proposed mechanism is too simplistic (see Moczydlowski and Schild, 1994).

μ-Conotoxins derived from *C. geographus* (μ-CTX-GIIIB and μ-CTX-GIIIC) are highly selective inhibitors of skeletal muscle Na$^+$-channels (West *et al.*, 1996). Like tetrodotoxin, the μ-conotoxins are thought to interact at site 1 on the channel (Catterall, 1996: *Table 6.2*). However, although μ-conotoxins interfere with saxitoxin binding in systems which express the NaSk1 channel, their channel-blocking effect is not modified by a channel mutation which abolishes the action of tetrodotoxin. It thus appears that the skeletal muscle Na$^+$-channel μ-CTX and tetrodotoxin binding sites are not identical, but may overlap (Stephan *et al.*, 1994).

Another group of conotoxins (μO-conotoxins), with inhibitory actions on both mammalian and molluskan neuronal Na$^+$-channels was recently isolated from the venom of *C. marmoreus* (McIntosh *et al.*, 1995).

Toxin openers. Scorpion α-toxin (α-ScTX) enhances Na$^+$-currents by inhibiting channel inactivation, whereas a similar effect is achieved by β-ScTX which shifts the threshold voltage for channel activation in a hyperpolarizing direction such that the channels can open closer to the resting potential of the cell (Catterall, 1994; Kirsch, 1994). These effects are produced by the interaction of α-ScTX and β-ScTX with sites 3 and 4, respectively (see *Table 6.2*). In the case of site 3, this is located on the extracellular loop between S5 and S6 in domain I and on the extracellular side of S5 in domain IV (Catterall, 1994, 1996). Furthermore, the observation that depolarization reduces the effectiveness of α-ScTX but potentiates that of β-ScTX suggests that each binds to a different state of the channel (Kirsch, 1994).

α-ScTX has been isolated from the venom of a variety of scorpions, including *Androctonus*, *Buthotus* and *Leiurus*. β-ScTX is found in the venom of *T. serrulatus* as well as that of several species of the genus *Centruroides* (Kirsch, 1994). Scorpion venom also contains other toxins which enhance the opening of insect or molluskan Na$^+$-channels, but which have little effect on vertebrate Na$^+$-channels (Stankiewicz *et al.*, 1996).

Batrachotoxin (*Figure 6.9*), originally isolated from the skin of the Columbian poison arrow frog *Phyllobates aurotaneia*, enhances Na$^+$-currents by suppressing both fast and slow channel inactivation and shifting the voltage-dependence of activation in a hyperpolarizing direction (Wang and Wang, 1994). It also reduces the Na$^+$:K$^+$ selectivity of the channel. Competition binding studies have demonstrated that this toxin binds to the same site on the channel (site 2) as do veratridine, aconitine and grayanotoxin (*Table 6.2*; see Moczydlowski and Schild, 1994). Recent studies have indicated the importance of the S6 region of the α-subunit domain I in the binding of batrachotoxin (Trainer *et al.*, 1996).

Properties similar to those of batrachotoxin are shared by δ-conotoxin GmVIA, recently isolated from the venom of the mollusk *C. gloriamaris* (Hasson *et al.*, 1995). Unlike the μ-conotoxin (see above), this *Conus* toxin suppresses Na$^+$-channel inacti-

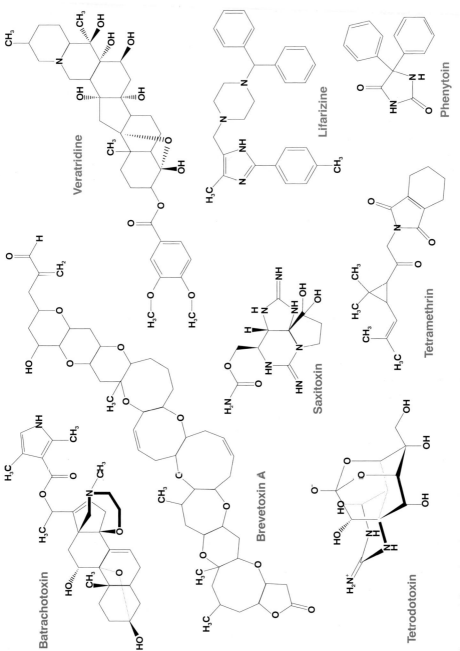
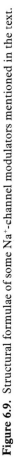

Figure 6.9. Structural formulae of some Na⁺-channel modulators mentioned in the text.

vation and shifts the voltage threshold for activation in a negative direction, effectively enhancing the Na^+-current after only a small depolarizing stimulus. In *Aplysia*, the toxin is selectively active at Na^+-channels with no effect on Ca^{2+}- or K^+-channels. The δ-conotoxin VIA and δ-conotoxin VIB (from *C. textile*) as well as δ-conotoxin GmVIA are selective for molluskan Na^+-channels whereas the toxin from *C. nigropunctatus* (NgVIA) is effective on both vertebrate and molluskan neurons. To date, only one vertebrate-selective form, δ-conotoxin PVIA from *C. purpurascens*, has been described (see West *et al.*, 1996).

The brevetoxins, which are produced by the marine dinoflagellate *Ptychodiscus brevis* (Baden, 1989), activate voltage-sensitive Na^+-channels in a manner similar to the other toxins which act at site 2 (see *Table 6.2*). However, they do not modify batrachotoxin binding and are thus thought to act at an independent site on the channel (see Baden, 1989). Another group of toxins, the ciguatoxins, which originate from the protozoon *Gambierdiscus toxicus* (Brock *et al.*, 1995) inhibit brevetoxin binding and probably act at the same site (site 5; see Catterall, 1992). By shifting the voltage-dependence of activation of Na^+-channels in a hyperpolarizing direction, brevetoxins and ciguatoxins cause the channels to open at resting membrane potentials, resulting in depolarization and action potential generation in both myelinated and unmyelinated neurons (Catterall, 1992).

Nontoxin Na^+-channel modulators. Both DDT and pyrethroid insecticides, such as tetramethrin (*Figure 6.9*), prolong the opening of neuronal Na^+-channels. This effect is attributed to stabilization of the gating charges (which move within the membrane in response to depolarization and which are thought to reflect movement of the S4 voltage sensor), an action which effectively traps the channel in a voltage-insensitive, stable open state (Salgado and Narahashi, 1993). Thus, after termination of an action potential by K^+-channel opening, the Na^+-channel may remain open and trigger a further action potential. Since pyrethroids have a higher affinity for the channel open state than for the closed or inactivated states they demonstrate use-dependence (i.e. the more frequently the channel opens, the greater the drug effect). Thus these compounds induce repetitive discharges, the frequency of which increases with time (Narahashi, 1992; Narahashi *et al.*, 1995). The action of pyrethroids is temperature-dependent and increases as the temperature is lowered, a property which probably contributes to their greater potency in insects in comparison to mammals.

'Local' anesthetics, such as procaine or lidocaine, are inhibitors of all types of Na^+-channel. Since local anesthetics preferentially bind to the open or inactivated states of the channel, they are more potent in the rapidly firing sensory neurons than in motor neurons which fire action potentials at a lower rate. Since these compounds are not neuronally selective, their clinical usefulness results from their injection into the vicinity of the appropriate neuron.

Class I cardiac antiarrhythmic agents such as lidocaine are, by definition, Na^+-channel inhibitors which exhibit some selectivity for cardiac rather than skeletal or neuronal Na^+-channels. Lidocaine binds selectively to inactivated Na^+-channels. Since the duration of the action potential in cardiac muscle is greater than that in neurons, the time during which the Na^+-channel is in the inactivated (rather than the open or closed) state and thus capable of binding lidocaine is greater in the heart than in neurons (Wang *et al.*, 1996).

The anticonvulsant and antiarrhythmic agent phenytoin (*Figure 6.9*) is another Na^+-channel inhibitor which also preferentially binds to inactivated Na^+-channels where it slows recovery from inactivation (Urenjak and Obrenovitch, 1996). Its anticonvulsant effects are presumably favored in rapidly firing neurons in which the time for which a channel will exist in an inactivated state will increase. However, other compounds such as lifarizine (*Figure 6.9*) or riluzole, which also appear only to act on the inactivated channel, are somewhat neuroprotective and the basis for this is unknown (MacKinnon *et al.*, 1995; Urenjak and Obrenovitch, 1996).

The site of action of local anesthetics and related agents is not fully understood. These agents do not modify channel block by either tetrodotoxin or saxitoxin. This lack of effect, combined with experiments using quaternary derivatives, suggests a site of action within the pore but close to its intracellular mouth. Current views favor the involvement of the intracellular margins of segments S4, S5 and S6 (Kirsch, 1994).

6.7 Conclusions

The study of voltage-sensitive channels has reached a fascinating stage. Never before has so much been known about the structure–function relationships of individual channel subunits and the diversity with which organisms have evolved channel modulators for use in stings and venoms continues to amaze. Ion channels are already drug targets of considerable clinical significance but existing agents are essentially the result of serendipitous discovery. The challenge now is to use current knowledge of channel structure and diversity to design even more useful and selective agents. Fascinating developments can confidently be expected.

Acknowledgment

Gillian Edwards was supported by the Medical Research Council.

References

Atkinson NS, Robertson GA, Ganetzky B. (1991) A component of calcium-activated potassium channels encoded by the *Drosophila slo* locus. *Science* 253: 551–555.

Baden DG. (1989) Brevetoxins: unique polyether dinoflagellate toxins. *FASEB J.* 3: 1807–1817.

Bagetta G, Nistico G, Dolly JO. (1992) Production of seizures and brain damage in rats by α-dendrotoxin, a selective K$^+$ channel blocker. *Neurosci. Lett.* 139: 34–40.

Bean BP, Mintz IM. (1994) Pharmacology of different types of calcium channels in rat neurons. In: *Handbook of Membrane Channels: Molecular and Cellular Physiology* (ed. C. Peracchia). Academic Press, London, pp. 199–210.

Brock JA, McLachlan EM, Jobling P, Lewis RJ. (1995) Electrical activity in rat tail artery during asynchronous activation of postganglionic nerve terminals by ciguatoxin-1. *Br. J. Pharmacol.* 116: 2213–2220.

Butler A, Tsunoda S, McCobb DP, Wei A, Salkoff L. (1993) *mSlo*, a complex mouse gene encoding maxi calcium-activated potassium channels. *Science* 261: 221–224.

Carbone E, Wanke E, Prestipino G, Possani L D, Maelicke A. (1982) Selective blockage of voltage-dependent K$^+$ channels by a novel scorpion toxin. *Nature* 296: 90–91.

Catterall WA. (1992) Cellular and molecular biology of voltage-gated sodium channels. *Physiol. Rev.* 72: S15-S48.

Catterall WA. (1994) Molecular properties of a superfamily of plasma-membrane cation channels. *Curr. Opin. Cell Biol.* 6: 607-615.

Catterall WA. (1995) Structure and function of voltage-gated ion channels. *Annu. Rev. Biochem.* 64: 493–531.

Catterall WA. (1996) Molecular properties of sodium and calcium channels. *J. Bioenerg. Biomembr.* 28: 219–230.

Chandy KG, Gutman GA. (1995) Voltage-gated potassium channel genes. In: *Handbook of Receptors and Channels: Ligand- and Voltage-Gated Ion Channels* (ed. RA North). CRC Press, London, pp.1–71.

Chernevskaya NI, Obukhov AG, Krishtal OA. (1991) NMDA receptor agonists selectively block N-type calcium channels in hippocampal neurons. *Nature* 349: 418–420.

Constanti A, Galvan M. (1983) Fast inward-rectifying current accounts for anomalous rectification in olfactory corted neurones. *J. Physiol.* 335: 153–178.

Coulter DA, Huguenard JP, Prince DA. (1989) Characterization of ethosuximide reduction of low-threshold calcium current in thalamic relay neurons. *Ann. Neurol.* 25: 582–593.

Cox DH, Dunlap K. (1992) Pharmacological discrimination of N-type from L-type calcium current and its selective modulation by transmitters. *J. Neurosci.* 12: 906–914.

Crest M, Jacquet G, Golas M, Zerrouk H, Benslimane A, Rochat H, Mansuelle P, Martin-Eauclaire M-F. (1992) Kaliotoxin, a novel peptidyl inhibitor of neuronal BK-type Ca^{2+}-activated K^+ channels characterized from *Androctonus mauretanicus mauretanicus* venom. *J. Biol. Chem.* 267: 1640-1647.

de Leon M, Wang Y, Jones L, Perez-Reyes E, Wei X, Soong TW, Snutch TP, Yue DT. (1995) Essential Ca^{2+}-binding motif for Ca^{2+}-sensitive inactivation of L-type Ca^{2+} channels. *Science* 270: 1502–1506.

Dolly JO, Parcej DN. (1996) Molecular properties of voltage-gated K^+ channels. *J. Bioenerg. Biomembr.* 28: 231–253.

Doupnik CA, Davidson N, Lester HA. (1995) The inward rectifier potassium channel family. *Curr. Opin. Neurobiol.* 5: 268–277.

Drewe J, Verma S, Frech G, Joho R. (1992) Distinct spatial and temporal expression patterns of K^+ channels mRNAs from different subfamilies. *J. Neurosci.* 12: 538–548.

Dreyer, F. (1990) Peptide toxins and potassium channels. *Rev. Physiol. Biochem. Pharmacol.* 115: 93–136.

Dunlap K, Luebke JI, Turner TJ. (1995) Exocytotic Ca^{2+} channels in mammalian central neurons. *Trends Neurosci.* 18: 89–98.

Dworetzky SI, Trojnacki JT, Gribkoff VK. (1994) Cloning and expression of a human large-conductance calcium-activated potassium channel. *Mol. Brain Res.* 27: 189–193.

Edwards G, Weston AH. (1993) The pharmacology of ATP-sensitive potassium channels. *Annu. Rev. Pharmacol.* Toxicol. 33: 597–637.

Edwards G, Weston AH. (1996) The pharmacology of potassium channel superfamilies: modulation of K_{ATP} and BK_{Ca}. In: *Molecular and Cellular Mechanisms of Cardiovascular Regulation* (eds M Endoh, M Morad, H Scholz, T Iijima). Springer-Verlag, Tokyo, pp. 93–109.

Edwards G, Niederste-Hollenberg A, Schneider J, Noack Th, Weston AH. (1994) Ion channel modulation by NS 1619, the putative BK_{Ca} channel opener, in vascular smooth muscle. *Br. J. Pharmacol.* 113: 1538–1547.

Galvez A, Gimenez-Gallego G, Reuben JP, Roy-Contancin L, Feigenbaum P, Kaczorowski GJ, Garcia ML. (1990) Purification and characterization of a unique, potent, peptidyl probe for the high conductance calcium-activated potassium channel from venom of the scorpion *Buthus tamulus*. *J. Biol. Chem.* 265: 11 083–11 090.

Garcia ML, Garcia-Calvo M, Hidalgo P, Lee A, MacKinnon R. (1994) Purification and characterization of three inhibitors of voltage-dependent K^+ channels from *Leiurus quinquestriatus* var. *hebraeus* venom. *Biochemistry* 33: 6834-6839.

Garcia ML, Knaus HG, Munujos P, Slaughter RS, Kaczorowski GJ. (1995) Charybdotoxin and its effects on potassium channels. *Am. J. Physiol.* 38: C1-C10.

Goldin AL. (1995) Voltage-gated sodium channels. In: *Handbook of Receptors and Channels: Ligand- and Voltage-Gated Ion Channels* (ed. RA North). CRC Press, London, pp.73–111.

Gottfried JA, Chesler M. (1995) Benzolamide inhibits low-threshold calcium currents in hippocampal pyramidal neurons. *J. Neurophysiol.* 74: 2774–2777.

Grissmer S, Nguyen AN, Aiyar J, Hanson DC, Mather RJ, Gutman GA, Karmilowicz MJ, Auperin DD, Chandy KG. (1994) Pharmacological characterization of five cloned voltage-gated K^+ channels, types Kv1.1, 1.2, 1.3, 1.5, and 3.1, stably expressed in mammalian cell lines. *Mol. Pharmacol.* 45: 1227–1234.

Gutman GA, Chandy KG. (1993) Nomenclature of mammalian voltage-dependent potassium channel genes. *Sem. Neurosci.* 5: 101–106.

Hasson A, Shon KJ, Olivera BM, Spira ME. (1995) Alterations of voltage-activated sodium current by a novel conotoxin from the venom of *Conus gloriamaris*. *J. Neurophysiol.* 73: 1295–1301.

Heinemann SH, Terlau H, Stuhmer W, Imoto K, Numa S. (1992) Calcium channel characteristics conferred on the sodium channel by single mutations. *Nature* 356: 441–443.

Heinemann S, Rettig J, Scott VES, Parcej DN, Lorra C, Dolly J, Pongs O. (1994) The inactivation behaviour of voltage-gated K^+-channels may be determined by association of α- and β-subunits. *J. Physiol. Paris.* 88: 173–180.

Heinemann SH, Rettig J, Wunder F, Pongs O. (1995) Molecular and functional characterization of a rat brain Kvβ3 potassium channel subunit. *FEBS Lett.* **377**: 383–389.

Higgins CF. (1995) The ABC of channel regulation. *Cell* **82**: 693–696.

Hille B. (1992) Na and K channels of axons. In: *Ionic Channels of Excitable Membranes.* Sinauer Associates, Sunderland, MA, pp. 59–82.

Hillyard DR, Monje VD, Mintz IM et al. (1992) A new *Conus* peptide ligand for mammalian presynaptic Ca^{2+} channels. *Neuron* **9**: 69–77

Inagaki N, Gonoi T, Clement JP, Namba N, Inazawa J, Gonzalez G, Aguilar-Bryan L, Seino S, Bryan J. (1995) Reconstitution of I_{KATP}: an inward rectifier subunit plus the sulfonylurea receptor. *Science* **270**: 1166–1170.

Isacoff EY, Jan YN, Jan LY. (1990) Evidence for the formation of heteromultimeric potassium channels in *Xenopus* oocytes. *Nature* **345**: 530–534.

Isom LL, De Jongh KS, Catterall WA. (1994) Auxiliary subunits of voltage-gated ion channels. *Neuron* **12**: 1183–1194.

Isom LL, Ragsdale DS, De Jongh KS, Westenbroek RE, Reber BF, Scheuer T, Catterall WA. (1995) Structure and function of the β2 subunit of brain sodium channels, a transmembrane glycoprotein with a CAM motif. *Cell* **83**: 433–442.

Jan LY, Jan YN. (1992) Tracing the roots of ion channels. *Cell* **69**: 715–718.

Johnston D, Williams S, Jaffe D, Gray R. (1992) NMDA-receptor independent long-term potentiation. *Annu. Rev. Physiol.* **54**: 489–505.

Kaczorowski GJ, Knaus HG, Leonard RJ, McManus OB, Garcia ML. (1996) High-conductance calcium-activated potassium channels; structure, pharmacology, and function. *J. Bioenerg. Biomembr.* **28**: 255–267.

Kamb A, Iverson, LE, Tanouye MA. (1987) Molecular characterization of *Shaker*, a *Drosophila* gene that encodes a potassium channel. Cell **50**: 405–413.

Kirkup AJ, Edwards G, Green ME, Miller M, Walker SD, Weston AH. (1996) Modulation of membrane currents and mechanical activity by niflumic acid in rat vascular smooth muscle. *Eur. J. Pharmacol.*, in press.

Kirsch GE. (1994) Na^+ channels: structure, function, and classification. *Drug Dev. Res.* **33**: 263–276.

Knaus HG, Garcia-Calvo M, Kaczorowski GJ, Garcia ML. (1994a) Subunit composition of the high conductance calcium-activated potassium channel from smooth muscle, a representative of the *mSlo* and *slowpoke* family of potassium channels. *J. Biol. Chem.* **269**: 3921–3924.

Knaus HG, McManus OB, Lee SH et al. (1994b) Tremorgenic indole alkaloids potently inhibit smooth muscle high-conductance calcium-activated potassium channels. *Biochemistry* **33**: 5819–5828.

Köhler M, Hirschberg B, Bond CT, Kinzie JM, Marrion NV, Maylie J, Adelman JP. (1996) Small-conductance, calcium-activated potassium channels from mammalian brain. *Science* **273**: 1709–1714.

Kubo Y. (1994) Towards the elucidation of the structural–functional relationship of inward rectifying K^+ channel family. *Neurosci. Res.* **21**: 109–117.

Kubo Y, Baldwin TJ, Jan, YN, Jan LY. (1993) Primary structure and functional expression of a mouse inward rectifier potassium channel. *Nature* **362**. 127–133.

Lee SH, Hensens OD, Helms GL et al. (1995) L-735,334, a novel sesquiterpenoid potassium channel-agonist from *Trichoderma virens*. *J. Nat. Prod.* **58**: 1822–1828.

Llinás R, Sugimori M, Lin JW, Cherksey B. (1989) Blocking and isolation of a calcium channel from neurons in mammals and cephalopods utilizing a toxin fraction (FTX) from funnel-web spider poison. *Proc. Natl Acad. Sci. USA* **86**: 1689–1693.

MacKinnon R, Heginbotham L, Abramson T. (1990) Mapping the receptor site for charybdotoxin, a pore-blocking potassium channel inhibitor. *Neuron* **5**: 767–771.

MacKinnon AC, Wyatt KM, McGivern JG, Sheridan RD, Brown CM. (1995) [³H]-lifarizine, a high affinity probe for inactivated sodium channels. *Br. J. Pharmacol.* **115**: 1103–1109.

Magee JC, Johnston D. (1995) Characterization of single voltage-gated Na^+ and Ca^{2+} channels in apical dendrites of rat CA1 pyramidal neurons. *J. Physiol.* **487**: 67–90.

Malouf NN, McMahon DK, Hainsworth CN, Kay BK. (1992) A two-motif isoform of the major calcium channel subunit in skeletal muscle. *Neuron* **8**: 899–906.

McBurney RN, Daly D, Fischer JB et al. (1992) New CNS-specific calcium antagonists. *J. Neurotrauma* **9** (suppl. 2): S531–S543.

McIntosh JM, Hasson A, Spira ME, Gray WR, Li W, Marsh M, Hillyard DR, Olivera B M. (1995) A new family of conotoxins that blocks voltage-gated sodium channels. *J. Biol. Chem.* **270**: 16 796–16 802.

McManus OB, Harris GH, Giangiacomo KM, Feigenbaum P, Reuben JP, Addy ME, Burka JF, Kaczorowski GJ, Garcia ML. (1993) An activator of calcium-dependent potassium channels isolated from a medicinal herb. *Biochemistry* 32: 6128–6133.

McManus OB, Helms LMH, Pallanck L, Ganetzky B, Swanson R, Leonard RJ. (1995) Functional role of the β subunit of high conductance calcium-activated potassium channels. *Neuron* 14: 645–650.

Miljanich GP, Ramachandran J. (1995) Antagonists of neuronal calcium channels: structure, function, and therapeutic implications. *Annu. Rev. Pharmacol. Toxicol.* 35: 707–734.

Miller C. (1995) The charybdotoxin family of K$^+$ channel-blocking peptides. *Neuron* 15: 5–10

Mintz IM, Bean BP. (1993) GABAB receptor inhibition of P-type Ca^{2+} channels in central neurons. *Neuron* 10: 889–898.

Mintz IM, Adams ME, Bean BP. (1992a) P-type calcium channels in rat central and peripheral neurons. *Neuron* 9: 85–95.

Mintz IM, Venema VJ, Swiderek KM, Lee TD, Bean BP. (1992b) P-type calcium channels blocked by the spider toxin ω-AGA-IVA. *Nature* 355: 827–829.

Moczydlowski E, Schild L. (1994) Unitary properties of the batrachotoxin-trapped state of voltage-sensitive sodium channels. In: *Handbook of Membrane Channels: Molecular and Cellular Physiology* (ed. C Peracchia). Academic Press, London, pp.137–160.

Nakahira K, Shi GY, Rhodes KJ, Trimmer JS. (1996) Selective interaction of voltage-gated K$^+$ channel β-subunits with α-subunits. *J. Biol. Chem.* 271: 7084–7089.

Narahashi T. (1992) Nerve membrane Na$^+$ channels as targets of insecticides. *Trends Pharmacol. Sci.* 13: 236–241.

Narahashi T, Carter DB, Frey J, Ginsburg K, Hamilton BJ, Nagata K, Roy ML, Song JH, Tatebayashi H. (1995) Sodium channels and GABA$_A$ receptor-channel complex as targets of environmental toxicants. *Toxicol. Lett.* 82–83: 239–245.

Newman EA. (1993) Inward-rectifying potassium channels in retinal glial (Muller) cells. *J. Neurosci.* 13: 3333–3345.

Norris PJ, Smith CT, DeBelleroche J, Bradford HF, Mantle PG, Thomas AJ. (1980) Actions of tremorgenic fungal toxins on neurotransmitter release. *J. Neurochem.* 34: 33–42.

Olesen SP, Munch E, Moldt P, Drejer J. (1994a) Selective activation of Ca^{2+}-dependent K$^+$ channels by novel benzimidazolone. *Eur. J. Pharmacol.* 251: 53–59.

Olesen SP, Munch E, Watjen F, Drejer J. (1994b) NS 004-an activator of Ca^{2+}-dependent K$^+$ channels in cerebellar granule cells. *Neuroreport* 5: 1001–1004.

Olivera BM, Miljanich GP, Ramachandran J, Adams ME. (1994) Calcium channel diversity and neurotransmitter release: the ω-conotoxins and ω-agatoxins. *Annu. Rev. Biochem.* 63: 823–867.

Panchenko VA, Pintor J, Tsyndrenko AY, Miras-Portugal MT, Krishtal OA. (1996). Diadenosine polyphosphates selectively potentiate N-type Ca^{2+} channels in rat central neurons. *Neuroscience* 70: 353–360.

Patton DE, West JW, Catterall WA, Goldin AL. (1993) A peptide segment critical for sodium channel inactivation functions as an inactivation gate in a potassium channel. *Neuron* 11: 967–974.

Perez-Reyes E, Schneider T. (1994) Calcium channels: structure, function, and classification. *Drug Dev. Res.* 33: 295–318.

Perney TM, Hiroring LD, Leeman SE, Miller RJ. (1986) Multiple neurotransmitter release from peripheral neurons. *Proc. Natl Acad. Sci. USA* 83: 6655–6659.

Pongs O. (1992) Molecular biology of voltage-dependent potassium channels. *Physiol. Rev.* 72: S69–S88.

Pongs O. (1995) Regulation of the activity of voltage-gated potassium channels by β subunits. *Sem. Neurosci.* 7: 137–146.

Randall AD, Tsien R. (1995) Pharmacological dissection of multiple types of Ca^{2+} channel currents in rat cerebellar granule neurons. *J. Neurosci.* 15: 2995–3012.

Reinhart PH, Tseng-Crank J, Krause JD, Mertz R, Godinot N, DiChiara TJ, Foster CD. (1995) Cloning, expression and distribution of human Ca^{2+}-activated K$^+$ channel α- and β-subunits. *Biophys. J.* 68: 270a.

Rogowski RS, Krueger BK, Collins JH, Blaustein MP. (1994) Tityustoxin Kα blocks voltage-gated noninactivating K$^+$ channels and unblocks inactivating K$^+$ channels blocked by α-dendrotoxin in synaptosomes. *Proc. Natl Acad. Sci. USA.* 91: 1475–1479.

Sah P. (1996) Ca^{2+}-activated K$^+$-currents in neurones: types, physiological roles and modulation. *Trends Neurosci.* 19: 150–154.

Salgado VL, Narahashi T. (1993) Immobilization of sodium channel gating charge in crayfish giant axons by the insecticide fenvalerate. *Mol. Pharmacol.* 43: 626–634.

Shi GY, Nakahira K, Hammond S, Rhodes KJ, Schechter LE, Trimmer JS. (1996) β subunits promote K$^+$ channel surface expression through effects early in biosynthesis. *Neuron.* **16**: 843–852.

Singh SB, Goetz MA, Zink DL, Dombrowski AW, Polishook JD, Garcia ML, Schmalhofer W, McManus OB, Kaczorowski GJ. (1994) Maxikdiol: a novel dihydroxyisoprimane as an agonist of maxi-K channels. *J. Chem. Soc. Perkin Trans.* **1**: 3349–3352.

Small RC, Isaac LM, McArdle S, Pocock TM. (1996) Relaxation of airways smooth muscle induced by agonists at beta-adrenoceptors: signal transduction pathways and role of plasmalemmal K$^+$-channel opening. In: *Sympathomimetic Enantiomers in the Treatment of Asthma* (ed. J Costello). Parthenon Publishing, London, pp. 11–41.

Snutch TP, Leonard JP, Gilbert MM, Lester HA, Davidson N. (1990) Rat brain expresses a heterogeneous family of calcium channels. *Proc. Natl Acad. Sci. USA* **87**: 3391–3395.

Spedding M, Paoletti R. (1992) Classification of calcium channels and the sites of action of drugs modifying channel function. *Pharmacol. Rev.* **44**: 363–376.

Stankiewicz M, Grolleau F, Lapied B, Borchani L, Elayeb M, Pelhate M. (1996) Bot IT$_2$, a toxin paralytic to insects from the *Buthus occitanus tunetanus* venom modifying the activity of insect sodium channels. *J. Insect Physiol.* **42**: 397–405.

Stea A, Dubel SJ, Pragnell M, Leonard JP, Campbell KP, Snutch TP. (1993) A β-subunit normalizes the electrophysiological properties of a cloned N-type Ca^{2+} channel α$_1$-subunit. *Neuropharmacology* **32**: 1103–1116.

Stephan MM, Potts JF, Agnew WS. (1994) The μI skeletal muscle sodium channel: mutation E403Q eliminates sensitivity to tetrodotoxin but not to μ-conotoxins GIIIA and GIIIB. *J. Membr. Biol.* **137**: 1–8.

Strong M, Chandy KG, Gutman GA. (1993) Molecular evolution of voltage-sensitive ion channel genes: on the origins of electrical excitability. *Mol. Biol. Evol.* **10**: 221–242.

Swarz KJ, Bean BP. (1992) Inhibition of calcium channels in rat CA3 pyramidal neurones by metabotropic glutamate receptor. *J. Neurosci.* **12**: 4358–4371.

Takahashi K, Akaike N. (1991) Calcium antagonist effects on low-threshold (T-type) calcium current in rat isolated hippocampal CA1 pyramidal neurons. *J. Pharmacol. Exp. Ther.* **256**: 169–175.

Trainer VL, Brown GB, Catterall WA. (1996) Site of covalent labeling by a photoreactive batrachotoxin derivative near transmembrane segment IS6 of the sodium channel alpha subunit. *J. Biol. Chem.* **271**: 11 261–11 267

Triggle DJ. (1994) Molecular pharmacology of voltage-gated calcium channels. *Ann. NY Acad. Sci.* **747**: 267–281.

Triggle DJ, Hawthorn M, Gopalakrishnan M, Minarini A, Avery S, Rutledge A, Bangalore R, Zheng W. (1991) Synthetic organic ligands active at voltage-gated calcium channels. *Ann. NY Acad. Sci.* **635**: 123–138.

Tytgat J, Vereecke J, Carmeliet E. (1994) Reversal of rectification and alteration of selectivity and pharmacology in a mammalian Kv1.1 potassium channel by deletion of domains S1 to S4. *J. Physiol.* **481**: 7–13.

Urenjak J, Obrenovitch TP. (1996) Pharmacological modulation of voltage-gated Na$^+$ channels: a rational and effective strategy against ischemic drain damage. *Pharmacol. Rev.* **48**: 21–67.

Varadi G, Mori Y, Mikala G, Schwartz A. (1995) Molecular determinants of Ca^{2+} channel function and drug action. *Trends Pharmacol. Sci.* **16**: 43–49.

Wallner M, Meera P, Ottolia M, Kaczorowski GJ, Latorre R, Garcia ML, Stefani E, Toro L. (1995) Characterization of and modulation by a β-subunit of a human maxi K$_{Ca}$ channel cloned from myometrium. *Recep. Chann.* **3**: 185–199.

Wang GK, Wang SY. (1994) Modification of cloned brain Na$^+$ channels by batrachotoxin. *Pflügers Arch.* **427**: 309–316.

Wang DW, Nie L, George AL, Bennett PB. (1996) Distinct local anesthetic affinities in Na$^+$ channel subtypes. *Biophys. J.* **70**: 1700–1708.

Weiser M, Vega-Saenz de Miera E, Kentros C, Moreno H, Franzen L, Hillman D, Baker H, Rudy B. (1994) Differential expression of Shaw-related K$^+$ channels in the rat central nervous system. *J. Neurosci.* **14**: 949–972.

West DJ, Andrews EB, Bowman D, McVean AR, Thorndyke MC. (1996) Toxins from some poisonous and venomous marine snails. *Comp. Biochem. Physiol. C – Pharmacol. Toxicol. Endocrinol.* **113**: 1–10.

Wheeler PJ, Randall AD, Tsien R. (1994) Roles of N-type and Q-type Ca^{2+} channels in supporting hippocampal synaptic transmission. *Science* **264**: 107–111.

Yellen G, Sodickson D, Chen TY, Jurman ME. (1994) An engineered cysteine in the external mouth of a K$^+$ channel allows inactivation to be modulated by metal binding. *Biophys. J.* **66**: 1068–1075.

G protein-coupled receptors

Jennifer A. Koenig

7.1 Introduction

G protein-coupled receptors reside in the plasma membrane of neuronal cells and transduce the binding of extracellular neurotransmitters or hormones to the receptor into changes in the activity of intracellular effectors. The G protein is the intermediary in this process. After binding of the ligand, the receptor catalyzes the exchange of GTP for GDP on the G protein causing it to dissociate from the receptor–G protein complex to receptor, activated α-subunit and βγ dimer (*Figure 7.1*). Both the activated α subunit bearing GTP and the βγ dimer can act upon one or more of a variety of effector molecules which may result in changes in the intracellular levels of second messengers such as cyclic AMP, cyclic GMP, inositol phosphates, calcium and arachidonic acid. These second messengers can generate changes in neurotransmitter release, hormone secretion, protein phosphorylation, cytoskeletal structure and gene transcription. G proteins also regulate the function of ion channels including voltage-gated calcium channels, potassium channels and ligand-gated ion channels such as the nicotinic acetylcholine receptor. G protein-coupled receptors have been implicated in the regulation of growth, synaptogenesis and differentiation. The activity of the G protein α-subunit is terminated by its intrinsic GTPase activity which converts the GTP back to GDP. Reassociation of the α-GDP and βγ-subunits with the unliganded receptor allows the cycle to begin again.

The G protein-coupled receptor family contains receptors for molecules as diverse as small neurotransmitters, neuropeptides and large glycoprotein hormones. Many of these receptors comprise a number of subtypes which have been defined by their pharmacological, structural and functional characteristics. Some G protein-coupled receptors exist in different splice variants which often show identical ligand binding properties but different G protein coupling or regulatory properties (reviewed in Milligan, 1995). G protein-coupled receptors can couple to one or more different types of G proteins, including G_s, G_i, G_o, G_q, G_{11}, G_{12}, G_{13}, G_t and G_{olf}. G_t and G_{olf} are found predominantly in visual and olfactory systems respectively. Generally, activation of G_s causes stimulation of adenylate cyclase and regulation of calcium channels via α_s. Activation of G_q causes stimulation of phospholipase C via α_q. In contrast, activation of G_i or G_o can influence multiple second messenger systems, including inhi-

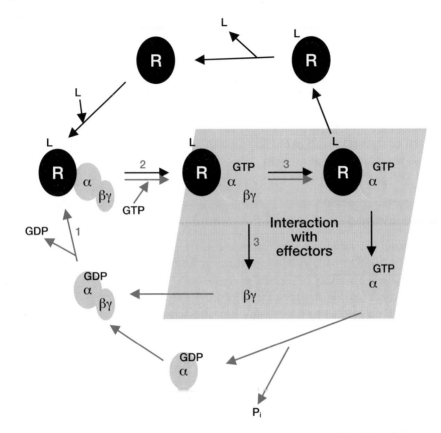

Figure 7.1. Activation of G proteins by liganded receptor. Formation of the liganded receptor–G protein complex catalyzes the following steps: (1) exchange of GTP for GDP, (2) a conformational change from inactive to activated α-GTP, and (3) the dissociation of βγ from α-GTP. The release of βγ and α-GTP allows them to interact with effectors. The activity of α-GTP is terminated by its intrinsic GTPase which converts the bound GTP to GDP. The activity of βγ is terminated by reassociation with α-GDP. There is still some debate as to whether the predominant inactive form is the unliganded receptor–G protein complex with GDP bound or with no nucleotide bound. It is also possible that the predominant inactive form is the unliganded receptor not complexed with G protein. L, agonist ligand; R, receptor. Adapted from Birnbaumer *et al.* (1990).

bition of adenylate cyclase, activation of cyclic GMP phosphodiesterase and regulation of potassium and calcium channels.

In many cases it is not entirely clear whether it is the α- or the βγ-subunits which are effective. This complexity has been partly resolved by the observation that there are different effector subtypes which are differentially regulated by α- and βγ-subunits. For example, different adenylate cyclase subtypes are differentially regulated by α- and βγ-subunits (Tang and Gilman, 1992) whereas phospholipase C-β can be independently activated by either α- or βγ-subunits while phospholipase C-γ is apparently unaffected by G proteins (Smrcka and Sternweis, 1993). (There are a number of excellent, recent reviews encompassing the field of receptor–G protein interactions including Birnbaumer *et al.*, 1990; Conklin and Bourne, 1993; Milligan, 1995; Neer, 1995; Simon *et al.*, 1991; Wickman and Clapham, 1995.) Recent information regarding the characteristics that define individual receptor subtypes can be found in the *Trends in Pharmacological Science Receptor Nomenclature Supplement* which is updated every year. *Tables 7.1–7.4* show some of the members of the G protein-coupled receptor superfamily.

7.2 Overall structural features

Over 200 types of G protein-coupled receptors have now been cloned and all share a common seven-transmembrane structure. Structural modeling has been based on the structure of bacteriorhodopsin, a light-activated proton pump found in photosynthetic bacteria, which also has a seven-transmembrane structure. However, bacteriorhodopsin is not a G protein-coupled receptor and there is little sequence homology between bacteriorhodopsin and G protein-coupled receptors. There is a 9 Å resolution structure for bovine rhodopsin, a light-activated G protein-coupled receptor which shows a similar

Table 7.1. Small molecule neurotransmitter rhodopsin-like G protein-coupled receptors and their associated G protein

Receptor	Subtype	G_s	G_q G_{11}	G_i G_o	Receptor	Subtype	G_s	G_q G_{11}	G_i G_o
Acetylcholine	M_1		✓		GABA	$GABA_B$			✓
(muscarinic)	M_2			✓	Histamine	H_1		✓	
	M_3		✓			H_2	✓		
	M_4			✓		H_3			
	M_5		✓		5-HT (serotonin)	$5\text{-}HT_{1A}$			✓
Adenosine	A_1			✓		$5\text{-}HT_{1B}$			✓
	A_{2A}	✓				$5\text{-}HT_{1D}$			✓
	A_{2B}	✓				$5\text{-}HT_{1E}$			✓
	A_3			✓		$5\text{-}HT_{1F}$			✓
Adrenergic-α_1	α_{1A}		✓			$5\text{-}HT_{2A}$		✓	
	α_{1B}		✓			$5\text{-}HT_{2B}$		✓	
	α_{1D}		✓			$5\text{-}HT_{2C}$		✓	
Adrenergic-α_2	α_{2A}			✓		$5\text{-}HT_4$	✓		
	α_{2B}			✓		$5\text{-}HT_6$	✓		
	α_{2C}			✓		$5\text{-}HT_7$	✓		
Adrenergic-β	β_1	✓			Leukotriene	BLT		✓	
	β_2	✓				CysLT		✓	
	β_3	✓			Melatonin	ML			✓
Cannabinoid	CB_1			✓	Prostanoid	DP	✓		
	CB_2					FP		✓	
Chemokine	CC CK1			✓		IP	✓		
	CC CK2			✓		TP		✓	
	CC CK3			✓		EP_1		✓	
	CC CK4			✓		EP_2	✓		
	$IL8_A$[a]			✓		EP_3		✓	✓
	$IL8_B$			✓		EP_4	✓		
Dopamine	D_1	✓			Purinergic	P_{2T}			✓
	D_2			✓		P_{2U}		✓	
	D_3			✓		P_{2Y}		✓	
	D_4			✓					
	D_5	✓							

Source: *Trends in Pharmacological Sciences Receptor Nomenclature Supplement* (1996). Note this table shows coupling that is generally observed, less specificity is often seen in transfected cell systems. [a]IL8, interleukin 8.

Table 7.2. Peptide and hormone rhodopsin-like G protein-coupled receptors and their associated G proteins

Receptor	Subtype	G_s	G_q G_{11}	G_i G_o	Receptor	Subtype	G_s	G_q G_{11}	G_i G_o
Angiotensin	AT_1		✓		Somatostatin	SST_1			✓
	AT_2					SST_2			✓
Atrial	ANP_A					SST_3			✓
natriuretic	ANP_B					SST_4			✓
peptide						SST_5			✓
Bombesin/	BB_1		✓		Neurokinin	NK_1		✓	
GRP[a]	BB_2		✓			NK_2		✓	
Bradykinin	B_1		✓			NK_3		✓	
	B_2		✓		Thyrotropin-	TRH		✓	
Cholecystokinin	CCK_A		✓		releasing				
/gastrin	CCK_B		✓		hormone				
Endothelin	ET_A		✓		Vasopressin	V_{1A}		✓	
	ET_B		✓			V_{1B}		✓	
Neuropeptide Y	Y_1			✓		V_2	✓		
	Y_2			✓	Oxytocin	OT		✓	
Neurotensin			✓						
Opioid	μ			✓					
	δ			✓					
	κ			✓					

Derived from *Trends in Pharmacological Sciences Receptor Nomenclature Supplement* (1996).
[a] GRP, gastrin-releasing peptide.

Table 7.3. Glucagon-like G protein-coupled receptors and their associated G proteins

Receptor	Subtype	G_s	G_q G_{11}	G_i G_o
Calcitonin		✓	✓	
Calcitonin gene-related peptide		✓		
Corticotropin-releasing hormone		✓		
Growth hormone-releasing hormone		✓	✓	
Glucagon		✓	✓	
Parathyroid hormone		✓	✓	
Secretin		✓		
Vasoactive intestinal peptide	VIP_1	✓		
	VIP_2	✓		
	PACAP	✓		

Derived from Segre and Goldring (1993).

Table 7.4. Metabotropic glutamate G protein-coupled receptors and their associated G proteins

Receptor	Subtype	G_s	G_q G_{11}	G_i G_o
Glutamate	$mGLU_1$		✓	
	$mGLU_2$			✓
	$mGLU_3$			✓
	$mGLU_4$			✓
	$mGLU_5$		✓	
	$mGLU_6$			✓
	$mGLU_7$			✓
	$mGLU_8$			✓

Derived from Pin and Duvoisin (1995).

arrangement of transmembrane helices to bacteriorhodopsin but with differences in the degree of tilt of the helices from the membrane (*Figure 7.2*; Schertler *et al.*, 1993). More recently a 6 Å structure for frog rhodopsin has been published (Schertler and Hargrave, 1995). While it is generally accepted that the transmembrane segments are largely α-helical and these α-helices may extend out of the membrane, there is still a lot of debate as to the three-dimensional arrangement of the α-helices (reviewed in Donnelly and Findlay, 1994; Hibert *et al.*, 1993). Computer modeling studies suggest that helix 3 is most deeply buried while helices 1, 4 and 5 are most exposed to lipid (Baldwin, 1993; Donnelly *et al.*, 1994). More recent mutagenesis studies have taken an alternative approach to determining the arrangement of helices in individual receptor types (e.g Liu *et al.*, 1995; Mizobe *et al.*, 1996). Rapid progress in large-scale expression and purification may mean that higher resolution structures will soon be available and many of these questions regarding the three-dimensional structure will be answered.

The G protein-coupled receptor superfamily has been divided into three main

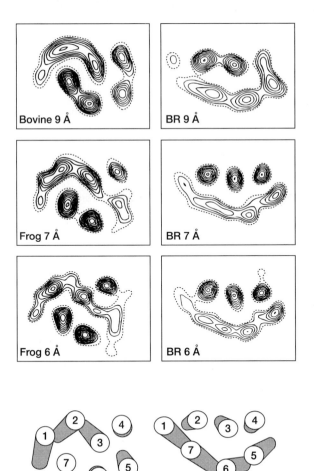

Figure 7.2. Comparison of bovine and frog rhodopsin and bacteriorhodopsin (BR) projection structures with a postulated diagrammatic arrangement of helices. Reproduced from Schertler and Hargrave (1995) with permission from the National Academy of Sciences.

groups. There are firstly the rhodopsin-like group which includes the majority of the G protein-coupled receptors, secondly the glucagon-like group, which includes receptors for glucagon, vasoactive intestinal peptide, secretin, corticotropin-releasing hormone, growth hormone-releasing hormone, calcitonin and parathyroid hormone (Segre and Goldring, 1993), and thirdly the metabotropic glutamate and calcium sensor receptors (Pin and Duvoisin, 1995). There is no sequence homology between the sub-families and relatively little is known about the second and third groups compared to the rhodopsin-like receptors. In general, the sequence similarity between the different G protein-coupled receptors is in the transmembrane segments while most of the variability resides in the size of the N-terminal extracellular domain, the third intracellular loop and the C-terminal domain. G protein-coupled receptors do not contain particular stretches of amino acids (domains) which can be linked to a particular aspect of their function; rather there are amino acids from different parts of the primary sequence which act in concert. The main structural features of a 'generic' G protein-coupled receptor are illustrated in *Figure 7.3* with the helices displayed in a two-dimensional format for clarity.

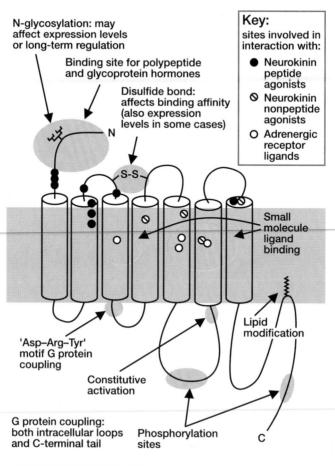

EXTRACELLULAR

N-glycosylation: may affect expression levels or long-term regulation

Binding site for polypeptide and glycoprotein hormones

Disulfide bond: affects binding affinity (also expression levels in some cases)

Key:
sites involved in interaction with:

● Neurokinin peptide agonists

⊘ Neurokinin nonpeptide agonists

○ Adrenergic receptor ligands

S-S

N

Small molecule ligand binding

Lipid modification

'Asp–Arg–Tyr' motif G protein coupling

Constitutive activation

G protein coupling: both intracellular loops and C-terminal tail

Phosphorylation sites

C

INTRACELLULAR

7.3 Receptor–ligand interactions

7.3.1 Small molecule neurotransmitters – rhodopsin-like subfamily

The ligand binding site for small molecule neurotransmitters is in a pocket in the transmembrane region and involves amino acids from several helices (reviewed by Hibert *et al.*, 1993; Ostrowski *et al.*, 1992; Savarese and Fraser, 1992; Strader *et al.*, 1994). The first evidence for this came from mutagenesis studies that showed that large portions of the extracellular and intracellular hydrophilic regions of the catecholamine (noradrenaline, dopamine) receptors can be deleted without markedly altering the binding of agonists and antagonists (e.g. Dixon *et al.*, 1987). In the case of the β-adrenergic receptor, mutagenesis studies have identified a small number of transmembrane residues that are important in catecholamine binding (shown diagrammatically in *Figure 7.4*) including Asp113 in transmembrane region 3, two

---

Figure 7.3. Structural features of a 'generic' G protein-coupled receptor. G protein-coupled receptors comprise seven transmembrane helices with an extracellular N-terminal domain and an intracellular C-terminal domain. *N-terminal domain.* The extracellular N-terminal region is glycosylated and this area may comprise the binding site for large polypeptide and glycoprotein hormones. Receptors for polypeptide and glycoprotein hormones have a large extracellular N-terminal domain (up to 350 amino acids) which has been proposed to be involved in the binding site for these receptors. Indeed the N-terminal extracellular domain of the luteinizing hormone receptor binds hormone with the same affinity as the entire receptor (Tsai-Morris *et al.*, 1990). The extracellular N-terminal domain is also the binding site for the metabotropic glutamate and calcium sensor receptors. The glycosylation sites in the N-terminal extracellular domain do not appear to affect ligand binding or functional responses but can affect the level of expression of some receptor types at the cell surface and may be involved in long-term regulation of surface receptor number (reviewed in Savarese and Fraser, 1992; see also Section 7.5.3). *Transmembrane regions.* The binding site for small molecule neurotransmitters is primarily located within the transmembrane regions; amino acids from several of the transmembrane helices contribute towards ligand binding. Small neuropeptides such as somatostatin and substance P are thought to bind to residues both within the transmembrane helices and parts of the extracellular loops (reviewed in Strader *et al.*, 1994). Small molecule neurotransmitters such as acetylcholine and noradrenaline bind exclusively within the transmembrane region (see Section 7.3.1. Also reviewed in Dohlman *et al.*, 1991; Savarese and Fraser, 1992). Some small molecule antagonists are thought to have additional interaction sites on the sixth and seventh transmembrane helices (Kobilka *et al.*, 1988; Osenberg *et al.*, 1992). In most receptors there is a *disulfide bridge* connecting extracellular loops 2 and 3 which may affect ligand binding affinity (Sidhu *et al.*, 1994) and/or expression levels (Savarese and Fraser, 1992). *Intracellular loops.* The main regions involved in interactions with G proteins are the intracellular loops and the C terminus with the particular regions varying between receptor types (reviewed in Strader *et al.*, 1994; Wess *et al.*, 1995; see also Section 7.4.2). Peptides derived from sequences in the third intracellular loop can activate purified G proteins *in vitro* (Dalman and Neubig, 1991; Okamoto *et al.*, 1991). The 'Asp-Arg-Tyr' motif at the intracellular face of the third transmembrane segment is thought to be involved in G protein coupling but is not found in the glucagon receptor-like family (Birnbaumer, 1995). There are a number of phosphorylation sites in the third intracellular loop and C terminus which may be involved in desensitization. Mutations in the C-terminal end of the third intracellular loop can lead to constitutive activation, allowing the receptor to activate G proteins without requiring binding of ligand. *Lipid modification* of highly conserved cysteine residue(s) within the C terminus occurs in some receptors and may anchor part of the C-terminal domain to the bilayer thus controlling tertiary structure in this region, in effect creating an additional intracellular loop (Milligan *et al.*, 1995b).

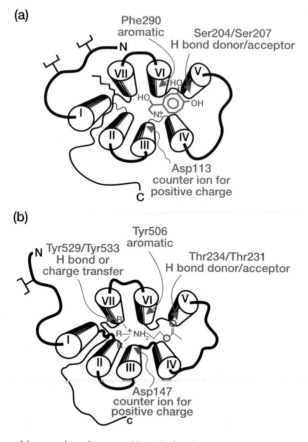

Figure 7.4. Proposed interactions between ligands for the β₂-adrenergic receptor and the muscarinic receptor. (a) β₂-Adrenergic receptor. Asp113 of the third transmembrane helix is a counter ion for the positive charge of the amine group of catecholamines. Two serines in transmembrane regions 5 (Ser204 and Ser207) are involved in hydrogen bonding with the hydroxyl groups of the catechol ring. Phe290 in the sixth transmembrane region is involved in stabilizing the interaction of the aromatic catechol ring with the receptor (reviewed in Savarese and Fraser, 1992; Strader *et al.*, 1994). (b) Muscarinic receptor. Asp147 of the third transmembrane helix forms an ion pair with the amine group of acetylcholine. Threonines in the fifth transmembrane helix may form hydrogen bonds with the ester group (reviewed in Wess *et al.*, 1995).

serines in transmembrane regions 5 (Ser204 and Ser207) and Phe290 in the sixth transmembrane region. These serines and phenylalanine residues are present in all G protein-coupled receptors that bind catecholamines but not in other G protein-coupled receptors. In contrast, the histamine receptor contains an Asp186 and Thr190 in analogous positions to the Ser204 and Ser207 of the β-adrenergic receptor and an interaction of these residues with the imidazole ring of histamine has been suggested. The muscarinic receptor contains an analogous Asp to Asp113 and in addition, Thr231 and Thr234 in the analogous part of the fifth transmembrane region which might interact with the ester group of acetylcholine (reviewed in Wess *et al.*, 1995; *Figure 7.4b*).

Although this simplistic picture holds for the well-studied β-adrenergic and muscarinic receptors, the binding sites for other neurotransmitters and peptides clearly do not involve the same distribution of amino acids (Hunyady *et al.*, 1996; Strader *et al.*, 1994). In the neurokinin receptor, peptide agonists bind to extracellular loops 1 and 2 and within the transmembrane region of the second and seventh transmembrane helices (reviewed in Gether *et al.*, 1995; Strader *et al.*, 1994). However, nonpeptide agonists do not require residues in the extracellular loops. Furthermore, the picture becomes much more complex when looking at the effect of mutagenesis on the binding of different classes of nonpeptide agonist drugs to the same receptor. These studies have shown that the binding sites for a number of different classes of drugs at the same receptor do not necessarily include the same set of amino acids (Neve and Wiens, 1995; Woodward *et al.*, 1995). In some cases, a single amino acid substitution can decrease the binding affinity for one class of drugs but not another (Strader *et al.*, 1994). This implies that several different combinations of interactions with different parts of the transmembrane region can collectively induce a conformational change sufficient to activate a G protein.

Similarly, there are no hard and fast rules as to which residues are important in antagonist binding. It is clear from both mutagenesis (Gether *et al.*, 1993) and fluorescence (Turcatti *et al.*, 1995) studies that agonists and antagonists do not interact with the same set of amino acids, particularly in the case of peptide agonists and nonpeptide antagonists of the NK1 receptor and the angiotensin receptor (Ji *et al.*, 1994; Strader *et al.*, 1994). Given that at least part of the agonist binding site is located in a pocket in the bilayer region, it is likely that binding of antagonists while not inducing a conformational change, could sterically block access of the agonist to its binding site. It is also possible that agonists and antagonists could exclude each other from binding by a very strong negative co-operativity (Gether *et al.*, 1995). Even more complex is the binding of drugs to allosteric sites. There are a number of drugs which act allosterically at the muscarinic acetylcholine receptor and it has been suggested that these drugs bind to a site more extracellular to the agonist binding site causing steric hindrance although still allowing the agonist to bind (reviewed in Tucek and Proska, 1995).

7.4 Receptor–G protein interactions

An emerging theme from mutagenesis and modeling studies is that some amino acids are not involved in the agonist binding site but are important in transmitting the binding event into a conformational change sufficient to activate G proteins. Before addressing the question of which areas of the protein are involved, we need to understand how this shift in conformation can be measured, albeit indirectly.

7.4.1 Effect of G proteins on agonist binding

The receptor exists in a number of dynamic states which are reflected by different affinities for agonist. Generally though, experimental limitations allow only the resolution of two different affinity sites (discussed in more detail in Birnbaumer *et al.*, 1990). The receptor–G protein complex has a high affinity for agonist. Once the G protein is activated and released from the receptor, the receptor converts to a conformation with low affinity for agonists. This conversion requires the presence of magnesium ions and GTP to allow activation of the G protein. Ligand binding assays are usually done with well-washed membrane preparations under equilibrium conditions so that, in the absence of GTP, both high and low affinity states are measured. In the presence of GTP and magnesium, only the low-affinity state is measured since binding of agonist rapidly induces the change from high to low affinity. Binding of agonists to intact cells generally shows only low affinity characteristics since intracellular levels of GTP are naturally high.

The interaction of G proteins with the receptor can be mimicked by the action of synthetic peptides based on regions of the α-subunit of G_s (Rasenick *et al.*, 1994). In ligand binding assays of β-adrenergic receptors in permeabilized cells, agonist displacement of antagonist binding showed two sites of different affinity. One site, with K_d in the nanomolar range, corresponds to the receptor coupled to G protein. The lower affinity site, with K_d in the micromolar range, corresponds to the receptor uncoupled from G protein. In the presence of a nonhydrolyzable analog of GTP (GTPγS), only a low affinity site was observed, suggesting that the agonist had promoted dissociation of the G protein from the receptor, converting all the receptors to a low affinity conformation:

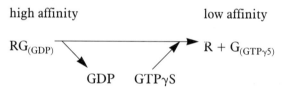

When the G protein peptide mimic was added, the high affinity site predominated. In this situation, when GTPγS was added, the high affinity state was maintained, since GTPγS could not initiate dissociation of the peptide mimic from the receptor. This effect was specific for peptides derived from G_s and did not occur with peptides derived from G_i or G_o.

7.4.2 Structural features involved in G protein activation

Regions of the receptor's intracellular loops and C-terminus are involved in G protein activation (reviewed in Conklin and Bourne, 1993; Strader *et al.*, 1994). Several models have been proposed to explain the transmission of information from the ligand binding event to activation of G proteins. A number of studies have identified a highly conserved aspartate in transmembrane region 2 (Asp79 in the β-adrenergic receptor), located near the intracellular end of the second transmembrane region which is thought to be involved in transmitting conformational changes in the binding site to activation of G proteins (e.g. Fraser *et al.*, 1989). This aspartate is involved in allosteric regulation by sodium and/or hydrogen ions (Horstman *et al.*, 1990; Neve *et al.*, 1991). Modeling studies have proposed that, upon binding of agonist, a conformational change induces an interaction between a tyrosine in the seventh transmembrane region with the aspartate in the second transmembrane region (Hibert *et al.*, 1993). The highly conserved 'Asp-Arg-Tyr' motif at the intracellular end of the third transmembrane region may also be involved (Birnbaumer, 1995).

A number of studies have identified mutations of particular amino acids that lead to reduced ability of the receptor to activate G proteins (reviewed in Strader *et al.*, 1994). However, this has not produced a clear picture of exactly which amino acids in the receptor are responsible for activation of G proteins (e.g. Savarese and Fraser,

1992). Regions of the third intracellular loop that are involved in G protein activation are amphipathic helices and mutational analysis has shown that insertion and substitution of residues that would disrupt this arrangement will disrupt receptor–G protein coupling (Strader *et al.*, 1994). Therefore, in the unstimulated receptor, these helices are conformationally constrained and the conformational change that occurs on agonist binding serves to remove this restraint. This underlines the idea that the secondary structure is as important as individual residues.

Specificity of coupling. To go further and determine which regions are involved in specificity of coupling for different types of G protein-coupled receptors is to enter a deep and murky quagmire of confusion. One reason for this is that some receptors show apparent selectivity for different G protein subtypes and others do not. The mechanisms involved in determining this selectivity are extremely complex and may be determined by factors other than the structure of the receptor itself (see Section 7.4.4). Having said that, some studies have identified particular regions thought to determine specificity (reviewed in Savarese and Fraser, 1992). However, it is possible that combination(s) of multiple regions of intracellular loops could define G protein binding specificity or that certain regions of the intracellular structure influence the availability of appropriate recognition sequences for G protein binding (Strader *et al.*, 1994; Wong and Ross, 1994).

7.4.3 Constitutive activation

A number of mutated receptors have been described which can activate G proteins without agonist being present (reviewed in Hwa *et al.*, 1996; Milligan *et al.*, 1995a; Perez *et al.*, 1996; Strader *et al.*, 1994). These constitutively active mutants must adopt one or more conformations which expose the intracellular sequences capable of activating G proteins. In the two-state receptor model (described in more detail by Leff, 1995) the receptor exists in equilibrium between two states R (inactive) and R* (active). An agonist has greater affinity for the R* state, pushing the equilibrium towards the R* state, which results in activation of the G protein and stimulation of effectors. Antagonists have no preference in affinity for either state and so do not alter the activity of G proteins and effectors but do prevent agonists from binding. Inverse agonists have preferential affinity for the inactive state, thereby decreasing basal levels of activity of the G protein. Presumably, constitutively active mutants exist in equilibrium further towards the R* state than the R state. A number of naturally occurring receptor mutations show clinical symptoms (reviewed by Clapham, 1993). There are at present a few examples of inverse agonists acting specifically at various receptors including opiate receptor ligands, 5-hydroxytryptamine (5-HT) ligands and a β-adrenergic receptor ligand (reviewed by Milligan, 1995a); their potential therapeutic benefit is not yet known.

7.4.4 Diversity of G proteins: signal sorting

The great diversity of receptor, G protein and effector subtypes has the potential to generate a complex diversity of signaling pathways and networks. It is impossible to review this enormous field here and only the aspects central to understanding the function of G protein-coupled receptors will be discussed. Structural and regulatory aspects of G proteins have been reviewed elsewhere (Birnbaumer *et al.*, 1990; Conklin and Bourne, 1993; Neer, 1995; Simon *et al.*, 1991). The relevance of different effector isoforms is reviewed in Milligan (1995).

The central question considered here is how cells, which might contain multiple receptor subtypes and G proteins (α and $\beta\gamma$) control the ultimate functional response which is produced. At first glance, one could expect to answer this by finding out which receptor subtypes activate which G proteins and which G proteins activate which effectors. However, this approach was stymied by the finding that in purified systems, the receptor–G protein interactions are remarkably nonspecific. This has led to the realization that there are more subtle controls within the cell that determine the signaling pathway(s) which respond to activation of a given receptor and that these controls will vary from one cell to another. Some examples to illustrate this are given below and are most certainly not exhaustive.

Selective or nonselective? There are many instances where selectivity of receptor–G protein interactions is not observed, that is one receptor type is able to activate multiple G protein subtypes in one cell, for example, opioid receptors in neuroblastoma cells and in transfected cells (Prather *et al.*, 1994, and references therein) and the thyrotropin receptor (reviewed in Milligan, 1995). One complicating factor in this case is that, although the agonists stimulate G proteins with the same potency, the concentration of drug required to activate the different effectors is different. This requires the postulation of different rates of GTP hydrolysis which may be controlled by $\beta\gamma$-subunits, by effectors or GAP (GTPase activating protein)-like proteins (Prather *et al.*, 1994):

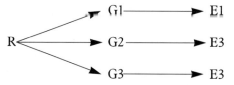

In the contrasting scenario, some receptors can show selectivity for a certain α-subtype. If a cell line does not contain the subtype required then the appropriate response will not be seen even though it might be present in another cell type. For example, somatostatin receptors transfected into CHO-DG44 cells do not show inhibition of adenylate cyclase whereas their transfection in CHO-K1 cells does reveal the appropriate response (Patel *et al.*, 1994).

Strength of coupling. Apparently variable specificities can be due to differences in coupling strength between receptor and G protein. For example, muscarinic m$_2$ receptors generally couple only in a negative manner to adenylate cyclase via G$_i$. However, when the receptor is expressed at high levels, stimulation of phospholipase C is also observed (Offermanns *et al.*, 1994; Vogel *et al.*, 1995, and references therein). This suggests that, although the receptor is actually able to couple to both, at normal expression levels only the stronger signal is observed:

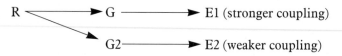

The strength of coupling could also be determined by the efficacy of the agonist (Kenakin, 1995). In this case, if a receptor has a greater ability to stimulate one G pro-

tein (G1) than another (G2) then an agonist of high efficacy could theoretically produce enough activated G1 and G2 to activate both pathways whereas an agonist of low
efficacy might only produce enough G1 to produce a measurable response. An even
more complex proposition is that the receptor may exist in a number of different conformations which each activate different G proteins with different efficacy (Kenakin,
1995). Much current work is aimed at identifying different agonists which are able to
promote the formation of particular conformations. In this case, the agonist could be
the determinant of which G protein-effector pathway is activated in a given cell type.
This has been termed agonist trafficking (Kenakin, 1995). Recent work has suggested
that there are some mutations in the third cytoplasmic loop of the m_2 muscarinic
receptor which confer differences in agonist potencies (Bulscco and Schimerlik,
1996).

Cross-talk and coincidence detection. If receptors are indeed promiscuous in their
G protein coupling then cross-talk between the receptors might be expected. Cross-
talk is generally defined as an effect of one agonist on the response to another either
at the level of the GTPase activity, effector response or regulation of receptor
response. One example of this is heterologous regulation where activation of one
receptor causes decreasing response to another receptor (see Section 7.5; Lee and
Fraser, 1993). Effector molecules can act as coincidence detectors, for example, observation of a rise in intracellular calcium resulting from muscarinic m_4 receptor activation is conditional on simultaneous, sub-maximal activation of purinergic receptors
(Carroll *et al.*, 1995). Adenylate cyclase type II can also act as a coincidence detector of
signals from β-adrenergic and $GABA_B$ (γ-aminobutyric acid) receptors (reviewed in
Bourne and Nicoll, 1993).

The opposite situation also occurs, where two different receptors appear to activate
the same effector via the same G protein subtype yet show no cross-talk (e.g. Graeser
and Neubig, 1993). This could be explained by physical compartmentation (see
below) or the kinetics of receptor–G protein coupling (Graeser and Neubig, 1993).
However at least in some situations, there are more subtypes or splice variants of G
proteins than was originally appreciated. For example, both somatostatin and muscarinic receptors regulate calcium channel function in GH_3 cells via different variants
of the same G protein subtype (Kleuss *et al.*, 1992):

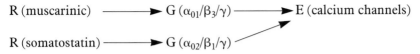

$$R \text{ (muscarinic)} \longrightarrow G\,(\alpha_{01}/\beta_3/\gamma) \longrightarrow E \text{ (calcium channels)}$$
$$R \text{ (somatostatin)} \longrightarrow G\,(\alpha_{02}/\beta_1/\gamma)$$

Compartmentation. There is some evidence for the restriction of receptors and/or G
proteins to particular domains within the cell. For example, Strittmatter *et al.* (1990)
showed that G_o is concentrated in growth cones. In addition, polarized cells show different localization of different α-subunits. In some epithelial cells, $G_{i\alpha2}$ is localized to
the basal lateral membrane while $G_{i\alpha3}$ is found in Golgi and apical membranes
(Ercolani *et al.*, 1990). Li *et al.* (1995) have noted that G proteins are localized within
caveolar membranes and suggested a regulatory interaction with caveolin. Studies of
N-formyl peptide receptors in neutrophils have demonstrated aggregation and immobilization of receptors in the plasma membrane which is enhanced in the presence of
agonist (Johansson *et al.*, 1993). It is not known if this is a general mechanism for all
cell types and receptor types. If the hypothesis of compartmentation is accepted then

the results obtained from transfected cells with high receptor density must be treated with caution. The control on receptor–G protein interactions may not be so restricted and decreased specificity may be observed.

Some unanswered questions. One problem which has not been resolved is why, in some cases, only the response to the α-subunit is observed and an effect of the βγ-subunits is not seen even though the appropriate effector exists:

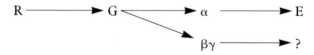

Another unanswered question is whether signal amplification does occur in intact cells. The amount of signal amplification will be determined by the relative number of G proteins compared to receptors and by the lifetime of the activated G protein. Simple quantification by immunochemical methods gives the total amount of the relevant components in a cell but cytoskeletal constraints (compartmentation) could mean that these measurements are of dubious value. Heterotrimeric G proteins are also found in intracellular compartments and control intracellular trafficking of proteins in the Golgi and in endosomes and are not necessarily only coupled to receptors (Nuoffer and Balch, 1994).

The lifetime of the activated G protein is determined by the rate of hydrolysis of GTP. Estimation of GTP hydrolysis rates have been attempted with purified proteins but data from G protein stimulation of atrial potassium channels show that hydrolysis is much faster than that predicted from information on purified proteins (reviewed in Birnbaumer *et al.*, 1990). This may be due to the action of GTPase-activating proteins. Indeed, effectors may act as GTPase-activating proteins and decrease the lifetime of the activated G protein (Birnbaumer *et al.*, 1990).

7.5 Regulation of G protein-coupled receptor function

The activity of G protein-coupled receptors is regulated by a number of mechanisms which exist to prevent excessive stimulation, to allow recovery after overstimulation and to modulate the response of the cell over time. Understanding these processes is fundamental to our understanding of the mechanisms of adaptation to stimuli. In the continued presence of agonist, the receptor response is decreased, a phenomenon known as desensitization. After removal of drug, the receptor activity recovers, although the speed and extent of this resensitization can depend on the duration of agonist activation. Desensitization can either be homologous, where only the response to activated receptor is reduced, or heterologous, where agonist activation of one receptor can lead to desensitization of other receptors which act on similar effector molecules. Heterologous desensitization can involve both changes in the receptor–G protein coupling and changes in the activity or number of the downstream effector molecules. Homologous desensitization is thought to involve decreased coupling of the receptor to its G protein. The mechanisms of homologous desensitization can be distinguished temporally. Rapid desensitization, which occurs within seconds or minutes may involve phosphorylation of the receptor and its internalization into an intracellular compartment. Long-term desensitization, or down-regulation, may involve changes in receptor and/or G protein levels. There may also be changes in the expression and stability of mRNA (Fraser and Lee, 1995). Long-term changes in the levels of G protein-coupled receptors and their accessory proteins are known to be induced by chronic drug treatment and are involved in a number of pathological states (Sleight et al., 1995).

7.5.1 Rapid desensitization

Rapid desensitization of the β_2-adrenergic receptor is correlated with phosphorylation. Much of our understanding of the mechanisms of rapid desensitization comes from studies of the β_2-adrenergic receptor transfected into nonneuronal cell lines (reviewed in Lefkowitz et al., 1990). The β_2-adrenergic receptor is coupled to stimulation of adenylate cyclase via G_s. Agonist binding results in an increase in cAMP levels which activates protein kinase A which, in turn, phosphorylates the receptor on serine residues located in the third intracellular loop and the C-terminal tail (Clark et al., 1989; Hausdorff et al., 1989). The concentration of agonist required to phosphorylate a substantial proportion of receptors will reflect the concentration required to maximally activate adenylate cyclase (Hausdorff et al., 1989), which will depend on both the receptor density and the coupling efficiency. This concentration may be quite low. Protein kinase A-mediated desensitization is an example of heterologous desensitization since stimulation of other receptors that activate G_s will also activate protein kinase A (Clark et al., 1989). Protein kinase C is also able to phosphorylate the same serine (261) in the third intracellular loop. Desensitization of the β-adrenergic receptor by protein kinase C activation has also been demonstrated (Yuan et al., 1994) suggesting that concomitant activation of a receptor which activates protein kinase C is also likely to induce heterologous desensitization. Whether this is the mechanism of rapid desensitization which occurs in intact cells under physiological levels of stimulation is unknown.

The β_2-adrenergic receptor is also phosphorylated by a specific receptor kinase known as βARK or, more recently GRK2 or GRK3 (G protein receptor kinase). These receptor kinases specifically recognize the agonist-occupied form of the receptor (Benovic et al., 1986) and phosphorylate serine residues in the carboxyl-terminal tail (reviewed in Dohlman et al., 1991; Premont et al., 1995). The agonist-dependent nature of this phosphorylation could explain homologous desensitization.

How does phosphorylation cause rapid desensitization? Involvement of arrestin. Mutagenesis of phosphorylation sites on the intracellular loops and C-terminal domain and the use of inhibitors of protein kinase A and βARK have demonstrated that phosphorylation plays an important role in desensitization of the β-adrenergic receptor (Hausdorff et al., 1989; Lohse et al., 1990a; Premont et al., 1995; see *Figure 7.5*). Phosphorylation of the purified β_2-adrenergic receptor by βARK does not decrease the GTPase activity stimulated by activated receptor (Lohse et al., 1990b). However, addition of cytosol from cells transfected with β-arrestin did decrease the GTPase activity of G_s stimulated by agonist suggesting that agonist occupation of the receptor allows phosphorylation of the receptor by βARK, and that this enhances the binding of β-arrestin to the receptor complex thereby preventing interaction between the receptor and G protein. There are a number of splice variants of arrestins which suggests that there may be specific arrestin molecules interacting with different receptors. Visual arrestin showed the greatest affinity for phosphorylated rhodopsin with very little binding to the adrenergic or muscarinic receptors; β-

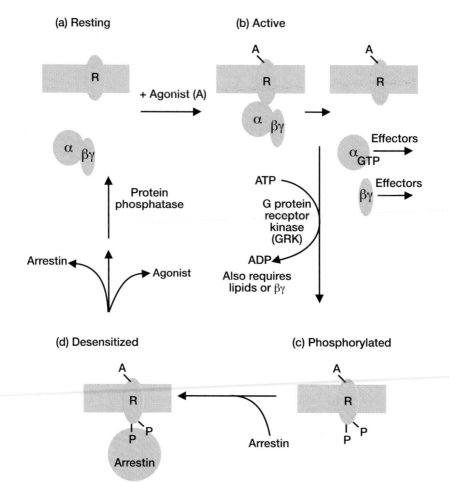

Figure 7.5. Regulation of receptor function by phosphorylation. (a) The receptor is converted from its resting state by binding of ligand and G protein. (b) After dissociation of the G protein α- and βγ-subunits, the receptor can be phosphorylated by G protein receptor kinase and/or by protein kinase A and/or protein kinase C. (c) There is some debate as to whether the phosphorylated state is actually desensitized or not. (d) In the case of the β-adrenergic receptor and rhodopsin, it has been shown that arrestin can bind to the phosphorylated receptor and may cause desensitization by preventing access of G proteins to the intracellular loops and C-terminus of the receptor. The receptor is resensitized by dissociation of arrestin and ligand and dephosphorylation by protein phosphatases.

arrestin had greater affinity for the adrenergic than the muscarinic receptor while arrestin-3 had similar affinity for these two receptors (Gurevich et al., 1995).

The physiological importance of GRKs and arrestin action in neuronal cells has not been widely demonstrated. In β₂-adrenergic receptor transfected cells, desensitization is more extensive in cells overexpressing βARK and β-arrestin (Pippig et al., 1993). At high levels of receptor expression, βARK and β-arrestin become limiting for desensitization: this represents further evidence for a role of β-arrestin in homologous desensitization and suggests that differences in desensitization between the same receptor type in different cell types could be due to varying levels of βARK and β-arrestin expression. In the case of *Drosophila* rhodopsin, the rate of inactivation is mirrored by the rate of arrestin binding (Ranganathan and Stevens, 1995); it will be interesting to find out if this holds true for neurotransmitter receptors.

Is arrestin involved with other receptors? Although the picture is now much clearer for the β_2-adrenergic receptor, the evidence for a similar mechanism occurring with other receptor types is now increasing. Recent studies using overexpression of GRKs suggest a role for GRKs in desensitization of the delta opioid receptor (Pei *et al.*, 1996), the α_{1A} adrenergic receptor (Diviani *et al.*, 1996) and the dopamine 1A receptor (Tiberi *et al.*, 1996). Injection of purified GRKs into sensory neurons enhances the desensitization of α_2-adrenergic receptor-mediated calcium channel inhibition (Diverse-Pierlussi *et al.*, 1996). Direct *in vitro* demonstration of phosphorylation of a receptor by a GRK requires that the receptor either be purified and reconstituted or overexpressed to densities above 5 pmol mg^{-1} protein although the reason for this remains unclear (Premont *et al.*, 1995). This has limited the identification of GRK substrates to a small group of receptors (reviewed in Haga *et al.*, 1994; Premont *et al.*, 1995) which includes receptors coupled to $G_{q/11}$ (e.g. m_1 muscarinic, Haga *et al.*, 1996; m_3 muscarinic, Hosey *et al.*, 1995; substance P, Kwatra *et al.*, 1993) and those coupled to G_o or G_i (e.g. α_2-adrenergic receptor, Benovic *et al.*, 1987; m_2 muscarinic receptors, Hosey *et al.*, 1995). With the exception of m_2 muscarinic receptors where phosphorylation of the receptor does decrease agonist-stimulated GTPase activity, the effect of phosphorylation on G protein coupling is generally unknown (Hosey *et al.*, 1995). The relative contributions of phosphorylation alone or arrestin binding to overall observed desensitization is still unknown.

The role of other kinases is also a matter of debate. In the case of $G_{q/11}$-linked receptors functional correlation of phosphorylation with agonist-induced desensitization has been demonstrated only for the neurokinin-2 receptor (Alblas *et al.*, 1995) and the α_1-adrenergic receptor (Leeb-Lundberg *et al.*, 1987); however the kinase(s) involved have not been identified. A number of studies have shown that activation of protein kinase C with phorbol esters induces agonist-independent phosphorylation of the receptor (e.g. muscarinic m_3 receptor, Haga *et al.*, 1993; CCK receptor, Klueppelberg *et al.*, 1991). Whether protein kinase C-mediated phosphorylation is generally associated with desensitization is still a matter for debate since in some studies it is associated with desensitization (e.g. Orellana *et al.*, 1985) whilst in other studies it is not (e.g. Eva *et al.*, 1990; Kanba *et al.*, 1990).

Similarly for G_i/G_o linked receptors, the role of phosphorylation in rapid desensitization is unclear. α_2-Adrenergic receptors lacking a large portion of the third intracellular loop containing potential phosphorylation sites do not undergo rapid desensitization (Liggett *et al.*, 1992). Circumstantial evidence for the involvement of βARK is that somatostatin induces translocation of βARK to the plasma membrane (presumably to the somatostatin receptor) with a similar time course to that of desensitization of somatostatin inhibition of adenylate cyclase (Mayor *et al.*, 1987). A major difficulty in elucidating the relative importance of each kinase is the lack of selective inhibitors. Heparin has been used to inhibit G protein receptor kinase (e.g. Lohse *et al.*, 1990a) and has been shown to decrease agonist-induced desensitization of the α_{2A}-adrenergic receptor (Liggett *et al.*, 1992). However, heparin is not very selective for GRKs and is believed to interact with a number of growth factor receptors and extracellular matrix proteins (among others) due to its strongly anionic nature (reviewed in Tyrrell *et al.*, 1995).

There are a number of instances where the same receptor appears to undergo desensitization in some cell types or tissues but not others. It has been postulated that this may be due to the presence of previously unrecognized receptor subtypes (e.g. α_{2A} receptor, Liggett *et al.*, 1992) or splice variants (e.g. somatostatin receptor, Vanetti *et al.*, 1993). However evidence is accumulating that the level of desensitization can be determined by the cell type in which the particular receptor subtype is expressed (e.g. β-adrenergic receptor, Chaudry and Granneman, 1994; thyrotropin-releasing hormone, Falck-Pedersen *et al.*, 1994). Furthermore, the time course of phosphorylation of cholecystokinin receptors is very different in native tissue compared to tranfected fibroblast cells (Ozcelebi *et al.*, 1996). Further information on the levels and subcellular distribution of accessory proteins such as GRKs and arrestin-like proteins will be necessary to answer this question.

7.5.2 Internalization/recycling of receptors

Most G protein-coupled receptors undergo agonist-induced internalization of receptor (and possibly ligand) into an endosomal compartment. Significant reduction in surface receptor numbers can occur within a few minutes for some receptors, while other receptors show much slower kinetics. After removal of agonist, receptors are recycled back to the plasma membrane (e.g. muscarinic receptors, Koenig and Edwardson, 1994a). The extent of the decrease of surface receptor numbers varies between receptors and cell types but in all cases depends on both the rate of internalization and the rate of recycling (see *Figure 7.6*). Kinetic analysis of the trafficking of muscarinic receptors in neuroblastoma cell lines (Koenig and Edwardson, 1994b) has shown that 12% of surface receptors are internalized in the first minute. After 20–30 min of incubation with agonist, when a steady state has been reached, the rates of internalization and recycling almost balance each other, with a turnover of 5% of receptors min^{-1}. The difference between the numbers of receptors recycled and internalized accounts for the number degraded (see *Figure 7.6*). The physiological relevance of this process most probably varies from one cell to the next but may involve one or more of the following: (i) short-term desensitization, (ii) an initial step in long-term down-regulation, (iii) retrograde signaling, where the internalized receptor–ligand complex is transported down the axon and acts as a signaling mechanism, (iv) a mechanism for dephosphorylation, and (v) a mechanism for inducing morphological changes.

Molecular mechanisms of internalization. For small molecule G protein-coupled receptors such as the adrenergic and muscarinic receptors, internalization is usually measured as a loss of hydrophilic antagonist ligand binding (e.g. Koenig and Edwardson, 1994b). On the other hand, the internalization of peptide receptors is usually demonstrated as internalization of a labeled agonist ligand into an acid-wash resistant internal compartment (e.g. Beaudet, *et al.*, 1994; Wiley, 1988). It is assumed that the receptor and ligand are internalized together in a one-to-one ratio but this has not been directly demonstrated. Receptors are generally thought to be internalized via clathrin-coated pits since internalization is blocked by agents which inhibit the formation of clathrin-coated pits such as hyperosmolar sucrose (e.g. substance P

(a) Movement of receptors to and from the plasma membrane

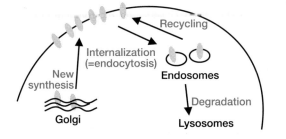

(b) Change in surface receptor number   (c) Rate of receptor movement

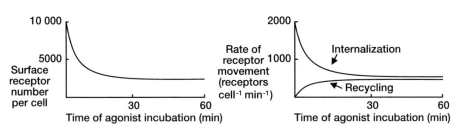

Figure 7.6. Regulation of surface receptor number by internalization and recycling of receptors.(a) Movement of receptors to and from the plasma membrane. Newly synthesized receptors are continuously delivered to the cell surface. In the absence of ligand there is a basal internalization of receptors which maintains the surface receptor number at a constant level. Generally, in the unstimulated state, most of the receptors are found at the plasma membrane rather than at intracellular sites. Upon addition of ligand, the rate of internalization is increased and a substantial proportion of receptors are internalized and are associated with the endosomal compartment. From the endosomes, the receptor can be recycled back to the plasma membrane, or sorted to lysosomes where it is degraded. (b) Change in surface receptor number. A significant reduction of surface receptor numbers generally occurs within 10 min of agonist application. The extent of surface receptor loss can vary between cell types and receptor subtypes. (c) Rate of receptor movement. The reduction in surface receptor numbers depends on the rates of both internalization and recycling. The rate of internalization is proportional to the number of receptors at the surface. The rate of recycling is proportional to the number of receptors in endosomes. Analysis of the rates of internalization and recycling can give an estimation of the rate of receptor turnover at steady state.

receptor, Garland *et al.*, 1994; neurotensin receptor, Chabry *et al.*, 1995; β₂-adrenergic receptor, Pippig *et al.*, 1995; gastrin-releasing peptide receptor, Slice *et al.*, 1994). Involvement of the cytoskeleton also appears to be important since, in some cells, internalization can be blocked by agents which disrupt the cytoskeleton, for example, colchicine (e.g. substance P receptor, Garland *et al.*, 1994 and references therein). Also, internalization of receptors in adherent cells is often much greater than for the same cell type in suspension (Kanba *et al.*, 1990, Slowiejko *et al.*, 1994). Roettger *et al.* (1995) have shown that the cholecystokinin (CCK) receptor can be internalized via both clathrin-coated and smooth pits although quantitative estimation of the importance of each mechanism is unknown. Interaction of G protein-coupled receptors with clathrin adaptor proteins has not yet been demonstrated but analogy with the epidermal growth factor (EGF) receptor (Sorkin and Carpenter, 1993) suggests that this is a likely mechanism. After internalization, receptors have been observed in clathrin-coated vesicles (e.g. muscarinic receptor, Silva *et al.*, 1986) and in the same endosomal compartment as transferrin (α_{1B}-adrenergic receptor, Fonseca *et al.*, 1995; substance P receptor, Garland *et al.*, 1994; thyrotropin-releasing hormone receptor, Ashworth *et al.*, 1995) suggesting that G protein-coupled receptors undergo trafficking similar to a number of other cell surface proteins. Recently, stimulation of the yeast α-factor receptor resulted in ubiquitination of the receptor at the plasma membrane raising the possibility of a role for ubiquitination in the control of plasma membrane density of G protein-coupled receptors (Hicke and Riezman, 1996).

Structural determinants. Aromatic residues in various sequence motifs, particularly the 'NPXY' sequence, have been implicated in the cellular recycling of low density lipoprotein, EGF and insulin receptors (Trowbridge, 1991). However, the structural requirements for agonist-induced internalization appear to vary between receptors. Tyr326 of the human β_2-adrenergic receptor at the junction of the seventh transmembrane domain and the C-terminal may be part of an 'NPXY' general internalization-determining sequence in G protein-coupled receptors since it is highly conserved and is required for internalization of β_2-adrenergic receptor (Barak *et al.*, 1994). However, mutation of the analogous residue does not affect internalization of gastrin-releasing peptide receptors (Slice *et al.*, 1994) or angiotensin receptors (Laporte *et al.*, 1996). A variety of mutations in the second intracellular loop, the C-terminal tail and the third intracellular loop have been implicated in internalization (Chabry *et al.*, 1995; Jockers *et al.*, 1996; Liggett *et al.*, 1992). It might be expected though, that mutations of some residues could have more subtle effects on trafficking of the receptor, for example through changes in both internalization and recycling, rather than a simple on or off mechanism (see below).

It is likely that there are a number of distinct mechanisms underlying internalization. The basal half-time of internalization (i.e. without agonist) has been estimated at greater than 1 h (muscarinic m_4 receptor, Koenig and Edwardson, 1994b; β_2-adrenergic receptor, von Zastrow and Kobilka, 1994). Agonist activation clearly increases the rate of internalization of m_4 muscarinic receptors, rising from a basal value of approximately 20 receptors per cell min^{-1}, to an initial rate of 1400 receptors per cell min^{-1} in the presence of a saturating concentration of agonist in a neuroblastoma cell line containing 11 500 receptors per cell (Koenig and Edwardson, 1994b). A number of factors including cytoskeletal interactions, agonist binding kinetics and phosphorylation by different kinases could be expected to influence the internalization rate to different extents. Tsuga *et al.* (1994) showed that phosphorylation by GRK2 facilitated the internalization of the m_2 muscarinic receptor by decreasing the concentration of carbachol required for maximal internalization. No effect was observed at saturating concentrations of agonist. It has to be noted that many studies of internalization have been carried out with receptors transfected at high density in nonneuronal cells. The effect of receptor density on internalization has not been examined for G protein-coupled receptors although it might be expected to be important since high levels of EGF receptor expression in A431 cells does lead to saturation of the endocytotic apparatus (Wiley, 1988). Furthermore, the molecular mechanisms of protein trafficking are likely to vary between cell types and the implications of this have not yet been addressed. The activation of protein kinase C with phorbol esters can mimic agonist-induced internalization (α_{1B}-adrenergic receptors, Fonseca *et al.*, 1995; muscarinic receptors, Eva *et al.*, 1990) although the physiological relevance of this is unclear. It is possible that the underlying mechanism may involve phosphorylation of accessory proteins in the endocytotic machinery as well as the receptor itself.

Is a functionally activated receptor a necessary prerequisite for internalization? Studies with mutant receptors have provided conflicting information as to whether activation of G proteins is necessary for agonist-induced internalization. Some mutant receptors which show normal G protein coupling and desensitization do not internalize (e.g. angiotensin$_{1A}$ receptor, Hunyady *et al.*, 1994; Thomas *et al.*, 1995) whereas there are some mutants which do not couple to G proteins but can be internalized (β_2-adrenergic receptor, Campbell *et al.*, 1991; neurotensin receptor, Chabry *et al.*, 1995). There are yet other examples where impairment of G protein coupling and internalization occur together (muscarinic m_3 receptor, Thompson *et al.*, 1991; m_1 muscarinic receptor, Lameh *et al.*, 1992). Given the dependence of both G protein coupling and internalization on cell type and in particular the presence of accessory proteins, it is unrealistic to expect a clear-cut effect of different structural elements of the receptor.

Is internalization involved in desensitization? The question of whether internalization can account partly or fully for the observed rapid or long-term desensitization has been hotly debated for a number of years. The short answer is probably that it is partly responsible for short-term desensitization for some receptors under certain conditions but it is not the primary mechanism in most cases. A more complete answer involves understanding some of the following issues. Is the receptor separated from G protein upon internalization? Under what circumstances is the ligand internalized with the receptor and, if the ligand is internalized with the receptor, does the receptor continue to generate a signal whilst in endosomes? How quickly is the internalized receptor recycled? When the recycled receptor reaches the cell surface again, is there a delay before recoupling to G protein and effector? At what stage is the phosphorylated receptor dephosphorylated?

Answers to most of these questions are at best sketchy. Recent attention has focused on the observation that there is greater phosphatase activity in isolated light vesicles containing sequestered receptor (Sibley *et al.*, 1986). A number of groups have now shown that receptors which are not internalized, as a result of either mutation or prevention of clathrin-coated pit formation, also show an inability to recover from desensitization (β_2-adrenergic receptor, Yu *et al.*, 1993; α_{1B}-adrenergic receptor, Fonseca *et al.*, 1995; neurokinin receptors, Garland *et al.*, 1996). Further, inhibition of phosphatases with calyculin A blocked β_2-adrenergic receptor resensitization (Pippig *et al.*, 1995).

Simultaneous translocation of receptor and G protein has been demonstrated for at least the muscarinic receptor in cultured astrocytoma cells (Harden *et al.*, 1985) and in rat brain (Ho *et al.*, 1991). It remains debatable whether the internalized receptor does still generate second messengers in endosomes. There is evidence that neuropeptide receptor–ligand complexes (e.g. Beaudet *et al.*, 1994, and references therein) and G proteins (e.g. Hendry and Crouch, 1991) undergo retrograde axonal transport but the functional significance remains unknown. In the case of neuropeptides, a perinuclear localization of the ligand has been demonstrated (Beaudet *et al.*, 1994) which may reflect accumulation in late endosomes (Gruenberg and Maxfield, 1995). A role in the nucleus has been suggested; alternatively, internalization may be involved in the removal and degradation of neuropeptide transmitters (Beaudet *et al.*, 1994, and references therein). Recently, Mantyh *et al.* (1995) have shown that internalization of substance P receptors in rat spinal cord neurons occurs in response to stimulation of primary afferent neurons. This was accompanied by morphological changes in dendrites which occurred on the same timescale as internalization; reversal showed a similar time-course to recycling of receptors back to the surface.

7.5.3 Mechanisms of long-term down-regulation

What is the role of internalization in down-regulation? It is clear that long-term (>1 h) treatment with agonist induces the loss of total cellular receptor numbers in addition to the decrease in surface receptor numbers. In the case of muscarinic receptors, the rate of receptor degradation increased three-fold in the presence of agonist compared to basal levels (Koenig and Edwardson, 1994b). This is an important mechanism in the response to chronic drug treatment. For example chronic treatment with antidepressants such as fluoxetine, which elevate synaptic levels of 5-HT, induces a decrease in the density of 5-HT receptors (Sleight *et al.*, 1995). Amino-terminal (i.e. extracellular) polymorphisms of the human β_2-adrenergic receptor lead to increased down-regulation (Green *et al.*, 1994). This was proposed to be due to an increased degradation rate rather than effects on synthesis or agonist-induced internalization. It is possible that these residues may be involved in sorting of the receptors in the endosomal compartment.

7.6 Conclusions

G protein-coupled receptors transduce extracellular signals into a multitude of intracellular changes including changes in electrical activity, levels of second messengers, secretion, morphology, growth and differentiation. Understanding how the common structural features of these receptors allow such controlled yet complex signaling patterns is a fundamental question in neurobiology. Over the last few years most of these receptors and their intracellular effector enzymes have been identified and cloned. Now the challenge is two-fold. First to understand how the receptor changes its conformation in order to transmit the signal. This will await a full three-dimensional structure of a number of different receptors along with further mutagenesis experiments and structural modeling. The second, and arguably more difficult challenge, is to understand the cell biology involved. We need to know how the direction and amplification of signal transmission is controlled by different cells under different conditions and how the receptors interact with the rest of the cellular machinery.

Acknowledgments

The author would like to thank her colleagues from the Department of Pharmacology and the Glaxo Institute of Applied Pharmacology at Cambridge University for helpful discussions and comments on the manuscript: Dr Mike Edwardson, Professor P. Humphrey, Dr Ruth Murrell-Lagnado, Dr Peter Richardson, Dr Philip Szekeres, Dr Richard Thurlow, Dr Graeme Wilkinson, Ms Andrea Williams, Dr Robert Woodward and Dr Mike Young.

References

Alblas J, van Etten I, Khanum A, Moolenaar WH. (1995) C terminal truncation of the neurokinin 2 receptor causes enhanced and sustained agonist-induced signaling. *J. Biol. Chem.* **270:** 8944–8951.

Ashworth R, Yu R, Nelson EJ, Dermer S, Gerschengorn MC, Hinkle PM. (1995) Visualization of the thyrotropin-releasing hormone receptor and its ligand during endocytosis and recycling. *Proc. Natl Acad. Sci.* **92:** 512–516.

Baldwin JM. (1993) The probable arrangement of helices in G protein-coupled receptors. *EMBO J.* **12:** 1693–1703.

Barak LS, Tiberi M, Freedman NJ, Kwatra MM, Lefkowitz RJ, Caron MG. (1994) A highly conserved tyrosine residue in G protein-coupled receptors is required for agonist-mediated β_2-adrenergic receptor sequestration. *J. Biol. Chem.* **269:** 2790–2795.

Beaudet A, Mazella J, Nouel D, Chabry J, Castel M-N, Laduron P, Kitabgi P, Faure M-P. (1994) Internalization and intracellular mobilization of neurotensin in neuronal cells. *Biochem. Pharmacol.* **47:** 43–52.

Benovic JL, Strasser RH, Caron MG, Lefkowitz RJ. (1986) Beta-adrenergic receptor kinase: identification of a novel protein kinase that phosphorylates the agonist-occupied form of the receptor. *Proc. Natl Acad. Sci.* **83:** 2797–2801.

Benovic JL, Regan JW, Matsui H, Mayor F, Cotecchia S, Leeb-Lundberg LMF, Caron MG, Lefkowitz RJ. (1987) Agonist-dependent phosphorylation of the α_2-adrenergic receptor by the β-adrenergic receptor kinase. *J. Biol. Chem.* **262:** 17251–17253.

Birnbaumer L, Abramowitz J, Brown AM. (1990) Receptor–effector coupling by G proteins. *Biochim. Biophys. Acta* **1031:** 163–224.

Birnbaumer, M. (1995) Mutations and diseases of G protein coupled receptors. *J. Rec. Signal Transd. Res.* **15:** 131–160.

Bourne HR, Nicoll R. (1993) Molecular machines integrate coincident synaptic signals. *Cell* **72:,** 65–75.

Bulseco DA, Schimerlik MI. (1996) Single amino acid substitutions in the pm2 muscarinic receptor alter receptor/G protein coupling without changing physiological responses. *Mol. Pharmacol.* **49:** 133–141.

Campbell PT, Hnatovich M, O'Dowd BF, Caron MG, Lefkowitz RJ. (1991) Mutations of the human beta-2 adrenergic receptor that impair coupling to Gs interfere with receptor down-regulation but not sequestration. *Mol. Pharmacol.* **39:** 192–198.

Carroll RC, Morielli AD, Peralta EG. (1995) Coincidence detection at the level of phospholipase C activation mediated by the m4 muscarinic acetylcholine receptor. *Curr. Biol.* **5:** 536–544.

Chabry J, Botto J-M, Nouel D, Vincent J-P, Mazella J. (1995) Thr-422 and Tyr-424 residues in the carboxyl terminus are critical for the internalization of the rat neurotensin receptor. *J. Biol. Chem.* **270:** 2439–2442.

Chaudry A, Granneman JG. (1994) Influence of cell type upon the desensitization of the β_3-adrenergic receptor. *J. Pharmacol. Exp. Ther.* **271:** 1253–1258.

Clapham DE. (1993) Mutations in G protein-linked receptors: novel insights on disease. *Cell* **75:** 1237–1239.

Clark RB, Friedman J, Dixon RAF, Strader CD. (1989) Identification of a specific site required for rapid heterologous desensitization of the β-adrenergic receptor by cAMP-dependent protein kinase. *Mol. Pharmacol.* **36:** 343–348.

Conklin BR, Bourne HR. (1993) Structural elements of G_α subunits that interact with $G_{\beta\gamma}$, receptors and effectors. *Cell* **73:** 631–641.

Dalman HM, Neubig RR. (1991) Two peptides from the α_{2A} adrenoceptor alter G protein coupling by distinct mechanisms. *J. Biol. Chem.* **266:** 11 025–11 029.

Dixon RAF, Sigal IS, Rands E. (1987) Ligand binding to the beta-adrenergic receptor involves its rhodopsin-like core. *Nature* **326:** 73–77.

Diverse-Pierluissi M, Inglese J, Stoffel RH, Lefkowitz RJ, Dunlap K. (1996) G protein-coupled receptor kinase mediates desensitization of norepinephrine-induced Ca^{2+} channel inhibition. *Neuron* **16:** 579–585.

Diviani D, Lattion A-L, Larbi N, Kunapuli P, Pronin A, Benovic JL, Cotecchia S. (1996) Effect of different G protein-coupled receptor kinases on phosphorylation and desensitisation of the α_{1B} adrenergic receptor. *J. Biol. Chem.* **271:** 5049–5058.

Dohlman HG, Thorner J, Caron MG, Lefkowitz RJ. (1991) Model systems for the study of seven-transmembrane-segment receptors. *Annu. Rev. Biochem.* **60:** 653–688.

Donnelly D, Findlay JBC. (1994) Seven-helix receptors: structure and modelling. *Curr. Opin. Struct. Biol.* **4:** 582–589.

Donnelly D, Findlay JBC, Blundell TL. (1994) The evolution and structure of aminergic G protein coupled receptors. *Recept. Chann.* **2:** 61–78.

Ercolani L, Stow JL, Boyle JF, Holtzman EJ, Lin H, Grove JR, Ausiello DA. (1990) Membrane localization of the pertussis toxin-sensitive G protein subunits α_{i2} and α_{i3} and expression of a metallothionein-α_{i2} fusion gene in LLC-PK1 cells. *Proc. Natl Acad. Sci. USA* **87:** 4635–4639.

Eva C, Gamalero SR, Genazzani E, Costa E. (1990) Molecular mechanisms of homologous desensitization and internalization of muscarinic receptors in primary cultures of neonatal corticostriatal neurons. *J. Pharmacol. Exp. Ther.* **253:** 257–265.

Falck-Pedersen E, Heinflink M, Alvira M, Nussenzveig DR, Gershengorn MC. (1994) Expression of thyrotropin-releasing hormone receptors by adenovirus-mediated gene transfer reveals that thyrotropin-releasing hormone desensitization is cell specific. *Mol. Pharmacol.* **45:** 684–689.

Fonseca MI, Button DC, Brown RD. (1995) Agonist regulation of α_{1B}-adrenergic receptor subcellular distribution and function. *J. Biol. Chem.* **270:** 8902–8909.

Fraser CM, Lee NH. (1995) Regulation of muscarinic receptor expression by changes in mRNA stability. *Life Sci.* **56:** 899–906.

Fraser CM, Wang C-D, Robinson DA, Gocayne JD, Venter JC. (1989) Site-directed mutagenesis of m1 muscarinic acetylcholine receptors: conserved aspartic acids play important roles in receptor function. *Mol. Pharmacol.* **36:** 840–847.

Garland AM, Grady EF, Payan DG, Vigna SR, Bunnett NW. (1994) Agonist-induced internalization of the substance P (NK1) receptor expressed in epithelial cells. *Biochem. J.* **383:** 177–186.

Garland AM, Grady EF, Lovett M, Vigna SR, Frucht MM, Krause JE, Bunnett NW. (1996). Mechanisms of desensitization and resensitization of G protein-coupled neurokinin1 and neuronkinin2 receptors. *Mol. Pharmacol.* **49:** 438–446.

Gether U, Johansen TE, Snider MR, Lowe JA, Nahanishi S, Schwartz TW. (1993) Different binding epitopes in the NK1 receptor for substance P and a non-peptide antagonist. *Nature* **362:** 345–348.

Gether U, Lower JA, Schwartz TW. (1995) Tachykinin non-peptide antagonists: binding domain and molecular mode of action. *Biochem. Soc. Trans.* **23:** 96–102.

Graeser D, Neubig RR. (1993) Compartmentation of receptors and guanine nucleotide-binding proteins in NG108-15 cells: lack of cross-talk in agonist binding among the α_2-adrenergic, muscarinic, and opiate receptors. *Mol. Pharmacol.* **43:** 434–443.

Green SA, Turki J, Innis M, Liggett SB. (1994) Amino-terminal polymorphisms of the human β_2-adrenergic receptor impart distinct agonist-promoted regulatory properties. *Biochemistry* **33:** 9414–9419.

Gruenberg J, Maxfield FR. (1995) Membrane transport in the endocytic pathway. *Curr. Biol.* **7:** 552–563.

Gurevich VV, Dixon SB, Onorato JJ, Ptasienski J, Kim CM, Sterne-Marr R, Hosey M, Benovic JL. (1995) Arrestin interactions with G protein-coupled receptors. *J. Biol. Chem.* **270:** 720–731.

Haga T, Haga K, Kameyama K, Nakata H. (1993) Phosphorylation of muscarinic receptors: regulation by G proteins. *Life Sci.* **52:** 421–428.

Haga T, Haga K, Kameyama K. (1994) G protein-coupled receptor kinases. *J. Neurochem.* **63:** 400–412.

Haga K, Kameyama K, Haga T, Kikkawa U, Shiozaki K, Uchiyama H. (1996) Phosphorylation of human m1 muscarinic acetylcholine receptors by G protein-coupled receptor kinase 2 and protein kinase C. *J. Biol. Chem.* **271:** 2776–2782.

Harden TK, Petch LA, Traynelis SF, Waldo GL. (1985) Agonist-induced alteration in the membrane form of muscarinic cholinergic receptors. *J. Biol. Chem.* **260:** 13 060–13 066.

Hausdorff WP, Bouvier M, O'Dowd BF, Irons G, Caron MG, Lefkowitz RJ. (1989) Phosphorylation sites on two domains of the β_2-adrenergic receptor are involved in distinct pathways of receptor desensitization. *J. Biol. Chem.* **264:** 12 657–12 665.

Hendry IA and Crouch MF (1991) Retrograde axonal transport of the GTP-binding protein $G_{i\alpha}$: a potential neurotrophic intra-axonal messenger. *Neurosci. Lett.* **133:** 29–32.

Hibert MF, Trumpp-Kallmeyer S, Hoflack J, Bruinvels A (1993) This is not a G protein-coupled receptor. *Trends Pharmacol. Sci.* **14:** 7–12.

Hicke L, Riezman H. (1996) Ubiquitination of a yeast plasma membrane receptor signals its ligand-stimulated endocytosis. *Cell* **84:** 277–287.

Ho AKS, Zhang Y-J, Duffield R, Zheng G-M. (1991) Evidence for the simultaneous translocation of muscarinic acetylcholine receptor and G protein by carbachol. *Cell Signal.* **3:** 587–598.

Horstman DA, Brandon S, Wilson AL, Guyer CA, Cragoe EJ, Limbird LE. (1990) An aspartate conserved among G protein receptors confers allosteric regulation of α_2-adrenergic receptors by sodium. *J. Biol. Chem.* **265:** 21 590–2 1595.

Hosey MM, Benovic JL, DebBurman SK, Richardson RM. (1995) Multiple mechanisms involving protein phosphorylation are linked to desensitization of muscarinic receptors. *Life Sci.* **56:** 951–955.

Hunyady L, Baukal AJ, Balla T, Catt KJ. (1994) Independence of type I angiotensin II receptor endocytosis from G protein coupling and signal transduction. *J. Biol. Chem.* **269:** 24 798–24 808.

Hunyady L, Balla T, Catt KJ. (1996). The ligand binding site of the angiotensin AT1 receptor. *Trends Pharmacol. Sci.* **17:** 135–140.

Hwa J, Graham RM, Perez DM. (1996) Chimeras of α_1-adrergic receptor subtypes identify critical residues that modulate active state isomerization. *J. Biol. Chem.* **271:** 7956–7964.

Ji H, Leung M, Zhang Y, Catt KJ, Sandberg K. (1994) Differential structural requirements for specific binding of non-peptide and peptide antagonists to the AT1 angiotensin receptor. *J. Biol. Chem.* **269:** 16 533–16 536.

Jockers R, Da Silva A, Strosberg AD, Bouvier M, Marullo S. (1996) New molecular and structural determinants involved in β_2-adrenergic receptor desensitization and sequestration. *J. Biol. Chem.* **271:** 9355–9362.

Johansson B, Wymann MP, Holmgren-Peterson K, Magnusson K-E. (1993) N-Formyl peptide receptors in human neutrophils display distinct membrane distribution and lateral mobility when labeled with agonist and antagonist. *J. Cell Biol.* **121:** 1281–1289.

Kanba S, Kanba KS, McKinney M, Pfenning M, Abraham R, Nomura S, Enloes L, Mackey S, Richelson E. (1990) Desensitization of muscarinic M1 receptors of murine neuroblastoma cells (clone N1E-115) without receptor down-regulation and protein kinase C activity. *Biochem. Pharmacol.* **40:** 1005–1014.

Kenakin T. (1995) Agonist-receptor efficacy II: agonist trafficking of receptor signals. *Trends Pharmacol. Sci.* **16:** 232–238.

Kleuss C, Scherubl H, Hescheler J, Schultz G, Wittig B. (1992) Different β-subunits determine G protein interactions with transmembrane receptors. *Nature* **358:** 424–426.

Klueppelberg UG, Gates LK, Gorelick FS, Miller LJ. (1991) Agonist-regulated phosphorylation of the pancreatic cholecystokinin receptor. *J. Biol. Chem.,* **266:** 2403–2408.

Kobilka BK, Kobilka TS, Daniel K, Regan JW, Caron MG, Lefkowitz RJ. (1988) Chimeric α_2/β_2 adrenergic receptors: delineation of domains involved in effector coupling and ligand binding specificity. *Science* **240:** 1310–1316.

Koenig JA, Edwardson JM. (1994a) Routes of delivery of muscarinic receptors to the plasma membrane in NG108-15 cells. *Br. J. Pharmacol.* **111:** 1023–1028.

Koenig JA, Edwardson JM. (1994b) Kinetic analysis of the trafficking of muscarinic acetylcholine receptors between the plasma membrane and intracelullar compartments. *J. Biol. Chem.* **269:** 17174–17182.

Kwatra MM, Schwinn DA, Screurs J, Blank JL, Kim CM, Benovic JL, Krause JE, Caron MG, Lefkowitz RJ. (1993) The substance P receptor, which couples to $G_{q/11}$ is a substrate of β-adrenergic receptor kinase 1 and 2. *J. Biol. Chem.* **268:** 9161–9164.

Lameh J, Philip M, Sharma WK, Moro O, Ramachandran J, Sadee W. (1992) Hm1 muscarinic cholinergic receptor internalization requires a domain in the third cytoplasmic loop. *J. Biol. Chem.* **267:** 13 406–13 412.

Laporte SA, Servant G, Richard DE, Escher E, Guillemette G, Leduc R. (1996) The tyrosine within the NPX_nY motif of the human angiotensin II type I receptor is involved in mediating signal transduction but is not essential for internalization. *Mol. Pharmacol.* **49:** 89–95.

Lee N, Fraser CM. (1993) Cross-talk between m_1 muscarinic acetylcholine and β_2-adrenergic receptors. *J. Biol. Chem.* **268:** 7949–7957.

Leeb-Lundberg LMF, Cotecchia S, DeBlasi A, Caron MG, Lefkowitz RJ. (1987) Regulation of adrenergic receptor function by phosphorylation. *J. Biol. Chem.* **262:** 3098–3105.

Leff P (1995) The two-state model of receptor activation. *Trends Pharmacol. Sci.* **16:** 89–97.

Lefkowitz RJ, Hausdorff WP, Caron MG. (1990) Role of phosphorylation in desensitization of the β-adrenoceptor. *Trends Pharmacol. Sci.* **11:** 190–194.

Liggett SB, Ostrowski J, Chesnut LC, Kurose H, Raymond JR, Caron MG, Lefkowitz RJ. (1992) Sites in the third intracellular loop of the α_{2A}-adrenergic receptor confer short term agonist-promoted desensitization. *J. Biol. Chem.* **267:** 4740–4746.

Li S, Okamoto T, Chun M, Sargiocomo M, Casanova JE, Hansen SH, Nishimoto I, Lisanti MP. (1995) Evidence for a regulated interaction between heterotrimeric G proteins and caveolin. *J. Biol. Chem.* **270:** 15 693–15 701.

Liu J, Schoneberg T, van Rhee M, Wess J. (1995) Mutational analysis of the relative orientation of transmembrane helices I and VII in G protein-coupled receptors. *J. Biol. Chem.* **270:** 19 532–19 539.

Lohse MJ, Benovic JL, Caron MG, Lefkowitz RJ. (1990a) Multiple pathways of rapid β_2-adrenergic receptor desensitization. *J. Biol. Chem.* **265:** 3202–3209.

Lohse MJ, Benovic JL, Codina J, Caron MG, Lefkowitz RJ. (1990b) β-arrestin: a protein that regulates β-adrenergic receptor function. *Science* **248:** 1547–1550.

Lutz MP, Pinon DI, Gates LK, Shenolikar S, Miller LJ. (1993) Control of cholecystokinin receptor dephosphorylation in pancreatic acinar cells. *J. Biol. Chem.* **268:** 12 136–12 142.

Mantyh PW, DeMaster E, Malhotra A et al. (1995) Receptor endocytosis and dendrite reshaping in spinal neurons after somatosensory stimulation. *Science* **268:** 1629–1632.

Mayor F, Benovic JL, Caron MG, Lefkowitz RJ. (1987) Somatostatin induces translocation of the β-adrenergic receptor kinase and desensitizes somatostatin receptors in S49 lymphoma cells. *J. Biol. Chem.* **262:** 6468–6471.

Milligan G. (1995) Signal sorting by G-protein-linked receptors. *Adv. Pharmacol.* **32:** 1–29.

Milligan G, Bond RA, Lee M. (1995a) Inverse agonism: pharmacological curiosity or potential therapeutic strategy? *Trends Pharmacol. Sci.* **16:** 10–13.

Milligan G, Parenti M, Magee AI. (1995b) The dynamic role of palmitoylation in signal transduction. *Trends Biochem Sci.* **20:** 181–186.

Mizobe T, Maze M, Lam V, Suryanarayana S, Kobilka BK. (1996) Arrangement of transmembrane domains in adrenergic receptors. *J. Biol. Chem.* **271:** 2387–2389.

Neer EJ. (1995) Heterotrimeric G proteins: organizers of transmembrane signals. *Cell* **80:** 249–257.

Neve KA, Wiens BL. (1995) Four ways of being an agonist: multiple sequence determinants of efficacy at D2 dopamine receptors. *Biochem. Soc. Trans.* **23:** 112–116.

Neve KA, Cox BA, Hennigsen RA, Spanoyannis A, Neve RL. (1991) Pivotal role for aspartate-80 in the regulation of dopamine D2 receptor affinity for drugs and inhibition of adenylyl cyclase. *Mol. Pharmacol.* **39:** 733–739.

Nuoffer C, Balch WE. (1994) GTPases: multifunctional molecular switches regulating vesicular traffic. *Annu. Rev. Biochem.* **63:** 949–990.

Offermanns S, Wieland T, Homann D, Sandmann J, Bombien E, Spicher K, Schultz G, Jakobs KH. (1994) Transfected muscarinic acetylcholine receptors selectively couple to Gi-type G proteins and $G_{q/11}$. *Mol. Pharmacol.* **45:** 890–898.

Okamoto T, Murayama Y, Hayashi Y, Inagaki M, Ogata E, Nishimoto I. (1991) Identification of a G_s activator region of the β_2-adrenergic receptor that is autoregulated via protein kinase A dependent phosphorylation. *Cell* **67:** 723–730.

Orellana SA, Solski PA, Brown JH. (1985) Phorbol ester inhibits phosphoinositide hydrolysis and calcium mobilization in cultured astrocytoma cells. *J. Biol. Chem.* **260:** 5236–5239.

Oksenberg D, Marsters SA, O'Dowd BF, Jin H, Havlik S, Peroutka SH, Ashkenazi A. (1992) A single amino acid difference confers major pharmacological variation between human and rodent $5HT_{1B}$ receptors. *Nature* **360:** 161–163.

Ostrowski J, Kjelsberg MA, Caron MG, Lefkowitz RJ. (1992) Mutagenesis of the β_2 adrenergic receptor: how structure elucidates function. *Annu. Rev. Pharmacol. Toxicol.* **32:** 167–183.

Ozcelebi F, Rao RV, Holicky E, Madden BJ, McCormick DJ, Miller LJ. (1996) Phosphorylation of cholecystokinin receptors expressed on chinese hamster ovary cells. *J. Biol. Chem.* **271:** 3750–3755.

Patel YC, Greenwood MT, Warszynska A, Panetta R, Srikant CB. (1994) All five cloned human somatostatin receptors (hSSTR1–5) are functionally coupled to adenylyl cyclase. *Biochem. Biophys. Res. Commun.* **198:** 605–612.

Pei, G, Kieffer BL, Lefkowitz RJ, Freedman NJ. (1995) Agonist-dependent phosphorylation of the mouse δ-opioid receptor: involvement of G protein-coupled receptor kinases but not protein kinase C. *Mol. Pharmacol.* **48:** 173–177.

Perez DM, Hwa J, Gaivin R, Mathur M, Brown F, Graham RM (1996) Constitutive activation of a single effector pathway: evidence for multiple activation states of a G protein-coupled receptor. *Mol. Pharmacol.* **49:** 112–122.

Pin J-P, Duvoisin R. (1995) The metabotropic glutamate receptors: structure and function. *Neuropharmacology* **34:** 1–26.

Pippig S, Andexinger S, Daniel K, Puzicha M, Caron MG, Lefkowitz RJ, Lohse MJ. (1993) Overexpression of β-arrestin and β-adrenergic receptor kinase augment desensitization of β₂-adrenergic receptors. *J. Biol. Chem.* **268:** 3201–3208.

Pippig S, Andexinger S, Lohse MJ. (1995) Sequestration and recycling of β₂-adrenergic receptors permit receptor resensitization. *Mol. Pharmacol.* **47:** 666–676.

Prather PL, McGinn TM, Erickson LJ, Evans CJ, Loh HH, Law P-Y. (1994) Ability of delta-opioid receptors to interact with multiple G-proteins is independent of receptor density. *J. Biol. Chem.* **269:** 21 293–21 302.

Premont RT, Inglese J, Lefkowitz RJ. (1995) Protein kinases that phosphorylate activated G protein-coupled receptors. *FASEB J.* **9:** 175–182.

Ranganathan R, Stevens, CF. (1995) Arrestin binding determines the rate of inactivation of the G protein-coupled receptor rhodopsin *in vivo. Cell* **81:** 841–848.

Rasenick MM, Watanabe M, Lazarevic MB, Hatta S, Hamm HE. (1994) Synthetic peptides as probes for G protein function. *J. Biol. Chem.* **269:** 21 519–21 525.

Roettger BF, Rentsch RU, Pinon D, Holicky E, Hadac E, Larkin J, Miller LJ. (1995) Dual pathways of internalization of the cholecystokinin receptor. *J. Cell. Biol.* **128:** 1029–1041.

Savarese TM, Fraser CM. (1992) *In vitro* mutagenesis and the search for structure–function relationships among G protein-coupled receptors. *Biochem. J.* **283:** 1–19.

Schertler GFX, Hargrave PA. (1995) Projection structure of frog rhodopsin in two crystal forms. *Proc. Natl Acad. Sci.* **92:** 11 578–11 582.

Schertler GFX, Villa C, Henderson R. (1993) Projection structure of rhodopsin. *Nature* **362:** 770–772.

Segre GV, Goldring SR. (1993) Receptors for secretin, calcitonin, parathyroid hormone (PTS)/PTH related peptide, vasoactive intestinal peptide, glucagon like peptide 1, growth hormone-releasing hormone, and glucagon belong to a newly discovered G-protein-linked receptor family. *Trends Endocrinol. Metab.* **4:** 309–314.

Sibley DR, Strasser RH, Benovic JL, Daniel K, Lefkowitz RJ. (1986) Phosphorylation/dephosphorylation of the β-adrenergic receptor regulates its functional coupling to adenylate cyclase and subcellular distribution. *Proc. Natl Acad. Sci.* **83:** 9408–9412.

Sidhu A, Kimura K, Vachvanishsanong P. (1994) Induction of G protein independent agonist high-affinity binding sites of D-1 dopamine receptors by β-mercaptoethanol. *Biochemistry* **33:** 11 246–11 253.

Silva WI, Andres A, Schook W, Puszkin S. (1986) Evidence for the presence of muscarinic acetylcholine receptors in bovine brain coated vesicles. *J. Biol. Chem.* **261:** 14 788–14 796.

Simon MI, Strathmann MP, Gautam N. (1991) Diversity of G proteins in signal transduction. *Science* **252:** 802–808.

Sleight AJ, Carolo C, Petit N, Zwingelstein C, Bourson A. (1995) Identification of 5-hydroxytryptamine 7 receptor binding sites in rat hypothalamus: sensitivity to chronic antidepressant treatment. *Mol. Pharmacol.* **47:** 99–103.

Slice LW, Wong HC, Stermini C, Grady EF, Bunnett NW, Walsh JH. (1994) The conserved NPXnY motif present in the gastrin-releasing peptide receptor is not a general sequestration sequence. *J. Biol. Chem.* **269:** 21 755–2 1762.

Slowiejko DM, Levey AI, Fisher SK. (1994) Sequestration of muscarinic cholinergic receptors in permeabilized neuroblastoma cells. *J. Neurochem.* **62:** 1795–1803.

Smrcka AV, Sternweis PC. (1993) Regulation of purified subtypes of phosphatidylinositol-specific phospholipase Cβ by G protein α and βγ subunits. *J. Biol. Chem.* **268:** 9667–9674.

Sorkin A, Carpenter G. (1993) Interaction of activated EGF receptors with coated pit adaptins. *Science* **261:** 612–615.

Strader CD, Fong TM, Tota MR, Underwood D. (1994) Structure and function of G protein-coupled receptors. *Annu. Rev. Biochem.* **63:** 101–132.

Strittmatter SM, Valenzuela D, Kennedy TE, Neer EJ, Filman MC. (1990) G_o is a major growth cone protein subject to regulation by GAP-43. *Nature* **344:** 836–841.

Tang W-J, Gilman AG. (1992) Adenylyl cyclases. *Cell* **70:** 869–872.

Thomas WG, Thekkumkara TJ, Motel TJ, Baker KM. (1995) Stable expression of a truncated AT_{1A} receptor in CHO-K1 cells. *J. Biol. Chem.* **270:** 207–213.

Thompson AK, Mostafapour, Denlinger LC, Bleasdale JE, Fisher SK. (1991) The aminosteroid U73122 inhibits muscarinic receptor sequestration and phosphoinositide hydrolysis in SK-N-SH neuroblastoma cells. *J. Biol. Chem.* **266:** 23 856–23 862.

Tiberi M, Nash SR, Bertrand L, Lefkowitz RJ, Caron MG. (1996). Differential regulation of dopamine D1A receptor responsiveness by various G protein-coupled receptor kinases. *J. Biol. Chem.* **271**: 3771–3778.

Trowbridge IS. (1991) Endocytosis and signals for internalization. *Curr. Biol.* **3**: 634–641.

Tsai-Morris CH, Buczko E, Wang W, Dufau ML. (1990) Intronic nature of the rat luteinizing hormone receptor gene defines a soluble receptor subspecies with hormone binding activity. *J. Biol. Chem.* **265**: 19 385–19 388.

Tsuga H, Kameyama K, Haga T, Kurose H, Nagao T. (1994) Sequestration of muscarinic acetylcholine receptor m2 subtypes. *J. Biol. Chem.* **269**: 32 522–32 527.

Tucek S, Proska J (1995) Allosteric modulation of muscarinic acetylcholine receptors. *Trends Pharmacol. Sci.* **16**: 205–212.

Turcatti G, Vogel H, Chollet A. (1995) Probing the binding domain of the NK2 receptor with fluorescent ligands: evidence that heptapeptide agonists and antagonists bind differently. *Biochemistry* **34**: 3972–3980.

Tyrrell DJ, Kilfeather S, Page CP. (1995) Therapeutic uses of heparin beyond its traditional role as an anticoagulant. *Trends Pharmacol. Sci.* **16**: 198–204.

Vanetti M, Vogt G, Hollt V. (1993) The two isoforms of the mouse somatostatin receptor (mSSTR2A and mSSTR2B) differ in coupling efficiency to adenylate cyclase and in agonist-induced receptor desensitization. *FEBS Lett.* **331**: 260–266.

Vogel WK, Mosser VA, Bulseco DA, Schimerlik MI. (1995) Porcine m2 muscarinic acetylcholine receptor–effector coupling in Chinese hamster ovary cells. *J. Biol. Chem.* **270**: 15 485–15 493.

von Zastrow M, Kobilka BK. (1994) Antagonist-dependent and -independent steps in the mechanism of adrenergic receptor internalization. *J. Biol. Chem.* **269**: 18 448–18 452.

Wess J, Blin N, Mutschler E, Bluml K. (1995) Muscarinic acetylcholine receptors: structural basis of ligand binding and G protein coupling. *Life Sci.* **56**: 915–922.

Wickman KD, Clapham DE. (1995) G protein regulation of ion channels. *Curr. Opin. Neurobiol.* 5. 278–285.

Wiley SH. (1988) Anomalous binding of epidermal growth factor to A431 cells is due to the effect of high receptor densities and a saturable endocytic system. *J. Cell Biol.*, **107**: 801–810.

Wong S K-F, Ross EM. (1994) Chimeric muscarinic cholinergic:β-adrenergic receptors that are functionally promiscuous among G proteins. *J. Biol. Chem.* **269**: 18 968–18 976.

Woodward R, Coley C, Daniell S, Naylor LH, Strange PG. (1995) Investigation of the role of conserved serines residues in the long form of the rat D_2 dopamine receptors using site-directed mutagenesis. *J. Neurochem.* **66**: 394–402.

Yu SS, Lefkowitz RJ, Hausdorff WP. (1993) β-adrenergic receptor sequestration: a potential mechanism of receptor resensitization. *J. Biol. Chem.* **268**: 337–341.

Yuan N, Friedman J, Whaley BS, Clark RB. (1994) cAMP-dependent protein kinase and protein kinase C consensus site mutations of the β-adrenergic receptor. *J. Biol. Chem.* **269**: 23 032–23 038.

Molecular biology of neurotransmitter-gated ion channel receptors

Thora A. Glencorse and R. Wayne Davies

8.1 Introduction

The sophistication of neuronal communication and synaptic diversity is determined, to a large extent, at the molecular level by the diversity of neuronal receptors. Rapid information flow between neurons is crucial for real-time functioning of the brain. All the receptor molecules that mediate fast synaptic transmission events are also transmembrane ion channels, which undergo allosteric structural changes on binding a particular neurotransmitter, resulting in the opening of the channel and the entry of selected ions into the neuron. These neurotransmitter-gated ion channel receptors (NGICR: they are also referred to as extracellular ligand-gated ion channels, as distinct from channels such as cyclic nucleotide-gated (CNG) channels which are gated by intracellular ligands) are distinguished from other ion channels by their responsiveness to small molecule transmitters and not to voltage states (or in some cases to both) and by distinctive molecular properties. The primary role of most NGICR is receiving input at postsynaptic membranes, but they are also involved in presynaptic and extrasynaptic functions. The neurotransmitters currently known to act at such receptors are γ-aminobutyric acid (GABA), glycine, acetylcholine, serotonin (5HT), glutamate and adenosine triphosphate (ATP). Most of these transmitters also act at G protein-linked receptors, which are termed metabotropic, while the NGICR are termed ionotropic. The major inhibitory and excitatory transmission systems of the brain depend on GABA$_A$ receptors (GABA$_A$R) and glutamate receptors (GluR) respectively, with glycine receptors (GlyR) fulfilling the major inhibitory transmission role in the spinal cord. The other types of receptors have more restricted distributions. It has been proposed that neural nicotinic acetylcholine receptors (nAChR), which are present at levels several orders of magnitude below the numbers of GABA$_A$R and GluR but are nevertheless found in many types of central nervous system (CNS) neuron, are involved in modifying rather than mediating synaptic transmission (Role and Berg, 1996). This may well also apply to many 5HT- and ATP-gated receptors.

We now know that there are three distinct molecular groups of NGICRs, distinguished at present by distinct polypeptide topologies within each subunit, and by primary sequence. These are: the nAChR group, consisting of all nAChR, GABA$_A$R,

Molecular Biology of the Neuron, edited by R.W. Davies and B.J. Morris.

GlyR and the 5HT3 receptor (5HT3R); the GluR group [α-amino-3-hydroxy-5-methylisoxazole-4-propionate receptor (AMPAR), kainate receptor (KAINR) and N-methyl-D-aspartate receptor (NMDAR)]; and the ATP P2XR. Within each group there is clear conservation of primary sequence, and evolutionary relationships can be calculated. For example, GABA$_A$R subunit isoforms (e.g. α1, α2) exhibit >70% sequence identity. This decreases to between 35 and 50% identity between the GABA$_A$R subunits (α, β, γ). Other members of this family, for example the GlyR α1-subunit (Grenningloh et al., 1987) and the nAChR α1-subunit (Noda et al., 1983a), exhibit about 34% and 20% identity, respectively, to the GABA$_A$R subunits. Each of these families of genes is thought to have evolved via gene duplication and sequence drift from a common ancestor (Schofield et al., 1987). Arbas et al. (1991) proposed that the ancestor of the nAChR family was a molecule that could interact with acetylcholine, GABA and glycine. The first to diverge, and therefore the most ancient member of this family, was the acetylcholine-gated ion channel. This was followed by GABA$_A$/glycine receptor divergence. Subsequently, the primordial GABA-gated ion channel subunit has evolved to give the present five GABA$_A$R subunit classes; α, β, γ, δ and ρ. Homology comparisons show that the α- and γ-subunits are more similar to each other than either is to the β-subunits: likewise, the β- and δ-subunits are more similar to each other than either is to the α-subunits. Further divergence has occurred within these subunit classes to produce receptor subunit isoforms (Section 8.4).

As might be expected by their frequency of occurrence, many of these receptors are implicated in the etiology of neurological disease. For example, the GABA$_A$ receptor–transmitter system has been implicated in the etiology of epilepsy, panic disorder, anxiety and depression (Matsumoto, 1989). GABA$_A$R, which occur in one form or another in 30% of synapses, are also well known as the target molecules for clinically relevant (and abused) benzodiazepines (e.g. Temazepam™), barbiturates and ethanol. The excitatory GluR (particularly NMDAR) play central roles in the spread of neuronal cell death after ischemic damage (stroke), and have therefore become the objects of intense molecular study. Inappropriate stimulation of GluR can lead to 'excitotoxic' cell death due to high Ca^{2+} influx through the channels, and this may occur in other neurodegenerative diseases. GluR are also important in neuronal plasticity [long-term potentiation (LTP) and long-term depression (LTD)], learning and memory acquisition. A prerequisite for understanding the essential role of these receptor–transmitter systems in brain function and dysfunction, is a comprehensive investigation of normal and pathological gene regulation and receptor function.

The application of molecular biology to the study of mammalian NGICR resulted in the rapid identification of a large number of different subunits and subunit isoforms for each of the different receptors (Table 8.1. For recent reviews see: nAChR, Lindstrom et al., 1995: GABA$_A$R, Sieghart, 1995; Stephenson, 1995; McKernan and Whiting, 1996: GlyR, Kuhse et al., 1995; 5HT3R, Boess and Martin, 1995: ATPR, Fredholm, 1995: GluR, Hollmann and Heinemann, 1994; Seeburg, 1996). Several different molecular approaches have been used in the isolation of cDNAs encoding these NGICR subunits, including hybridization with degenerate oligonucleotide probes, degenerate polymerase chain reaction (PCR) and expression cloning. The distinct subunit classes and subunit isoforms of the mammalian NGICRs that have been identified to date are shown in Table 8.1, together with typical pharmacological agents specific for each receptor type and their clinical relevance. Space limitations preclude a comprehensive listing of all references for every subunit and subunit isoform isolated to date

Table 8.1. The neurotransmitter-gated ion channel superfamily

Family	Number of genes	Selectivity and ions gated	Natural ligand	Pharmacology Agonist	Pharmacology Antagonist	Associated disease(s) and/or therapeutics
nAChR (neuronal)	α2–9 β2–4	Nonselective cation channel $Na^+ K^+$ Ca^{2+}	Acetylcholine	Nicotine Cytesine	α-Bungarotoxin Atropine (+)tubocurarine (channel block)	Targets for local anesthetics, sedatives and hallucinogenic drugs Nicotine enhances attention, diminishes anxiety, improves acquisition and retention of short-term memory
GABA$_A$R	α1–6 β1–3(4) γ1–3(4) δ ρ1–2	Anion channel Cl^- HCO_3^-	γ-Aminobutyric acid (GABA)	Muscimol Flunitrazepam Diazepam Clonazepam Zolpidem Alfaxalone Pentobarbital Zn^{2+} sensitive	Bicuculline Flumazenil Ro15–4513 (partial inverse agonist) TBPS and picrotoxin (channel block)	Targets for anesthetics and sedatives Anxiety Epilepsy (generalized Cleft palate/Prader–Willi
GlyR	α1–4 β	Anion channel Cl^- HCO_3^-	Glycine	β-Alanine taurine, proline	Strychnine	Deficiency in GlyR leads to spasticity and loss of motor control Strychnine poisoning mimics spastic mice Spastic mice exhibit severe motor disease after birth Hyperekplexia, spastic paraplegia
5HT$_3$R	5HT$_3$	Nonselective cation channel $Na^+ K^+$ Ca^{2+}	Serotonin	2-Methyl-5-hydroxy tryptamine, 1-phenylbiguandine mCPBG	Zacopride Ondansetron Granisetron Tropisetron (+)tubocurarine (channel block)	Emesis (general) Anxiety Anti-nociceptive Anti-psychotic

(continued)

Table 8.1. (*Continued*)

Family	Number of genes	Selectivity and ions gated	Natural ligand	Pharmacology		Associated disease(s) and/or therapeutics
				Agonist	Antagonist	
ATP R	P2X1–7	Nonselective cation channel Na$^+$ K$^+$ Ca^{2+}	ATP	2-Methyl-thioATP, αβ methylene ATP; Zn^{2+} sensitive	Suramin Stilbene isothiocyanate; (+) tubocurarine (nonselective block)	Nociception Primary afferent neurotransmission
GluR:NMDAR)	NMDAR1 NMDAR2A–2D	Cation channel Na$^+$ K$^+$ Ca^{2+}; Mg^{2+} voltage dependent channel block	Glutamate; Glycine=co-agonist	NMDA Aspartate; Zn^{2+} sensitive	D-AP5 MK-801	LTP/LTD Learning and memory Neuronal plasticity Epilepsy (kindling) Anxiogenesis Ischemia (local)
GluR:AMPAR	GluR1–4	Cation channel Na$^+$ K$^+$ (Ca^{2+})	Glutamate	AMPA Domoate Quisqualate Kainate	NBQX CNQX; Potentiators: Cyclothiazide Concanavalin A	LTP/LTD Learning and memory Neuronal plasticity Epilepsy (kindling) Anxiogenesis Ischemia (global)
GluR:KAINR	GluR5–7 KA1–2	Cation channel Na$^+$ K$^+$ (Ca^{2+})	Glutamate	Kainate Domoate Quisqualate	NBQX CNQX NS-102; Potentiator: Concanavalin A	LTP/LTD Learning and memory Neuronal plasticity Epilepsy (kindling) Anxiogenesis Ischemia (global)

CNQX, 6-cyano-7-nitroquinoxaline-2,3-dione; D-AP5, D-2-amino-5-phosphopentanoic acid; mCPBG, *meta*-chloro-phenylbiguanide; MU-801, dizocilpine; NBQX, 6-nitro-7-sulfamobenzo-*f*-quinoxaline-2,3-dione; R.15-4513, ethyl-8-azido, 5,6-dihydro-5-methyl-6-oxo-4H-imidazo [1,5-a][1,4]benzodiazepine-3-carboxylate; TBPS, *t*-butylbicyclophosphorothionate.

– these can be identified by computer searches of the Entrez, MGD and OMIM data-bases (see Chapter 1; Mouse Genome Database, 1996; Online Mendelian Inheritance in Man, 1996) and by reference to Conley (1996) which provides a complete collection of NGICR facts up to 1994, with updates on the Web site. A great deal is known about the occurrence of various NGICR receptor subtypes in the developing and adult brain, and this, together with other special features and functions of each receptor type and subunit are summarized in *Tables 8.2–8.7* at the end of this chapter.

We present an overview of the current state of knowledge of the molecular biology of these receptors. The descriptive phase of molecular characterization is well advanced in some areas, and provides a base for exciting progress to be made in understanding how these molecules work, and how their action relates to neuronal and brain function. Since we intend to illuminate principles and the present status, rather than give exhaustive detail, we will use examples primarily from $GABA_AR$ mol-ecular biology, except where knowledge of another receptor is significantly more advanced, or provides a unique insight.

8.2 Genes and gene structure

The availability of sequenced cDNA clones encoding the various subunits of NGICR has permitted the isolation and characterization of many of the corresponding genes (*Tables 8.1–8.7*). Not surprisingly, they are exemplars of standard eukaryotic genes containing introns. Further, the genomic organization can be conserved between genes encoding different members of the same family. For example, the gene struc-tures of three $GABA_AR$ subunit genes have been characterized to date. Comparison of the organization of the murine δ-subunit gene (Sommer *et al.*, 1990a), the human β1-subunit gene (Kirkness *et al.*, 1991) and the murine α6-subunit gene (Glencorse *et al.*, unpublished) demonstrates a conserved gene structure, organized into nine distinct exons with identical patterning of the intron–exon boundaries. Although the genes encoding the α6- and δ-subunits are about 14 kb long and that of the β1-subunit gene is 65 kb long there is complete conservation of exon–intron structure. The chicken β4-subunit gene, also 65 kb in size, exhibits a similar structure with five of the eight intron–exon boundaries conserved with the murine δ-subunit gene (Lasham *et al.*, 1991) with the other three in comparable positions. In addition, the $GABA_AR$ subunit genes appear to always have one, sometimes two, extremely large introns while the other introns are much smaller in size. However, there is no conservation in the size of each intron in any given position within the gene. For example, the smallest intron is 70 bp in size and is present as the third intron of the δ-subunit gene while the first, and largest intron is about 8 kb (Sommer *et al.*, 1990a). In contrast, the smallest intron of the β1-subunit gene is 103 bp between exons six and seven, while the third and largest intron is 19.4 kb long (Kirkness *et al.*, 1991).

Comparison of the genomic organization of the inhibitory $GABA_AR$ and GlyR shows remarkable conservation between gene families (Kirkness *et al.*, 1991; Lasham *et al.*, 1991; Matzenbach *et al.*, 1994; Sommer *et al.*, 1990a). Only one of the intron positions is radically different; in $GABA_AR$, unlike GlyR, the second transmem-brane domain (TM2) is composed of two exons separated by an intron. This is unusual given the predicted importance of this domain in channel function (Section 8.6). In contrast the positions of the intron–exon boundaries in $GABA_AR$ subunits do not correspond with those in nAChR genes (Buonanna *et al.*, 1989). This is con-sistent with the proposition that the $GABA_AR$ and GlyR subunit encoding genes are evolutionarily more closely related to each other than either set is to AChR encoding genes. Interestingly, however, gene structure within the nAChR family differ: while the intron–exon patterning of the $\alpha2$- to $\alpha5$- and $\beta1$- to $\beta3$-subunit genes (six exons) are conserved, this is not true of the $\alpha7$- (10 exons, the first four conserved) and $\alpha9$- (five exons, patterning quite distinct) subunit genes. Of interest, the genomic organization of the 5HT3R gene most closely resembles that of the nAChR $\alpha7$-subunit gene, suggesting that the 5HT3R and nAChR gene families are more closely related than either is to the GlyR or GABA$_A$R gene families.

Most of the genes encoding NGICR have been genetically mapped in man and the mouse. The map locations are given in *Tables 8.2–8.7*, with the mouse location below the human. GABA$_A$R subunit genes have been found to be clustered on chromosomes in both species: for example, in man the $\alpha1$-, $\alpha6$-, $\beta2$- and $\gamma2$-subunit genes are all located on chromosome 5 close together at q31–35, the $\alpha5$, $\beta3$ and $\gamma3$ genes are on chromosome 15 in a group at q11–13, and the $\alpha2$, $\alpha4$, $\beta1$ and $\gamma1$ genes are clustered on chromosome 4 (*Table 8.3*). Gene clustering has also been shown for other genes encoding members of other NGICR families (Conley, 1996).

8.3 Gene expression

Given the complexity of the mammalian CNS, mechanisms must exist to ensure that the correct numbers and types of receptors are present in neurons in the correct spatiotemporal pattern. Regulation of gene expression can be achieved at several different levels [i.e. gene copy number, DNA methylation, initiation, elongation and termination of transcription, mRNA stability, RNA editing, and translational efficiency (reviewed by Winnacker, 1989)]. However, transcriptional regulation has been implicated as the major mechanism by which eukaryotic gene regulation is achieved (He and Rosenfeld, 1991; Struhl, 1991), particularly in neurons (Mandel and McKinnon, 1993). The expression of NGICR genes is regulated during synapse formation in response to axonal arrival at a target neuron or muscle cell, during adaptive synaptic change in LTP and probably learning and memory (Armstrong and Montminy, 1993; Goelet *et al.*, 1986), and in response to long-term exposure to commonly encountered artificial agonists or potentiator compounds, such as alcohol and benzodiazepine tranquillizers for GABA$_A$R and nicotine for nAChR. Alteration in gene expression is certainly a component of the mechanism of addiction to such compounds. The expression of many NGICR-encoding genes is highly controlled during development (Section 8.3.2), and the great majority of NGICR are expressed in sharply defined subsets of neurons. Understanding neuronal NGICR promoters and the protein factors that act on them is a prerequisite to analysis of these important phenomena.

8.3.1 Promoter characterization

The characterization of vertebrate neuronal promoters and of the transcription factors that act upon them is at an early stage of investigation (see Chapter 3). The factors and DNA sequences involved in NGICR cell-type specific gene expression are almost unknown. Studies of the regulation of neuronal NGICR gene expression has been limited by the lack of a suitable *in vitro* system. However, the development of new techniques for the culturing of primary and transformed neuronal cells (Levine and Manley, 1989) and transgenic mouse analysis (Grosveld and Kollias, 1992) have led to progress in this field.

Most of the promoter characterization work on nAChR genes has been carried out in muscle-related cells, where an Sp-1 like factor, G-stretch binding factor and muscle-specific transcription factors have been shown to be involved in transcription control, and several *cis*-acting elements have been identified. The involvement of particular sequence elements in expression of the gene encoding nAChR subunit α/ has been demonstrated (Matter-Sadinski *et al.*, 1992). Relatively little is known about the regulation of GABA$_A$R gene expression other than: (a) all genes exhibit regional-, developmental- and cell-specific expression patterns (*Table 8.3*); and (b) expression patterns can be altered in response to chronic receptor activation. Recently a few reports describing the characterization of GABA$_A$R gene 5′ ends have been published, but only three of these have demonstrated promoter function. The first two groups used cell transfection/chloramphenicol acetyltransferase assay techniques. Kirkness and Fraser (1993) showed that the 5′ ends of the human and rat GABA$_A$R β3-subunit genes are conserved and demonstrated strong promoter activity of this region (proximal and distal elements) in neuronal cells. They further identified *cis*-acting sequence elements that bind nuclear protein factors near the transcription initiation sites. Kang and colleagues (1994) similarly demonstrated a strong proximal promoter activity near the transcription initiation site of the GABA$_A$R α1-subunit gene. They further demonstrated that transcriptional activity of this promoter construct was strongly repressed by chronic administration of the benzodiazepine lorazepam. The third group of Lüscher and co-workers (1993) employed the use of transgenic mouse lines carrying a *lacZ* gene driven by δ-subunit gene sequences to analyze promoter activity. They demonstrated faithful neuron-specific expression in most regions of the CNS but were unable to show the correct developmental profile of the native gene. Thus the construct used in these experiments lacked sequences essential for the inherent developmental expression profile of the rat GABA$_A$R δ-subunit gene. During this work, a novel *cis* sequence element and associated novel DNA binding protein, brain-specific factor 1 (BSF1), was identified (Motejlek *et al.*, 1994). However, this *cis* element cannot be found so far in extensive sequence analysis of the mouse δ-subunit gene (A.B. Roberts and R.W. Davies, unpublished observations). Clearly, much remains to be learned about the regulation of GABA$_A$R and other NGICR genes in neurons.

8.3.2 Developmental regulation

The expression of all NGICR subunit genes is regulated to give very specific spatio-temporal patterns of subunit occurrence and level. The functional significance of most of these regulatory phenomena remains unknown, but it is generally held that NGICR play special roles in development distinct from their adult roles; an example is that modulation of Ca^{2+} levels by NMDAR is essential for granule cell neuron migration in the developing cerebellum. Two particularly dramatic shifts in subunit expression and incorporation into NGICR are known. One is the gene expression switch that leads to the replacement of nAChR fetal γ-subunits by functionally homologous ε-subunits in muscle cells. The second is the switch from fetal expression of only GlyR α2-subunits to adult expression of only GlyR α1- and α3-subunits in spinal cord neurons in early postnatal life, which explains the differential strychnine sensitivity of neonates and adults in terms of the different strychnine-binding affinities of the respective GlyR subtypes. The regulatory mechanisms involved are not known.

A particularly important stage in nervous system development is the formation of functional synapses, and the induction of NGICR gene expression in response to growth cone arrival is an important component of synapse development. This has been most clearly demonstrated by the failure of neuronal and muscle AChR gene expression in mice lacking a functional agrin gene (Gautam *et al.*, 1996). Agrin is secreted by the incoming neuron and stimulates many aspects of AChR synapse formation. Synapse-specific expression of AChR genes is also known to be dependent on peptides known as ARIA or neuregulin, which are members of the glial growth factor peptides and act via ErbB family receptors (reviewed by Carraway and Burden, 1995): however, it appears that agrin-signaled establishment of a properly differentiated synapse is a prerequisite for this, so that agrin mutations are epistatic to the neuregulin control. This is an important area of future investigation for all NGICRs.

8.4 RNA processing

Generation of isoform diversity by RNA processing delineates an additional level of post-transcriptional regulation of NGICR within the CNS. The most frequent RNA processing which occurs within the NGICR families is alternative splicing of the primary gene transcript (*Tables 8.2–8.7*).

Alternative splicing can affect almost all aspects of gene/protein function (Smith *et al.*, 1989). Within NGICR, alternatively spliced transcripts have been shown to have differential localization within the vertebrate CNS (Glencorse *et al.*, 1992) and it has been shown that such variant gene products can be functionally distinct. For example, variant gene products which differ solely by the inclusion or exclusion of a short exon that consists almost entirely of a putative PKC (protein kinase C) phosphorylation site have been observed to be differentially phosphorylated (Section 8.5; Moss *et al.*, 1992a,b), thus acquiring different electrophysiological properties. Further, developmental switches from one alternatively spliced isoform to another, with corresponding differences in localization of gene products and functional properties of glutamate-activated channels, have been observed for the flip and flop variants of the AMPAR subunits (GluR1–GluR4: Monyer *et al.*, 1991; Sommer *et al.*, 1990b). In this case, one of two adjacent exons is selected, which encode 38 amino acids closely related but of different sequences.

The mechanism of alternative splicing is currently under intensive investigation in nonneural systems. Recent work on alternative splicing of adenovirus L1 pre-mRNA (Kanopka *et al.*, 1996) indicates that the determining factors are the set of SR proteins present in a cell (SR proteins are a class of essential splicing factors necessary for early steps in spliceosome formation), and the locations of specific binding sites for particular SR proteins within the pre-mRNA. SR protein binding at 5′ splice sites or within exons enhances the efficiency of splicing, whereas SR protein bound to an intron just downstream of the branch-point inhibits splicing. It is likely that the same principles will operate in neurons, with the addition of neuron-specific splicing factors, one of which has been described (SmN; McAllister *et al.*, 1988) and shows greatly increased expression postnatally (Grimaldi *et al.*, 1993).

Another type of RNA processing, namely RNA editing, has been observed solely in the GluR family (reviewed by Seeberg, 1996). RNA editing affects several sites in five of the 16 GluR subunit mRNAs (*Table 8.7*). *In vitro* experiments have shown that adenosines in pre-mRNAs are converted to inosines by oxidative deamination, this conversion depending on the presence of short double-stranded RNA structures within the pre-mRNA, as shown in *Figure 8.1*. Editing of a particular CAG codon encoding glutamine (Q) to produce a CIG codon encoding arginine (R) results in the incorporation of R instead of Q at the Q/R site of protein segment M2 (the proposed channel lining domain; Section 8.6) of the GluR2, GluR5 and GluR6 pre-mRNAs. This results in drastically lowered calcium permeability and altered current rectification properties of receptors edited. Further RNA editing occurs in the GluR6 pre-mRNA to generate receptor polypeptides edited at the isoleucine/valine (I/V) and tyrosine/cysteine (Y/C) sites of M1, the putative first transmembrane domain, further altering and fine-tuning the regulation of channel function. Another site known to be edited in GluR2 is the R/G (G=glycine) site, where receptors containing the edited subunit recover faster from channel desensitization.

It is known that double-stranded RNA adenosine deaminase (dsRAD), an enzyme first encountered as part of cellular antiviral defence mechanisms, can carry out the deamination reaction involved in neuronal RNA editing. Whether it is actually the enzyme that does this is not clear. Recent work has shown that dsRAD can edit the R/G site of GluR2 pre-mRNA efficiently *in vitro* (Melcher *et al.*, 1996), and that no other proteins are required (Polson *et al.*, 1996). However, dsRAD edits the Q/R site of GluR2 pre-mRNA very poorly, and a second enzyme RED1 (dsRNA-specific editase 1) with some homology to dsRAD has been identified that can carry out Q/R editing efficiently (Melcher *et al.*, 1996). Neither enzyme is brain-specific, being expressed in many tissues including brain, and it remains possible that a family of such enzymes may exist, some of which may be brain specific. Whatever the proteins responsible for neuronal RNA editing of GluR subunit pre-mRNAs are, it is clear that RNA editing increases the molecular complexity and functional capacity of this receptor family.

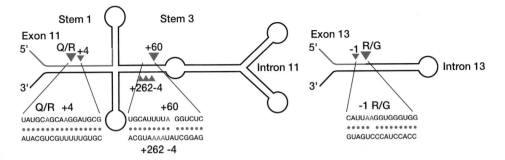

(a) GluR Q/R editing

(b) GluR R/G editing

Figure 8.1. RNA editing of the GluR2 pre-mRNA. (a) Q/R editing. The pre-mRNA is edited at the Q/R and other sites (+4, +60 and +262–4) in exon 11 and intron 11. (b) R/G editing at this and the -1 site in exon 13. Editing at all sites involves the oxidative deamination of adenosine to inosine. Editing frequencies at the sites shown and other low-frequency sites varies with experimental conditions. Edited As are indicated by triangles and by bold letters in the corresponding nucleotide sequence. Dots indicate Watson–Crick or G:U base-pairing. Exon sequences are shown in orange and intron sequences in gray. Reprinted with permission from *Nature*, vol. 380, pp. 391–392. ©1996 Macmillan Magazines Ltd.

8.5 Post-translational modification

The central role of the NGICRs in mammalian neurotransmission makes them a likely site for regulation of neuronal activity by post-translational modification mechanisms: for example, acetylation, carboxylation, glycosylation, methylation and phosphorylation (reviewed by Han and Martinage, 1992). In the molecular era in NGICR research, glycosylation and phosphorylation sites are predicted on the basis of consensus sequences found within the protein sequence. All NGICR family members contain predicted phosphorylation sites and glycosylation sites (Conley, 1996, and references therein). However, the presence of these sites in the primary sequence does not mean that they are actually modified *in vivo* or that the glycosylation or phosphorylation is a requirement for receptor functionality. However, there is evidence that the phosphorylation state of NGICRs affects desensitization, subunit assembly and receptor aggregation at the neuronal synapse (Swope *et al.*, 1992) and that the glycosylation state of NGICR may affect assembly and cell-surface expression (Connolly *et al.*, 1996; Hollmann *et al.*, 1994; Sumikawa and Miledi, 1989).

8.5.1 Phosphorylation

Protein phosphorylation is one of the most widespread and effective ways of modulating protein activity (Nestler and Greengard, 1984) and there is evidence for a role for phosphorylation in regulating certain potassium and calcium channels (Browning *et al.*, 1985) as well as the nAChR (Huganir *et al.*, 1986). GluR phosphorylation has also been shown to occur widely, and to modify the properties of resulting channels. PKC phosphorylates Ser831 and PKA phosphorylates Ser845 of GluR1 in neurons in culture. The PKA modification results in a 40% potentiation of the peak current through GluR1 homomeric channels, which may relate to the known PKA-induced potentiation of AMPAR in neurons (Roche *et al.*, 1996). As is the case for all NGICRs, there is no direct evidence for phosphorylation as a means of regulating GABA$_A$R activity *in vivo*, but a series of recent experiments (Moss *et al.*, 1995) have shown both that GABA$_A$R can be phosphorylated by PKC [and by PKA, calmodulin kinase II (CaMKII) and PKG], and that the phosphorylation state alters the electrophysiological properties of GABA$_A$R channels. In the brain, a variety of kinases are found and the relative activity and localization of these in particular neurons, combined with the structural specificity and stoichiometry of phosphorylation sites on those GABA$_A$R subunits expressed in the neuron, will combine to determine the phosphorylation state of GABA$_A$R subtypes.

Considerable experimental evidence exists showing that GABA$_A$R can be phosphorylated by the action of known protein kinases (reviewed by Rabow *et al.*, 1995). Highly purified GABA$_A$R proteins can be phosphorylated by exogenously added PKA and PKC. Purified fusion proteins of the intracellular domains of GABA$_A$R subunits are also phosphorylated by various kinases. These experiments allowed the identification of the residues phosphorylated by phosphopeptide analysis and elimination of consensus recognition sequences by site-directed mutagenesis. All β-subunits have a conserved PKA phosphorylation site, a PKC phosphorylation site, a PKG phosphorylation site and CaMKII can also phosphorylate β-subunits (McDonald and Moss, 1994; Moss *et al.*, 1992a,b; Swope *et al.*, 1992). Phosphorylation of α-subunits by an unknown protein kinase has also been observed (Sweetnam *et al.*, 1988). In addition, the γ2L and γ2L forms of the γ2-subunit, derived from alternatively spliced mRNAs with an extra short exon being incorporated into the γ2L mRNA, are phosphorylated by PKC but not by PKA (Moss *et al.*, 1992b) or PKG (McDonald and Moss, 1994), one of the PKC sites being present only in the γ2L variant (Moss *et al*, 1992a). In addition, CaMKII phosphorylates Ser343 in γ2L only, and Ser348 and Thr350 in γ2L and γ2S (McDonald and Moss, 1994).

Effects of PKC phosphorylation on GABA$_A$R channel properties have been observed. Krishek *et al.* (1994) studied the effects of phorbolesters on electrophysiological properties of recombinant GABA$_A$R expressed in HEK293 cells co-transfected with the α isoform of PKC. They concluded that increased PKC phosphorylation caused a reduction in the amplitudes of GABA-activated currents without affecting the time constants for current decay. Similar inhibitory effects on GABA-activated currents of phorbolester stimulation have also been found previously (Leidenheimer *et al.*, 1992). Krishek *et al.* (1994) also showed that the most important PKC phosphorylation site was Ser343, in the extra amino acid sequence of γ2L. Thus extensive phosphorylation of GABA$_A$R subtypes occurs in the CNS. It is clear from the recent work on both GABA$_A$R and GluR that phosphorylation represents another important level of regulation of NGICR function.

Tyrosine phosphorylation sites are also found on NGICR, and the *Torpedo* nAChR has been shown to be highly phosphorylated on tyrosine residues in postsynaptic membranes (Hopfield *et al.*, 1988; Wagner *et al.*, 1991), which have been shown to contain a protein tyrosine kinase that phosphorylates the β-, γ- and δ-subunits. Tyrosine phosphorylation of muscle AChR has been shown to be dependent on agrin stimulation (Wallace *et al.*, 1991), and it may play a part in the aggregation of AChR at synapses, possibly by leading to enhanced association with rapsyn and thus to the cytoskeleton (although, mutations that remove the β-subunit tyrosine phosphorylation site do not block receptor clustering; Yu and Hall, 1994a). Tyrosine phosphorylation of the δ-subunit has also been suggested to be involved in the assembly of the SH2 domain proteins Fyk and Fyn into a signaling complex. Tyrosine phosphorylation may play a similar role for other NGICRs.

8.5.2 Glycosylation

Glycosylation is one of the most common and extensive modifications of extracellular proteins (Han and Martinage, 1992). Glycosylation events within the cell have been implicated to play an important role in receptor assembly and cell-surface expression (Connolly *et al.*, 1996; Hollmann *et al.*, 1994; Sumikawa and Miledi, 1989).

Biochemical analysis of purified receptor populations from brain membranes indicated heterogeneity of receptor polypeptides – a result of differentially glycosylated forms of the same protein. Analysis of GABA$_A$R subunit polypeptides has highlighted extensive glycosylation of α- and β-subunit proteins. These were initially believed to indicate the possible existence of receptor subunit isoforms generated by alternative-splicing events. However, the molecular cloning of receptor subunit genes and their transcripts (cDNAs) has demonstrated the existence of few such alternatively spliced transcripts (*Table 8.3*). Further, the GABA$_A$R α5-subunit has been shown to be both N- and O-glycosylated, giving rise to two distinct α5-subunit isoforms differing in O-linked carbohydrate content (Sieghart *et al.*, 1993). Both differentially glycosylated forms are present in rat membranes but the exact localization and functional role(s) of these two differentially glycosylated forms of α5-subunit protein are not currently known. However, recent research has shown that whilst N-glycosylation is not essential for GABA$_A$R assembly, it may be important for efficient (and accurate) transport of receptors to the plasma membrane (Buller *et al.*, 1994; Connolly *et al.*, 1996).

Effects of differential glycosylation on receptor trafficking and assembly are also observed for other NGICRs. Glycosylation of the nAChR is also not a prerequisite for receptor assembly, but is required for efficient insertion into the plasma membrane (Gehle and Sumikawa, 1991). Thus, the heterogeneity, assembly and functionality of all NGICR are likely to be affected by differential glycosylation events. It is to be expected that glycosylation in neurons may involve some special neuronal enzymes, and may find uses beyond those encountered in other cell types.

8.6 Protein structure

8.6.1 Subunit composition

All ion-channel receptors are multimeric transmembrane proteins, with subunit polypeptides surrounding a central pore through which ions can pass. In most cases, naturally occurring receptors are predominantly heteromeric (i.e. are made up of more than one of the known subunits). Exceptions to this are the 5HT3R, for which only one subunit has been discovered, and possibly the GABA$_C$R (Cutting et al., 1991). When expressed by themselves in *Xenopus* oocytes, some subunits of other receptors also form homooligomeric channels (e.g. rat nAChR α9), but the significance of this in their natural context is unclear. The NMDA subclass of GluR always contains the NMDAR1 subunit, together with any of the NMDAR2, -3 or -4 subunits. Similarly, the AMPA class of GluR probably mostly have a GluR2 subunit, with various combinations of GluR1, GluR3 and GluR4. The β2-subunit of nAChR is a component of all nicotine-binding nAChR (Picciotto et al., 1995) and the β subunit of GlyR is ubiquitously expressed (Malosio et al., 1991). There do not appear to be ubiquitous subunits of GABA$_A$R, although certain subunits are expressed at higher levels and/or more widely. The subunit composition of ATPR is unknown. It is known (Unwin, 1989) that the nAChR has five subunits in the mature channel, and by analogy to these data together with various indirect experiments, other ion channel receptors are tentatively regarded as being pentameric. The five subunits are thought, in accord with nAChR data, to be in a quasi-symmetrical arrangement (*Figure 8.2*).

The assembly of any five of a large number of available subunits into the mature receptor potentially provides a source of very high levels of receptor diversity. This is in fact constrained to varying extents by molecular rules for successful assembly, restrictions on the positioning of subunits around the channel (e.g. in GABA$_A$R an α- and a γ-subunit both contribute to the binding site for benzodiazepines and must be nearest neighbors), and by the expression pattern of subunits in particular differentiated neurons. Nevertheless, a large number of different receptor subtypes (molecules with a particular subunit composition and arrangement) must occur. For example, experimental evidence for GABA$_A$R of over 20 different compositions is available, and many more probably exist. Most of these are, however, relatively rare. The predominant GABA$_A$R are α1β2γ2, followed by α2βnγ2, α3βnγ2 and α2βnγ1 (Whiting et al., 1995). A general or predominant GABA$_A$R stoichiometry of 2α-, 1β-, 2γ-subunits is likely, and two different α-subunits and/or two different γ-subunits have been shown to coexist in the same receptor molecule. Since each receptor subtype can differ in pharmacology and electrophysiology, some of them dramatically, it is clear that establishing which subtype is used at each site, and the relationship between receptor subtype and function is an important but complex task.

8.6.2 3-D structure and allostery

It is known that there are at least three distinct functional states of NGICR which must reflect alternative protein structures with different intrinsic stabilities. These are the resting ('closed') state, which predominates in the absence of neurotransmitter, the active ('open') state(s) which occurs transiently after neurotransmitter binding and the desensitized state(s) with a closed channel but high affinity for neurotransmitter. These protein structural states differ dramatically in the probability of the channel being open. A major challenge for NGICR molecular biology is to describe these protein structures and understand the mechanism of allosteric transitions between them.

The only ion channel receptor for which 3-D structure data have been obtained is the postsynaptic nAChR of *Torpedo marmorata*. The structure of this molecule has been determined to 9Å resolution using electron microscopy and 3-D image reconstruction, in both the closed (Unwin, 1993) and the open (Unwin, 1995) states, providing information on the allosteric structural changes occurring within the molecule on binding ligand as well as on the structure *per se*. Data on this molecule can probably be extrapolated to varying extents to mammalian nAChR, GABA$_A$R, GlyR and 5HT3R, but not to other NGICRs.

The overall structure and dimensions of the closed nAChR are shown in *Figure 8.2a*. The five subunits of the *Torpedo* nAChR are clearly arranged quasi-symmetrically in the arrangement $\alpha\beta\alpha\gamma\delta$ (note that mammalian neuronal nAChR are made up of α- and β-subunits). Most details of secondary structure cannot be resolved, but four dense rods presumed to be α-helices can be discerned in each subunit. Three of these are in the large extracellular N-terminal domain. The α-subunits also show a central cavity which may connect to the surface and has been proposed to represent the ACh-binding pocket. The fourth rod structure occurs within the transmembrane region of each subunit, and forms the lining of the transmembrane pore. These putative transmembrane α-helices form a 'barrel' with a pronounced right-handed twist. The remainder of the transmembrane region external to these rods is a star-shaped region of diffuse density which most likely corresponds to β-sheets (*Figure 8.2b*). A striking feature of the single transmembrane α-helix is that it is kinked, coming closest to the center of the pore at a point just below the middle of the bilayer. Unwin (1993) proposed that this may correspond to the position of Leu251, and that this may act as a pore closing residue via a leucine-zipper sidechain interaction.

When the open structure is compared to the closed structure, they are seen to be most alike at the extracellular mouth of the channel. Elsewhere in the molecule, small net rotational displacements around the channel axis occur. The twisting of the extracellular domains is likely to be central to the co-operative mechanism of channel opening. Most striking, however, are the effects of the rotational displacements of the pore-lining α-helix, resulting in the helices now coming closest to the axis not at their central kinks but close to the lower face of the bilayer. *Figure 8.2c* shows these changes in orientation of the helix diagrammatically. This suggests a molecular mechanism for the connection between ACh binding within the extracellular domains of α-subunits, and the opening of the ion channel (Unwin, 1995). ACh binding induces local twisting within α-subunits, co-ordinated allosterically by the intervening β-subunit which moves away from one α-subunit instead of changing shape. These deformations are communicated to the membrane segment, where the pore-lining helices transmit the rotations to the gate-forming Leu251 side-chains, pulling them away from the axis. This destabilizes the leucine-zipper, and the helices switch to side-to-side interactions, leaving the pore open. However, the proposal that Leu251 forms the gate of the channel is in some doubt, since the results of cysteine-substitution experiments (Akabas *et al.*, 1994) indicate a more cytoplasmic location for the gate, and data from mutant 5HT3R and muscle AChR appear inconsistent with the Leu251 hypothesis (reviewed by Karlin and Akabas, 1995). An alternative model of the opening and closing of the gate (Karlin and Akabas, 1995) is shown in *Figure 8.2d*.

Unfortunately, the resolution of the electron microscopic analysis of the nAChR to date is inadequate to determine the polypeptide folding within the extracellular or intracellular domains. These regions of the nAChR family of NGICR do not show

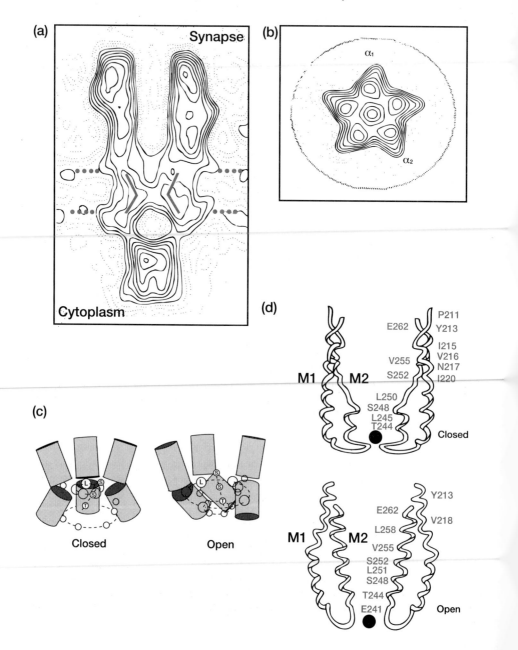

posed (Imoto *et al.*, 1988) that rings of charged M2 residues around the channel determined ion selectivity and conductance; subsequent studies with mutant NGICR have shown that these charged residues alone do not determine ion selectivity (reviewed by Karlin and Akabas, 1995). The residues in two of these rings do have strong effects on channel conductance.

The M2 segment of GluR has also been thought to be the pore-lining segment by analogy with the nAChR model, and is still regarded as the primary candidate despite being clearly bilayer re-entrant rather than transmembrane; re-entrant membrane segments are involved in pore formation in voltage-gated ion channels. There is at least good evidence that the GluR M2 segment plays an important role in determining ion permeability. Site-directed mutagenesis of the M2 residue at which arginine is introduced into AMPAR subunit GluR2 by RNA editing changes the ion permeability and I/V relationships of glutamate channels. However, amino acid exchanges caused by RNA editing of the KAINR GluR6 subunit in both M1 as well as M2 affect ion permeability.

8.7 Assembly and subcellular localization

Mature NGICR are complex molecules that carry out an essential function. The information for the correct assembly of the desired receptor subtype at the correct cellular location must be encoded within the subunit protein sequences and structures. Moreover, once assembled, NGICR need to be concentrated close to the sites of transmitter release in order for interneuronal communication to be effective. Some of the rules and mechanisms governing these important phenomena are just beginning to become known.

Knowledge of how NGICR subunits assemble into mature receptors and are transported to their sites of action (primarily postsynaptic membranes at synapses, but also extrasynaptic sites) is fragmentary, and some general principles have emerged for the nAChR family. Little is known for GluR, and nothing for ATP P2XR. All subunit polypeptides have a standard N-terminal signal sequence. Subunit polypeptides are inserted into the endoplasmic reticulum (ER) membrane and protein folding proceeds with the assistance of chaperones such as BiP and calnexin, which have been found associated with $GABA_A R$ subunits (Connolly *et al.*, 1996). Protein folding continues for some time after subunits begin to associate. The subunits of each receptor follow a complex and strict set of rules for association, which occurs in the ER as calnexin dissociates from the subunits (Gelman *et al.*, 1995). The first stage is the formation of intracellular dimer or trimer intermediates (Green and Millar, 1995). For example, the *Torpedo* nAChR subunits α, δ and γ form a trimer very rapidly, which is joined by a β-subunit after an hour, and a second α-subunit after several hours. Intersubunit associations are very specific and preferential. GlyR subunits always assemble as $2(\alpha\beta) + \alpha$, giving 3α:2β stoichiometry. Another crucial level of sorting occurs between the ER and the plasma membrane: only certain combinations of subunits are able to make this passage. When α-, β2- and γ2L-subunits of $GABA_A R$ are co-expressed in A293 cells the αγ2L and βγ2L combinations form, but are retained in the ER; only receptors containing α1β2 and α1β2γ2L appear at the surface. The mechanism of this transport selectivity is unknown. Glycosylation can modulate transport, but is not essential, since tunicamycin treatment does not prevent $GABA_A R$ reaching the plasma membrane (Connolly *et al.*, 1996).

Receptors with particular subunits in a particular arrangement within the pentamer can emerge preferentially from more complex mixtures. Although 30 different arrangements of pentameric channels containing all three of GABA$_A$R α1-, β1- and γ2-subunits are possible after co-expression, the conductance and gating properties of the resulting receptors were homogeneous, suggesting that one subunit arrangement predominates (Angelotti and Macdonald, 1993). In another case, a homogeneous population of GABA$_A$R occurred when six subunits were co-expressed (Sigel *et al.*, 1990). In chick ciliary ganglion neurons, an nAChR containing α3-, α5- and β4- (and other) subunits predominates at synapses, but the same cells express an extrasynaptic receptor that contains none of these subunits. Given this level of precision, it is not surprising that there is little evidence for the occurrence of hybrid receptors with subunits of mixed origin, despite frequent co-expression in neurons. Even AMPA and KAIN GluR subunits segregate completely when co-expressed (Partin *et al.*, 1993).

The information for subunit association is primarily encoded in the 3-D structure of the N-terminal domain(s) (Verrall and Hall, 1992), but a sequence within the intracellular M3–M4 'loop' structure of certain subunits (e.g. nAChR α- but not β-subunits), has also been shown to play a role in later stages of assembly or transport including specific association with accessory proteins (Yu and Hall, 1994b). In GlyR, four amino acid motifs termed assembly boxes have been identified (Kuhse *et al.*, 1993). In the wild-type these sequences appear to prevent the formation of α–α or β–β homodimers.

Assembled NGICR become located in particular regions of the neuron. Those receptors at synapses can also aggregate into very dense clusters. It is clear that specific association of these receptors with accessory proteins that in turn connect to cytoskeletal proteins (particularly tubulin) underlies these phenomena. For nAChR and GlyR, the mediating accessory proteins have been identified and named rapsyn and gepharin respectively. They interact with specific sequences in the M3–M4 loop of certain subunits, and are present at equimolar amounts in purified receptor complexes. The intracellular density of the nAChR complex in *Figure 8.2a* is primarily rapsyn. Gepharin has been shown to be important in subcellular localization of GlyR.

All the available evidence indicates that rapsyn plays a critical role in ACh receptor clustering. Rapsyn (also called 43 kDa) co-localizes with AChR from the earliest time that clusters of receptors are detectable, and rapsyn expression leads to AChR clustering in cell lines. Mice lacking rapsyn are incapable of clustering AChR in response to agrin (Gautam *et al.*, 1995). Rapsyn regulates the subcellular localization and clustering of MuSK, a muscle receptor tyrosine kinase, and stimulates the kinase activity of this protein, leading to the phosphorylation of tyrosine in the β-subunit of the AChR (Gillespie *et al.*, 1996). Rapsyn clearly plays a key role in clustering AChR and elements of the agrin signaling pathway, which is essential for synaptic differentiation at the neuromuscular junction. Since agrin is certainly expressed in the CNS, a similar system may operate in CNS neuronal synapse formation.

8.8 Future prospects

Molecular cloning of subunit genes has provided the key molecular definition of the components of NGICR transmission systems. On this base further molecular characterization using combined molecular biology and pharmacological tools has provided at least some insight into all important aspects of NGICR biology. The field has become much more complex than could have been envisaged a decade ago, and the future of the field will become increasingly dependent on combining molecular and genetic technology with neurophysiological and pharmacological analysis. Determination of high resolution 3-D structures of domains of these receptors at least, with and without bound neurotransmitter, is essential for further progress in understanding the molecular mechanisms underlying their action and interaction with drugs. Progress here is likely to depend upon expression of protein domains and structures determination by 3-D nuclear magnetic resonance spectroscopy or crystallography, unless considerable advances are made in studying membrane protein structure. The regulation of receptor number and activity is a second key area where relatively little is known, but where the present tools of molecular biology and biochemistry should allow rapid progress to be made. Further data in this area are needed to increase our understanding of the role of these receptors in addiction, learning and memory. Finally, gene targeting technology can provide a link between the receptor genes and subunits and actual biological function. Several simple gene elimination experiments have been reported (Culiat *et al.*, 1994; Forrest *et al.*, 1994; Günther *et al.*, 1995; Ikeda *et al.*, 1995; Kashiwabuchi *et al.*, 1995; Kutsuwada *et al.*, 1996; Li *et al.*, 1994; Picciotto *et al.*, 1995; Sakimura *et al.*, 1995; Treinin and Chalfie, 1995). As expected, loss of function effects were observed in most knockout transgenic mice, with some more drastic than others. Viability problems were observed with NGICR major subunit knockouts of the GABA$_A$R γ2-subunit, the NMDARA1 and the NMDAR2B subunits. Mice lacking NMDAR2B had impaired suckling response but could be hand reared. All NGICR transgenic animals exhibited some form of abnormal phenotype either structural, behavioral, motor or cognitive (learning and memory), both predicted and unexpected. For example, while null mutations of the NMDAR1 and nAChR β2-subunits caused the loss of the entire complement of NMDA and nACh receptors, respectively, this was not true of the null mutation in the GABA$_A$R γ2-subunit gene. One of the most interesting points to note about these NGICR knockout transgenic animals is that the anticipated up-regulation of other receptor subunit(s) to compensate for the loss of functional receptors containing the deleted subunit was not observed. In those cases, most notably the GABA$_A$R α5 and γ3 loss-of-function mutations, where no clear phenotypic difference has been observed, it remains to be seen whether closer investigation will reveal phenotypic effects, or whether in the case of these minor subunits compensation by other subunits has indeed occurred. The potential for mouse mutants, both spontaneously occurring and those derived by experimental manipulation, as animal models for human disease is vast. Transgene rescue experiments have demonstrated the ability to restore normal phenotypes from disease states. Cleft palate, caused by deficiency of the GABA$_A$R β3-subunit gene, can be rescued by transgene expression of the GABA$_A$R β3-subunit (Culiat *et al.*, 1995), while phenotypic correction of the spastic mouse can be achieved by transgene expression of the glycine receptor β-subunit (Hartenstein *et al.*, 1996). The wider application of this technology and its sophisticated variants will provide information about the role of these receptors during development, in particular neuronal circuits and in whole animal behavior, and provide cells lacking particular NGICR subunits as hosts for work on receptor structure–function and molecular cell biology. Novel functions for neurotransmitters and their receptors, such as the recently proposed role for GABA and glutamate in cortical neurogenesis (LaMantia, 1995) and ACh in the modulation of synaptic transmission (Role and Berg, 1996) and neuronal degeneration (Treinin and Chalfie, 1995) in the brain will become apparent. A great leap forward in understanding NGICR transmission systems is required if we are to comprehend and effectively treat human pathological conditions in which they play a role; the molecular tools are now available to achieve this.

Table 8.2. The neuronal nicotinic acetylcholine receptor family

nACh	Gene		Distribution	Special features and/or functions
	Name	Map		
nAChR general			CNS, widely distributed but at much reduced levels compared to GluR and GABA$_A$R Present at the neuromuscular junction PNS, especially autonomic neurons	Excitatory neurotransmission Pre- and postsynaptic receptors Presynaptic receptors mediate release of several different neurotransmitters and may modulate CNS synapses Postsynaptic receptors mediate and modulate ionotropic neurotransmission Possible role in neuronal pathfinding and target selection Pentametric receptor structure: stoichiometry: $\alpha_2\beta_3$ 11 distinct genes encoding: eight α-subunits three β-subunits
$\alpha 2$	CHRNA2 Acra2	8q24 14D1–D3 (19)	Embryonic through neonate Restricted expression Relatively high levels in lateral spiriform nucleus, Purkinje cells of cerebellum, cochlea	Component of αBgt insensitive nAChRs
$\alpha 3$	CHRNA3 Acra3	15q24 9B–E3 (31)	Embryonic through adult Brain and retina Autonomic ganglia Postsynaptic localization	Major component of αBgt insensitive nAChRs $\alpha 3\beta 4$ receptors (?) with associated populations of $\alpha 5$- and $\beta 2$-subunit containing receptors
$\alpha 4$	CHRNA4 Acra4	20q13.2–13.3 2H3–H4 (91)	Adult Widespread within CNS, especially cerebellum, optic lobe, cochlea Pre- and postsynaptic localization Not present in periphery	Major component of αBgt insensitive nAChRs $\alpha 4\beta 2$ nAChRs comprise 90% of high-affinity nicotine binding sites in mammalian brain Mis-sense mutation associated with autosomal dominant nocturnal frontal-lobe epilepsy
$\alpha 5$	CHRNA5 Acra5	15q24 9B–E3 (34)	Embryonic Widespread within CNS, especially hipocampus and substantia nigra, but more restricted than $\alpha 3$, $\alpha 4$ and $\beta 2$ Not expressed in amygdala, septum, thalamus or cerebellum	Component of αBgt insensitive nAChRs Found associated with minor fraction of $\alpha 4\beta 2$ receptors Homomeric $\alpha 5$ receptors do not form functional channels
$\alpha 6$	? ?	? ?	? Isolated/cloned from substantia nigra	Component of αBgt insensitive nAChRs Homomeric $\alpha 5$ receptors do not form functional channels

(continued)

Table 8.2. (*Continued*)

nACh	Gene Name	Map	Distribution	Special features and/or functions
α7	CHRNA7 Acra7	15q13–14 7C–D3 (28)	Widely distributed in adult CNS but in discrete neuronal populations Embryonic through adult CNS Highly expressed in sensory/motor and olfactory regions, brainstem, retina, hippocampus Extrasynaptic localization	Major component of brain αBgt binding nAChRs (except retina) Highly permeable to Ca^{2+}, more so than NMDAR Insensitive to voltage block by Mg^{2+} Minority population contain both α7- and α8-subunits Can form homomeric receptors Expressed in all components of the limbic system Possible role in cell proliferation
α8	? ?	? ?	Embryonic through adult CNS Cochlear localization High levels of expression in retina	Highly permeable to Ca^{2+} Mixed nicotinic/muscarinic pharmacological profile Minor component of brain αBgt binding nAChRs Major component of αBgt receptors in retina Possible role in modulation of auditory stimuli Minority population contain both α7- and α8-subunits
α9	? ?	? ?	Embryonic, not expressed in adult brain Relatively high levels in retina and cochlea	Homomeric receptors Mixed nicotinic/muscarinic pharmacological profile Receptors containing the α9-subunit are αBgt sensitive Probably modulate the encoding of auditory stimuli
β2	CHRNB2 Acrb2	1p21 3F1–F3 (58)	Embryonic through adult Widespread within CNS Distribution same as α2, α3 and α4 combined	Major component of αBgt insensitive nAChRs α4β2 nAChRs comprise 90% of high-affinity nicotine binding sites in mammalian brain
β3	CHRNB3 Acrb3	8p11.2 9	Restricted expression in adult brain Relatively high levels in cochlea	Component of αBgt insensitive nAChRs Unable to form functional channels with α2, α3 or α4
β4	CHRNB4 ?	15q24 ?	Widespread within CNS, especially ciliary and cervical ganglia, Purkinje cells Expression levels between those of β2 and β3	Component of αBgt insensitive nAChRs

CNS, central nervous system; PNS, peripheral nervous system; αβgt, α-bungarotoxin.

Table 8.3. The GABA$_A$ receptor family

GABA	Gene		Distribution	Special features and/or functions
	Name	Map locus		
GABA$_A$R general			CNS, widely distributed Postsynaptic receptors	Inhibitory neurotransmission → neuronal hyperpolarization Heterogeneous receptor population Pentameric receptor stucture 17 distinct genes encoding: six α-subunits four β-subunits four γ-subunits one δ-subunit two ρ-subunits Three distinct gene clusters α(α)βγ Alternative splicing
α1	GABRA1 Gabra1	5q34–35 11A2–B1 (19)	Postnatal to adult Expressed throughout the brain	Most abundant α-subunit Component of major GABA$_A$R subtype (α1β2γ2) GABA$_A$R containing the α1-subunit exhibit BZI pharmacology
α2	GABRA2 Gabra2	4p13-12 5C-E2 (35)	Embryonic to neonatal Peak expression throughout the brain Adult expression restricted to telencephalic and hippocampal regions	Component of major developmental isoform of GABA$_A$R (α2β2/3γ2) GABA$_A$R containing the α2-subunit exhibit BZII pharmacology
α3	GABRA3 Gabra3	Xq28 XA6–B (32)	Embryonic to neonatal Peak expression throughout the brain Limited adult expression in the cortex and hippocampus	GABA$_A$R containing the α3-subunit exhibit BZII pharmacology
α4	GABRA4 Gabra4	4p14–q12 7	Onset of expression E15 Peak levels of expression in the neonate Restricted expression in the cerebellum	GABA$_A$R containing the α4-subunit are BZ 'insensitive'
α5	GABRA5 Gabra5	15q11–13 7C–D3 (29)	Neonatal to adult Widely expressed throughout the brain Highest levels found in hippocampus	GABA$_A$R containing the α5-subunit exhibit unique BZII pharmacology (distinct from GABA$_A$R containing either the α2- or α3-subunits
α6	GABRA6 Gabra6	5q31.1–35 11 (23)	Expressed only in cerebellar granule cells Birth to adult Two alternatively spliced transcripts	GABA$_A$R containing the α6-subunit are BZ 'insensitive' but will bind Ro15-4513 with high affinity Ethanol sensitive Alternatively spliced variants α6s and α6L differ by 10αα in the extracellular domain (rat)

(continued)

Table 8.3. (*Continued*)

GABA	Gene Name	Map locus	Distribution	Special features and/or functions
β1	GABRB1 Gabrb1	4p13–12 5C–E2 (35)	Neonatal to adult Highest levels found in the hippocampus No expression in the cerebellum	Structural, involved in agonist binding
β2	GABRB2 Gabrb2	5q34–35 ?	Embryonic through to adult Complex regulation through development Alternatively spliced variants show little difference in expression patterns	Most abundant β-subunit Component of major GABA$_A$R subtype (α1β2γ2) Structural, involved in agonist binding
β3	GABRB3 Gabrb3	15q11.2–12 7C–D3 (30)	Tight control of expression in diencephalon and thalamic regions Expressed throughout the brain	Least abundant β-subunit Structural, involved in agonist binding Possible role in cleft palate (Culiat *et al.*, 1995)
β4	? ?	? ?	Low levels of expression throughout the neuroaxis Embryonic Alternatively spliced variants show predominantly overlapping expression patterns	To date, only isolated from chick brain Alternative splice variants β4 and β4′ differ by 4$\alpha\alpha$ in the intracellular domain No functional information available
γ1	GABRG1 ?	4p14–q21.1 ?	Primarily embryonic to neonatal Adult expression limited to cortical telencephalic regions	Pharmacology and functionality of GABA$_A$R containing γ1-subunits are quite distinct Presence of a γ-subunit is an absolute requirement for BZ pharmacology
γ2	GABRG2 Gabrg2	5q31.1–33.2 11A2–B1 (19)	Widely expressed throughout neuroaxis, alternatively spliced variants differentially expressed	Most abundant γ-subunit Component of major GABA$_A$R subtype (α1β2γ2) Alternative splice variants γ2S and γ2L differ by 8aa in the intracellular domain: the exclusion/inclusion of a PKC phosphorylation site Ethanol sensitive Presence of a γ-subunit is an absolute requirement for BZ pharmacology
γ3	GABRG3 Gabrg3	15q11.2–12 7	Expresion restricted to late embryonic/ neonatal stages Transient expression in cerebellum	Least abundant γ-subunit Pharmacology and functionality of receptors containing γ3-subunits are quite distinct Presence of a γ-subunit is an absolute requirement for BZ pharmacology

(continued)

Table 8.3. (*Continued*)

GABA	Gene		Distribution	Special features and/or functions
	Name	Map locus		
γ4	? ?	? ?	Low levels of expression throughout neuroaxis in the chick	To date, only isolated from chick brain No functional information
δ	GABRD ?	1p ?	Neonatal to adult Expressed throughout the brain Highest levels in cerebellum	GABA$_A$R containing the δ-subunit are BZ 'insensitive' May replace the γ-subunit in some receptor combinations, but more closely resembles β-subunit(s) in sequence
ρ1	GABRR1 Gabrr1	6q14–21 4A1–A5 (13)	Retinal specific Low level expression within CNS	Classic GABA$_C$R BIC/BAC insensitive
ρ2	GABRR2 Gabrr2	6q14–21 4A1+A5 (13)	Retinal specific Low level expression within CNS	Classic GABA$_C$R BIC/BAC insensitive

BZ, benzodiazepine; BZI, benzodiazepine type I; BZII, benzodiazepine type II.

Table 8.4. The glycine receptor family

Glycine	Gene		Distribution	Special features and/or functions
	Name	Map		
GlyR general			CNS, especially the lower neuroaxis including brainstem and spinal cord Involved in regulation of motor and sensory functions Postsynaptic receptors	Inhibitory neurotransmission Heterogeneous receptor population Invariant 3α:2β stoichiometry Five distinct genes Alternative splicing GlyR co-precipitate with gephyrin, a peripheral membrane bound protein
α1	GLRA1 Glra1	5q32 11B1–B5 (33)	Adult brain and spinal cord High levels of expression Especially in superior and inferior colliculi Two transcripts	Major component of adult GlyR Alternative-splice variant α1$_{ins}$ contains an 8aa insertion between M3 and M4 encoding a potential phosphorylation site
α2 α2*	GLRA2 Glra2	Xp22.2–22.1 XF3–ter (73)	Fetal through neonatal brain and spinal cord High levels of expression especially in cortex, thalamus, hippocampus Two alternatively spliced transcripts (alternate exon 3/3a) which appear to be isofunctional when expressed	Major component of fetal GlyR α2/α2* differ by 5aa in N-terminal domain GlyR containing the α2-subunit exhibit 500-fold lower sensitivity to the antagonist strychnine Developmental switch from α2- to α1-subunit containing receptors occurs within 3 weeks of birth

(*continued*)

Table 8.4. (*Continued*)

Glycine	Gene Name	Map	Distribution	Special features and/or functions
α3	GLRA3 Glra3	? ?	Adult brain Low levels of expression. Greatest expression in cerebellum, hippocampus and olfactory bulb	Major component of cerebellar GlyR
α4	GLRA4 Glra4	? X	? developmental stage Low levels of expression and/or restricted to limited set of neurons Closest in aa homology to the α2-subunit	No functional data No cDNA clone isolated to date
β1	GLRB Glrb	? ?	Constitutive expression throughout development Brain and spinal cord High levels of expression	β-Subunit not required for agonist or antagonist binding Contain 'assembly domains' involved in the assembly of receptors Predominantly structural Required for picrotoxin resistance

Table 8.5. The seratonin ($5HT_3$) receptor

$5HT_3$	Gene Name	Map	Distribution	Special features and/or functions
$5HT_3$	HTR3 Htr3	? ?	Two transcripts, differentially expressed Poorly expressed in brain compared to periphery CNS: cortical, limbic and brainstem structures including, ventral hippocampus, amygdala, olfactory bulb, dorsal ganglia, brainstem motor neurons PNS: enteric, autonomic and primary sensory neurons Neuronal cell lines (NG108-15, N1E-115, NCB20)	RNA splicing mechanisms Pre- and postsynaptic receptors Presynaptic receptors mediate the release of several neurotransmitters (GABA, dopamine, 5HT, acetylcholine, noradrenalin) Postsynaptic receptors mediate ionotropic neurotransmission Function of central receptors: mediate pain reception, cognition, sensory processing, cranial motor neuron activity, modulation of effect

Table 8.6. The purinoceptor (P2X) family

ATP	Gene		Distribution	Special features and/or functions
	Name	Map		
P2XR general			CNS and peripheral neurons (cell bodies and nerve termini) Located in most tissues of the body including heart, liver, spleen, spinal cord, vas deferens and urinary bladder	Central: control fast sensory, motor and cognitive functions Periphery: control of effector structures (heart, autonomic sensory neurons, vas deferens, smooth muscles) Distinct structure: • two proposed transmembrane domains • ATP receptor domain • pore forming motif • intracellular N- and C-termini
P2X1	? ?	17 ?	Low levels in adult brain compared to neonate Poorly expressed in brain (cerebellum, stratium, dentate gyrus, hippocampus, cortex) compared to periphery (vas deferens, urinary bladder), also expressed in spinal cord Four transcripts, each differentially expressed Relative expression levels in the brain 4.2 kb > 2.6 kb >1.8 kb and 3.6 kb	P2X1R are predominantly neonatal RNA splicing mechanisms Potential role in apoptosis Agonist sensitivity of recombinant P2X1R resemble that of native receptors on vascular smooth muscle, vas deferens and some CNS neurons: 2-methylthioATP $\geq$ ATP $\geq$ α,β-meATP $>>$ ADP α,βmeATP full agonist at recombinant P2X1 receptors
P2X2	? ?	? ?	Low levels in adult brain compared to neonate Poorly expressed in brain (stratium, hippocampus, dentate gyrus, amygdala, cortex, cerebellum) compared to periphery Relatively high levels found in the pituitary, vas deferens, spinal cord and PC12 cells Single transcript, ~2 kb	P2X2R are predominantly neonatal Agonist sensitivity resembles that of native receptors on PC12 cells and certain sensory and autonomic neurons: 2-methyl thioATP = ATP = ATP-γ-S α,βmeATP is inactive at this receptor Co-expression of P2X2 and P2X3 can account for ATP-gated currents in sensory neurons
P2X3	? ?	? ?	Expression restricted to sensory neurons, in particular dorsal root ganglia	Possible role in nociception Agonist sensitivity resembles that of native receptors on sensory neurons: 2-methylthioATP $>>$ ATP $>>$ α,βmeATP $>>$ ADP Co-expression of P2X2 and P2X3 can account for ATP gated currents in sensory neurons

(continued)

Table 8.6. (*Continued*)

ATP	Gene		Distribution	Special features and/or functions
	Name	Map		
P2X4	? ?	? ?	Widespread distribution in brain (similar to P2X6) – highest levels in cerebellum Widespread distribution in periphery (including the heart and epithelia)	One of the major P2X subunits in brain P2X4R may have a role in hormone secretion/release P2X4R exhibit a novel pharmacology: • α,βmeATP is not effective • P2X4R are insensitive to antagonists suramin and PPADS
P2X5	? ?	? ?	Low levels of transcript in brain, spinal cord and adrenal gland More restricted than P2X1, 2, 4, 6, 7 Predominant form found in heart	α,βmeATP not effective at recombinant P2X5R Recombinant P2X5R are sensitive to antagonists suramin and PPADS P2X5R resemble P2X2R
P2X6	? ?	? ?	Widespread distribution in brain (similar to P2X4 but more restricted) Mainly located in secretory tissues	One of the major P2X subunits in brain P2X6R homomeric channels are nonfunctional/not activated by ATP P2XR containing the P2X6 subunit may have a role in hormone secretion
P2X7	? ?	? ?	Distributed both centrally and peripherally Strongly expressed in macrophage, brain, spinal cord, lung and spleen	Novel pharmacology: α,βmeATP not effective at recombinant P2X7 receptors Recombinant P2X7R are sensitive to PPADS, and only slightly sensitive to suramin Unique carboxyl-terminal domain involved in lytic actions of ATP Bifunctional P2X7 receptors involved in fast synaptic transmission and ATP-induced lysis of antigen-presenting cells

Table 8.7. The glutamate receptor family

	Gene		Distribution	Special features and/or
	Name	Map		functions
(a) AMPAR				
GluR1	GRIA1	5q33	CNS, widespread	Subject to alternate splicing → flip
	Gria1	11 (30)	distribution	and flop variants
			Differential	Can form functional homomeric
			distribution of flip	receptors (inwardly rectifying)
			and flop isoforms	
GluR2	GRIA2	4q32–33	CNS, widespread	Major component of neuronal
	Gria2	3(33.6)	distribution	AMPAR (few neuronal receptors
			Differential	lack the GluR2 subunit)
			distribution of flip	Subject to alternate splicing → flip
			and flop isoforms	and flop variants
				Can form functional homomeric
				receptors
				Subject to RNA editing at Q/R site
				in M2 (exists solely in the
				edited form)
				GluR2 containing receptors
				exhibiting weak Ca^{2+} flux
				(mediated by arginine residue in
				M2)
GluR3	GRIA3	Xq25–26	CNS, widespread	Subject to alternate splicing → flip
	Gria3	X	distribution	and flop variants
			Differential	Can form functional homomeric
			distribution of flip	receptors (inwardly rectifying)
			and flop isoforms	
GluR4	GRIA4	11q22–23	CNS, widespread	Subject to alternate splicing → flip
	Gria4	9 (8)	distribution	and flop variants
			Differential	Can form functional homomeric
			distribution of flip	receptors (inwardly rectifying)
			and flop isoforms	
			PNS, low levels	
(b) KAINR				
GluR5	GRIK1	21q22	CNS, widespread	Subject to alternate splicing (two
	Grik1	16 (58)	distribution (lower	sites → three variants)
			levels than GluR6)	Subject to RNA editing at Q/R site
			Differential	in TM2 (both forms expressed)
			distribution of	GluR5(Q) can form functional
			alternate splice	homomeric channels which
			variants	resemble KAINR on dorsal root
			PNS low levels	ganglia
				GluR5R are sensitive to AMPA
GluR6	GRIK2	6	CNS, widespread	Subject to RNA editing at Q/R site
	Grik2	?	distribution	in M2, I/V and Y/C sites in
			High levels present in	M1
			cerebellar granule	All eight possible combinations of
			cells	edited/unedited transcript variants
				are expressed
				Can form functional homomeric
				channels
GluR7	GRIK3	1p34–p33	CNS, widespread	GluR7 homomeric recptors are
	Grik3	4 (57.7)	distribution	nonfunctional
			High levels present in	GluR7 is one of the most
			neocortex, caudate-	abundant KAINR subunits in the
			putamen, and stellate	adult CNS
			cells in cerebellum	

(continued)

Table 8.7. (*Continued*)

Gene Name	Gene Map	Distribution	Special features and/or functions
KA-1 GRIK4 Grik4	11q23 9 (23.5)	CNS, localized distribution High levels present in hippocampal CA3 and dentate gyrus regions	KA-1 homomeric receptors are nonfunctional but when co-expressed with GluR5 or GluR6 functionally novel receptors are formed
KA-2 GRIK5 Grik5	19q13.2 7 (6.5)	CNS, widespread distribution High levels present in neocortex, dentate gyrus, hippocampus Also present in the pineal gland	KA-2 homomeric receptors are nonfunctional but when co-expressed with GluR5 or GluR6 functionally novel receptors are formed KA-2 is one of the most abundant KAINR subunits in the adult CNS

(c) *NMDAR*

Gene Name	Gene Map	Distribution	Special features and/or functions
NMDAR1 GRIN1 Grin1	9q34.3 2 (13)	CNS, widely distributed NMDAR1 solely expressed in hypothalamus Alternatively spliced variants differentially expressed	Most abundant NMDAR subunit within CNS Present in all NMDAR (essential for activity of NMDAR) Subject to extensive alternate splicing (three sites → eight variants) Can form functional homomeric receptors
NMDAR2A GRIN2A Grin2A	16p13 ?	CNS, widely distributed similar to NMDAR1	Functional only when expressed with NMDAR1
NMDAR2B GRIN2B Grin2B	12p12 6 (64.5)	CNS, distribution more restricted than NMDAR2A Predominant in adult forebrain regions, widespread during embryonic development	Functional only when expressed with NMDAR1 Critical role in trigeminal neuronal pattern formation and hippocampal LTD in neonate
NMDAR2C GRIN2C Grin2C	17q25 ?	CNS, localized expression Highest levels of expression in the cerebellum Not expressed in amygdala or caudate nuclei	Functional only when expressed with NMDAR1
NMDAR2D GRIN2D Grin2D	? ?	CNS distribution, especially diencephalon and lower brainstem Predominantly embryonic expression	Functional only when expressed with NMDAR1

References

Akabas MH, Kaufmann C, Archdeacon P, Karlin A. (1994) Identification of acetylcholine receptor channel-lining residues in the entire M2 segment of the α subunit. *Neuron* **13**: 919–927.

Angelotti TP, Macdonald RL. (1993) Assembly of GABA$_A$ receptor subunits: α1 β1 and α1 β1 γ2S subunits produce unique ion channels with dissimilar single-channel properties. *J. Neurosci.* **13**: 1429–1440.

Arbas EA, Meinertzhagen IA, Shaw SR. (1991) Evolution in nervous systems. *Annu. Rev. Neurosci.* **14**: 9–38.

Armstrong RC, Montminy MR. (1993) Transsynaptic control of gene expression. *Annu. Rev. Neurosci.* **16**: 17–29.

Benne R. (1996) The long and the short of it. *Nature* **380**: 391–392.

Bennett JA, Dingledine R. (1995) Topology profile for a glutamate receptor: three transmembrane domains and a channel-lining reentrant membrane loop. *Neuron* **14**: 373–384.

Boess FG, Martin IL. (1995) Molecular biology of 5-HT receptors. *Neuropharmacology* **33**: 275–317.

Browning MD, Huganir RL, Greengard P. (1985) Protein phosphorylation and neuronal function. *J. Neurochem.* **45**: 11–23.

Buller AL, Hastings GA, Kirkness EF, Fraser CM. (1994) Site-directed mutagenesis of N-linked glycosylation sites on the gamma-aminobutyric acid type A receptor alpha 1 subunit. *Mol. Pharmacol.* **46**: 858–865.

Buonanno A, Mudd J, Merlie JP. (1989). Isolation and characterisation of the β genes of mouse muscle acetylcholine receptor. *J. Biol. Chem.* **264**: 7611–7617.

Carraway KL, Burden SJ. (1995) Neuregulins and their receptors. *Curr. Opin. Neurobiol.* **5**: 606–612.

Chavez RA, Hall ZW. (1991) The transmembrane topology of the amino terminus of the α subunit of the nicotinic acetylcholine receptor. *J. Biol. Chem.* **266**: 15 532–15 538.

Chavez RA, Hall ZW. (1992) Expression of fusion proteins of the nicotinic acetylcholine receptor from mammalian muscle identifies the membrane-spanning regions in the α and δ subunits. *J. Cell Biol.* **116**: 385–393.

Claudio T, Ballivet M, Patrick J, Heinemann S. (1983) Nucleotide and deduced amino acid sequences of *Torpedo californica* acetylcholine receptor γ subunits. *Proc. Natl Acad. Sci. USA* **80**: 1111–1115.

Conley EC. (1996) *The Ion Channel Facts Book*, Vol. I, *Extracellular Ligand-Gated Channels*. Academic Press, London.

Connolly CN, Krishek BJ, McDonald BJ, Smart TG, Moss SJ. (1996) Assembly and cell surface expression of heteromeric and homomeric γ-aminobutyric acid type A receptors. *J. Biol. Chem.* **271**: 89–96.

Culiat CT, Stubbs LJ, Montgomery CS, Russell LB, Rinchik EM. (1994) Phenotypic consequences of deletion of the γ3, α5, or β3 subunit of the type A γ-aminobutyric acid receptor in mice. *Proc. Natl Acad. Sci. USA* **91**: 2815–2818.

Culiat CT, Stubbs LJ, Woychik RP, Russell LB, Johnson DK, Rinchik EM. (1995) Deficiency of the β3 subunit of the type A γ-aminobutyric acid receptor causes cleft palate in mice. *Nature Genetics*, **11**: 344–346.

Cutting GR, Lu L, O'Hara BF et al. (1991) Cloning of the gamma-aminobutyric acid rho1 cDNA: a GABA receptor subunit highly expressed in retina. *Proc. Natl Acad. Sci. USA* **88**: 2673–2677.

DiPaola M, Czaikowski C, Karlin A. (1989) The sidedness of the C-terminus of the acetylcholine receptor delta subunit. *J. Biol. Chem.* **264**: 15 457–15 463.

Forrest D, Yuzaki M, Soares HD et al. (1994) Targeted disruption of NMDA receptor 1 gene abolishes NMDA response and results in neonatal death. *Neuron* **13**: 325–338.

Fredholm BB. (1995) Purinoceptors in the nervous system. *Pharmacol. Toxicol.* **76**: 228–239.

Galzi J-L, Changeux J-P. (1994) Neurotransmitter-gated ion channels as unconventional allosteric proteins. *Curr. Opin. Struct. Biol* **4**: 554–565.

Galzi J-L, Deviliers-Thierry A, Hussy N, Bertrand S, Changeux J-P, Bertrand D. (1992) Mutations in the channel domain of a neuronal nicotinic receptor convert ion selectivity from cationic to anionic. *Nature* **359**: 500–505.

Gautam M, Noakes PG, Mudd JM, Nichol M, Chu GC, Sanes JR, Merlie, JP. (1995) Failure of postsynaptic specialization to develop at the neuromuscular junction of rapsyn-deficient mice. *Nature* **377**: 232–236.

Gautam M, Noakes PG, Moscaso L, Rupp F, Scheller RH, Merlie JP, Sanes, JR. (1996) Defective neuromuscular synaptogenesis in agrin-deficient mutant mice. *Cell* **85**: 525–535.

Gehle VM, Sumikawa K. (1991) Site-directed mutagenesis of the conserved N-glycosylation site on the nicotinic acetylcholine receptor subunits. *Mol. Brain Res.* **11**: 17–25.

Gelman MS, Chang W, Thomas DY, Bergeron JJ, Prives JM. (1995) Role of the endoplasmic reticulum chaperone calnexin in subunit folding of nicotinic acetylcholine receptors. *J. Biol. Chem.* **270**: 15 085–15 092.

Gillespie SKH, Balasubramanian S, Fung ET, Huganir RL. (1996) Rapsyn clusters and activates the synapse-specific receptor tyrosine kinase MuSK. *Neuron* **16**: 953–962.

Glencorse TG, Bateson AN, Darlison MG. (1992) Differential localization of two alternatively-spliced GABA$_A$ receptor γ2-subunit mRNAs in the chick brain. *Eur. J. Neurosci.* **4**: 271–277.

Goelet P, Castellucci VF, Schacher S, Kandel ER. (1986) The long and the short of long-term memory – a molecular framework. *Nature* **322**: 419–422.

Green WN, Millar NS. (1995) Ion channel assembly. *Trends Neurosci.* **18**: 280–287.

Grenningloh G, Rienitz A, Schmitt B, Methfessel C, Zensen M, Beyreuther K, Gundelfinger ED, Betz H. (1987) The strychnine-binding subunit of the glycine receptor shows homology with nicotinic acetylcholine receptors. *Nature* **328**: 215–220.

Grimaldi K, Horn DA, Hudson LD, Terenghi G, Barton P, Polak JM, Latchman DS. (1993) Expression of the SmN splicing protein is developmentally regulated in the rodent brain but not in the rodent heart. *Devel. Biol.* **156**: 319–323.

Grosveld F, Kollias G. (1992) *Transgenic Animals.* Academic Press, London.

Günther U, Benson J, Benke D *et al.* (1995) Benzodiazepine-insensitive mice generated by targeted disruption of the γ2 subunit gene of γ-aminobutyric acid type A receptors. *Proc. Natl Acad. Sci. USA* **92**: 7749–7753.

Han KK, Martinage A. (1992) Post-translational chemical modification(s) of proteins. *Int. J. Biochem.* **24**: 19–28.

Hartenstein B, Schenkel J, Kuhse J, Besenbeck B, Kling C, Becker CM, Betz H, Weiher H. (1996) Low level expression of glycine receptor beta subunit transgene is sufficient for phenotype correction in spastic mice. *EMBO J.* **15**: 1275–1282.

He X, Rosenfeld MG. (1991) Mechanisms of complex transcriptional regulation: implications for brain development. *Neuron* **7**: 183–196.

Hirai H, Kirsch J, Laube B, Betz H, Kuhse J. (1996) The glycine binding site of the N-methyl-D-aspartate receptor subunit NR1: identification of novel determinants of co-agonist potentiation in the extracellular M3-M4 loop region. *Proc. Natl Acad. Sci. USA* **93**: 6031–6036.

Hollmann M, Heinemann S. (1994) Cloned glutamate receptors. *Annu. Rev. Neurosci.* **17**: 31–108.

Hollmann M, O'Shea-Greenfield A, Rogers SW, Heinemann S. (1989) Cloning by functional expression of a member of the glutamate receptor family. *Nature* **342**: 643–648.

Hollmann M, Maron C, Heinemann S. (1994) N-glycosylation site tagging suggests a three transmembrane domain topology for the glutamate receptor GluR1. *Neuron* **13**: 1331–1343.

Huganir RL, Delcour AH, Greengard P, Hess GP. (1986) Phosphorylation of the nicotinic acetylcholine receptor regulates its rate of desensitization. *Nature* **321**: 774–776.

Hopfield JF, Tank DW, Greengard P, Huganir RL. (1988) Functional modulation of the nicotinic acetylcholine receptor by tyrosine phosphorylation. *Nature* **336**: 677–680.

Ikeda K, Araki K, Takayama C, Inoue Y, Yagi T, Aizawa S, Mishina M. (1995) Reduced spontaneous activity of mice defective in the ε4 subunit of the NMDA receptor channel. *Mol. Brain Res.* **33**: 61–71.

Imoto K, Busch C, Sakmann B *et al.* (1988) Rings of negatively charged amino acids determine the acetylcholine receptor channel conductance. *Nature* **335**: 645–648.

Kang I, Lindquist DG, Kinane TB, Ercolani L, Pritchard GA, Miller LG. (1994) Isolation and characterization of the promoter of the human GABA$_A$ receptor α1 subunit gene. *J. Neurochem.* **62**: 1643–1646.

Kanopka A, Mühlemann O, Akusjärvi G. (1996) Inhibition by SR proteins of splicing of a regulated adenovirus pre-messenger-RNA. *Nature* **381**: 535–538.

Karlin A. (1993) Structure of nicotinic acetylcholine receptors. *Curr. Opin. Neurobiol.* **3**: 299–309.

Karlin A, Akabas MH. (1995) Toward a structural basis for the function of nicotinic acetylcholine receptors and their cousins. *Neuron* **15**: 1231–1244.

Kashiwabuchi N, Ikeda K, Araki K *et al.* (1995) Impairment of motor co-ordination, Purkinje cell synapse formation, and cerebellar long-term depression in GluRδ2 mutant mice. *Cell* **81**: 245–252.

Keinänen K, Wisden W, Sommer B, Werner P, Herb A, Verdoorn TA, Sakmann B, Seeburg PH. (1990) A family of AMPA-selective glutamate receptors. *Science* **249**: 1203–1211.

Kirkness EF, Fraser CM. (1993) A strong promoter element is located between alternative exons of a gene encoding the human γ-aminobutyric acid-type A receptor β3 subunit (GABRB3). *J. Biol. Chem.* **268**: 4420–4428.

Kirkness EF, Kusiak JW, Fleming JT, Menninger J, Gocayne JD, Ward DC, Venter JC. (1991) Isolation, characterization, and localization of human genomic DNA encoding the β1 subunit of the GABA_A receptor (GABRB1). *Genomics* **10**: 985–995.

Krishek BJ, Wie XM, Blackstone C, Huganir RL, Moss SJ, Smart TG. (1994) Regulation of GABA_A receptor function by protein kinase C phosphorylation. *Neuron* **12**: 1081–1095.

Kuhse J, Laube B, Magalei D, Betz H. (1993) Assembly of the inhibitory glycine receptor: identification of amino acid sequence motifs governing subunit stoichiometry. *Neuron* **11**: 1049–1056.

Kuhse J, Betz H, Kirsch J. (1995) The inhibitory glycine receptor – architecture, synaptic localization and molecular pathology of a post-synaptic ion channel complex. *Curr. Opin. Neurobiol.* **5**: 318–323.

Kuryatov A, Laube B, Betz H, Kuhse J. (1994) Mutational analysis of the glycine-binding site of the NMDA receptor: structural similarity with bacterial amino acid-binding proteins. *Neuron* **12**: 1291–1300.

Kutsuwada T, Sakimura K, Manabe T et al. (1996) Impairment of suckling response, trigeminal neuronal pattern formation, and hippocampal LTD in NMDA receptor ε2 subunit mutant mice. *Neuron* **16**: 333–344.

LaMantia A-S. (1995) The usual suspects: GABA and glutamate may regulate proliferation in the neocortex. *Neuron* **15**: 1223–1225.

Lasham A, Vreugdenhil E, Bateson AN, Barnard EA, Darlison MG. (1991) Conserved organization of γ-aminobutyric acid_A receptor genes: cloning and analysis of the chicken β4-subunit gene. *J. Neurochem.* **57**: 352–355.

Leidenheimer NJ, McQuilkin SJ, Hahner LD, Whiting P, Harris RA. (1992) Activation of protein kinase C selectively inhibits the γ-aminobutyric acid_A receptor: role of desensitization. *Mol. Pharmacol.* **41**: 1116–1123.

Levine M, Manley JL. (1989) Transcriptional repression of eukaryotic promoters. *Cell* **59**: 405–408.

Li Y, Erzurumlu RS, Chen C, Jhaveri S, Tonegawa S. (1994) Whisker-related neuronal patterns fail to develop in the trigeminal brainstem nuclei of NMDAR1 knockout mice. *Cell* **76**: 427–437.

Lindstrom J, Anand R, Peng X, Gerzanich V, Wang F, Li Y. (1995) Neuronal nicotinic receptor subtypes. *Ann. N.Y. Acad. Sci.* **757**: 100–116.

Lüscher B, Motejlek K, Fritschy J-M, Häuselmann R, Rülicke T. (1993) Analysis of neuron-specific GABA_A receptor gene promoters *in vitro* and in transgenic mice. *Soc. Neurosci. Abstracts* **19**: 35.13, p.67.

Malosio ML, Marqueze-Pouey B, Kuhse J, Betz H. (1991) Widespread expression of glycine receptor subunit mRNAs in the adult and developing brain. *EMBO J.* **10**: 2401–2409.

Mandel G, McKinnon D. (1993) Molecular basis of neural-specific gene expression. *Annu. Rev. Neurosci.* **16**: 323–345.

Matsumoto RR. (1989) GABA receptors: are cellular differences reflected in function? *Brain Res.* **14**: 203–225.

Matter-Sadinski L, Hernandez M-C, Roztocil T, Ballivet M, Matter JM. (1992) Neuronal specificity of the α7 nicotinic acetylcholine receptor promoter develops during morphogenesis of the central nervous system. *EMBO J.* **11**: 4529–4538.

Matzenbach B, Maulet Y, Sefton L, Courtier B, Avner P, Guenet JL, Betz H. (1994) Structural analysis of mouse glycine receptor alpha subunit genes. Identification and chromosomal localization of a novel variant. *J. Biol. Chem.* **269**: 2607–2612.

McAllister G, Amara SG, Lerner MR. (1988) Tissue-specific expression and cDNA cloning of small nuclear ribonucleoprotein associated polypeptide N. *Proc. Natl Acad. Sci. USA* **85**: 5296–5300.

McDonald BJ, Moss SJ. (1994) Differential phosphorylation of intracellular domains of γ-aminobutyric acid type A receptor subunits by calcium/calmodulin type 2-dependent protein kinase and cGMP-dependent protein kinase. *J. Biol. Chem.* **269**: 18 111–18 117.

McKernan RM, Whiting PJ. (1996) Which GABA_A-receptor subtypes really occur in the brain? *Trends Neurosci.* **19**: 139–143.

Melcher T, Maas S, Herb A, Sprengel R, Seeburg PH, Higuchi, M. (1996) A mammalian RNA editing enzyme. *Nature* **379**: 460–464.

Molnar E, McIlhinney J, Baude A, Nusser Z, Somogyi P. (1994) Membrane topology of the GluR1 glutamate receptor subunit: epitope mapping by site-directed antipeptide antibodies. *J. Neurochem.* **63**: 683–693.

Monyer H, Seeburg PH, Wisden W. (1991) Glutamate-operated channels: developmentally early and mature forms arise by alternative splicing. *Neuron* **6**: 799–810.

Moss SJ, Doherty CA, Huganir RL. (1992a) Identification of the cAMP-dependent protein kinase and protein kinase C phosphorylation sites within the major intracellular domains of the beta 1, gamma 2S, and gamma 2L subunits of the gamma-aminobutyric acid type A receptor. *J. Biol. Chem.* **267**: 14 470–14 476.

Moss SJ, Smart TG, Blackstone CD, Huganir RL. (1992b) Functional modulation of GABA$_A$ receptors by cAMP-dependent protein phosphorylation. *Science* **257**: 661–665.

Moss SJ, Gorrie GH, Amato A, Smart TG. (1995) Modulation of GABA$_A$ receptors by tyrosine phosphorylation. *Nature* **377**: 344–348.

Motejlek K, Häuselmann R, Leitgeb S, Lüscher B. (1994) BSF-1, a novel brain-specific DNA-binding protein recognizing a tandemly repeated purine DNA element in the GABA$_A$ receptor δ subunit gene. *J. Biol. Chem.* **269**: 15 265–15 273.

Mouse Genome Database (MGD) 3.1. *Mouse Genome Informatics*, The Jackson Laboratory, Bar Harbor, ME. World Wide Web (URL: http: //www.informatics.jax.org/). (February, 1996.)

Nakanishi N, Shneider NA, Axel R. (1990) A family of glutamate receptor genes: evidence for the formation of heteromultimeric receptors with distinct channel properties. *Neuron* **5**: 569–581.

Nestler EJ, Greengard P. (1984) *Protein Phosphorylation in the Nervous System.* Wiley Press, New York.

Noda M, Furutani Y, Takahashi H et al. (1983a) Cloning and sequence analysis of calf cDNA and human genomic DNA encoding α-subunit precursor of muscle acetylcholine receptor. *Nature* **305**: 818–823.

Noda M, Takahashi H, Tanabe T et al. (1983b) Structural homology of *Torpedo californica* acetylcholine receptor subunits. *Nature* **302**: 528–532.

O'Hara PJ, Sheppard PO, Thøgersen H et al. (1993) The ligand-binding domain in metabotropic glutamate receptors is related to bacterial periplasmic binding proteins. *Neuron* **11**: 41–52.

Online Mendelian Inheritance in Man, OMIM (TM). Center for Medical Genetics, Johns Hopkins University (Baltimore, MD) and National Center for Biotechnology Information, National Library of Medicine (Bethesda, MD), 1996. World Wide Web (URL: http: //www3.ncbi.nlm.nih.gov/omim/).

Partin KM, Patneau DK, Winters CA, Mayer ML, Buonanno A. (1993) Selective modulation of desensitization at AMPA versus kainate receptors by cyclothiazide and concanavalin A. *Neuron* **11**: 1069–1082.

Picciotto MR, Zoli M, Léna C et al. (1995) Abnormal avoidance learning in mice lacking functional high-affinity nicotine receptor in the brain. *Nature* **374**: 65–67.

Polson AG, Bass BL, Casey JL. (1996) RNA editing of hepatitis-delta virus antigenome by dsRNA-adenosine deaminase. *Nature* **380**: 460–464.

Rabow LE, Russek SJ, Farb DH. (1995) From ion currents to genomic analysis: recent advances in GABAA receptor research. *Synapse* **21**: 189–274.

Roche KW, O'Brien RJ, Mammen AL, Bernhardt J, Huganir RL. (1996) Characterization of multiple phosphorylation sites on the AMPA receptor GluR1 subunit. *Neuron* **16**: 1179–1188.

Role LW, Berg DK. (1996) Nicotinic receptors in the development and modulation of CNS synapses. *Neuron* **16**: 1077–1085.

Sakimura K, Kutsuwada T, Ito I et al. (1995) Reduced hippocampal LTP and spatial learning in mice lacking NMDA receptor ε1 subunit. *Nature* **373**: 151–155.

Schofield PR, Darlison MG, Fujita N et al. (1987) Sequence and functional expression of the GABA$_A$ receptor shows a ligand-gated receptor super-family. *Nature* **328**: 221–227.

Seeburg PH. (1996) The role of RNA editing in controlling glutamate receptor channel properties. *J. Neurochem.* **66**: 1–5.

Sieghart W. (1995) Structure and pharmacology of γ-aminobutyric acid$_A$ receptor subtypes. *Pharmacol. Rev.* **47**: 181–234.

Sieghart W, Item C, Buchstaller A, Fuchs K, Höger H, Adamiker D. (1993) Evidence for the existence of differential O-glycosylated α5-subunits of the γ-aminobutyric acid$_A$ receptor in rat brain. *J. Neurochem.* **60**: 93–98.

Sigel E, Baur R, Trube G, Möhler H, Malherbe P. (1990) The effect of subunit composition of rat brain GABA$_A$ receptor on channel function. *Neuron* **5**: 703–711.

Smith GB, Olsen RW. (1995) Functional domains of GABA$_A$ receptors. *Trends Pharmacol. Sci.* **16**: 162–168.

Smith CWJ, Patton JG, Nadal-Grinard B. (1989) Alternative splicing in the control of gene expression. *Annu. Rev. Genet.* **23**: 527–577.

Sommer B, Poustka A, Spurr NK, Seeburg PH. (1990a) The murine GABA$_A$ receptor δ-subunit gene: structure and assignment to human chromosome 1. *DNA Cell Biol.* **9**: 561–568.

Sommer B, Keinänen K, Verdoorn TA *et al.* (1990b) Flip and flop: a cell-specific functional switch in glutamate-operated channels of the CNS. *Science* **249**: 1580–1585.

Stephenson FA. (1995) The GABA$_A$ receptors. *Biochem. J.* **310**: 1–9.

Struhl K. (1991) Mechanisms for diversity in gene expression patterns. *Neuron* **7**: 177–181.

Sumikawa K, Miledi R. (1989) Assembly and N-glycosylation of all ACH receptor subunits are required for their efficient insertion into plasma membranes. *Mol. Brain Res.* **5**: 183–192.

Sweetnam PM, Lloyd J, Gallombardol R, Madison RT, Gallager DW, Tallman JF, Nestler EJ. (1988) Phosphorylation of the GABA$_A$/benzodiazepine receptor alpha subunit by a receptor-associated protein kinase. *J. Neurochem.* **51**: 1274–1284.

Swope SL, Moss SJ, Blackstone CD, Huganir RL. (1992) Phosphorylation of ligand-gated ion channels: a possible mode of synaptic plasticity. *FASEB J.* **6**: 2514–2523.

Treinin M, Chalfie M. (1995) A mutated acetylcholine receptor subunit causes neuronal degeneration in *C. elegans*. *Neuron* **14**: 871–877.

Unwin N. (1989) The structure of ion channels in the membranes of excitable cells. *Neuron* **3**: 565–575.

Unwin N. (1993) Nicotinic acetylcholine receptor at 9Å resolution. *J. Mol. Biol.* **229**: 1101–1124.

Unwin N. (1995) Acetylcholine receptor channel imaged in the open state. *Nature* **373**: 37–43.

Verrall S, Hall Z-W. (1992) The N-terminal domains of acetylcholine receptor subunits contain recognition signals for the initial steps of receptor assembly. *Cell* **68**: 23–31.

Wagner K, Eson K, Heginbotham L, Post M, Huganir RL, Czernik AJ. (1991) Determination of the tyrosine phosphorylation sites of the nicotinic acetylcholine receptor. *J. Biol. Chem.* **266**: 23 784–23 789.

Wallace BG, Qu Z, Huganir RL. (1991) Agrin induces phosphorylation of the nicotinic acetylcholine receptor. *Neuron* **6**: 869–878.

Whiting P, McKernan RM, Wafford KA. (1995) Structure and pharmacology of vertebrate GABA$_A$ receptor subtypes. *Int. Rev. Neurobiol.* **38**: 95–137.

Winnacker EL. (1989) Tissue specific gene expression: a summary. In: *Tissue Specific Gene Expression* (ed. R Renkawitz). VCH Publishers, New York.

Yu X-M, Hall ZW. (1994a) The role of the cytoplasmic domains of individual subunits of the acetylcholine receptor in 43 kDa protein-induced clustering in COS cells. *J. Neurosci.* **14**: 785–795.

Yu X-M, Hall ZW. (1994b) A sequence in the main cytoplasmic loop of the α subunit is required for assembly of mouse muscle nicotinic acetylcholine receptor. *Neuron* **13**: 247–255.

Signaling pathways in neurons: focus on second messengers and protein phosphorylation

Michael R. Boarder

9.1 Introduction

In this chapter we address the question of the nature of second messenger pathways and protein phosphorylation cascades in neurons, and the role they play in neuronal function. We are concerned mainly with the seven-transmembrane receptors which are coupled to heterotrimeric G proteins. A role for receptors with intrinsic ion channels (ionotropic receptors) in controlling neuronal activity is well established. For example, the postsynaptic role of glutamatergic or cholinergic intrinsic ion channel receptors includes membrane depolarization and movement towards action potential (the ion channel receptors are discussed in Chapter 8). But what if the receptor is 'metabotropic', such as those receptors linked to second messenger formation through G proteins? Considering the two neurotransmitters mentioned above, this could be the action of glutamate at the metabotropic glutamate receptors (mGluR), acetylcholine (ACh) at the muscarinic ACh receptor (mAChR), or a plethora of other neurotransmitters of diverse chemical type which are believed to act in the brain in a predominantly 'metabotropic' manner. What role do these pathways play in the regulation of neuronal function?

The features of the G protein-coupling mechanism are discussed elsewhere (Chapter 7); in the first part of what follows the major players in the second messenger-linked systems will be introduced (Section 9.2). These are: Section 9.2.1 – the regulation of cyclic nucleotides (cAMP and cGMP); Section 9.2.2 – the phospholipid systems comprising phospholipase A_2 (PLA_2) phospholipase C (PLC), and phospholipase D (PLD) (with the consequent control of cytosolic Ca^{2+}, protein kinase C (PKC) and arachidonic acid metabolites such as prostaglandins); Section 9.2.3 – the tyrosine phosphorylation cascades (previously associated with growth factor receptors, but now known to be regulated by G protein-coupled receptors) such as the tyrosine kinase/mitogen-activated protein kinase (MAPK) cascade. Less emphasis in these sections will be placed on the cyclic nucleotides and PLC systems, since these are already widely discussed in the

Molecular Biology of the Neuron, edited by R.W. Davies and B.J. Morris.
© 1997 BIOS Scientific Publishers Ltd, Oxford.

neurochemical literature. In each case the discussion will outline the second messenger system in relation to its presence in neurons, and introduce its possible role in short-term neuronal regulation (long-term effects of this pathway and others on genomic expression and differentiation are found in Chapters 12–14). An integrated discussion of the functional consequences of these signaling pathways will follow (Section 9.3), using two examples: (i) the regulation of ion channels by G protein-coupled receptors, and (ii) their role in neuronal plasticity, as illustrated by long-term potentiation (LTP) and long-term depression (LTD), a subject discussed in a wider context in Chapter 12.

The role of second messenger-coupled receptors stimulated by neurotransmitters is most clearly understood when they are acting on nonneuronal cells. For example, we know a great deal about the mechanisms and functional consequences of noradrenaline and ACh acting at G protein-coupled receptors to control the heart, or the salivary glands, or the muscles of the eye. The studies with nonneuronal cells provide us with a vast amount of information about the signaling pathways themselves, and much light has thereby been cast on neuronal second messenger systems. Here, though, we are considering the case of neuron–neuron transmission, both in the peripheral nervous system and in the brain and spinal cord central nervous system (CNS). Unlike the cells of the heart, salivary glands or eye, our understanding of the consequences of control of neuronal function by G protein-coupled receptors is still very primitive. In considering this problem we start with two notions in mind. Firstly, that the role of second messenger based receptors will depend on their location; for example, those in the cell body are likely to play a different role from those in the terminals. Secondly, the recognition that the second messenger based systems are slower than intrinsic ion channel signaling.

The relationship between G proteins, second messengers and ion channels is particularly important when exploring the regulation of neuronal function by G protein-coupled receptors. For example, the second messenger system cannot be considered, in terms of functional consequences, separately from the ion channel receptors. There is an hierarchy of relationships between the two which must always be addressed. Furthermore, the G protein-coupled receptors are themselves linked to ion channel function, either by direct association of G protein components with ion channels, or downstream of the control of second messenger levels. This interaction of second messengers with ion channel function in neuronal regulation will be explored with specific examples in Section 9.3.1.

9.2. The major second messengers and protein phosphorylation cascades

9.2.1 Regulation of cyclic nucleotides

Regulation of cAMP synthesis. The enzyme which synthesizes cAMP in cells is adenylyl cyclase, an integral membrane glycoprotein comprising a single polypetide chain. This takes the form of two sequential cassettes, each of six transmembrane domains followed by a catalytic sequence (*Figure 9.1*). Receptors stimulate adenylyl cyclase directly by promoting the dissociation of G_s into the $\beta\gamma$ and α_s-GTP subunits. In the classical pathway for stimulation of cAMP levels the α_s-GTP subunit associates with adenylyl cyclase, which leads to the formation of an α_s-GTP–adenylyl cyclase–ATP complex and thus synthesis of cAMP from ATP. It is also well established that receptors coupled to G_i can control cAMP levels by inhibition of adenylyl cyclase; the formation of $\beta\gamma$ and α_i-GTP contribute to the inhibition of adenylyl cyclase in a manner dependent in part on the subtypes of adenylyl cyclase present. The target for cAMP is protein kinase A, which is a cytosolic enzyme comprising four subunits, two catalytic and two regulatory subunits. The latter inhibit enzyme activity, but on binding cAMP they dissociate from, and thereby activate, the catalytic subunits (*Figure 9.1*).

This conventional picture of G_s regulation of adenylyl cyclase is now deeply influenced by the presence of multiple forms of the enzyme. There are some apparently brain-specific forms (e.g. type I and type VIII). However, the brain also contains those found in other parts of the body. While some of these are widely distributed in the

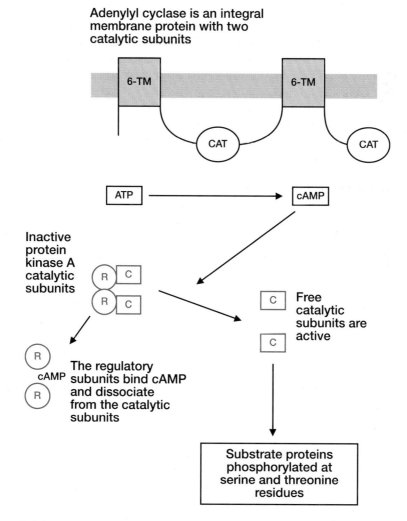

Figure 9.1. Adenylyl cyclase and protein kinase A. The repeats of six-transmembrane sequences (6-TM), each with a catalytic unit at the C-terminal aspect (CAT), are activated by the G protein subunit α_s binding to the N-terminal aspect. R = regulatory subunits of PKA, to which cAMP binds, freeing the catalytic subunits (C).

brain, other are restricted in their location. An example of the latter is type V, which in the brain is localized to the basal ganglia. The type of adenylyl cyclase contributing to any given response is important in understanding cell signaling, since they are not only distinct in distribution, but are also fundamentally different in modes of regulation (Cooper *et al.*, 1995; Mons *et al.*, 1995). Here two instances will be mentioned: regulation by Ca^{2+} and regulation by PKC. Of particular interest in the brain is type I adenylyl cyclase, which diverges from the pattern of G protein coupling described above in that it is principally activated by Ca^{2+}/calmodulin. This is of considerable importance, since it illustrates the principle that in neurons both receptors and ion channels may control cAMP levels by crosstalk with the Ca^{2+} signaling systems, independent of G protein-coupled events. This may be of significance in LTP (Section 9.3.2), as in the G protein-independent activation of type I adenylyl cyclase by Ca^{2+} influx through the *N*-methyl-D-aspartate (NMDA) class of ionotropic glutamate receptor. Furthermore, type V adenylyl cyclase may be under the inhibitory influence of elevated Ca^{2+}, resulting in a fall of cAMP levels as cytosolic Ca^{2+} rises. PKC has long been recognized as important in control of cAMP levels, providing early explanations for stimulations in cAMP seen in response to activation of receptors thought to be PLC linked. The nature of this regulation is now known to vary according to the participation of different adenylyl cyclase isoforms. For example, the widely distributed type II adenylyl cyclase is dramatically activated by PKC, apparently by direct phosphorylation; other isoforms show different, often less profound, modulations by PKC, which may in some cases involve modification of the interaction of adenylyl cyclase with G protein α-subunits. The examples given are sufficient to indicate that the recognition of adenylyl cyclase diversity has shown that this family of enzymes are a point of integration of multiple ion-channel and second messenger signaling inputs, with an output in the form of modulation of cAMP levels.

Regulation of cGMP synthesis. Guanylyl cyclase exists in both membrane-bound and soluble forms. Soluble guanylyl cyclase is principally regulated by NO, which activates the enzyme on association with its intrinsic heme moiety. NO acts as a neurotransmitter in all brain regions, although its synthesis is limited to a minority of neurons. NO can also be synthesized by nonneuronal cell types in the brain, such as astrocytes and endothelial cells, influencing the potential role of soluble guanylyl cyclase in the brain. One of the most exciting of the proposed roles for NO in the brain is its possible action as a retrograde transmitter, in which it is produced at the postsynaptic site in response to transmitter action. NO then diffuses 'backwards' to the presynaptic site, where it activates soluble guanylyl cyclase and regulates presynaptic function by elevating cGMP (*Figure 9.2*). Where the neurotransmitter is glutamate acting on postsynaptic NMDA receptors, the resultant Ca^{2+} entry into the postsynaptic site, activation of the Ca^{2+}/calmodulin-sensitive NO synthase, diffusion of NO back into the presynaptic site and facilitation of presynaptic events by cGMP, is a sequence of events which may play a role in LTP (see Section 9.3.2).

Particulate guanylyl cyclase is found in the plasmalemma, in the form of atrial natriuretic peptide (ANP) receptors with a catalytic domain in the cytosolic segment of the receptor protein. It is now known there are various forms of ANP receptor, including those known to occur in the brain; the consequences for neurotransmission remain obscure.

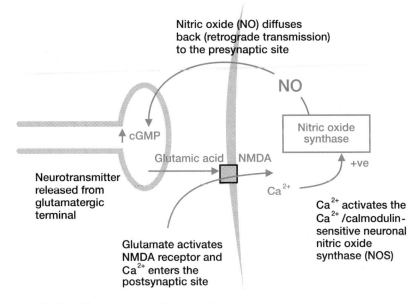

Figure 9.2. Nitric oxide as a retrograde transmitter.

Removal of cAMP and cGMP by phosphodiesterases. Second messengers, like neurotransmitters, must have efficient mechanisms for their removal if signaling with a high resolution with respect to time is to be achieved. It is apparent that the enzymic breakdown of cAMP and cGMP is by a family of enzymes called phosphodiesterases. These enzymes show varying degrees of selectivity between the two cyclic nucleotides, and differ in their regulation. Two types abundant in the brain illustrate these issues. Type I is a Ca^{2+}/calmodulin-independent enzyme with a relatively low but equal affinity for both cGMP and cAMP. Under the conditions found in most cells, where the level of cGMP is likely to be an order of magnitude lower than that of cAMP, we can expect this to result in an activity mainly directed at cAMP. Type II similarly has low and equal affinity for the two cyclic nucleotides, but has the interesting characteristic that it is activated by cGMP (but not by cAMP). Of particular importance in the brain is type IV, which has the characterisitic of high affinity and selectivity for cAMP; this enzyme is deficient in the *Dunce* mutant of *Drosophila* (Davis, 1996) stimulating interest in its role in brain function.

The presence of phosphodiesterase activities which are limiting and of equal affinity for cGMP and cAMP raises the possibility that there could be competition between the two cyclic nucleotides, such that an increase in one might reduce the breakdown of the other. There is evidence that in certain cells this does take place, indicating that crosstalk between cGMP and cAMP may occur at the level of phosphodiesterase activity.

Targets for cAMP and cGMP. The target for cAMP in signaling pathways is the cAMP-dependent family of protein kinases (protein kinase A). In neurons cAMP controls many events in cell body function, as widely discussed in nonneuronal cells. Of specific interest in neuronal function are the down-regulation of certain receptors by protein kinase A and the regulation of ion channels, a theme developed in Section

9.3.1. It is worth noting here that this gives cAMP a potential role to play in the regulation of postsynaptic events, and possibly in synaptic plasticity (Section 9.3.2). In addition to these events, cAMP is able to exert a long-term influence over transcriptional events by control of the cAMP responsive elements in the genome.

cGMP exerts many of its influences through cGMP-dependent kinases, thereby directly controlling protein phosphorylation cascades. There is some crosstalk at this level of the two cyclic nucleotide signaling pathways, in that cGMP may activate certain cAMP-dependent kinases; it seems, by contrast, that cAMP cannot activate cGMP-dependent kinases. An effect of cGMP that is independent of kinase activity is on certain cyclic nucleotide phosphodiesterases, as indicated above. A further pathway for control of cellular events by cGMP independent of the kinase is a direct influence of the nucleotide on ion channels. The best known and understood example is in phototransduction in the retina, whereby activation of rhodopsin by light leads, via the G protein transducin, to the activation of phosphodiesterase, reduction of cGMP levels, and the closure of cGMP-dependent cation channels. This leads in turn to reduction in Na^+ entry and hyperpolarization. In this way changes in cGMP levels can lead directly to changes in the membrane potential of an excitable cell. It is now known that this mechanism has widespread significance in neuronal function.

9.2.2 Phospholipases

Phospholipase C. PLC is a family of enzymes which, acting on the inositol phospholipids (phosphoinositides), activate a complex cascade of signaling events dominated, in their outcome, by elevations in intracellular Ca^{2+} and the activation of protein kinases. A scheme comparing PLC with PLD and PLA_2 hydrolysis of phospholipids is presented in *Figure 9.3*. The PLC family comprises PLCβ, PLCγ and PLCδ, with

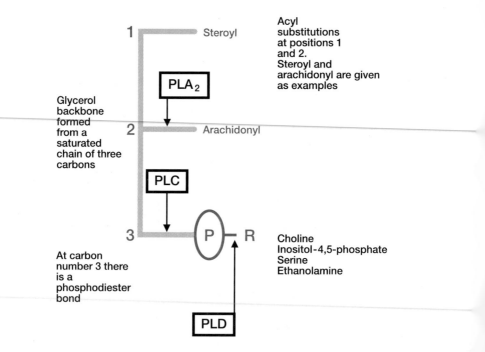

Figure 9.3. The sites of action of PLA_2, PLC and PLD.

further subdivisions in each of these classifications. The predominant forms coupled to heterotrimeric G proteins are the β isoforms. An outline scheme of the central events is presented in *Figure 9.4*. PLC hydrolysis of phosphatidylinositol-4,5-bisphosphate leads to the production of cytosolic inositol-1,4,5-trisphosphate [$Ins(1,4,5)P_3$] and membrane bound diacylglycerol (DAG). $Ins(1,4,5)P_3$ causes mobilization of intracellular calcium from stores associated with the endoplasmic reticulum, depleting these stores and transiently raising cytosolic Ca^{2+}. Associated with these events entry of Ca^{2+} also occurs, contributing a characteristically more sustained rise in cytosolic Ca^{2+}. These changes in Ca^{2+} show complex time courses (e.g. oscillations) and a high degree of spatial localization (e.g. waves, or very high levels at specific subplasmalemma sites) within the cytosolic compartment of a cell. Both these are lost when, as is common, the cytosolic Ca^{2+} is measured as a fluorescent signal from populations of cells. $Ins(1,4,5)P_3$ is only transiently raised, since it is metabolized by a 3-kinase to $Ins(1,3,4,5)P_4$ [and subsequently to $Ins(1,3,4)P_3$] or by a 5-phosphatase to $Ins(1,4)P_2$.

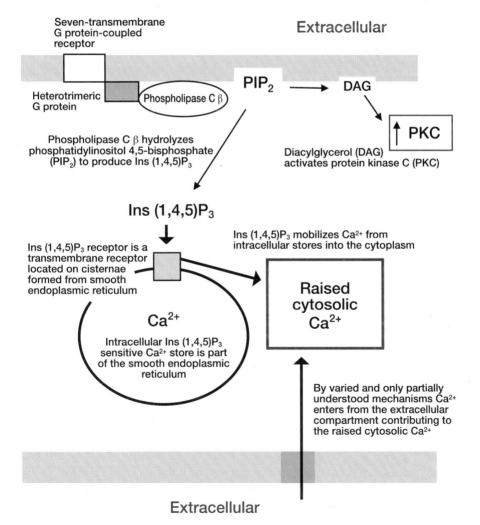

Figure 9.4. The PLC, $Ins(1,4,5)P_3$, Ca^{2+} system.

Concomitant with the formation of Ins(1,4,5)P$_3$, DAG is produced. This may have a variety of acyl substitutions on the 1 and 2 positions of the glycerol backbone; a common example is 1-steroyl, 2-arachidonyl. DAG remains in the membrane and causes the activation of the major classes of PKC, leading to a variety of messenger and protein phosphorylation cascades, some of which are indicated elsewhere in this chapter.

These events have been the subject of an enormous volume of research and numerous recent reviews, some of which deal specifically with the nervous system (e.g. Berridge, 1993; Furuichi and Mikoshiba, 1995; Nishizuka, 1992; Simpson et al., 1995). While this subject will not be reviewed here it should be recalled that the events downstream of PLC hydrolysis of PIP$_2$ are intrinsically related to the other processes described in this chapter. It is clear from these studies that Ins(1,4,5)P$_3$ and Ca^{2+} mobilization occur in both cell body and, in at least some cases, in the nerve terminal, although the role these processes play in terminal function is far from clear.

PKC has also been extensively studied in the nervous system, and here there are clearer indications of a role in the terminal. Indeed, it may be that the major role that the PLC signaling system has in terminal function is the regulation of PKC. PKC is a family of serine/threonine kinases with diverse regulatory characteristics (Nishizuka, 1992) and diverse localization in the brain at both presynaptic and postsynaptic sites (e.g. Suzuki et al., 1993). Certain PKCs (e.g. the γ subtype) appear to be selectively located within the CNS. There is considerable evidence in many neuronal systems that PKC is involved in the exocytotic process, and both the ϵ and the α subtypes are implicated in this process (Turner et al., 1994). Interestingly, the γ subtype appears not to be involved in this aspect of presynaptic function, and it is of interest to speculate that its role may be in postsynaptic densities (Oda et al., 1991; Suzuki et al., 1993). It is known that PKCα is localized to postsynaptic densities, where its function may be related to its participation in postsynaptic scaffolding (see Section 9.2.4).

Phospholipase D. PLD cleaves phospholipids on the distal side of the phosphodiester bond, forming as the lipid fragment phosphatidic acid (in place of the DAG formed by PLC). The general case is illustrated in *Figure 9.3*, where the reaction is compared with PLC and PLA$_2$. A more detailed account of the action of PLD on phosphatidylcholine, its major substrate, is shown in *Figure 9.5*. Two reactions catalyzed by PLD are shown; the reaction in the presence of H$_2$0, generates phosphatidic acid and choline, while the reaction in the presence of butanol generates phosphatidylbutanol and choline. In the native system the first reaction occurs. The second reaction, the transphosphatidylation reaction, is unique to PLD and has been widely used to estimate the PLD activity in intact cells and other systems. The difficulties inherent in the various procedures for PLD measurement, in particular in neuronal preparations, have recently been discussed (Boarder and Purkiss, 1993); they have contributed to the relatively low profile of PLD in neurochemical investigations. This low profile is curious considering that studies on transphosphatidylation using brain-derived PLD provide one of the first demonstrations of this activity in animal tissues. Many subsequent studies have investigated the presence of receptor-regulated PLD in neuronally related preparations, notably broken cell preparations, cells in culture and brain slices, as reviewed in Klein et al. (1995). Each of these has its own well known limitations. The majority of broken cell preparations are not neuron-specific, and will therefore be largely nonneuron-derived material. There has not been widespread use of highly purified synaptosomal material, which may provide a route around this problem. Similarly, brain slices con-

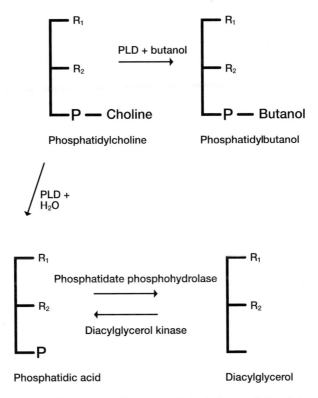

Figure 9.5. Phospholipase D, phosphatidate phosphohydrolase and diacylglycerol kinase. In the presence of butanol the product, phosphatidylbutanol, is unique to the PLD reaction. In the absence of alcohols the product of PLD, phosphatidic acid, is enzymatically interchangeable with DAG, the product of the PLC reaction.

tain more nonneuronal cells than neurons, and many receptors are known to be located on abundant glial cells. The cells used in culture in the published PLD studies are mainly dividing cells, and PLD activity may be closely related to the control of cell division in these cells (Boarder, 1994), and not to the function of differentiated neurons. It is of interest to note, in this context, that receptor-regulated PLD is not found in nondividing cultured adrenal chromaffin cells, but it is found in the chromaffin-derived PC12 cell line which does proliferate in culture (Purkiss *et al.*, 1991). These problems are held in common in the study of other neurochemical functions, but they assume particular importance in the assessment of our neurochemical knowledge of PLD.

The role of PLD in the nervous system has recently been reviewed (Klein *et al.*, 1995), and here we shall consider only some implications of some of the latest observations to emerge in the literature. The two issues underlying this brief discussion are the mechanisms of PLD activation, and the role PLD plays in the function of the nervous system.

Studies on pathways for the activation of PLD are mainly on nonneuronal systems, with some work with neuron-like cells in culture. The conclusions are dominated by three issues: firstly, observations going back some years that PLD activation is downstream of receptor regulation of PLC, in particular mediated by PKC activation; secondly, evidence exists in some cases that receptor regulation of PLD requires a tyrosine kinase step; thirdly, that there is direct G protein coupling to PLD, an idea initially developed with respect to heterotrimeric G protein, and latterly with important studies implicating a small G protein called ADP-ribosylating factor (ARF).

The first two issues have been discussed previously (Boarder, 1994), and will only be touched upon here. It is clear that in many systems the activation of PLD by receptors occurs concomitantly with PLC activation, and that the PLD response can be mimicked by PKC-stimulating phorbol esters and attenuated by inhibitors of PKC, or by down-regulation of PKC following prolonged exposure to phorbol esters. When this pattern of events is seen, it is concluded that the receptor activates PLC, leading to sequential activation of PKC and PLD. While implicating PKC in these events, it is important to note that the involvement of other mechanisms is not excluded. For example, tyrosine kinase activation may occur downstream of PKC (see below). Furthermore, G protein involvement may co-operate with PKC in the regulation of PLD (see below). It is not always the case that studies confirm a PKC involvement. For example, in PC12 cells muscarinic activation of PLD is not inhibited by staurosporine (Kanoh et al., 1992), from which the authors conclude that there is a PKC-independent pathway. Conversely, investigating the regulation of PC12 cells by P_2-purinoceptors, Murrin and Boarder (1992) showed that the more selective PKC inhibitor, Ro 31-8220, was able to inhibit receptor-stimulated PLD activity, concluding that receptor stimulation of PLD was downstream of PLC and PKC.

In brain slice preparations it has been shown that agonists acting at various receptor types (e.g. histamine H_1 and endothelin ET_B: Sarri et al., 1995), and phorbol esters acting directly at the level of PKC (Sandemann et al., 1990), can stimulate PLD. While not directly investigating a role for PKC, Holler et al. (1994) concluded that stimulation of PLD in hippocampal slices was independent of PLC and inositol (poly)phosphate production. This is consistent with other studies indicating two pathways for receptor regulation of PLD in hippocampal slices, PKC-dependent and PKC-independent (Klein et al., 1994). However, there is no evidence to tell us whether in native neurons (as opposed to cultured neuron-like cells and the mainly nonneuronal cells in brain slices) the activation of PLD is related to PLC and PKC activation. Studies are needed with primary cultures of pure neurons, and with highly purified synaptosomal preparations to investigate a role for PLD in nerve terminal function.

There is clear evidence in some systems that PLD activation by receptors is downstream of tyrosine phosphorylation. This is true with both heterotrimeric G protein-coupled and intrinsic tyrosine kinase growth factor receptors (see Boarder, 1994, review). It is not known whether this mechanism operates in neurons.

The most significant observation in recent years concerning PLD regulation is the recognition of the involvement of ARF, a small G protein with a role in the control of intracellular membrane trafficking (Brown et al., 1993; Cockroft et al., 1994). Attempts have been made to integrate this mechanism with that involving PKC (Whatmore et al., 1994). However, it is perhaps relevant to note that the relationship between the PLD regulated by ARF and the PLD regulated by cell-surface receptors in the work discussed above is unclear. The role of an ARF mechanism in neurons is unknown.

Nevertheless the involvement of ARF has generated the hypothesis that PLD plays a role in the regulation of membrane traffic (Kahn et al., 1993). Whether or not this PLD is controlled by receptors for neurotransmitters, this provides a potentially important role for PLD in neurons, cells in which the control of vesicle traffic (and thus membrane kinetics) is particularly complex.

In nonneuronal cells the most widely proposed role for PLD is in control of mitogenesis (Boarder, 1994). PLD is a putative component in one of many pathways to mitogenesis, and it is not known whether it has any role to play in the control of the cell cycle in either the developing or the mature brain. Another widely discussed role for receptor-regulated PLD is the control of DAG levels, by sequential PLD and phosphatidate phosphohydrolase (*see Figure 9.5*). The formation of phosphoinositide-derived DAG by PLC is often described as being short lived, with more sustained rises being derived from other phospholipids, such as the more abundant phosphatidylcholine, a substrate for receptor-regulated PLD. In 1321N1 astrocytoma cells, for example, it has been shown that PLD leads to a delayed DAG formation (Martinson *et al.*, 1990). The potential to provide a pathway for the formation of DAG by activation of heterotrimeric G protein-coupled receptors leads to a possible wide-ranging role for PLD involving all those aspects of neuronal function which have been shown to be modulated by PKC. In general this is a hypothesis which remains untested. An example is in the short feedback regulation of PLC responses by PKC activation. In neuroblastoma-derived SK-N-MC stimulated with endothelin-1, evidence has been presented that PLD plays an important role in activation of PKC and the attenuation of the receptor stimulation of PLC (Challiss *et al.*, 1993).

A further putative role for PLD emerges from the generation of free choline. PLD acting on phosphatidylcholine generates not only the lipid moiety, phosphatidic acid, but also free choline. It has been suggested that this may play a role in choline mobilization as a prerequisite for acetylcholine synthesis, as discussed in Klein *et al.* (1995). While there are arguments in favor of this notion, it presumably plays a limited role in the significance of PLD in neuronal function, an issue which remains largely unresolved.

Phospholipase A$_2$. PLA$_2$ cleaves phospholipids at the middle carbon (the number 2 position) of the glycerol backbone, removing the acyl group to form the corresponding fatty acid (*Figure 9.3*). PLA$_2$ has been intensively studied, more because of its role in inflammatory responses than for its role in neuronal processes. PLA$_2$ is a family of enzymes, but for the present purposes it is sufficient to note that two forms, cytosolic PLA$_2$ (cPLA$_2$) and secreted PLA$_2$ (sPLA$_2$), have been cloned and distinguished on structural grounds as well as the mechanisms of activation and substrate specificity (Glaser *et al.*, 1993). Both forms are of significance in inflammation, but for the role in short-term second messenger responses we need consider only cPLA$_2$. This is because it is this form which is present in the cytosol, is activated by receptor stimulation, and which displays a substrate preference for those phospholipids with an arachidonyl substitution at the number 2 position. This latter point means that the fatty acid product of the cleavage will be arachidonic acid, which may be an active second messenger itself but which is metabolized to form the prostaglandin-related family of products collectively referred to as the eicosanoids. This is a complex and diverse family of structurally related compounds with a largely uninvestigated influence on neuronal function. The two most studied pathways for arachidonic acid metabolism in cellular regulation are the cyclooxygenase pathway and the lipoxygenase pathway, generating a complex cascade of active metabolites, including prostaglandins, thromboxanes and leukotrienes. Only an indication of the products of these pathways is given; PLA_2 is widely regarded as the rate-limiting step in the synthesis of these active products in the inflammatory process and in response to receptor activation.

Another feature of the PLA_2 pathway which has assumed prominence in studies on inflammatory processes but played little role in investigations of neuronal function is that where the substrate phospholipid is phosphatidylcholine, cleavage by PLA_2 produces *lyso*-phosphatidylcholine in addition to arachidonic acid. *Lyso*-phosphatidylcholine is the remaining phospholipid with the 2-acyl group removed, and is a precursor for platelet-activating factor, known to be an active second messenger controlling many aspects of cellular function. Its role in events related to neurotransmission are largely unknown. A notable exception to this is the demonstration (Kato *et al.*, 1994) that platelet-activating factor plays a role in the retrograde signaling cascade involved in hippocampal LTP (see Section 9.3.2). This highlights the point that demonstration of a role for PLA_2 in functional studies, often by the outcome of PLA_2 inhibition, may indicate a role for the *lyso*-phospholipid products as well as for arachidonic acid and metabolites.

There are two salient issues when considering PLA_2 as a second messenger cascade in events related to neurotransmission. Firstly, how is its activity controlled? Secondly, how does activation of PLA_2 influence short-term neuronal events?

The principles underlying control of PLA_2 activity have been elucidated in some considerable detail in nonneuronal systems. This work will be briefly summarized, followed by an indication of what we know about the situation in neurons. Studies on activation of PLA_2 have, until recently, been dominated by a role for elevated cytosolic Ca^{2+}. This has included the interpretation of the outcome of cloning studies which established the $cPLA_2$ and $sPLA_2$ forms of the enzyme, with the demonstration that $cPLA_2$ is activated by micromolar levels of Ca^{2+} while $sPLA_2$ requires millimolar Ca^{2+} (Glaser *et al.*, 1993). This suggests that $cPLA_2$ may be activated *in situ* by levels of cytosolic Ca^{2+} achieved by agonist stimulation, consistent with the interpretation put on many earlier studies on nonneuronal cells where PLA_2 controls the production of prostacyclin (e.g. Carter *et al.*, 1988). In recent work however it has been shown that in these cells the control of PLA_2 by receptors is dependent on a series of interconnected protein kinase cascades involving PKC, tyrosine kinases and MAPK (Bowden *et al.*, 1995; Patel *et al.*, 1996a,b; Sa *et al.*, 1995). This follows the demonstration that recombinant $cPLA_2$ is phosphorylated and activated by MAPK (Lin *et al.*, 1993). A model for integration of the MAPK and Ca^{2+} involvement in control of $cPLA_2$ activation is now possible (Schalkwijk *et al.*, 1996; Schievella *et al.*, 1995): PLA_2 is activated by MAPK phosphorylation, but only has access to its substrate when elevated cytosolic Ca^{2+} causes translocation to the membrane. Phosphorylation itself does not cause translocation, but the translocated enzyme is not active if unphosphorylated. Thus phosphorylation (by MAPK) and translocation (by Ca^{2+}) are necessary and independent events for a PLA_2-mediated arachidonic acid response, although the phosphorylation must precede translocation since the membrane-bound enzyme is not a substrate for MAPK. We can expect the elements of this model to regulate PLA_2 in neurons in response to receptor activation and depolarization, but it should be emphasized that there are clear indications of other influences controlling PLA_2, and these may also be involved in neuronal function.

A variety of neurotransmitters are known to have the potential to stimulate arachidonic acid release. For example, when applied to cultures of striatal neurons, glutamate causes the release of arachidonic acid by a mechanism requiring the associative activation of both ionotropic D,L-amino-3-hydroxy-5-methyl-4-isoxalone propionic acid (AMPA) receptors and NMDA or metabotropic receptors (Dumuis *et al.*, 1988, 1990, 1993). This enhanced arachidonic acid release does not necessarily mean that PLA$_2$ was activated since receptor-regulated arachidonic acid release can come from routes other than PLA$_2$, notably sequential PLC and DAG lipase activities. In some neuronal studies there is direct evidence that PLA$_2$ activation does occur. In the case of cultured cortical neurons, it is apparent that stimulation with glutamate leads to stable activation of cPLA$_2$ in cell-free assays. This is a consequence of increases in Ca^{2+} and PKC (Kim *et al.*, 1995). The regulation of neuronal PLA$_2$ by PKC may be widespread, since other receptors on neurons, such as muscarinic receptors in striatum, are linked to PLA$_2$ by PKC (Tence *et al.*, 1994). This is possibly due to phosphorylation by MAPK, since in many cell types PKC activation leads to MAPK activation. Neuronal cPLA$_2$ may be controlled in part by the same joint MAPK phosphorylation and Ca^{2+} processes investigated in nonneuronal studies and described above. However, there is currently no direct evidence implicating MAPK in the glutamate receptor stimulation of neuronal cPLA$_2$. In their studies on cultured striatal neurons Dumuis *et al.* (1993) show that depolarization, and Ca^{2+} entry through calcium channels, is not sufficient to stimulate arachidonic acid release. This may be because another pathway in addition to Ca^{2+} must be simultaneously activated (e.g. MAPK), although it could equally reflect a spatial requirement if the Ca^{2+} rise is to stimulate PLA$_2$, with the calcium channels being in the wrong place.

These reports serve to illustrate that cPLA$_2$ may play an important role in the consequences of glutamate neurotransmission in the brain; this may extend beyond arachidonic acid and its metabolites to include platelet-activating factor. The proposed roles for arachidonic acid and its products in neurotransmission are diverse, and have been reviewed recently (Piomelli, 1994; Shimizu and Wolfe, 1990).

9.2.3 Growth factor-associated pathways: tyrosine kinases and MAPK

Figure 9.6 shows a conventional picture for signaling pathways involving seven-transmembrane G protein-coupled receptors and growth factor receptors with intrinsic tyrosine kinase activity, in the same cell. In this representation there are cascades associated with G protein-coupled receptors (illustrated in *Figure 9.6* by the PLC cascade and K$^+$ channels, although others such as cAMP should also be included) and a separate tyrosine kinase/MAPK cascade associated with growth factor receptors. The former has been generally associated with short-term events, such as neurosecretion, while the latter has been associated with longer term transcriptional events, such as differentiation and proliferation. It has been recognized that some events show overlap. For example, the growth factor receptor link to tyrosine phosphorylation and activation of PLCγ, producing many events parallel to activation of the G protein-coupled PLCβ. Furthermore, certain events, such as neurite outgrowth, have been widely recognized as controlled by both receptor types. Recently, however, there has been a fundamental change in our understanding of the relationship between these types of signaling. The initiating studies were in nonneuronal cells, establishing that enhanced tyrosine phosphorylations in response to activation of seven-transmembrane receptors are widespread and central to many responses. This was rapidly followed by the establishment that the MAPK cascade is also commonly activated by G protein-coupled receptors, and that in at least some cases this could be by activation of upstream Ras and Raf mechanisms previously elucidated for the growth factor

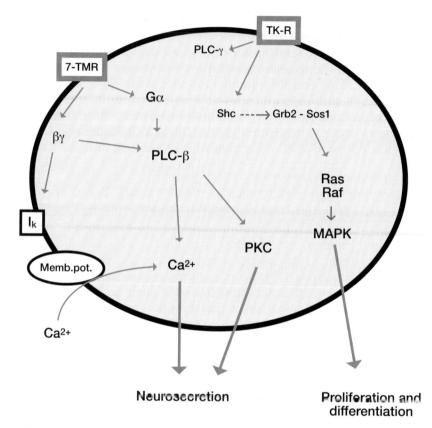

Figure 9.6. Pathways conventionally associated with cell surface receptors. The heterotrimeric G protein-coupled seven-transmembrane receptors (7-TMR) signaling is illustrated by the PLC cascade, although it could equally well include other pathways, such an adenylyl cyclase and cAMP. Direct G protein links to K⁺ channels (I_K) are also shown. The intrinsic tyrosine kinase, single membrane-spanning, growth factor receptors (TK-R) are shown linked to the formation of the Shc-Grb2-Sos 1 complex, which leads to the exchange of GDP for GTP at the small G protein Ras, and the recruitment of the Raf/MAPK cascade.

receptors. The mechanisms by which heterotrimeric G proteins couple to these upstream components may include both α-GTP and $\beta\gamma$-subunits. The detailed description of these events is beyond the scope of this chapter, but is summarized in Bourne (1995), and has resulted in the integration of the tyrosine kinase/MAPK cascade into schema for the G protein stimulated events, as in *Figure 9.7*.

Developing parrallel with these studies has been a body of evidence implicating tyrosine kinases in neuronal function, beyond that associated with growth factor receptors. This work started with a body of observations that the nervous system is well endowed with tyrosine phosphorylated proteins, and various protein tyrosine kinases and phosphatases (Wagner *et al.*, 1991). Subsequent studies established that neuronal stimulations of various kinds, including depolarization and the action of both metabotropic and ionotropic glutamate receptor agonists, stimulate neuronal protein tyrosine phosphorylation (e.g. Siciliano *et al.*, 1994). These observations, that tyrosine phosphorylations could be stimulated by ion fluxes, were interpreted with

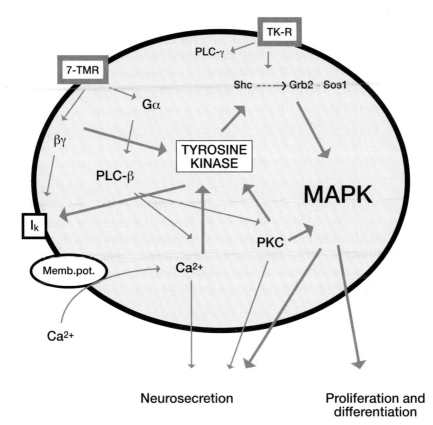

Figure 9.7. Integration of the Raf/MAPK cascade into the signaling cascades controlled by heterotrimeric G protein-coupled receptors. The activation of tyrosine kinases (e.g. PYK2) by the seven-transmembrane receptors (7-TMR) provides a mechanism for activation of the Raf/MAPK cascade upstream at the level of Shc phosphorylation and guanine nucleotide exchange factor recruitment.

emerging evidence that ion channels were themselves subject to regulation by tyrosine phosphorylation. More recent studies have enabled the integration of these observations with the mechanisms by which G protein-coupled receptors regulate tyrosine kinase/MAPK cascades in neurons, and the role this may play in controlling neuronal function. In an important paper, Lev *et al.* (1995) identified a protein tyrosine kinase called PYK2 which is highly expressed in the CNS. This kinase is activated by elevated Ca^{2+} and by PKC, and is a link between these and the stimulation of the events upstream of MAPK. Lev *et al.* (1995) go on to show that PYK2 regulates, not only this MAPK cascade, but also independently the tyrosine phosphorylation and kinetics of a delayed rectifier K^+ channel.

It is apparent that tyrosine phosphorylation is involved in early responses, such as neuronal excitability and neurosecretion, as well as long-term events such as neuronal survival, development and differentiation. Further work is establishing a specific role for MAPK in early responses of neurons to stimulation. A requirement for sequential tyrosine kinase/MAPK in stimulus-evoked noradrenaline release from chromaffin cells has been proposed (Cox *et al.*, 1996), possibly involving the MAPK activation of

PLA$_2$ (established in nonneuronal cell types: Lin *et al.*, 1993; Patel *et al.*, 1996a,b), and the activation of MAPK in hippocampal neurons in response to depolarization has been demonstrated (Baron *et al.*, 1996). The consequences of the involvement of the tyrosine kinase/MAPK cascade in responses to depolarization and activation of ionotropic and metabotropic receptors for neuronal function is not clear, but will be the subject of intensive future research.

9.2.4 Protein kinases, phosphatases and molecular scaffolding in neurons

One of the difficult problems in signaling pathways is understanding the mechanisms for maintaining specificity of protein phosphorylations in the face of a diversity of sub-strates for many of the kinases, such as PKC and protein kinase A (PKA), which are found in cells. This is related to the question of how different neurotransmitters which stimulate the same kinase lead to a different outcome. An emerging contribution to these issues, which is likely to have profound consequences for how we understand functioning of the neuron, is the formation of molecular scaffolds. These scaffolds include in their structures various kinases and phosphatases, and are strategically located so as to anchor signaling enzymes in apposition to substrate proteins as well as incoming signals. This creates a microdomain within the neuron, and has so far been successfully studied in postsynaptic densities and in dendrites. The concept is essen-tially related to the anchoring of tyrosine kinases to activating and substrate molecules by SH2 and SH3 domains. The formation of a scaffold depends on the presence of anchoring proteins. Scaffolds are then formed by associations of these anchoring pro-teins with signaling proteins, such as PKA and PKC (Mochly-Rosen *et al.*, 1995). In hip-pocampal postsynaptic densities and dendrites it has been shown that an anchoring pro-tein forms a scaffold of PKC-α, PKA and calcineurin, the neuronal Ca^{2+}-regulated phosphatase (Klauck *et al.*, 1996). This structure is itself associated with, for example, NMDA receptors, which can act as activators of the protein phosphorylation scaffold and also be regulated by it (Cooper *et al.*, 1995; Klauck *et al.*, 1996). The scaffold itself responds to inputs activating PKC-α (e.g. DAG), PKA (e.g. cAMP) and calcineurin (e.g. Ca^{2+}), and is able to control both the rate of phosphorylation of associated substrates and the rate of dephosphorylation. The formation of the functional complex presumably confers co-ordination of control between the individual components, although the manner and consequences of this are poorly understood. These functional scaffolds therefore enable the integration of different inputs, and the specific regulation of pro-teins associated with a particular microdomain within a neuron. It seems very likely that future studies will reveal such molecular scaffolding in the nerve terminal.

9.3 Role of second messenger signaling pathways in neuronal function

Neuronal function is variously ascribed, depending on the bias of the laboratory from which the study originates, as being indicated by neuronal excitability (membrane potential, particularly relating to action potential frequency), cytosolic Ca^{2+} or neuro-transmitter release. In attempts to provide an integrated view of the regulation of neu-rons by second messenger signaling pathways, we shall consider how G protein-coupled receptors act through second messenger pathways to regulate ion channels, followed by some comments on second messengers and the development of LTP and LTD.

9.3.1 Control of neuronal ion channels by G protein-coupled receptors

There have been no unequivocal demonstrations that neuronal ion channels can be directly controlled by association with G protein subunits. In many cases where it has been shown that ion channel control is dependent on a G protein, it cannot be excluded that this control is via an intermediate, possibly a second messenger based pathway. Even when the experimental configuration shows the G protein–ion channel coupling to be restricted to the membrane (membrane delimited), it does not exclude mediation by a lipophilic second messenger or intermediate membrane-bound protein. However there is a widespread view that direct G protein regulation of neuronal ion channels does occur, in particular with respect to the regulation of Ca^{2+} channels by G_o, a protein of notable abundance in the brain.

Control of neuronal Ca^{2+} channels by G protein-coupled receptors. Using cell culture systems such as stimulation of α_2-adrenergic or $GABA_B$ (γ-aminobutyric acid) receptors of embryonic chick sensory neurons, it can be shown that receptor activation leads to inhibition of N-type Ca^{2+} currents (Cox and Dunlap, 1992; Dunlap and Fischbach, 1978). This inhibition is pertussis toxin-sensitive, telling us not only that it is mediated by G proteins, but also that the G protein is of the $G_{o/i}$ group (Kleuss et al., 1991). In an influential paper using neuroblastoma–glioma hybrid cells, Heschler et al. (1987) showed that G_o heterotrimers were able to restore inhibition of N-type Ca^{2+} currents which had been lost due to pertussis toxin pretreatment. It is studies of this type, combined with work which excludes likely candidates for second messenger mediation, which have led to the view that neuronal Ca^{2+} channel modulation may be by direct association with G protein subunits. Various research groups proceeded to show that an involvement of G_o in the receptor regulation of neuronal Ca^{2+} channels is widespread, including for example neuropeptide Y and $GABA_B$ receptors in sensory neurons (Campbell *et al.*, 1993; Ewald *et al.*, 1988). Caulfield *et al.* (1994) provide evidence that inhibition of ion-channel currents in sympathetic neurons can be via different G proteins for different receptors on the same cell, including G_o for α-adrenoceptor inhibition of Ca^{2+} currents. In further studies on chick sensory neurons Dunlap and colleagues have shown that multiple pathways are involved in the mediation of the α-adrenergic inhibition of N-type currents (Diverse-Pierluissi et al., 1995). They provide strong evidence that the $\beta\gamma$-subunits of heterotrimeric G proteins play an important role, but also confirm earlier reports of involvement of PKC with a model for two bifurcating pathways from the α-receptor, involving different G proteins and having different effects on the channel which have in common an attenuation of current. This introduces two important themes with respect to the role of second messengers and G protein regulation of ion channels: firstly, that the relationship between G proteins and channels is likely to be complex, perhaps involving multiple subunits; secondly, that this complexity may include both direct G protein regulation and second messenger involvement issuing simultaneously from the same receptor, and interacting with the same population of channels.

These and related studies have established that receptor regulation of neuronal Ca^{2+} channels may be dependent on PKC, and is therefore controlled by a second messenger-linked pathway. PKC influences on Ca^{2+} channels have been well established for some time as a result of direct activation of PKC with phorbol esters, although from the beginning there has been a diversity of effects, including for example an enhancement of calcium channel opening in *Aplysia* (De Riemer *et al.*, 1985), facilitation of depolarization-enhanced calcium flux in PC12 cells (Di Virgilio *et al.*, 1986; Harris *et al.*, 1986) and attenuation of calcium influx in neutrophils (McCarthy *et al.*, 1989). Advancing from this experimental approach to demonstrating the involvement of PKC in receptor regulation of neuronal Ca^{2+} channels is illustrated by the chick sensory neuron studies from Dunlap and colleagues described above. It seems likely that this is a widespread pathway for Ca^{2+} channel regulation in neurons. It is interesting to note that PKC is a family of enzymes with different regulatory characteristics. While in several nonneuronal systems there is accumulating evidence indicating which isoforms are responsible for individual responses to PKC activation, there is nothing known about which isoforms are involved in regulation of neuronal Ca^{2+} channels.

The other salient pathway for second messenger regulation of neuronal Ca^{2+} channels is by cAMP, acting to stimulate PKA and the direct phosphorylation of channels. L-, P- and N- channels are each known to have consensus sites for phosphorylation by PKA. Phosphorylation is at the α-subunit and dephosphorylation is by protein phosphatases 1 and 2A. However, the regulatory role played by phosphorylation of neuronal Ca^{2+} channels is poorly understood. The demonstration of PKA phosphorylation is best established in a nonneuronal system: the adrenergic regulation of cardiac L-type Ca^{2+} channels. It has been claimed that the influence of β-adrenergic agonists is exclusively due to cAMP-dependent phosphorylation of cardiac L-type channels (Hartzell *et al.*, 1991). This has been disputed as a result of evidence that there is a fast, membrane-delimited direct G protein activation (e.g. Yatani and Brown, 1989) in addition to the larger but slower influence via cAMP and PKA. This is reminiscent of the dual control exerted by α_2-adrenoceptors in chick sensory neurons described above (Diverse-Pierluissi *et al.*, 1995), and alerts us to the possibility that such dual control, both direct association with subunits and second messenger-mediated (involving PKA as well as PKC) may be widespread. On dissociation of the G protein into α_{GTP} and $\beta\gamma$-subunits, the α-subunits may provide a route for 'slow' regulation of the channels by activation of second messenger pathways (PLC and adenylyl cyclase cascades are illustrated), while the more direct $\beta\gamma$ interaction provides for a 'fast' route. We can expect models of this nature to be developed in future studies of integrated pathways for the control of neuronal Ca^{2+} channels.

With respect to the location of the channels, on cell body or nerve terminal, the major part of the studies undertaken relate to the modulation by phosphorylation of ion currents in the cell body, usually in cells in culture. In some cases it has been possible to make inferences about events occurring at the nerve terminal, which generally are not amenable to ion channel recording directly. This has been possible because, in some instances, the receptors are known to be restricted to the terminals, or because the receptors regulate neurotransmitter release from nerve terminals. The problem with the latter is that release of neurotransmitter may be modulated by action at sites other than Ca^{2+} influx, such as at the exocytotic mechanism. For example it is known that noradrenaline acts on prejunctional α_2-receptors to modulate neurotransmitter release. Adrenergic α_2-receptors are linked via G_i to the inhibition of adenylyl cyclase. The presynaptic inhibition of release has been described as being dependent or independent of cAMP in different studies, and could be due to an inhibitory influence on Ca^{2+} channels or direct inhibition of exocytosis. In an interesting study on noradrenaline release from sympathetic neurons Lipscombe *et al.*

(1989) reported that depolarization-stimulated release, but not ionomycin-stimulated release, can be inhibited by presynaptic α receptors. Ionomycin bypasses the Ca^{2+} channel by allowing Ca^{2+} directly into the terminal, whereas depolarization-stimulated Ca^{2+} entry is through voltage-sensitive channels. This study suggests that presynaptic α_2 receptors inhibit release by action at the Ca^{2+} channels, and not at the exocytotic process. They then showed that N-type, but not L-type, Ca^{2+} channels were inhibited by α_2-agonists in a G protein-dependent manner.

In the CNS, interest in both cell body and nerve terminal G protein receptors has been evoked by the regulation of channels by dopamine receptors. It is widely acknowledged that D1 receptors are linked to the stimulation, and D2 receptors to the inhibition, of adenylyl cyclase. D1 receptors have been associated with postsynaptic, cell body, function, while D2 receptors are studied widely in terms of presynaptic influences, where in addition to inhibition of adenylyl cyclase their action is associated with Ca^{2+} and K^+ channel modulation (see below). The influence of $D1_a$ receptors on different Ca^{2+} channels has been shown to be a consequence of modulation of cAMP levels, but a recent study reveals a considerable degree of complexity in the relationship between the receptor and different types of Ca^{2+} channel. Surmeier et al. (1995) provide evidence that D1 receptors *enhance* L-type channel function by stimulation of cAMP levels and consequent phosphorylation of the channel by PKA. However, the same receptors *reduce* N- and P- type currents, again following the elevation of cAMP and activation of PKA. This inhibitory effect is due to the activation (by PKA) of protein phosphatase 1. The action of this enzyme is controlled by inhibitory phosphoproteins, such as DARPP-32, which is in turn subject to control by PKA phosphorylation. This complex pattern of control illustrates an important notion, that bifurcation of control, and the differential regulation of channel activity, can occur at the level of a single second messenger pathway, downstream of G proteins.

The notion that nerve terminal Ca^{2+} channels can be regulated by second messenger pathways raises the possibility that neurotransmitter release could be stimulated by the action of second messenger-linked receptors acting locally to open Ca^{2+} channels and allow Ca^{2+} influx at the exocytotic site.

Control of neuronal K^+ channels by G protein-coupled receptors. The regulation of K^+ channels is also of considerable importance in neurons, although with respect to G protein-coupled channels there is little information as to the importance in nerve terminals versus cell bodies. The major advances in understanding were, as with the Ca^{2+} channels, first provided by studies on cardiac function. The pacemaker I_{KACh}, regulated by G protein-coupled muscarinic ACh receptors, is dependent for its regulation on G protein activation, providing a classic example of 'membrane delimited' regulation (Sakmann et al., 1983) by G proteins (Breitwieser and Szabo, 1985; Pfaffinger et al., 1985). Despite controversy for the role of G_α, strong evidence has been presented that the effect is mediated by $\beta\gamma$-subunits (Logothetis et al., 1987; Reuveny et al., 1994; Wickman et al., 1994). Recent studies have shown that $\beta\gamma$-subunits associate directly with the I_{KACh} channel protein, providing the best evidence yet for direct G-protein regulation of ion channels (Krapivinsky et al., 1995) This background is important because it is clear that G protein-coupled receptors are linked to K^+ channels in neurons. In the examples to be considered it is apparent that this is a second messenger/protein phosphorylation-mediated regulation, distinct from the direct effect of G proteins proposed in the cardiac studies. This regulation of

K^+ currents is widely seen to be inhibitory, and may therefore be expected to increase neuronal activity and neurotransmitter release (but see below for possible facilitation of K^+ currents by presynaptic D2 receptors).

There are numerous examples of this type of control of neuronal K^+ channels, in the CNS and periphery, although in the majority of instances the nature of involvement of second messengers is unclear. For example, it is known that in frog sympathetic ganglion neurotransmission, activation of mAChR attenuates the K^+ channels, and that this can be mimicked by direct activation of PKC (Brown and Adams, 1987). This leads to the proposal that the mAChR effect is due to formation of DAG and activation of PKC. However, it has proved difficult to confirm that this second messenger pathway is how the receptor exerts its influence, since PKC inhibitors failed to block the effect; an alternative pathway from receptor to channel therefore cannot be excluded (Bosma *et al.*, 1990). Further evidence has been provided for a mACh effect on K^+ channels which is second messenger-dependent and mediated by a pertussis toxin-insensitive pathway involving $G_{q/11}$ (Caulfield *et al.*, 1994; Selyanko *et al.*, 1992). In a similar vein it has been known for some time that bradykinin can excite rat sympathetic neurons, and it has recently been shown that this is a result of a $Gq_{/11}$-dependent closure of K^+ channels (Jones *et al.*, 1995). The second messenger responsible for these effects remains unclear.

Earlier studies from the same group, on neuroblastoma cells in culture, have investigated two second messenger-linked responses to bradykinin, which serve to illustrate both the nature of second messenger links to K^+ channels which may control neuronal function, and also the complexity of interacting pathways to ion channel regulation, as we have already seen for the Ca^{2+} channels. Using both NG 108-15 cells and N1E-115 cells a model for bradykinin regulation has been developed in which the activation of PLC and generation of $Ins(1,4,5)P_3$ is followed by an initial hyperpolarization, caused by the stimulation of Ca^{2+}-activated K^+ channels, followed by a depolarization, mediated by activation of PKC (Higashida and Brown, 1986, 1987). The example of regulation of K^+ channels by Ca^{2+} is particularly important, since this is likely to be a very common mechanism whereby second messenger-linked responses are able to regulate neuronal excitability.

An interesting and potentially very important example in the CNS of K^+ channel regulation by second messenger pathways is the role of 5-hydroxytryptamine 5-HT_4 receptors in controlling neurons in various locations in the brain. The 5-HT_4 receptor is currently considered to act by stimulation of adenylyl cyclase, increased accumulation of cAMP and activation of PKA. In brain neurons with these receptors this results in inhibition of both voltage-sensitive and Ca^{2+}-sensitive K^+ currents, and a consequent increase in neuronal excitability and neurotransmitter release. This effect can be long-lasting, persisting beyond the period of agonist action, probably because the effect of stimulation of adenylyl cyclase is accompanied by an inhibition of phosphatase activity, resulting in a persistent protein phosporylation (Ansanay *et al.*, 1995).

These studies are all essentially looking at the postsynaptic site, the regulation of K^+ channels at cell bodies, and they illustrate a very simple and yet important principle about the role of second messenger systems in neurons: *receptors are able to regulate neuronal excitability by second messenger pathways*. The example of the 5-HT_4 receptors shows that in some cases this effect on neuronal excitability may be very long lasting, and possibly therefore with a role to play in neuronal plasticity and learning.

Having established this important principle, it is reasonable to ask whether control over K^+ channels occurs with G protein-coupled receptors located on the nerve terminal, and if so whether this can be seen to involve second messenger pathways. Here evidence is very sparse. Perhaps one of the most importance examples is that of presynaptic D2 receptors for dopamine, which exert an inhibitory influence on dopamine release in the brain, and are likely to be important sites in the action of neuroleptic drugs used in the treatment of schizophrenia. Initially described as being linked to inhibition of adenylyl cyclase, these receptors were also shown to cause inhibition of Ca^{2+} channels and opening of K^+ channels (Vallar and Meldolesi, 1989). The recognition that D2 receptors are found in multiple forms, and that there is a larger family of D2-like receptors, has led to studies which have revealed a partial dissociation of the inhibition of adenylyl cyclase and opening of K^+ channels associated with a differential coupling to G proteins (Castro and Strange, 1993; Montmayeur *et al.*, 1993; Vallar *et al.*, 1990). The nature of the link between D2 receptors and K^+ channels in the presynaptic environment remains an important area for further study.

In addition to the well established regulation of K^+ channels by PLC and cAMP second messengers, further pathways of importance in neuronal systems are PLA_2 and tyrosine kinases. There is convincing evidence that PLA_2 and arachidonic acid are of importance in regulating K^+ conductances underlying neuronal excitability in a number of preparations. This effect can be inhibitory or excitatory, and involve arachidonic acid itself, or lipoxygenase or cyclooxygenase metabolites, depending on the examples chosen (e.g. Koyano *et al.*, 1994; Schweitzer *et al.*, 1993; Villarroel, 1994; Yu, 1995). The nature of the PLA_2 involved is not apparent from these studies, although $cPLA_2$ would seem most likely. It also remains for future research to resolve whether this influence of these eicosanoids is directly on the channel or via intermediates. An example of the latter might be the influence which arachidonic acid exerts in enhancing DAG stimulation of PKC, and the subsequent influence of this kinase on channel activity.

A recent observation of potentially wide impact is the regulation of K^+ channels by tyrosine kinase pathways. This is best seen in the study by Lev *et al.* (1995) in which a neuronal tyrosine kinase was cloned and named PYK2. This is a Ca^{2+}-activated tyrosine kinase which leads to activation of MAPK and to modulation of K^+ channel activity. In this case then the tyrosine kinase influence on K^+ channels provides an alternative route to the PLC cascade in the signaling pathways which regulate neuronal excitablity.

9.3.2 Second messengers and models of learning and plasticity: LTP and LTD

In one of the most influential pieces of writing in brain research, D.O. Hebb described a model for plasticity in neural networks, in which within a web of interconnecting neurons transmission of the nervous impulse would be facilitated through those pathways most frequently excited. This proposal has, in its major recent manifestations of LTP and LTD, provided fertile ground for the development of biochemical models for plasticity and learning based upon events occurring at individual synapses. LTP and related phenomena have been the subject of recent review (Bliss and Collingridge, 1993) and can only be mentioned here to illustrate the studies implicating various second messenger systems in the processes involved. However, it is important to recognize the general point, that potentiation (or depression) of transmission across a synapse could be a result of presynaptic and postsynaptic events.

There is evidence that both are involved. There may be more dependence on presynaptic events in the establishment of the adaptive change, and more dependence on postsynaptic events in its long-term maintenance. Various biochemical changes have been proposed to contribute to these events. It is clear that LTP occurs at more than one site in the brain, and that the mechanisms involved are not the same at each site investigated. Having said this, it is of interest to look at some of the evidence for involvement of second messenger systems.

Numerous summaries of LTP, often based upon the example of the innervation of hippocampal CA1 pyramidal cells by CA3 Schaffer collaterals, have concluded that the facilitation of this glutamatergic neurotransmission is due to repeated high frequency stimulation of CA1 inputs, or coincidental activation of two converging inputs, causing the activation of AMPA receptors, and NMDA receptors, at the dendritic postsynaptic site. The action of glutamate at the AMPA site results in depolarization which, under conditions which generate LTP, is permissive of the action of glutamate at the dendritic NMDA receptors (attenuation of Mg^{2+} block), resulting in Ca^{2+} entry and the elevation of postsynaptic Ca^{2+}_i which is essential for the development of LTP. This postsynaptic model for LTP is not exclusive of presynaptic events. The involvement of second messenger systems then can be seen as firstly a role for second messengers in the central events which establish LTP and secondly as a role which modulates either the establishment of LTP or its consequences for synaptic transmission. The latter may be due to the control of second messenger pathways by local receptors not involved in the establishment of LTP.

The action of Ca^{2+}_i is likely to be dominated by the very high levels of Ca^{2+}/calmodulin kinase II (CaMKII) found at the immediate postsynaptic site, the postsynaptic density. Direct evidence for a role for postsynaptic CaMKII in LTP has been provided by studies in which transgenic mice lacking full CaMKII (Silva *et al.*, 1992), or introduction of constitutively active CaMKII into hippocampal slice preparations (Pettit *et al.*, 1994), prevented LTP. This also introduces the more general notion, that protein phosphorylations are involved in neuronal pasticity.

Various protein kinases have been implicated in LTP. One of the most widely studied has been the cAMP-dependent kinase PKA. cAMP has been implicated in the processes of plasticity by many studies; recently a role in LTP has been firmly established. cAMP has been shown to rise in the hippocampal CA1 area following NMDA receptor activation, and PKA is localized in the postsynaptic density (Carr *et al.*, 1992; Chetkovich and Sweatt, 1993). Firstly, we must ask how a rise in cAMP occurs, within the context of the essential NMDA-initiated events for establishing LTP. Here, we have a satisfyingly simple answer at hand. The central event of a spatially localized, NMDA receptor-mediated, rise in Ca^{2+} leads to the subsequent activation of CaMKII at the postsynaptic density. It is known that some isoforms of adenylyl cyclase are Ca^{2+}/calmodulin-sensitive (Cooper *et al.*, 1995). It has been shown that the NMDA-mediated rise in cAMP in the CA1 region is calmodulin dependent (Chetkovitch and Sweatt, 1993; Frey *et al.*, 1993). The suppression by LTP-inducing trains of stimulation of after hyperpolarization, one of the electrical correlates of early events in LTP, has been shown to require increased adenylyl cyclase activity. This suppression was blocked by a calmodulin-binding peptide (Blitzer *et al.*, 1995). These various observations support the hypothesis that cAMP rises associated with LTP are generated by NMDA-mediated increases in postsynaptic Ca^{2+} leading to CaMKII-dependent activation of adenylyl cyclase.

When LTP is considered in terms of initiating events (early phase) and maintaining events (late phase), we can find evidence for the involvement of cAMP in both. The longer term events have been associated with the regulation of transcription in the nucleus involving, in part, the cAMP-responsive element binding protein (Frey et al., 1993; Huang and Kandel, 1994; see Chapter 12). With respect to early LTP, Blitzer et al. (1995) have provided evidence that cAMP rises are necessary for the generation of LTP, but that cAMP alone is not sufficient for LTP. They propose that cAMP leads to inhibition of protein phosphatases, permitting the consequences of activation of CaMKII to be expressed as an increase in levels of phosphorylation of specific proteins and thereby an enhanced synaptic response. They express the relationships between these events as a gating role for cAMP, through which the signal pathway of CaMKII must pass. Two general themes can be pointed out here. Firstly, as in examples discussed above, functional roles for signaling pathways can only be understood when an attempt is made to integrate disparate cascades. Secondly, the functional response seen with LTP is finally expressed as a change in ion channel function, and therefore any discussion of second messengers and neuronal plasticity will merge with the discussion of second messengers and ion channels outlined above.

There is widespread evidence for a role for the PKC family of kinases in neuronal plasticity, and in LTP in particular. While a role for PKC has been well established, its relationship to other kinase pathways, and to the modification of ion channel function which will result in postsynaptic aspects of synaptic plasticity, remains to be clarified. A particularly interesting example of a class of kinases which will be the subject of future evaluation for a role in synaptic plasticity is the family of tyrosine kinases. It is already known (see above) that a tyrosine kinase called PY2 is localized in rat hippocampal pyramidal cell dendrites, and that this Ca^{2+}- and PKC-sensitive enzyme can modulate ion channel function and has the potential to control, perhaps by the activation of MAPK, long-term changes in expression of the genome. It is interesting to speculate that aspects of short- and long-term changes involved in LTP which are known to be mediated by PKC and Ca^{2+} may in part depend on downstream activation of the tyrosine kinase/MAPK pathway. This will be a fertile and demanding field for future research.

While MAPK and related events are widely interpreted as significant in the longer term aspects of cellular function (e.g. transcriptional regulation, differentiation, proliferation) there are examples emerging from nonneuronal studies which indicate a role in short-term events. Of particular relevance here is the demonstration that tyrosine kinases and MAPK are important in the control of PLA_2 and receptor-regulated control of arachidonic acid and its active metabolites (Bowden et al., 1995; Lin et al., 1993; Patel et al., 1996b). Dumuis et al. (1988) showed that arachidonic acid release occurs in striatal neurons in response to glutamate receptor activation, and proceeded to demonstrate a requirement for conjoint mGluR activation and depolarization by ionotropic AMPA receptors (Dumuis et al., 1990). This may reflect a requirement for multiple inputs into the PLA_2 activation process, such as Ca^{2+} and MAPK. If this is occurring in postsynaptic sites under conditions of establishment of LTP, then this may play a role in the generation of arachidonic acid and platelet-activating factor, which may contribute to LTP by acting as a 'retrograde transmitter'. In this manner messengers which can pass freely between the intracellular and extracellular compartments may play a role as second messengers and also as molecules communicating between cells. The 'retrograde transmitter' hypothesis is that the messenger is formed at the postsynaptic site and then passes in a retrograde manner to the postsynaptic site where it influences the subsequent release of neurotransmitter. In this way convergence of information at the postsynaptic site may lead to the modulation of presynaptic events, and thus contribute to presynaptic aspects of LTP (Herrero *et al.*, 1992). The recruitment of presynaptic events by retrograde transmitters is widely discussed in terms of arachidonic acid and NO. *Figure 9.2* illustrates the possible role of retrograde transmission by these two agents. Initial questions to ask on this issue are, what are the events which may stimulate the production of the retrograde transmitter at the postsynaptic site, and what are the second messenger systems at the presynaptic site which may bring about their effects? It seems likely that PLA_2 and arachidonic acid production are likely to play an increasing role in future models of neuronal plasticity (e.g. Linden, 1995). It is relevant to note that alternative receptor-regulated routes for the generation of arachidonic acid are known to be important, notably the sequential action of PLC and DAG. In addition, receptor-regulated DAG may derive from sequential PLD and phosphatidate phosphohydrolase activity, which combined with DAG lipase may provide a further route for arachidonic acid production, independent of both PLC and PLA_2. If arachidonic acid does have a role to play in neuronal plasticity, then the contribution of these alternative pathways to its synthesis should be considered.

References

Ansanay H, Dumuis A, Sebben M, Bockaert J, Fangi L. (1995) cAMP-dependent, long lasting inhibition of a K^+ current in mammalian neurons. *Proc. Natl Acad. Sci. USA* **92**: 6635–6639.

Baron C, Benes C, van Tan H, Fagard R, Roisin M-P. (1996) Potassium chloride pulse enhances mitogen activated protein kinase activity in rat hippocampal slices. *J. Neurochem.* **66**: 1005–1010.

Berridge MJ. (1993) Inositol trisphosphates and calcium signalling. *Nature* **361**: 315–325.

Bliss TVP, Collingridge GL. (1993) A synaptic model of memory: long term potentiation in the hippocampus. *Nature* **361**: 31–39.

Blitzer RD, Wong T, Noranifar R, Iyengar R, Landau EM. (1995) Postsynaptic cAMP pathway gates early LTP in hippocampal CA1 region. *Neuron* **15**: 1403–1414.

Boarder MR. (1994) A role for phospholipase D in control of mitogenesis. *Trends Pharmacol. Sci.* **15**: 57–62.

Boarder MR, Purkiss J. (1993) Assay of phospholipase D as a neuronal receptor–effector mechanism. *Neuroprotocols* **3**: 157–164.

Bosma M, Bernheim L, Leibowitz MD, Pfaffinger PJ, Hille B. (1990) Modulation of M current in frog sympathetic ganglion cells. In: *G Proteins and Signal Transduction* (eds NM Nathanson, TK Harden). Rockefeller University Press, New York, pp. 43–59.

Bourne HR. (1995) Team blue sees red. *Nature* **376**: 727–729.

Bowden A, Patel V, Brown C, Boarder MR. (1995) Evidence for requirement of tyrosine phosphorylation in endothelial P_{2Y}- and P_{2U}- purinoceptor stimulation of prostacyclin release. *Br. J. Pharmacol.* **116**: 2563–2568.

Breitwieser GE, Szabo G. (1985) Uncoupling of cardiac muscarinic and β-adrenergic receptors from ion channels by a guanine nucleotide analogue. *Nature* **317**: 538–540.

Brown DA, Adams PR. (1987) Effects of phorbol dibutyrate on M currents and M current inhibition in bullfrog sympathetic neurons. *Cell. Mol. Neurobiol.* **7**: 255–269.

Brown HA, Gutowski S, Moomaw CR, Slaughter C, Sternweiss PC. (1993) ADP-ribosylation factor, a small GTP-dependent regulatory protein, stimulates phopholipase D activity. *Cell* **75**: 1137–1144.

Campbell V, Berrow N, Dolphin AC. (1993) $GABA_B$ receptor modulation of Ca^{2+} currents in rat sensory neurons by the G protein Go: antisense oligonucleotide studies. *J. Physiol. (Lond.)* **470**: 1–11.

Carr DW, Stofko-Hahn RE, Fraser IDC, Cone RD, Scott JD. (1992) Localisation of the cAMP-dependent protein kinase to the postsynaptic densities by A-kinase anchoring proteins. *J. Biol. Chem.* **267**: 16 816–16 823.

Carter TD, Hallam TJ, Cusack NJ, Pearson JD. (1988) Regulation of P_{2Y}-purinoceptor-mediated prostacyclin release from human endothelial cells by cytoplasmic calcium concentration. *Br. J. Pharmacol.* **95:** 1181–1190.

Castro SW, Strange PG. (1993) Differences in the ligand binding properties of the short and long versions of the D2 dopamine receptor. *J. Neurochem.* **60:** 372–375.

Caulfield MP, Jones S, Vallis Y, Buckley NJ, Kim G-D, Milligan, G, Brown DA. (1994) Muscarinic M-current inhibition via $G_{\alpha q/11}$ and α-adrenoceptor inhibition of Ca^{2+} current via $G\alpha_o$ in rat sympathetic neurons. *J. Physiol. (Lond.)* **477:** 415–422.

Challiss RAJ, Wilkes LC, Patel V, Purkiss JR, Boarder MR. (1993) Phospholipase D activation regulates endothelin-1 stimulation of phosphoinositide-specific phospholipase C in SK-N-MC cells. *FEBS Lett.* **327:** 157–160.

Chetkovitch DM, Sweatt JD. (1993). NMDA receptor activation increases cAMP in area CA1 of the hippocampus via calcium/calmodulin stimulation of adenylyl cyclase. *J. Neurochem.* **61:** 1933–1942.

Cockroft S, Thomas GMH, Fensome A, Geny B, Cunningham E, Gout I, Hiles I, Totty NF, Truong O, Hsuan JJ. (1994) Phospholipase D: a downstream effector of ARF in granulocytes. *Science* **263:** 523–526.

Cooper DMF, Mons N, Karpen JW. (1995) Adenylyl cyclases and the interaction between calcium and cAMP signalling. *Nature* **374:** 421–424.

Cox DH, Dunlap K. (1992) Pharmacological discrimination of N-type from L-type calcium current and its selective modulation by neurotransmitters. *J. Neurosci.* **12:** 906–914.

Cox ME, Ely CM, Catling AD, Weber MJ, Parsons SJ. (1995) Tyrosine kinases are required for catecholamine secretion and mitogen activated protein kinase activation in bovine adrenal chromaffin cells. *J. Neurochem.* **66:** 1103–1112.

Davis RL. (1996) Physiology and biochemistry of drosophila learning mutants. *Physiol. Rev.* **76:** 299–317.

De Reimer SA, Strong JA, Albert KA, Greengard P, Kaczmarek LK. (1985) Enhancement of calcium current in *Aplysia* neurones by phorbol ester and protein kinase C. *Nature* **313:** 313–316.

Di Virgilio F, Pozzan T, Wollheim CB, Vincentini LM, Meldolesi J. (1986) Tumour promoter phorbol myristate acetate inhibits calcium influx through voltage gated calcium channels in two secretory cell lines, PC12 and RINm5F. *J. Biol. Chem.* **261:** 32–35.

Diverse-Pierluissi M, Goldsmith PK, Dunlap K. (1995) Transmitter mediated inhibition of N-type calcium channels in sensory neurons involves multiple GTP-binding proteins and subunits. *Neuron* **14:** 191–200.

Dumuis A, Sebben M, Haynes L, Pin J-P, Bockaert J. (1988) NMDA receptors activate the arachidonic acid cascade system in striatal neurons. *Nature* **336:** 68–70.

Dumuis A, Pin JP, Oomagari K, Sebben M, Bockaert J. (1990) Arachidonic acid release by joint stimulation of ionotropic and metabotropic quisqualate receptors. *Nature* **347:** 182–184.

Dumuis A, Sebben M, Fagni L, Prezeau L, Manzoni O, Cragoe EJ, Bockeart J. (1993) Stimulation by glutamate receptors of arachidonic acid release depends on the Na^+/Ca^{2+} exchanger in neuronal cells. *Mol. Pharmacol.* **43:** 976–981.

Dunlap K, Fishbach GD. (1987) Neurotransmitters decrease the calcium component of sensory neuron action potentials. *Nature* **319:** 670–672.

Ewald DA, Sternweiss PC, Miller RJ. (1988) Guanine nucleotide-binding protein G_0-induced coupling of neuropeptide Y receptors to Ca^{2+} channels in sensory neurons. *Proc. Natl Acad. Sci. USA* **85:** 3633–3637.

Frey U, Huang Y-Y, Kandel ER. (1993) Adenylyl cyclases and the interaction between calcium and cAMP signalling. *Nature* **374:** 421–424.

Furuichi T, Mikoshiba K. (1995) Inositol 1,4,5-trisphosphate receptor-mediated Ca^{2+} signalling in the brain. *J. Neurochem.* **64:** 953–960.

Glaser KB, Mobilio D, Chang JY, Senko N. (1993) Phospholipase A_2 enzymes: regulation and inhibition. *Trends Pharmacol. Sci.* **14:** 92–98.

Harris KM, Konsamut S, Miller RJ. (1986) Protein kinase C mediated regulation of calcium channels in PC-12 phaeochromocytoma cells. *Biochem. Biophys. Res. Commun.* **134:** 1298–1305.

Hartzell HC, Mery P-F, Fischmeister R, Szabo G. (1991) Sympathetic regulation of cardiac calcium current is due exclusively to cAMP-dependent phosphorylation. *Nature* **351:** 573–576.

Herrero I, Miras-Portugal MT, Sanchez-Prieto J. (1992) Positive feedback of glutamate exocytosis by metabotropic presynaptic receptor stimulation. *Nature* **360:** 163–166.

Heschler J, Rosenthal W, Trautwein W, Schultz G. (1987) The GTP binding protein, Go, regulates neuronal calcium channels. *Nature* **325:** 445–447.

Higashida H, Brown DA. (1986) Two polyphosphoinositol metabolites control two K^+ currents in a neuronal cell. *Nature* 323: 333–335.

Higashida H, Brown DA. (1987) Bradykinin inhibits potassium (M) currents in NIE-115 neuroblastoma cells. *FEBS Lett.* 220: 302–306.

Holler T, Klein J, Loffelholz K. (1994) Phospholipase C and phospholipase D are independently activated in rat hippocampal slices. *Biochem. Pharmacol.* 47: 411–414.

Huang YY, Kandel ER. (1994) Recruitment of long-lasting and protein kinase A dependent long-term potentiation in the CA1 region of hippocampus requires repeated tetanisation. *Learning Memory* 1: 74–82.

Jones S, Brown DA, Milligan G, Willer E, Buckley NJ, Caulfield MP. (1995) Bradykinin excites rat sympathetic neurons by inhibition of M current through a mechanism involving B2 receptors and $G_{\alpha q/11}$. *Neuron* 14: 399–405.

Kahn RA, Yucel JK, Malhotra V. (1993) ARF signalling: a potential role for phospholipase D in membrane traffic. *Cell* 75: 1045–1048.

Kanoh H, Kanaho Y, Nozawa Y. (1992) Pertussis-toxin-insensitive G protein mediates carbachol activation of phospholipase D in rat pheochromocytoma PC12 cells. *J. Neurochem.* B59B: 1786–1794.

Kato K, Clark GD, Bazan NG, Zorumski CF. (1994) Platelet activating factor as a potential retrograde messenger in CA1 hippocampal long-term potentiation. *Nature* 367: 175–179.

Kim DK, Rordorf G, Nemenoff A, Koroshetz WJ, Bonventre JV. (1995) Glutamate stably enhances the activity of two cytosolic forms of phospholipase A_2 in brain cortical cultures. *Biochem. J.* 310: 83–90.

Klauck, T.M., Faux M.C., Labudda K, Langeburg LK, Jaken S, Scott JD. (1996) Coordination of three signalling enzymes by AKAP79, a mammalian scaffold protein. *Science* 271: 1589–1592.

Klein J, Holler T, Koppen A, Loffelholz K. (1994) Two independent pathways of phospholipase D activation in rat hippocampal slices. *Nauyn Schmeideberg's Arch. Pharmacol.* (Suppl. 350): R9.

Klein K, Chalifa V, Licovitch M, Loffelholz K. (1995) Role of phospholipase D activation in nervous system physiology and pathophysiology. *J. Neurochem.* 65: 1445–1455

Kleuss, Hescheler J, Ewel C, Rosenthal W, Schultz G, and Wittig B. (1991) Assignment of G protein subtypes to specific receptors inducing inhibition of calcium currents. *Nature* 353: 43–48

Koyano K, Grigg JJ, Velimirovic BM, Nakajima S, Nakajima Y. (1994) The role of arachidonic acid metabolism in somatostatin and substance P effects on inward rectifier K conductance in rat brain neurons. *Neurosci. Res.* 20: 345–354.

Krapivinsky G, Krapivinsky L, Wichman K, Clapham DE. (1995) $G\beta\gamma$ binds directly to the G protein-gated K^+ channel, I_{KACh}. *J. Biol. Chem.* 27: 29 059–29 062.

Lev S, Moreno H, Matinez R, Canoll P, Peles E, Musacchio JM, Plowman GD, Rudy B, Schlesinger J. (1995) Protein tyrosine kinase PYK2 involved in Ca^{2+}-induced regulation of ion channel and MAP kinase functions. *Nature* 376: 737–745.

Lin LL, Wartmann M, Lin AY, Knopf JL, Seth A, Davis RJ. (1993) $cPLA_2$ is phosphorylated and activated by MAP kinase. *Cell* 72: 269–278.

Linden DJ. (1995) Phospholipase A_2 controls the induction of short-term versus long-term depression in the cerebellar Purkinje neuron in culture. *Neuron* 15: 1393–1401.

Lipscombe D, Kongsamut S, Tsien R. (1989) α-Adrenergic inhibition of sympathetic neurotransmitter release mediated by modulation of N-type calcium-channel gating. *Nature* 340: 639–642.

Logothetis DE, Kurachi Y, Galper J, Neer E, Clapham DE. (1987) Purified $\beta\gamma$ subunits of GTP-binding proteins regulate muscarinic K channel activity in heart. *Nature,* 325: 321–326.

Martinson EA, Trilivas I, Brown JH. (1990) Rapid protein-kinase C dependent activation of phopholipase D leads to delayed 1,2-diglyceride accumulation. *J. Biol. Chem.* 265: 22 282–22 287.

McCarthy SA, Halam TJ, Merritt JE. (1989) Activation of protein kinase C in human neutrophils attenuates agonist stimulated rises in cytosolic free Ca^{2+} release in addition to stimulating Ca^{2+} efflux. *Biochem. J.* 264: 357–364.

Mochly-Rosen D. (1995) Localisation of protein kinases by anchoring proteins: a theme in signal transduction. *Science* 268: 247–251.

Mons N, Harry A, Dubourg P, Premont RT, Iyengar R, Cooper DMF. (1995) Immunohistochemical localisation of adenylyl cyclase in rat brain indicates a highly selective concentration at synapses. *Proc. Natl Acad. Sci. USA* 92: 8473–8477.

Montmayeur J-P, Borelli E. (1991) Preferential coupling between dopamine D2 receptors and G-proteins. *Mol. Endocrinol.* 88: 3135–3139.

Murrin RJA, Boarder MR. (1992) Neuronal 'nucleotide' receptor linked to phospholipase C and phospholipase D? Stimulation of PC12 cells by ATP analogues and UTP. *Mol. Pharmacol.* 41: 561–568.

Nishizuka Y. (1992) Intracellular signalling by hydrolysis of phospholipids and activation of protein kinase C. *Science* **258:** 607–614.

Oda T, Shearman MS, Nishizuka Y. (1991) Synaptosomal protein kinase C subspecies: B. Downregulation promoted by phorbol ester and its effect on evoked norepinephrine release. *J. Neurochem.* **56:** 1263–1269.

Patel V, Brown C, Boarder MR. (1996a) Protein kinase C isoforms in bovine aortic endothelial cells: role of regulation of P_{2Y}- and P_{2U}- purinoceptor stimulated prostacyclin release. *Br. J. Pharmacol.* **118:** 123–130.

Patel V, Brown C, Goodwin A, Wilkie N, Boarder MR. (1996b) Phosphorylation and activation of p42 and p44 mitogen-activated protein kinase are required for the P2 purinoceptor stimulation of endothelial prostacyclin production. *Biochem. J.* **320:** 221–226.

Pettit DL, Perlman S, Manilow R. (1994). Potentiated transmission and prevention of further LTP by increased CaMKII activity on postsynaptic hippocampal slice neurons. *Science* **266:** 1881–1885.

Pfaffinger PJ, Martin JM, Hunter DD, Nathanson NM, Hille B. (1985) GTP-binding proteins couple cardiac muscarinic receptors to a K^+ channel. *Nature* **317:** 536–538.

Piomelli D. (1994). Eicosanoids in synaptic transmission. *Crit. Rev. in Neurobiol.* **8:** 65–83.

Purkiss JR, Murrin RA, Owen PJ, Boarder MR. (1991) Lack of phospholipase D activity in chromaffin cell: bradykinin-stimulated phosphatidic acid formation involves phospholipase C in chromaffin cells but phospholipase D in PC12 cells. *J. Neurochem.* **57:** 1084–1087.

Reveuny E, Slesinger PA, Inlese J, Morales JM, Iniguez-Lluhl JA, Lefkkowitz RJ, Bourne HR, Jan LY. (1994) Activation of the cloned muscarinic potassium channel by G protein $\beta\gamma$ subunits. *Nature* **370:** 143–146.

Sa G, Muragesan G, Jaye M, Ivashenko Y and Fox PL. (1995). Activation of cytosolic phospholipase A_2 by basic fibroblast growth factor via p42 mitogen activated protein kinase dependent phosphorylation pathway in endothelial cells. *J. Biol. Chem.* **270:** 2360–2366.

Sakmann B, Noma A, Trautwein W. (1983) Acetylcholine activation of single muscarinic K^+ channels in isolated pacemaker cells of the mammalian heart. *Nature* **303:** 250–253.

Sandmann J, Leissner J, Lindmar R, Loffelholz J. (1990) The effects of phorbol esters on choline phospholipid hydrolysis in heart and brain. *Eur. J. Pharmacol* **188:** 89–95.

Sari E, Picatoste F, Claro E. (1995) Histamine H_1 and endothelin ET_B receptors mediate phospholipase D stimulation in rat brain hippocampal slices. *J. Neurochem.* **65:** 837–841.

Schalkwijk CG, van der Heijden MAG, Bunt G, Maas R, Tertoolen LGJ. (1996) Maximal epidermal growth factor induced cytosolic phospholipase A_2 activation *in vivo* requires phosphorylation followed by an increased intracellular calcium concentration. *Biochem. J.* **313:** 91–96.

Schievella AR, Regier MK, Smith WL, Lin L-L. (1995) Calcium-mediated translocation of cytosolic phospholipase A_2 to the nuclear envelope and endoplasmic reticulum. *J. Biol. Chem.* **270:** 30 749–30 754.

Schweitzer P, Madamba S, Champagnat S, Siggins GR. (1993) Somatostatin inhibition of hippocampal CA1 pyramidal neurons: mediation by arachidonic acid and its metabolites. *J. Neurosci.* **13:** 2033–2049.

Selyanko AA, Stansfield CE, Brown, DA. (1992) Closure of potassium M-channels by muscarinic acetylcholine-receptor stimulation requires a diffusible messenger. *Proc. R. Soc. Lond. (B)* **250:** 119–125.

Shimizu T, Wolfe LS. (1990) Arachidonic acid cascade and signal transduction. *J. Neurochem.* **55:** 1–15.

Siciliano JC, Gelman M, Girault J-A. (1994) Depolarisation and neurotransmitters increase neuronal protein tyrosine phosphorylation. *J. Neurochem.* **62:** 950–959.

Silva AJ, Stevens CF, Tonegawa S, Wang Y. (1992) Deficient hippocampal long term potentiation in α-calcium calmodulin kinase II mutant mice. *Science* **257:** 201–206.

Simpson PB, Challiss RJ, Nahorski SR. (1995) Neuronal Ca^{2+} stores: activation and function. *Trends Neurosci.* **18:** 299–305.

Surmeier DJ, Bargas J, Hemming HC, Nairn AC, Greengard P. (1995) Modulation of calcium currents by a D1 dopaminergic protein kinase/phosphatase casdcade in rat neostriatal neurons. *Neuron* **14:** 385–397.

Suzuki T, Okumura-Noji K, Tanaka R, Ogura A, NakamuraK Kudo Y, Tada T. (1993) Characterisation of protein kinase C activities in post synaptic density fractions prepared from cerebral cortex, hippocampus and cerebellum. *Brain Res.* **619:** 69–75.

Tence M, Cordier J, Premont J, Glowinski J. (1994) Muscarinic cholinergic agonists stimulate arachidonic acid release from mouse neurons in primary culture. *J. Pharmacol. Exp. Therap.* **269:** 646–653.

Turner NA, Rumsby MG, Walker JH, McMorris FA, Ball SG, Vaughan PFT (1994) A role for protein kinase C subtypes α and ε in phorbol ester enhanced K^+- and charbachol-evoked noradrenaline release from the human neuroblastoma SH-SY5Y. *Biochem. J.* **297**: 407–413.

Vallar L, Meldolesi J. (1989) Mechanism of signal transduciton at the dopamine D2 receptor. *Trends Pharmacol. Sci.* **10**: 74–77.

Vallar L, Muca C, Magni M, Albert P, Bunzow JR, Meldolesi J, Civelli O. (1990) Differential coupling of dopaminergic D2 receptors expressed in different cell types. *J. Biol. Chem.* **265**: 10 320–10 326.

Villaroel A. (1994) On the role of arachidonic acid in M-current modulation by muscarine in bullfrog sympatheic neurons. *J. Neurosci.* **14**: 1053–7066.

Wagner JA, Cozens AL, Schulman H, Gruenert DC, Stryer L, Gardner P. (1991) Activation of airway chloride channels in normal and cystic fibrosis airway epithelial cells by multifunctional calcium/calmodulin-dependent protein kinase. *Nature* **349**: 793–796.

Whatmore J, Cronin P, Cockroft S. (1994) ARF1-regulated phospholipase D in human neutrophils is enhanced by PMA and MgATP. *FEBS Lett.* **352**: 113–117.

Wickman KD, Iniguez-Lluhl JA, Davenport PA, Taussig R, Krapivinsky GB, Linder ME, Gilman AG, Clapham DE. (1994) Recombinant protein βγ subunits activate the muscarinic gated atrial potassium channel. *Nature* **368**: 255–257.

Yatani A, Brown AM. (1989) Rapid β-adrenergic modulation of cardiac calcium currents by a fast G protein pathway. *Science* **245**: 71–74.

Yu SP. (1995) Role of arachidonic acid, lipoxygenases and phosphatases on calcium-dependent modulation of M-current in bullfrog sympathetic neurons. *J. Physiol. (Lond.)* **487**: 797–811.

Cell-surface and extracellular matrix glycoproteins implicated in the movements of growth cones and neural cells and in synaptogenesis in the vertebrate nervous system

Hansjürgen Volkmer and Fritz G. Rathjen

10.1 Introduction

The development of the highly ordered structure of the nervous system involves a variety of interactions between neural cells and their local environment. Many of these interactions occur with components of the extracellular matrix (ECM) which is composed of collagens, glycoproteins and proteoglycans (Reichardt and Tomaselli, 1991). In this review we concentrate on glycoproteins of the cell surface and of the ECM that participate in the regulation of key events of nervous system development: neural cell migration, axonal pathfinding and synapse formation.

During nervous system development neural cells are generated in a timely ordered sequence. After becoming postmitotic many neural cells migrate long distances from their birthplaces to their final positions where they form layered cell sheets or neuronal nuclei. Several studies have shown that the precise spatio–temporal distribution of specific ECM glycoproteins is most likely to be important for the pattern of paths neural cells take. Consistently several ECM glycoproteins have been identified that

Molecular Biology of the Neuron, edited by R.W. Davies and B.J. Morris.
© 1997 BIOS Scientific Publishers Ltd, Oxford.

are permissive for neural migration in *in vitro* monolayer or explant assays. In the past few years, however, it also became clear that some ECM glycoproteins are nonpermissive or inhibit cell migration and might therefore prevent cells from entering specific areas. Equally important in this context is the expression of the neural cell surface receptors that are capable of interacting with the different ECM components. Several of these cell surface receptors fall into structural subgroups, notably integrins (Reichardt and Tomaselli, 1991), and members of the immunoglobulin superfamily (Brümmendorf and Rathjen, 1995). The cadherins, a large family of cell surface adhesion proteins implicated in homophilic and heterophilic Ca^{2+}-dependent cell–cell adhesion, appear not to interact with ECM components in the nervous system (Takeichi, 1995).

Once a precursor cell has differentiated into a neuron and has migrated to its final position in the course of development it then extends an axon and dendrites to establish a complex pattern of connections that are the basis of neuronal transmission. Axon extension involves the formation of a specialized motile structure termed the growth cone. It is localized at the tip of the extending neurite and elongates the neurite predominantly by migration of its lamellipodia. The migrating growth cone explores its environment by fast extension and retraction of filopodia. It functions as a sensor that recognizes and integrates information from its environment. The growth cone reacts on external cues that guide the extending neurite along predetermined pathways to its target region where specific synapses should be formed.

Environmental cues may be provided by diffusible factors, the extracellular matrix or other cells encountered by the extending growth cone (Keynes and Cook, 1995). Diffusible factors synthesized by an intermediate target or by the final target area may provide long-range signaling that depends on the formation of a gradient. Components of the extracellular matrix or the surface of neighboring cells may contain local cues that permit short-range signaling on contact with the growth cone.

Depending on the kind of signal, the growth cone may change its shape, it may quickly extend to a certain, favorable direction or may stall, it may be deflected or even retracted. Presumably, the growth cone reads environmental signals with cellular receptors termed recognition molecules. Acquired signals are transduced into the interior of the growth cone and result in the activation of second messenger systems and in the rearrangement of cytoskeletal components. The latter is a prerequisite for the morphological response of the growth cone. The integration of external signals may account for the behavioral changes of a growth cone to different environments.

As for cell migration environmental cues that influence pathway choices of axons may be subdivided into promoting nonpermissive and repulsive signals. Promoting signals may be delivered by simply providing a permissive substrate for neurite outgrowth. This interaction may stabilize the adherence of the growth cone to the substrate and preformed permissive pathways may guide growth cones into a certain direction. In addition, guidance molecules may lead growth cones by attraction along a gradient or by displaying guide post signals. In contrast, nonpermissive or repulsive substrates may inhibit growth cone extension into a certain direction. In this case, growth cones retain their motility and continue to explore their environment in a more favorable direction. More drastically, certain signals lead to the repulsion of the growth cone. On contact with such a cue, growth cones collapse immediately and are retracted. The extending neurite is reversibly paralyzed and loses motility. Finally, a new growth cone is formed to extend to another direction. As a consequence, the neurite is deflected from its former direction (Luo and Raper, 1994).

After reaching the target cell, axons stop growing and a sequence of interactions between the presynaptic growth cone and the postsynaptic target regulate the formation of a synaptic connection. Our current knowledge on this complex process of development comes predominantly from studies on the vertebrate neuromuscular junction (Hall and Sanes, 1993). The initial contact between the motor neuron and muscle cell bears no signs of a synapse, although as synaptogenesis proceeds morphological and biochemical changes develop in the presynaptical nerve terminal and in the postsynaptic muscle cell (Hall and Sanes, 1993). These changes include aggregation of the acetylcholine receptor on the surface of the myotube which are evenly distributed along the muscle membrane and the accumulation of synaptic vesicles in the presynapse. Two of these signals, agrin and β2-laminin, that mediate interactions between the muscle cell and the motor neuron have been identified as ECM glycoproteins and will be discussed in this article.

10.2 The netrins: chemoattractants and chemorepellents of the ECM

In the past few years considerable progress has been made in the interpretation of neurite guidance mechanisms by proteins that act as chemoattractants and that are secreted into the ECM. As a surprise, different approaches in the *Caenorhabditis elegans* system and in vertebrates converged to a coherent view of the guidance of circumferentially outgrowing axons by both promoting and inhibitorial signals (Colamarino and Tessier-Lavigne, 1995a).

In the developing spinal cord of rat, dorsal commissural axons circumferentially grow out along the lateral margin of the spinal cord from dorsal to ventral, cross the floor plate and then turn rostrally into the longitudinal axis (*Figure 10.1*). It has been suggested that the floor plate may provide diffusible signals that guide commissural axons towards the ventral midline by attraction. This view is supported by the finding that a floor plate explant placed in the vicinity of a dorsal explant of the spinal cord in a less favorable collagen matrix, directs commissural axons to the floor plate explant (Tessier-Lavigne *et al.*, 1988). Furthermore, floor plate explants grafted laterally of the spinal cord of a developing chick *in ovo*, let commissural axons leave the spinal cord towards the ectopic graft (Placzek *et al.*, 1990).

It was then shown that floor plate extracts derived from membrane fractions promoted commissural axon outgrowth from dorsal explants *in vitro*. Subsequently, brain-derived protein fractions were screened for this activity and after several purification steps Serafini *et al.* (1994) ended up with two proteins of 78 and 75 kDa termed netrin-1 and netrin-2. Netrin cDNA was cloned and expressed in COS cells. High salt fractions of these transfected cells and, to a less extent, supernatant promoted commissural neurite outgrowth from dorsal explants and were able to supplement the function of floor plate extracts *in vitro* (Kennedy *et al.*, 1994). Although tight membrane or ECM association does not support the hypothesis that netrins are diffusible chemoattractants for commissural axons, the presence of a less abundant fraction of netrins in solution sustains this view. In fact, both netrin-1 and -2 promoted commissural axon outgrowth and deflection to netrin-expressing COS cells placed in some distance of a dorsal explant.

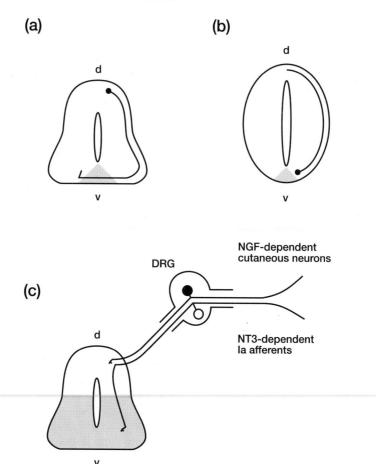

Figure 10.1. Action of two ECM proteins, collapsin-I/SemaIII and netrin-1, on the guidance of neurites. Netrin-1 expressing floor plate (a/b) or collapsinI/SemaIII expressing ventral spinal cord (c) are shown in orange. (a) Attraction by netrin-1: neurites of commissural axons grow out along the lateral margin of the spinal cord from dorsal to ventral, cross the floor plate and then turn rostrally into the longitudinal axis. (b) Repulsive action of netrin-1: the cell bodies of trochlear motor neurons are located ventrally near the floor plate at the junction between hindbrain and midbrain. Presumably, floor plate-derived netrin-1 drives trochlear motoneurons to project dorsally by repulsion. (c) Repulsive action of collapsin-I/SemaIII: Two classes of sensory neurons project from the dorsal root ganglia (DRG) to the spinal cord and can be distinguished on the basis of their response to certain neurotrophins. Cutaneous neurons depend on NGF and terminate in the dorsal spinal cord. In contrast, Ia afferents respond to NT-3 (neurotrophin 3) and project to ventral. In the presence of NGF, a ventral spinal cord explant placed some distance from the dorsal root ganglion inhibited axon outgrowth whereas outgrowth remained unaffected by dorsal spinal cord (Fitzgerald *et al.*, 1993). This indicates that ventral spinal cord may be inhibitory for NGF-dependent sensory axon outgrowth in comparison to dorsal spinal cord. This inhibitory effect is supplemented by COS or 293 cells expressing recombinant Sema III/collapsin I in the presence of NGF, but not of NT3 (Messersmith *et al.*, 1995; Püschel *et al.*, 1995). Therefore, Sema III/collapsin I may confine the projection of NGF-dependent sensory neurons but not of NT3 dependent sensory neurons to dorsal regions of the spinal cord. d, dorsal, v, ventral.

The amino acid sequences of netrin-1 and -2 are 72% identical: they comprise a signal peptide, but no additional hydrophobic sequence that might be used for membrane anchoring. Therefore, netrins share structural properties of secreted molecules. They are composed of three types of protein domains: at the N-terminus are two domains related to domains V and VI of the β2 chain of the ECM component laminin, and the C-terminus contains several positively charged amino acids that may contribute to the association with negatively charged membrane surfaces or ECM components (*Figure 10.2*). The highest degree of similarity between netrin-1 and -2 is found in one of the laminin-related domains (91%) which contains three EGF-like repeats.

In situ hybridization studies showed that netrin-1 is exclusively expressed in the floor plate of the spinal cord throughout the period of commissural axon growth (Kennedy *et al.*, 1994). In contrast, netrin-2 expression was found in the ventral two-thirds of the spinal cord except for the floor plate. Although data about the precise location of netrin protein are still lacking, it appears most likely that netrin-1 is expressed by the intermediate target region and netrin-2 by parts of the pathway of commissural axons. Therefore, netrins-1 and netrin-2 are strong candidates for secreted guidance cues of commissural axons.

Further sequence analysis revealed that netrins are related to a protein termed UNC-6 described in the nematode worm *C. elegans* (about 50% identity). UNC stands for uncoordinated movement and represents a group of *C. elegans* mutant phenotypes. In *C. elegans*, circumferential axons project along the embryonic epidermis either in the dorsal-to-ventral or ventral-to-dorsal direction (Culotti, 1994; Hedgecock *et al.*, 1990). Three phenotypes have been described affecting the migration of growth cones in either direction. The *unc-5* gene is required to direct neurites dorsally, *unc-40* for

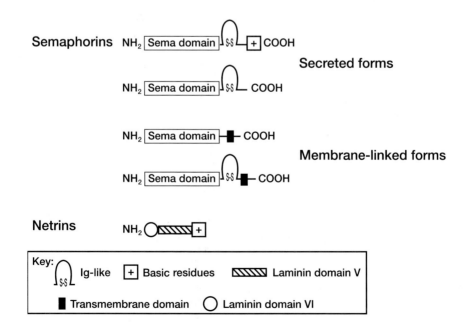

Figure 10.2. Netrins and semaphorins. Symbols for individual domains are shown below. The N-terminus is at the left. Ig, immunoglobulin-like domain.

migrations to the ventral aspect and *unc-6* affects pathfinding in both ventral and dorsal directions and accounts for the sum of UNC-5 and UNC-40 phenotypes. Both *unc-5* and *unc-40* depend on the function of *unc-6* and vice versa. Therefore, *unc-6* functions with *unc-5* and *unc-40* in a common pathway, perhaps by direct interaction and it has been discussed that the transmembrane protein UNC-5 is a receptor for UNC-6 (Culotti, 1994; Leung-Hagesteijn *et al.*, 1992). UNC-6, UNC-5 and UNC-40 are thought to be instructive rather than providing permissiveness because the outgrowth of axons is not reduced but misguided. Furthermore, ectopic expression of UNC-5 in touch receptor neurons that normally project longitudinally or ventrally resulted in a dorsal orientation of the touch receptor axons (Hamelin *et al.*, 1993). As it has been suggested that UNC-6 is expressed ventrally, a model was proposed that UNC-5 interacts with UNC-6 leading to the guidance of axons to the dorsal direction via repulsive mechanisms. On the other hand, UNC-40 may interact with UNC-6 in order to attract growth cones to the ventral direction. In summary, UNC-6 may be bifunctional in that it may exert both attractive and repulsive functions.

It was noted above that the vertebrate homolog of UNC-6, netrin-1 may provide chemoattractive cues for the orientation of commissural axons towards the floor plate. It was therefore tempting to speculate whether there is a parallel mechanism to the nematode UNC-5/UNC-6 interaction that may guide axons by repulsion. And indeed an axon system was found that provides evidence for a repulsive activity of netrin-1 in vertebrates (Colamarino and Tessier-Lavigne, 1995b). The cell bodies of trochlear motor neurons are located ventrally near the floor plate at the junction between hindbrain and midbrain. In contrast to motor neurons in other regions they circumferentially project dorsally. The ventral third of a transversely dissected explant was sufficient to allow motor axon bundles to grow out of the dorsal edge of the explant into a collagen matrix. If floor plate explants or netrin-1 expressing COS cells were placed adjacent to the dorsal edge of a ventral explant, bundle formation was virtually suppressed.

Therefore, the extracellular matrix proteins netrin-1 and -2 and UNC-6 are not only structurally, but also functionally conserved between nematode worms and vertebrates with respect to the guidance of circumferentially growing axons. They guide ventral axons to dorsal by a repulsive interaction and dorsal axons to ventral by attractive cues. This dual function relies on the nature of the receptor displayed by the respective axon.

10.3 Semaphorins guide axons to their target through repulsion

Within 3 years the semaphorin protein family comprising at least 14 members, emerged from G-Sema I (previously fasciclin IV, Dodd and Schuchardt, 1995; Kolodkin *et al.*, 1992) and collapsin. Originally, G-Sema I appeared from an antibody screen for the detection of antigenes in the grasshopper that may contribute to selective fasciculation. Independently, collapsin I was isolated as a growth cone collapsing activity of 100 kDa from chick brain (Luo *et al.*, 1993). Sequence analysis revealed that collapsin is structurally related to G-Sema I. Based on the sequence data of the prototype semaphorins, G-Sema I and collapsin I, a variety of new semaphorins were characterized from *Drosophila*, chick, mouse, human as well as two viral semaphorin-related sequences from vaccinia and variola (Kolodkin *et al.*, 1993; Luo *et al.*, 1995; Püschel *et al.*, 1995). Comparison of the expression pattern revealed that different members of the semaphorin/collapsin family in chick and mouse are differentially expressed in the developing spinal cord and contain both secreted ECM and transmembrane forms.

The main characteristic of the semaphorin/collapsin sequence is the presence of the so-called semaphorin domain that spans about 500 amino acids (*Figure 10.2*). Semaphorin domains in invertebrates and vertebrates share 14–16 conserved cysteine residues and contain no repeated elements (Kolodkin *et al.*, 1993). The semaphorins can be subdivided into two classes of either secreted or membrane-bound forms with a cytoplasmic domain that varies between 45 and 140 amino acid residues in length. The latter may contain an Ig-like domain between the hydrophobic transmembrane domain and the semaphorin domain. This Ig-like domain is also present in all secreted forms (Kolodkin, 1996). In addition, some secreted semaphorins contain a cluster of basic amino acids, a property shared with the netrins (Kolodkin *et al.*, 1993; Luo *et al.*, 1995; Püschel *et al.*, 1995). The positive charge may target semaphorins to negatively charged components of the ECM or of cell surfaces and may thereby limit free diffusion. As with netrins, recombinant collapsin is found in the supernatant and cell-associated after expression in COS cells (Luo *et al.*, 1993).

In situ hybridization showed that Sema III/collapsin I is specifically expressed in the ventral spinal cord, but not dorsally (Messersmith *et al.*, 1995). *In vitro* experiments revealed that the presence of recombinantly expressed Sema III/collapsin I collapses sensory but not retinal growth cones (Luo *et al.*, 1993). The contact of only a few filopodia with a localized collapsin source generated a signal that was strong enough to steer growth cones of sensory axons into other directions (Fan and Raper, 1995). Collapsin is therefore a strong candidate for the repulsive activity displayed by ventral spinal cord. And indeed, the inhibitory properties of ventral spinal cord explants to sensory neurons that depend on nerve growth factor (NGF) and project dorsally are supplemented by COS cells expressing recombinant Sema III/collapsin I (Messersmith *et al.*, 1995; Püschel *et al.*, 1995). In contrast, neurotrophin-3 (NT3)-dependent Ia afferents that project to the ventral motoneurons, do not respond to an inhibitory Sema III/collapsin signal (*Figure 10.1*). Therefore, Sema III/collapsin I may specifically confine the projection of NGF-responsive neurons to dorsal regions of the spinal cord.

As with netrins/UNC-6, the study of invertebrate members of the semaphorin family supplies additional information on the function of semaphorins. Branches of segmental nerve Snb in *Drosophila melanogaster* innervate ventral muscles. It contains the axons of motoneurons RP1 and RP3 (Matthes *et al.*, 1995). The RP1 growth cone synapses on muscle 13 whereas RP3 terminates on muscles 6 and 7. Ectopic expression of Sema II under the control of the *toll* enhancer leads to high Sema II levels in muscles 6 and 7 in comparison to lower levels in muscle 13. While innervation of muscle 13 remained unperturbed by RP1, innervation of muscles 6 and 7 was dramatically reduced. RP3 approaches these muscles, but fails to form synaptic arborizations. This finding is in accordance with a putative inhibitory activity of Sema II in *Drosophila* and parallels in this repect the observations obtained in vertebrate systems.

Several lines of evidence indicate that semaphorins are factors secreted into the ECM that guide axons by chemorepulsion. Together with netrins, semaphorins may establish a pattern of cues that are read by outgrowing neurites. The local composition of these cues as well as the differential expression of the corresponding receptors may contribute to determine the outgrowth direction of an extending neurite.

10.4 The tenascins: a family of proteins with complex functions during nervous system development

The tenascin family of extracellular matrix glycoproteins is currently composed of three members, notably tenascin-C (TN-C), tenascin-R (TN-R) and tenascin-X (TN-X). The tenascin family members are modular glycoproteins composed of four structural motifs (Bristow *et al.*, 1993; Chiquet-Ehrismann *et al.*, 1994; Erickson, 1993). The N-terminus contains a cysteine-rich segment which appears to be unique to members of the tenascin family. In the C-terminal direction, the cysteine-rich segment is followed by several epidermal growth factor (EGF)-like repeats and then by multiple consecutive motifs that are related to fibronectin type III (FNIII)-like domains. At the C-terminus, the tenascins contain a segment similar to the β and γ chains of fibrinogen including a calcium-binding stretch (*Figure 10.3*). TN-X is the largest of the currently known tenascin family members and has so far not been found in the nervous system (Matsumoto *et al.*, 1994) while TN-C and TN-R are expressed in the developing and adult brain. In contrast to TN-C which is localized in many tissues during development TN-R appears to be restricted to the central nervous system (Faissner *et al.*, 1994; Nörenberg *et al.*, 1996). Although TN-R and TN-C show a considerable amino acid sequence homology TN-C was found to form hexamers, while for TN-R only trimers, dimers and monomers could be visualized by electron microscopy (Erickson and Iglesias, 1984; Nörenberg *et al.*, 1992).

In the developing cerebellum TN-C was associated with premigratory granule cells and found later in the molecular layer on the surface of Bergmann glial cells. This localization of TN-C correlates with *in vitro* studies which showed that TN-C participates in the migration of cerebellar granule cells. In contrast to anti-thrombospondin (TSP) antibodies, antibodies to TN-C arrested granule cell migration primarily in the molecular layer, most likely by modulating the interactions with the Bergmann glial fibers (Bartsch *et al.*, 1992; Chuong *et al.*, 1987; Husmann *et al.*, 1992). TN-C has also

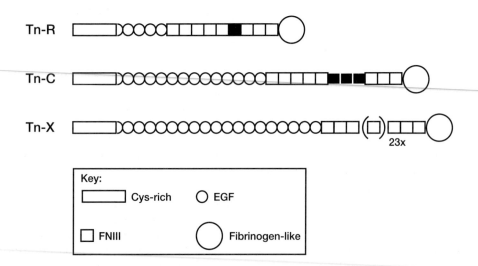

Figure 10.3. The tenascin (TN) family. Symbols for individual domains are shown below. The brackets mark fibronectin type III-like domains repeated 23 times. Alternatively spliced sequences are shown in black. The N-terminus is at the left. *EGF,* epidermal growth factor-like repeats; *FNIII,* fibronectin type III-like repeat.

the nervous system (Fearon *et al.*, 1990). In accordance with this assumption, neogenin has been localized on extending axons of the optic fiber layer (Vielmetter *et al.*, 1994) and DCC stimulates the outgrowth of PC12 cells independent of NGF pathways (Pierceall *et al.*, 1994).

10.9.5 OBCAM, LAMP, neurotrimin and CEPU-1

Another subgroup of GPI-linked molecules is formed by LAMP (limbic system-associated protein), neurotrimin, opioid-binding cell adhesion molecule (OBCAM) and cerebellar Purkinje cells (CEPU-1) which share only three extracellular Ig-like domains and have no FNIII-like modules. Within this subgroup only LAMP has been shown to promote neurite outgrowth of limbic neurons *in vitro* (Pimenta *et al.*, 1995). All other members of this subgroup, however, show an interesting tissue distribution arguing for a specific role in the establishment and maintenance of the nervous system. The most restricted expression pattern is found for CEPU-1 which was primarily localized on a single neuronal cell type, the cerebellar Purkinje cell (Spaltmann and Brümmendorf, 1996). LAMP expression is primarily expressed in limbic regions which is in accordance with its specific function (Pimenta *et al.*, 1995). After injection *in vivo*, antibodies to LAMP perturb the mossy fiber projection in the hippocampus. OBCAM expression is concentrated in the cortical plate and the hippocampus whereas neurotrimin is found more widespread in the developing brain (Stuyk *et al.*, 1995).

10.9.6 DM-GRASP and gicerin

DM-GRASP and gicerin differ from all other proteins described so far as they mix two N-terminal Ig-like domains of the V-type with three membrane proximal Ig-like domains of the C2-type which is predominantly used by other members of the IgSF. Expression of DM-GRASP on developing neurites in several neural tissues and of gicerin in the optic fiber layer of chick E8 retina suggests a role in axon outgrowth (Burns *et al.*, 1991; Pourquie *et al.*, 1990; Tanaka *et al.*, 1991; Taniura *et al.*, 1991). Within this subgroup only DM-GRASP has been shown to be a substrate for neurite outgrowth (DeBernardo and Chang, 1996).

10.9.7 Adhesion pathways of axonal IgSF members

Axonal IgSF members not only display structural diversity, they also show a high degree of complexity in the interaction either with other members of the IgSF or with members of other protein families. These can be classified with respect to different criteria and are summarized in *Figure 10.6*.

A CAM on one cellular surface may interact with an identical, second molecule on an opposing cell surface, a process termed homophilic interaction. An interaction is heterophilic if the second molecule is distinct from the first. Neurofascin and F11 undergo heterophilic interactions (*Figure 10.6*) while L1, axonin-1, NrCAM, NCAM, gicerin, and DM-GRASP interact homophilically and heterophilically (Brümmendorf *et al.*, 1993; DeBernardo and Chang, 1996; Grumet *et al.*, 1993; Hoffman and Edelman, 1983; Kuhn *et al.*, 1991; Lemmon *et al.*, 1989; Mauro *et al.*, 1992; Morales *et al.*, 1993; Taira *et al.*, 1994; Tanaka *et al.*, 1991; Volkmer *et al.*, 1996).

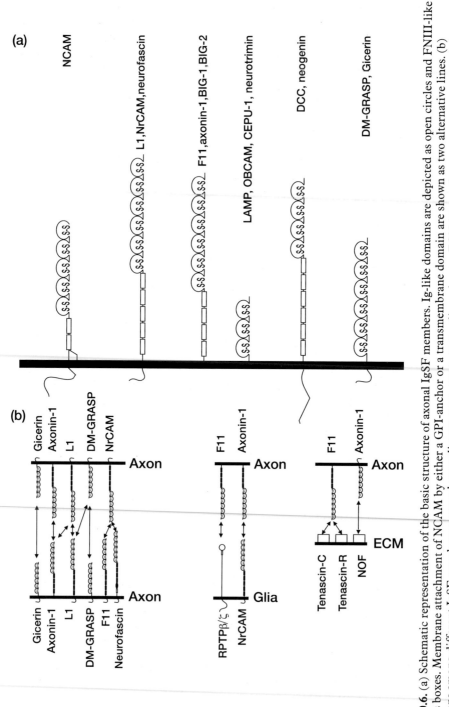

Figure 10.6. (a) Schematic representation of the basic structure of axonal IgSF members. Ig-like domains are depicted as open circles and FNIII-like repeats as boxes. Membrane attachment of NCAM by either a GPI-anchor or a transmembrane domain are shown as two alternative lines. (b) Interactions among different IgSF members grouped according to axon–axon, axon–glia and axon–ECM interactions.

These interactions may take place between different neuronal surfaces [L1–L1 (Lemmon *et al.*, 1989), L1–DM-GRASP (DeBernardo and Chang, 1996), axonin-1–axonin-1 (Felsenfeld *et al.*, 1994; Rader *et al.*, 1993), F11–NrCAM (Morales *et al.*, 1993), neurofascin–NrCAM (Volkmer *et al.*, 1996)], between neurons and glial cells [axonin-1–NrCAM (Suter *et al.*, 1995), F11–protein tyrosine phosphatase β/ζ (Peles *et al.*, 1995)] or between neurons and ECM components (F11–TN-C (Zisch *et al.*, 1992), F11–TN-R (Nörenberg *et al.*, 1995, Pesheva *et al.*, 1993), gicerin–neurite outgrowth-promoting center (Taira *et al.*, 1994)].

10.9.8 Signaling by axonal IgSF members

In order to regulate axon extension and cell migration, IgSF members must activate intracellular second messenger systems that might result in a reorganization of the cytoskeleton. Most of the axon-associated IgSF members do not reveal structural relationships to known signaling components suggesting that their effects on signal transduction must be exerted through associated proteins, either intracellularly or by extracellular *cis*-binding to receptor components. An approach using transgenic mice lacking nonreceptor tyrosine kinases pp60[c-src], pp59[c-fyn] and pp62[c-yes] led to the suggestion that L1-dependent neurite outgrowth is coupled to pp60[c-src] but not to pp59[c-fyn] and pp62[c-yes] whereas NCAM-dependent neurite outgrowth is coupled to pp59[c-fyn] but not pp60[c-src] or pp62[c-yes] (Beggs *et al.*, 1994; Ignelzi *et al.*, 1994). Furthermore, L1- and NCAM-induced neurite outgrowth was found to be inhibited by soluble peptides containing sequences of the fibroblast growth factor (FGF) receptor or by antibodies to the FGF receptor. These findings suggest that the neurite outgrowth response induced by L1 or NCAM involves the direct or indirect activation of neuronal FGF receptors which contain an intracellular tyrosine kinase domain. Based on studies relying on the application of divers inhibitors, the FGF receptor second messenger pathway finally results in the influx of calcium which is necessary and sufficient to promote neurite outgrowth (Williams *et al.*, 1992, 1994). Progress has also been made on the characterization of the signal transduction principles used by IgSF members which are GPI anchored. Co-precipitation studies revealed that pp59[c-fyn] complexes with the GPI-anchored F11 (Zisch *et al.*, 1995). However, a comprehensive understanding of direct intracellular interactions leading to neurite outgrowth remains to be derived by future investigations.

References

Adams J, Lawler J. (1993) The thrombospondin family: extracellular matrix molecules that are related to the adhesive glycoprotein thrombospodin and expressed in a variety of different tissues have recently been identified. *Curr. Biol.* **3**: 188–190.

Arber S, Caroni P. (1995) Thrombospondin-4, an extracellular matrix protein expressed in the developing and adult nervous system promotes neurite outgrowth. *J. Cell Biol.* **131**: 1083–1094.

Aukhil I, Joshi P, Yan Y, Erickson HP. (1993) Cell- and heparin-binding domains of the hexabrachion arm identified by tenascin expression proteins. *J. Biol. Chem.* **268**: 2542–2553.

Barnea G, Grumet M, Milev P, Silvennoinen O, Levy JB, Sap J, Schlessinger J. (1994) Receptor tyrosine phosphatase β is expressed in the form of proteoglycan and binds to the extracellular matrix protein tenascin. *J. Biol. Chem.* **269**: 14 349–14 352.

Barthels D, Vopper G, Boned A, Cremer H, Wille W. (1992). High degree of NCAM diversity generated by alternative RNA splicing in brain and muscle. *Eur. J. Neurosci.* **4**: 327–337.

Bartsch S, Bartsch U, Dörris U, Faissner A, Weller A, Ekblom P, Schachner M. (1992) Expression of tenascin in the developing and adult cerebellar cortex. *J. Neurosci.* **12**: 736–749.

Bartsch U, Pesheva P, Raff M, Schachner M. (1993) Expression of janusin (J1-160/180) in the retina and optic nerve of the developing and adult mouse. *Glia* **9**: 57–69.

Beggs HE, Soriano P, Maness PF. (1994) NCAM-dependent neurite outgrowth is inhibited in neurons from Fyn-minus mice. *J. Cell Biol.* **127**: 825–833.

Bixby JL, Pratt RS, Lilien J, Reichardt LF. (1987) Neurite outgrowth on muscle cell surfaces involves extracellular matrix receptors as well as Ca^{2+}-dependent and -independent cell adhesion molecules. *Proc. Natl Acad. Sci. USA.* **84**: 2555–2559.

Bowe MA, Fallon JR. (1995) The role of agrin in synapse formation. *Annu. Rev. Neurosci.* **18**: 443–462.

Bowe MA, Deyst KA, Leszyk JD, Fallon JR. (1994) Identification and purification of an agrin receptor from *Torpedo* postsynaptic membranes: a heteromeric complex related to the dystroglycans. *Neuron* **12**: 1173–1180.

Bristow J, Tee MK, Gitelman SE, Mellon SH, Miller WL. (1993) Tenascin-X: a novel extracellular matrix protein encoded by the human XB gene overlapping P450c21B. *J. Cell Biol.* **122**: 265–278.

Brümmendorf T, Rathjen, FG. (1995) Cell adhesion molecules 1: immunoglobulin superfamily. *Protein Profile.* **2**: 963–1108.

Brümmendorf T, Wolff JM, Frank R, Rathjen FG. (1989) Neural cell recognition molecule F11: homology with fibronectin type III and immunoglobulin type C domains. *Neuron* **2**: 1351–1361.

Brümmendorf T, Hubert M, Treubert U, Leuschner R, Tarnok A, Rathjen FG. (1993) The axonal recognition molecule F11 is a multifunctional protein: specific domains mediate interactions with Ng-CAM and restrictin. *Neuron.* **10**: 711–727.

Burg MA, Halfter W, Cole G. (1995) Analysis of proteoglycan expression in developing chicken brain: characterization of a heparan sulfate proteoglycan that interacts with the neural cell adhesion molecule. *J. Neurosci. Res.* **41**: 49–64.

Burns FR, von Kannen S, Guy L, Raper JA, Kamholz J. Chang S. (1991) DM-GRASP, a novel immunoglobulin superfamily axonal surface protein that supports neurite extension. *Neuron* **7**: 209–220.

Buskirk DR, Thiery JP, Rutishauser U, Edelman GM. (1980) Antibodies to a neural cell adhesion molecule disrupt histogenesis in cultured chick retinae. *Nature* **285**: 488–489.

Campagna JA, Rüegg MA, Bixby JL. (1995) Agrin is a differentiation-inducing 'Stop Signal' for motoneurons *in vitro*. *Neuron* **15**: 1365–1374.

Campanelli JT, Roberds SL, Campbell KP, Scheller RH. (1994) A role for dystrophin-associated glycoproteins and utrophin in agrin-induced AChR clustering. *Cell* **77**: 663–674.

Carey DJ, Evans DM, Stahl RC, Asundi VK, Conner KJ, Garbes P, Cizmeci-Smith G. (1992) Molecular cloning and characterization of *N*-Syndecan, a novel transmembrane heparan sulfate proteoglycan. *J. Cell Biol.* **117**: 191–201.

Chang S, Rathjen FG, Raper JA. (1987) Extension of neurites on axons is impaired by antibodies against specific neural cell surface glycoproteins *J. Cell. Biol.* **104**: 355–362.

Chiquet-M, Wehrle-Haller B. (1994) Tenascin-C in peripheral nerve morphogenesis. *Persp. Devel. Neurobiol.* **2**: 67–74.

Chiquet M, Vrucinic-Filipi N, Schenk S, Beck K, Chiquet-Ehrismann R. (1991) Isolation of chick tenascin variants and fragments. *Eur. J. Biochem.* **199**: 379–388.

Chiquet-Ehrismann R, Hagious C, Matsumoto K. (1994) The tenascin gene family. *Persp. Devel. Neurobiol.* **2**: 3–7.

Chung CY, Erickson HP. (1994) Cell surface annexin II is a high affinity receptor for the alternatively spliced segment of tenascin-C. *J. Cell Biol.* **126**: 539–548.

Chuong C-M, Edelman GM. (1984) Alterations in neural cell adhesion molecules during development of different regions of the nervous system. *J. Neurosci.* **4**: 2354–2368.

Chuong C-M, Crossin KL, Edelmann GM. (1987) Sequential expression and differential function of multiple adhesion molecules during the formation of cerebellar cortical layers. *J. Cell Biol.* **104**: 331–342.

Cohen MW, Godfrey EW. (1992) Early appearance of and neural contribution to agrin-like molecules at embryonic frog nerve–muscle synapses formed in culture. *J. Neurosci.* **12**: 2982–2992.

Colamarino C, Tessier-Lavigne MT. (1995a) The role of the floor plate in axon guidance. *Annu. Rev. Neurosci.* **18**: 497–529.

Colamarino SA, Tessier-Lavigne MT. (1995b) The axonal chemoattractant netrin-1 is also a chemorepellent for trochlear motor axons. *Cell* **81**: 621–629.

Corless CL, Mendoza A, Collins T, Lawler J. (1992) Colocalization of thrombospondin and syndecan during murine development. *Dev. Dyn.* **193**: 346–358.

Culotti J. (1994) Axon guidance mechanisms in *C. elegans. Curr. Opin. Gen. Dev.* **4**: 587–595.

Cunningham BA, Hemperly JJ, Murray BA, Prediger EA, Brackenbury R, Edelman GM. (1987) Neural cell adhesion molecule: structure, immunoglobulin-like domains, cell surface modulation, and alternative RNA splicing. *Science* **236**: 799–806.

Davis JQ, McLaughlin T, Bennett V. (1993) Ankyrin-binding proteins related to nervous system cell adhesion molecules: candidates to provide transmembrane and intercellular connections in adult brain. *J. Cell Biol.* **121**: 121–133.

DeBernardo AP, Chang S. (1996) Heterophilic interactions of DM-GRASP: GRASP-NgCAM interactions involved in neurite extension. *J. Cell Biol.* **133**: 657–666.

Debreuil RR, MacVicar G, Dissanayake S, Liu C, Homer D, Hortsch M. (1996) Neuroglian-mediated cell adhesion induces assembly of the membrane skeleton at cell contact sites. *J. Cell Biol.* **133**: 647–655.

DeFreitas MF, Yoshida CK, Frazier WA, Mendrick DL, Kypta RM, Reichardt LF. (1995) Identification of integrin $\alpha_3\beta_1$ as a neuronal thrombospondin receptor mediating neurite outgrowth. *Neuron* **15**: 333–343.

de la Rosa EJ, Kayyem JF, Roman JM, Stierhof YD, Dreyer WJ, Schwarz U. (1990) Topologically restricted appearance in the developing chick retinotectal system of Bravo, a neural surface protein: experimental modulation by environmental cues [published erratum appears in *J. Cell Biol.* 112: 1049 (1991)]. *J. Cell Biol.* **111**: 3087–3096.

Dodd J, Schuchardt A. (1995) Axon guidance: a compelling case for repelling growth cones. *Cell* **81**: 471–474.

Doherty P, Cohen J, Walsh FS. (1990a) Neurite outgrowth in response to transfected N-CAM changes during development and is modulated by polysialic acid. *Neuron* **5**: 209–219.

Doherty P, Fruns M, Seaton P, Dickson G, Barton CH, Sears TA, Walsh FS. (1990b) A threshold effect of the major isoforms of NCAM on neurite outgrowth. *Nature* **343**: 464–466.

Doherty P, Skaper SD, Moore SE, Leon A, Walsh FS. (1992a) A developmentally regulated switch in neuronal responsiveness to NCAM and N-cadherin in the rat hippocampus. *Development* **115**: 885–892.

Doherty P, Moolenaar CE, Ashton SV, Michalides RJ, Walsh FS. (1992b) The VASE exon downregulates the neurite growth-promoting activity of NCAM 140. *Nature* **356**: 791–793.

Drazba J, Lemmon V. (1990) The role of cell adhesion molecules in neurite outgrowth on muller cells. *Devel. Biol.* **138**: 82–93.

Erickson HP. (1993) Tenascin-C, tenascin-R and tenascin-X: a family of talented proteins in search of functions. *Curr. Opin. Cell Biol.* **5**: 869–876.

Erickson HP, Iglesias JL. (1984) A six-armed oligomer isolated from cell surface fibronectin preparations. *Nature* **311**: 267–269.

Faissner A, Kruse J. (1990) J1/tenascin is a repulsive substrate for central nervous system neurons. *Neuron* **5**: 627–637.

Faissner A, Scholze A, Götz B. (1994) Tenascin glycoproteins in developing neural tissues: only decoration? *Persp. Devel. Neurobiol.* **2**: 53–66.

Fan J. Raper JA. (1995) Localized collapsing cues can steer growth cones without inducing their full collapse. *Neuron* **14**: 263–274.

Fearon ER, Cho KR, Nigro JM et al. (1990) Identification of a chromosome 18q gene that is altered in colorectal cancers. *Science* **247**: 49–56.

Felsenfeld DP, Hynes MA, Skoler KM, Furley AJ, Jessell TM. (1994) TAG-1 can mediate homophilic binding, but neurite outgrowth on TAG-1 requires an L1-like molecule and β_1 integrins. *Neuron* **12**: 675–690.

Ferns M, Hoch W, Campanelli JT, Rupp F, Hall ZW, Scheller RH. (1992) RNA splicing regulates agrin-mediated acetylcholine receptor clustering activity on cultured myotubes. *Neuron* **8**: 1079–1086.

Ferns MJ, Campanelli JT, Hoch W, Scheller RH, Hall Z. (1993) The ability of agrin to cluster AChRs depends on alternative splicing and on cell surface proteoglycans. *Neuron* **11**: 491–502.

Fischer D, Chiquet-Ehrismann R, Bernasconi C, Chiquet M. (1995). A single heparin binding region within the fibrinogen-like domain is functional in chick tenascin-C. *J. Biol. Chem.* **270**: 3378–3384.

Fitzgerald M, Kwiat GC, Middleton J, Pini A. (1993) Ventral spinal cord inhibition of neurite outgrowth from embryonic rat dorsal root ganglia. *Development* **117**: 1377–1384.

Friedlander DR, Milev P, Karthikeyan L, Margolis RK, Margolis RU, Grumet M. (1994) The neural chondroitin sulfate proteoglycan neurocan binds to the neural cell adhesion molecules Ng-CAM/L1/NILE and N-CAM, and inhibits neuronal adhesion and neurite outgrowth. *J. Cell Biol.* **125**: 669–680.

Furley AJ, Morton SB, Manalo D, Karagogeos D, Dodd J, Jessell TM. (1990) The axonal glycoprotein TAG-1 is an immunoglobulin superfamily member with neurite outgrowth-promoting activity. *Cell* **61:** 157–170.

Fuss B, Wintergerst ES, Bartsch U, Schachner M. (1993) Molecular characterization and *in situ* mRNA localization of the neural recognition molecule J1-160/180: a modular structure similar to tenascin. *J. Cell Biol.* **120:** 1237–1249.

Gee S, Montaro F, Lindebaum M, Carbonetto S. (1994) The dystrophin associated glycoprotein, dystroglycan-α, is a functional agrin receptor. *Cell* **77:** 675–686.

Gesemann M, Denzer AJ, Ruegg MA. (1995) Acetylcholine receptor-aggregating activity of agrin isoforms and mapping of the active site. *J. Cell Biol.* **128:** 625–636.

Gower HJ, Barton CH, Elsom VL, Thompson J, Moore SE, Dickson G, Walsh FS. (1988) Alternative splicing generates a secreted form of N-CAM in muscle and brain. *Cell* **55:** 955–964.

Grumet M, Flaccus A, Margolis RU. (1993) Functional characterization of chondroitin sulfate proteoglycans of brain: interactions with neurons and neural cell adhesion molecules. *J. Cell Biol.* **120:** 815–824.

Grumet M, Milvee P, Sakurai T, Karthikeyan L, Bourdon M, Margolis RK, Margolis RU. (1994) Interactions with tenascin and differential effects on cell adhesion of neurocan and phosphacan, two major chondroitin sulfate proteoglycans of nervous tissue. *J. Biol. Chem.* **269:** 12 142–12 146.

Halfter W, Chiquet-Ehrismann R, Tucker RP. (1989) The effect of tenascin and embryonic basal lamina on the behavior and morphology of neural crest cells *in vitro. Devel. Biol.* **128:** 245–255.

Hall ZW, Sanes JR. (1993) Synaptic structure and development: the neuromuscular junction. *Cell* 72/*Neuron* 10 (Suppl.), 99–121.

Hamelin M, Zhou Y, Su M-W, Scott IM, Culotti JG. (1993) Expression of the UNC-5 guidance receptor in the touch neurons of *C. elegans* steers their axons dorsally. *Nature* **364:** 327–330.

Hardingham TE, Fosang AJ. (1992) Proteoglycans: many forms and many functions. *FASEB J.* **6:** 861–870.

Harpaz Y, Chothia C. (1994) Many of the immunoglobulin superfamily domains in cell adhesion molecules and surface receptors belong to a new structural set which is close to that containing variable domains. *J. Mol. Biol.* **238:** 528–539.

Hedgecock EM, Culotti JG, Hall DH. (1990) The unc-5, and unc-40 genes guide circumferential migrations of pioneer axons and mesodermal cells on the epidermis in *C. elegans. Neuron* **2:** 61–85.

Hoch W, Ferns M, Campanelli JT, Hall ZW, Scheller RH. (1993) Developmental regulation of highly active alternatively spliced forms of agrin. *Neuron* **11:** 470–490.

Hoch W, Campanelli JT, Harrison S, Scheller RH. (1994) Structural domains of agrin required for clustering of nicotinic acetylcholine receptors. *EMBO J.* **13:** 2814–2821.

Hoffman S, Edelman GM. (1983) Kinetics of homophilic binding by embryonic and adult forms of the neural cell adhesion molecule. *Proc. Natl Acad. Sci. USA* **80:** 5762–5766.

Hoffman S, Sorkin BC, White PC, Brackenbury R, Mailhammer U. (1982) Chemical characterization of a neural cell adhesion molecule purified from embryonic brain membranes. *J. Biol. Chem.* **257:** 7720–7729.

Hoffman JR, Dixit VM, O'Shea KS. (1994) Expression of thrombospondin in the adult nervous system. *J. Comp. Neurol.* **340:** 126–139.

Hu H, Tomasiewicz H, Magnuson T, Rutishauser U. (1996) The role of polysialic acid in migration of olfactory bulb interneuron precursors in the subventricular zone. *Neuron* **16:** 735–743.

Hunter DD, Shah V, Merlie JP, Sanes JR. (1989a) A laminin-like adhesive protein concentrated in the synaptic cleft of the neuromuscular junction. *Nature* **338:** 229–234.

Hunter DD, Porter BE, Bulock JW, Adams SP, Merlie JP, Sanes JR. (1989b) Primary sequence of a motor neuron-selective adhesive site in the synaptic basal lamina protein S-laminin. *Cell* **59:** 905–913.

Husmann K, Faissner A, Schachner M. (1992) Tenascin promotes cerebellar granule cell migration and neurite outgrowth by different domains in the fibronectin type III repeats. *J. Cell Biol.* **116:** 1475–1486.

Ignelzi MAJ, Miller DR, Soriano P, Maness PF. (1994) Impaired neurite outgrowth of src-minus cerebellar neurons on the cell adhesion molecule L1. *Neuron* **12:** 873–884.

Iruela-Arispe ML, Liska DJ, Sage EH, Bornstein P. (1993) Differential expression of thrombospondin 1, 2, and 3 during murine development. *Devel. Dyn.* **197:** 40–56.

Jaworski DM, Kelly GM, Hockfield S. (1994) BEHAB, a new member of the proteoglycan tandem repeat family of hyaluronan-binding proteins that is restricted to the brain. *J. Cell Biol.* **125:** 495–509.

Jaworski DM, Kelly GM, Hockfield S. (1995) The CNS-specific hyaluronan-binding protein BEHAB is expressed in ventricular zones coincident with gliogenesis. *J. Neurosci.* **15:** 1352–1362.

Kapfhammer JP, Raper JA. (1987) Collapse of growth cone structure on contact with specific neurites in culture. *J. Neurosci.* **7:** 201–212.

Kennedy TE, Serafini T, de la Torre JR, Lavigne MT. (1994) Netrins are diffusible chemotropic factors for commissural axons in the embryonic spinal cord. *Cell* **78:** 425–435.

Keynes R, Cook MW. (1995) Axon guidance molecules. *Cell* **83:** 161–169.

Klar A, Baldassare M, Jessell TM. (1992) F-spondin: a gene expressed at high levels in the floor plate encodes a secreted protein that promotes neural cell adhesion and neurite extension. *Cell* **69:** 95–110.

Kolodkin AL. (1996) Semaphorins: mediators of repulsine growth cone guidance. *Trends Cell Biol.* **6:** 15–22.

Kolodkin AL, Matthes DJ, O'Connor TP, Patel NH, Admon A, Bentley D, Goodman CS. (1992) Fasciclin IV: sequence, expression, and function during growth cone guidance in the grasshopper embryo. *Neuron* **9:** 831–845.

Kolodkin AL, Matthes DJ, Goodman CS. (1993) The semaphorin genes encode a family of transmembrane and secreted growth cone guidance molecules. *Cell* **75:** 1389–1399.

Krystosek A, Seeds, NW. (1984) Peripheral neurons and Schwann cells secrete plasminogen activator. *J. Cell Biol.* **98:** 773–776.

Kuhn TB, Stoeckli ET, Condrau MA, Rathjen FG, Sonderegger P. (1991) Neurite outgrowth on immobilized axonin-1 is mediated by a heterophilic interaction with L1(G4). *J. Cell Biol.* **115:** 1113–1126.

Kuhn TB, Schmidt MF, Kater SB. (1995) Laminin and fibronectin guideposts signal sustained but opposite effects to passing growth cones. *Neuron* **14:** 275–285.

Lawler J, Weinstein R, Hyness RO. (1988) Cell attachment to thrombospondin: the role of ARG-GLY-ASP, calcium, and integrin receptors. *J. Cell Biol.* **107:** 2351–2361.

Lawler J, Duquette M, Urry L, McHenry K, Smith TF. (1993) The evolution of the thrombospondin gene family. *J. Mol. Evol.* **36:** 509–516.

LeBaron RG, Zimmermann DR, Ruoslahti E. (1992) Hyaluraonate binding properties of versican. *J. Biol. Chem.* **267:**10 003–10 010.

Lemmon V, Farr KL, Lagenaur C. (1989) L1-mediated axon outgrowth occurs via a homophilic binding mechanism. *Neuron* **2:** 1597–1603.

Leung-Hagesteijn C, Spence AM, Stern BD, Zhou Y, Su M-W, Hedgecock EM, Culotti JG. (1992) UNC-5, a transmembrane protein with immunoglobulin and thrombospondin type 1 domains, guides cell and pioneer axon migration in *C. elegans*. *Cell* **71:** 289–299.

Liesi P. (1985) Laminin-immunoreactive glia distinguish regenerative adult CNS systems from nonregenerative ones. *EMBO J.* **4:** 2505–2511.

Lindner J, Rathjen FG, Schachner M. (1983) L1 mono- and polyclonal antibodies modify cell migration in early postnatal mouse cerebellum. *Nature* **305:** 427–430.

Luo Y, Raper JA. (1994) Inhibitory factors controlling growth cone motility and guidance. *Curr. Opin. Neurobiol.* **4:** 648–654.

Luo Y, Raible D, Raper JA. (1993) Collapsin: a protein in brain that induces the collapse and paralysis of neuronal growth cones. *Cell* **75:** 217–227.

Luo Y, Shepherd I, Li J, Renzi MJ, Chang S, Raper JA. (1995) A family of molecules related to collapsin in the embryonic chick nervous system. *Neuron* **14:** 1131–1140.

Martin PT, Ettinger AJ, Sanes JR. (1995) A synaptic localization domain in the synaptic cleft protein laminin β2 (s-Laminin). *Science* **269:** 413–416.

Matsumoto K, Saga Y, Ikemura T, Sakakura T, Chiquet-Ehresmann R. (1994) The distribution of tenascin-X is distinct and often reciprocal to that of tenascin-C. *J. Cell Biol.* **125:** 483–493.

Matsumura K, Ervasti JM, Ohlendieck K, Kahl SD, Campbell KP. (1992) Association of dystrophin-related protein with dystrophin-associated proteins in mdx muscle. *Nature* **360:** 588–591.

Matthes DJ, Sink H, Kolodkin AL. (1995) Semaphorin II can function as a selective inhibitor of specific synaptic arborizations. *Cell* **81:** 631–639.

Maurel P, Rauch U, Flad M, Margolis RK, Margolis RU. (1994) Phosphacan, a chondroitin sulfate proteoglycan of brain that interacts with neurons and neural cell-adhesion molecules, is an extracellular variant of a receptor-type protein tyrosine phosphatase. *Proc. Natl Acad. Sci. USA* **91:** 2512–2516.

Mauro VP, Krushel LA, Cunningham BA, Edelman GM. (1992) Homophilic and heterophilic binding activities of Nr-CAM, a nervous system cell adhesion molecule. *J. Cell Biol.* **119:** 191–202.

McGuire PG, Seeds NW. (1990) Degradation of underlying extracellular matrix by sensory neurons during neurite outgrowth. *Neuron* **4:** 633–642.

McMahan UJ, Horton SE, Werle MJ, Honig LS, Kröger S, Ruegg MA, Escher G. (1992) Agrin isoforms and their role in synaptogenesis. *Curr. Opin. Cell Biol.* **4**: 869–874.

Mercurio AM. (1995) Laminin receptors: achieving specificity through cooperation. *Trends Cell Biol.* **5**: 419–423.

Messersmith EK, Leonardo ED, Shatz CJ, Tessier-Lavigne M, Goodman CS, Kolodkin AL. (1995) Semaphorin III can function as a selective chemorepellent to pattern sensory projections in the spinal cord. *Neuron* **14**: 949–959.

Miller B, Sheppard AM, Bicknese AR, Pearlman AL. (1995) Chondroitin sulfate proteoglycans in the developing cerebral cortex: the distribution of neurocan distinguishes forming afferent and efferent axonal pathways. *J. Comp. Neurol.* **355**: 615–628.

Moonen G, Grau-Wagemans MP, Selak I. (1982) Plasminogen activator–plasmin system and neuronal migration. *Nature* **298**: 753–755.

Morales G, Hubert M, Brümmendorf T, Treubert U, Tárnok A, Schwarz U, Rathjen FG. (1993) Induction of axonal growth by heterophilic interactions between the cell surface recognition proteins F11 and Nr-CAM/Bravo. *Neuron* **11**: 1113–1122.

Morgelin M, Heinegard D, Engel J. Paulsson M. (1992) Electronmicroscopy of native cartilage oligomeric matrix protein purified from the Swarm rat chondrosarcoma reveals a five-armed structure. *J. Biol. Chem.* **267**: 6137–6141.

Murray BA, Owens GC, Prediger EA, Crossin KL, Cunningham BA, Edelman GM. (1986) Cell surface modulation of the neural cell adhesion molecule resulting from alternative mRNA splicing in a tissue-specific developmental sequence. *J. Cell Biol.* **103**: 1431–1439.

Neugebauer KM, Emmett CJ, Venstrom KA, Reichardt LF. (1991) Vitronectin and thrombospondin promote retinal neurite outgrowth: developmental regulation and role of integrins. *Neuron* **6**: 345–358.

Nishiyama A, Dahlin KJ, Prince JT, Johnstone SR, Stallcup WB. (1991) The primary structure of NG2, a novel membrane-spanning proteoglycan. *J. Cell Biol.* **114**: 359–371.

Noakes PG, Gautam M, Mudd J, Sanes JR, Merlie JP. (1995) Aberrant differentiation of neuromuscular junctions in mice lacking s-laminin/laminin β2. *Nature* **374**: 258–262.

Nörenberg U, Wille H, Wolff R, Frank R, Rathjen FG. (1992) The chicken neural extracellular matrix molecule restrictin: similarity with EGF-, fibronectin type III-, and fibrinogen-like motifs. *Neuron* **8**: 849–863.

Nörenberg U, Hubert M, Brümmendorf T, Tárnok A, Rathjen FG. (1995) Characterization of functional domains of the tenascin-R (Restrictin) polypeptide: cell attachment site, binding with F11, and enhancement of F11-mediated neurite outgrowth by tenascin-R. *J. Cell Biol.* **130**: 473–484.

Nörenberg U, Hubert M, Rathjen FG. (1996) Structural and functional characterization of tenascin-R (Restrictin), an extracellular matrix glycoprotein of glia cells and neurons. *Int. J. Devel. Neurosci.* **14**: 217–231.

Oakley RA, Tosney KW. (1991) Peanut agglutinin and chondroitin-6-sulfate are molecular markers for tissues that act as barriers to axon advance in the avian embryo. *Devel. Biol.* **147** 187–206.

Ono K, Tomasiewicz H, Magnuson T, Rutishauser U. (1994) N-CAM mutation inhibits tangential neuronal migration and is phenocopied by enzymatic removal of polysialic acid. *Neuron* **13**: 595–609.

O'Rourke KM, Laherty CD, Dixit VM. (1992) Thrombospondin 1 and thrombospondin 2 are expressed as both homo- and heterotrimers. *J. Biol. Chem.* **267**: 24 921–24 924.

O'Shea KS, Rheinheimer JST, Dixit VM. (1990) Deposition and role of thrombospondin in the histogenesis of the cerebellar cortex. *J. Cell Biol.* **110**: 1275–1282.

O'Shea KS, Liu L-H, Dixit VM. (1991) Thrombospondin and a 140 kd fragment promote adhesion and neurite outgrowth from embryonic central and peripheral neurons and from PC12 cells. *Neuron* **7**: 231–237.

Osterhout DJ, Frazier WA, Higgins D. (1992) Thrombospondin promotes process outgrowth in neurons from the peripheral and central nervous system. *Devel. Biol.* **150**: 256–265.

Peles E, Nativ M, Campbell PL *et al.* (1995) The carbonic anhydrase domain of receptor tyrosine phosphatase β is a functional ligand for the axonal cell recognition molecule contactin. *Cell* **82**: 251–260.

Perris R, Krotoski D, Lallier T, Domingo C, Sorell JM, Bronner-Fraser M. (1991) Spatial and temporal changes in the distribution of proteoglycans during avian neural crest development. *Development* **111**: 583–599.

Pesheva P, Spiess E, Schachner M. (1989) J1-160 and J1-180 are oligodendrocyte-secreted nonpermissive substrates for cell adhesion. *J. Cell Biol.* **109**: 1765–1778.

Pesheva P, Gennarini G, Goridis C, Schachner M. (1993) The F3/11 cell adhesion molecule mediates the repulsion of neurons by the extracellular matrix glycoprotein J1-160/180. *Neuron* **10:** 69–82.

Pierceall WE, Cho KR, Getzenberg RH, Reale MA, Hedrick L. Vogelstein B, Fearon ER. (1994) NIH3T3 cells expressing the deleted in colorectal cancer tumor suppressor gene product stimulate neurite outgrowth in rat PC12 pheochromocytoma cells. *J. Cell Biol.* **124:** 1017–1027.

Pimenta AF, Zhukareva V, Barbe MF, Reinoso BS, Grimley C, Henzel W, Fischer I, Lewitt P. (1995) The limbic system-associated membrane protein is an Ig superfamily member that mediates selective neuronal growth and axon targeting. *Neuron* **15:** 287–297.

Pindzola RR, Doller C, Silver J. (1993) Putative inhibitory extracellular matrix molecules at the dorsal root entry zone of the spinal cord during development and after root and sciatic nerve lesions. *Devel. Biol.* **156:** 34–48.

Placzek M, Tessier-Lavigne M, Yamada T, Dodd J, Jessell TM. (1990) Guidance of developing axons by diffusible chemoattractants. *Cold Spring Harbor Symposia* **LV:** 279–289.

Porter BE, Weis J, Sanes JR. (1995) A motoneuron-selective stop signal in the synaptic protein S-laminin. *Neuron* **14:** 549–559.

Pourquie O, Coltey M, Thomas J, Le Douarin N. (1990) A widely distributed antigen developmentally regulated in the nervous system. *Development* **109:** 743–752.

Prieto AL, Jones FS, Cunningham BA, Crossin KL, Edelman GM. (1990) Localization during development of alternatively spliced forms of cytotactin mRNA by *in situ* hybridization. *J. Cell Biol.* **111:** 685–698.

Prieto AL, Andersson-Fisone C, Crossin KL. (1992) Characterization of multiple adhesive and counteradhesive domains in the extracellular matrix protein cytotactin. *J. Cell Biol.* **119:** 663–678.

Prieto AL, Edelman GM, Crossin KL. (1993) Multiple integrins mediate cell attachment to cytotactin/tenascin. *Proc. Natl Acad. Sci. USA* **90:** 10154–10158.

Püschel AW, Adams RH, Betz H. (1995) Murine semaphorin D/collapsin is a member of a diverse gene family and creates domains inhibitory for axonal extension. *Neuron* **14:** 941–948.

Rader C, Stoeckli ET, Ziegler U, Osterwalder T, Kunz B, Sonderegger P. (1993) Cell–cell adhesion by homophilic interaction of the neuronal recognition molecule axonin-1. *Eur. J. Biochem.* **215:** 133–141.

Rathjen FG, Wolff JM, Chang S, Bonhoeffer F, Raper JA. (1987a) Neurofascin: a novel chick cell-surface glycoprotein involved in neurite-neurite interactions. *Cell* **51:** 841–849.

Rathjen FG, Wolff JM, Frank R, Bonhoeffer F, Rutishauser U. (1987b) Membrane glycoproteins involved in neurite fasciculation. *J. Cell Biol.* **104:** 343–353.

Rathjen FG, Wolff JM, Chiquet-Ehrismann R. (1991) Restrictin: a chick neural extracellular matrix protein involved in cell attachment co-purifies with the cell recognition molecule F11. *Development* **113:** 151–164.

Rauch U, Gao P, Janetzko A, Flaccus A, Hilgenberg L, Tekotte H, Margolis RK, Maargolis RU. (1991) Isolation and characterization of developmentally regulated chondrontin sulfate and chondroitin/keratin sulfate proteoglycans of brain identified with monoclonal antibodies. *J. Biol. Chem.* **266:** 14785–14801.

Rauch U, Karthikeyan L, Maurel P, Margolis RU, Margolis RK. (1992) Cloning and primary structure of neurocan, a developmentally regulated, aggregating chondroitin sulfate proteoglycan of brain. *J. Biol. Chem.* **267:** 19536–19547.

Reale MA, Hu G, Zafar AI, Getzenberg RH, Levine SM, Fearon ER. (1994) Expression and alternative splicing of the deleted in colorectal cancer (DCC) gene in normal and malignant tissues. *Cancer Res.* **54:** 4493–5001.

Reichardt LF, Tomaselli KJ. (1991) Extracellular matrix molecules and their receptors: functions in neural development. *Annu. Rev. Neurosci.* **14:** 531–570.

Reid RA, Bronson DD, Young KM, Hemperly JJ. (1994) Identification and characterization of the human cell adhesion molecule contactin. *Mol. Brain Res.* **21:** 1–8.

Reist NE, Werle MJ, McMahan UJ. (1992) Agrin released by motor neurons induces the aggregation of acetylcholine receptors at neuromuscular junctions. *Neuron* **8:** 865–868.

Rivas RJ, Burmeister DW, Goldberg DJ. (1992) Rapid effects of laminin on the growth cone. *Neuron* **8:** 107–115.

Ruegg MA, Tsim KWK, Horton SE, Kröger S, Escher G, Gensch EM, McMahan UJ. (1992) The agrin gene codes for a family of basal lamina proteins that differ in function and distribution. *Neuron* **8:** 691–699.

Ruthishauser U, Grumet M, Edelman GM. (1983) Neural cell adhesion molecule mediates initial interactions between spinal cord neurons and muscle cells in culture. *J. Cell Biol.* **97:** 145–152.

Ruthishauser U, Acheson A, Hall AK, Mann DM, Sunshine J. (1988) The neural cell adhesion molecule (NCAM) as a regulator of cell–cell interactions. *Science* **240**: 53–57.

Salmivirta M, Elenius K, Vainio S, Hofer U, Chiquet-Ehrismann F, Thesleff I, Jalkanen M. (1991) Syndecan from embryonic tooth mesenchyme binds tenascin. *J. Biol. Chem.* **266**: 7733–7739.

Sanes JR. (1989) Extracellular matrix molecules that influence neural development. *Annu. Rev. Neurosci.* **12**: 491–516.

Schachner M, Taylor JP, Bartsch U, Pesheva P. (1994) The perplexing multifunctionality of janusin, a tenascin-related molecule. *Persp. Devel. Neurobiol.* **2**: 33–41.

Schwab ME, Kapfhammer JP, Bandtlow CE. (1993) Inhibitors of neurite growth. *Annu. Rev. Neurosci.* **16**: 565–595.

Seilheimer B, Schachner M. (1988) Studies of adhesion molecules mediating interactions between cells of peripheral nervous system indicate a major role for L1 in mediating sensory neuron growth on Schwann cells in culture. *J. Cell Biol.* **107**: 341–351.

Seilheimer B, Persohn E, Schachner M. (1989) Antibodies to the L1 adhesion molecule inhibit Schwann cells ensheathment of neurons *in vitro. J. Cell Biol.* **109**: 3095–3103.

Serafini T, Kennedy TE, Galko MJ, Mirzayan C, Jessell TM, Tessier-Lavigne M. (1994) The netrins define a family of axon outgrowth-promoting proteins homologous to *C. elegans* unc-6. *Cell* **78**: 409–424.

Silverstein RL, Leung LLK, Harpel PC, Nachman RL. (1984) Complex formation of platelet thrombospondin and plasminogen. *J. Clin. Invest.* **74**: 1625–1633.

Silverstein RL, Harpel PC, Nachman RL. (1986) Tissue plasminogen activator and urokinase enhance the binding of plasminogen to TSP. *J. Biol. Chem.* **261**: 9959–9965.

Smith MA, O'Dowd DK. (1994) Cell-specific regulation of agrin RNA splicing in the chick ciliary ganglion. *Neuron* **12**: 795–804.

Snow DM, Lemmon V, Carrino DA, Caplan AI, Silver J. (1990) Sulfated proteoglycans in astroglial barriers inhibit neurite outgrowth *in vitro. Exp. Neurol.* **109**: 111–130.

Spaltmann F, Brümmendorf T. (1996) CEPU-1, a novel immunoglobulin superfamily molecule, is expressed by developing cerebellar Purkinje cells. *J. Neurosci.* **16**: 1770–1779.

Spring J, Beck K, Chiquet-Ehrismann R. (1989) Two contrary functions of tenascin: dissection of the active sites by recombinant tenascin fragments. *Cell* **59**: 325–334.

Sretavan D, Feng L, Puré E, Reichardt LF. (1994) Embryonic neurons of the developing optic chiasm express L1 and CD44, cell surface molecules with opposing effects on retinal axon growth. *Neuron* **12**: 957–975.

Steindler D. (1993) Glial boundaries in the developing nervous system. *Annu. Rev. Neurosci.* **16**: 445–470.

Steindler DA, Cooper NG, Faissner A, Schachner M. (1989) Boundaries defined by adhesion molecules during development of the cerebral cortex: the J1 tenascin glycoprotein in the mouse somatosensory cortical barrel field. *Devel. Biol.* **131**: 234–260.

Stoeckli ET, Landmesser LT. (1995) Axonin-1, Nr-CAM, and NgCAM play different roles in the *in vivo* guidance of chick commissural neurons. *Neuron* **14**: 1165–1179.

Stoeckli ET, Kuhn TB, Duc CO, Ruegg MA, Sonderegger P. (1991) The axonally secreted protein axonin-1 is a potent substratum for neurite growth. *J. Cell Biol.* **112**: 449–455.

Struyk AF, Canoll PD, Wolfgang MJ, Rosen CL, D'Eustachio P, Salzer JL. (1995) Cloning of neurotrimin defines a new subfamily of differentially expressed neural cell adhesion molecules. *J. Neurosci.* **15**: 2141–2156.

Sugiyama J, Bowen DC, Hall ZW. (1994) Dystroglycan binds nerve and muscle agrin. *Neuron* **13**: 103–115.

Suter DM, Pollerberg GE, Buchstaller A, Giger RJ, Dreyer WJ, Sonderegger P. (1995) Binding between the neural cell adhesion molecule axonin-1 and NrCAM/Bravo is involved in neuron–glia interaction. *J. Cell Biol.* **131**: 1067–1081.

Taira E, Takaha N, Taniura H, Kim CH, Miki N. (1994) Molecular cloning and functional expression of gicerin, a novel cell adhesion molecule that binds to neurite outgrowth factor. *Neuron* **12**: 861–872.

Takeichi M. (1995) Morphogenetic roles of classic cadherins. *Curr. Opin. Cell Biol.* **7**: 619–627.

Tan S-S, Crossin KL, Hoffman S, Edelman GM. (1987) Asymmetric expression in somites of cytotactin and its proteoglycan ligand is correlated with neural crest cell distribution. *Proc. Natl Acad. Sci. USA* **84**: 7977–7981.

Tanaka H, Matsui T, Agata A, Tomura M, Kubota I, McFarland KC, Kohr B, Lee A, Phillips HS, Shelton DL. (1991) Molecular cloning and expression of a novel adhesion molecule, SC1. *Neuron* **7**: 535–545.

Tang J, Landmesser L, Rutishauser U. (1992) Polysialic acid influences specific pathfinding by avian motoneurons. *Neuron* **8**: 1031–1044.

Tang J, Rutishauser U, Landmesser L. (1994) Polysialic acid regulates growth cone behavior during sorting of motor axons in the plexus region. *Neuron* **13**: 405–414.

Taniura H, Kuo CH, Hayashi Y, Miki N. (1991) Purification and characterization of an 82-kD membrane protein as a neurite outgrowth factor binding protein: possible involvement of NOF binding protein in axonal outgrowth in developing retina. *J. Cell Biol.* **112**: 313–322.

Taylor J, Pesheva P, Schachner M. (1993) Influence of janusin and tenascin on growth cone behavior *in vitro*. *J. Neurosci. Res.* **35**: 347–362.

Tessier-Lavigne M, Placzek M, Lumsden AGS, Dodd J, Jessell TM. (1988) Chemotropic guidance of developing axons in the mammalian central nervous system. *Nature* **336**: 775–778.

Theodosis DT, Rougon G, Poulain DA. (1991) Retention of embryonic features by an adult neuronal system capable of plasticity: polysialylated neural cell adhesion molecule in the hypothalamo-neurohypophysical system. *Proc. Natl Acad. Sci. USA* **88**: 5494–5498.

Tomaselli KJ, Hall DE, Flier LA, Gehlsen KR, Turner DC, Carbonetto S, Reichardt LF. (1990) A neuronal cell line (PC 12) expresses two β_1-class integrins-$\alpha_1\beta_1$, and $\alpha_3\beta_1$-that recognize different neurite outgrowth-promoting domains in laminin. *Neuron* **5**: 651–662.

Tomaselli KJ, Doherty P, Emmett CJ, Damsky CH, Walsh FS, Reichardt LF. (1993) Expression of $\beta1$ integrins in sensory neurons of the dorsal root ganglion and their functions in neurite outgrowth on two laminin isoforms. *J. Neurosci.* **13**: 4880–4888.

Tsen G, Halfter W, Kröger S, Cole GJ. (1995) Agrin is a heparan sulfate proteoglycan. *J. Biol. Chem.* **270**: 3392–3399.

Tsim KWK, Ruegg MA, Escher G, Kröger S, McMahan UJ. (1992) cDNA that encodes active agrin. *Neuron* **8**: 677–589.

Tucker RP. (1993) The *in situ* localization of tenascin splice variants and thrombospondin 2 mRNA in the avian embryo. *Development* **117**: 347–348.

Tuszynski GP, Karczewski J, Smith L, Murphy A, Rothman VL, Knudsen KA. (1989) The GPIIb–IIIa-like complex may function as a human melanoma cell adhesion receptor for thrombospondin. *Exp. Cell Res.* **182**: 473–481.

Varnum-Finney B, Venstrom K, Muller U, Kypta R, Backus C, Chiquet M, Reichardt LF. (1995) The integrin receptor $\alpha_8\beta_1$ mediates interactions of embryonic chick motor and sensory neurons with tenascin-C. *Neuron* **14**: 1213–1222.

Venstrom KA, Reichardt LF. (1993) Extracellular matrix 2: role of extracellular matrix molecules and their receptors in the nervous system. *FASEB J.* **7**: 996–1003.

Verrall S, Seeds NW. (1988) Tissue plasminogen activator release from mouse cerebellar granule neurons. *J. Neurosci. Res.* **21**: 420–425.

Verrall S, Seeds NW. (1989) Characterization of ^{125}I-tissue plasminogen activator binding to cerebellar granule neurons. *J. Cell Biol.* **109**: 265–271.

Vielmetter J, Kayyem JF, Roman J, Dreyer WJ. (1994) Neogenin, an avian cell surface protein expressed during terminal neuronal differentiation, is closely related to the human tumor suppressor molecule deleted in colorectal cancer. *J. Cell Biol.* **127**: 2009–2020.

Volkmer H, Hassel B, Wolff JM, Frank R, Rathjen FG. (1992) Structure of the axonal surface recognition molecule neurofascin and its relationship to a neural subgroup of the immunoglobulin superfamily. *J. Cell Biol.* **118**: 149–161.

Volkmer H, Leuschner R, Zacharias U, Rathjen FG. (1996) Neurofascin induces neurites by heterophilic interactions with axonal NrCAM while NrCAM requires F11 on the axonal surface to extend neurites. *J. Cell Biol.*, in press.

Wallace BG. (1994) Staurosporine inhibits agrin-induced acetylcholine receptor phosphorylation and aggregation. *J. Cell Biol.* **125**: 661–668.

Wallace BG. (1995) Regulation of the interaction of nicotinic acetylcholine receptors with the cytoskeleton by agrin-activated protein tyrosine kinase. *J. Cell Biol.* **128**: 1121–1129.

Wallace BG, Qu Z, Huganier RL. (1991) Agrin induces phosphorylation of the nicotinic acetylcholine receptor. *Neuron* **6**: 869–878.

Walter J. Allsopp TE, Bonhoeffer F. (1990) A common denominator of growth cone guidance and collapse. *Trends Neurosci.* **13**: 447–452.

Weber P, Zimmermann DR, Winterhalter KH, Vaughans L. (1995) Tenascin-C binds heparin by its fibronectin type III domain five. *J. Biol. Chem.* **270**: 4619–4623.

Wehrle B, Chiquet M. (1990) Tenascin is accumulated along developing peripheral nerves and allows neurite outgrowth *in vitro. Development* **110:** 401–415.

Wehrle-Haller B, Chiquet M. (1993) Dual function of tenascin: simultaneous promotion of neurite growth and inhibition of glial migration. *J. Cell Sci.* **106:** 597–610.

Wight TN, Kinsella MG, Qwarnstrom EE. (1992) The role of proteoglycans in cell adhesion, migration, and proliferation. *Curr. Opin. Cell Biol.* **4:** 793–801.

Williams AF, Barclay AN. (1988) The immunoglobulin superfamily – domains for cell surface recognition. *Annu. Rev. Immunol.* **6:** 381–405.

Williams EJ, Doherty P, Turner G, Reid RA, Hemperly JJ, Walsh FS. (1992) Calcium influx into neurons can solely account for cell contact-dependent neurite outgrowth stimulated by transfected L1. *J. Cell Biol.* **119:** 883–892.

Williams EJ, Furness J, Walsh FS, Doherty P. (1994) Activation of the FGF receptor underlies neurite outgrowth stimulated by L1, N-CAM, and N-cadherin. *Neuron* **13:** 583–594.

Wintergerst ES, Fuss B, Bartsch U. (1993) Localization of Janusin mRNA in the central nervous system of the developing and adult mouse. *Eur. J. Neurosc.* **5:** 299–310.

Yabkowitz R, Dixit VM, Guo N, Roberts DD, Shimizu Y. (1993) Activated T-cell adhesion to thrombospondin is mediated by the $\alpha 4\beta 1$ (VLA-4) and $\alpha 5\beta 1$ (VLA-5) integrins. *J. Immunol.* **151:** 149–158.

Yamada H, Watanabe K, Shimonaka M, Yamaguchi Y. (1994) Molecular cloning of brevican, a novel brain proteoglycan of the aggrecan/versican family. *J. Biol. Chem.* **269:** 10 119–10 126.

Yoshihara Y, Kawasaki M, Tani A, Tamada A, Nagata S, Kagamiyama H, Mori K. (1994) BIG-1 – a new TAG-1/F3-related member of the immunoglobulin superfamily with neurite outgrowth-promoting activity. *Neuron* **13:** 415–426.

Yoshihara Y, Kawasaki M, Tamada A, Nagata S, Kagamiyama H, Mori K. (1995) Overlapping and differential expression of Big-2, Big-1, Tag-1, and F3: four members of an axon-associated cell adhesion molecule subgroup of the immunoglobulin superfamily. *J. Neurobiol.* **28:** 51–69.

Zisch AH, D'Alessandri L, Ranscht B, Falchetto R, Winterhalter KH, Vaughan L. (1992) Neuronal cell adhesion molecule contactin/F11 binds to tenascin via its immunoglobulin-like domains. *J. Cell Biol.* **119:** 203–213.

Zisch AH, D'Alessandri L, Amrein K, Ranscht B, Winterhalter KH, Vaughan L. (1995) The glypiated neuronal cell adhesion molecule contactin/F11 complexes with src-family protein tyrosine kinase fyn. *Mol. Cell. Neurosci.* **6:** 263–279.

Zuellig RA, Rader C, Schroeder A et al. (1992) The axonally secreted cell adhesion molecule, axonin-1. *Eur. J. Biochem.* **204:** 453–463.

Genetic control of brain development

N.D. Allen, M.J. Skynner, H. Kato and J.N. Pratap

11.1 Introduction

Development of the vertebrate nervous system is highly complex, but can be broken down into a number of distinct phases. The first stages of neural development involve the specification of anterior versus posterior ectoderm in the primitive streak stage embryo. This involves the organizing activities of cells in the node, a group of about 20 cells at the most anterior end of the primitive streak (Hensen's node in the chick and the dorsal blastopore lip in *Xenopus*). When transplanted to an ectopic region of the epiblast, the organizing properties of cells in the node can induce the development of second neural axes (Beddington, 1994; Spemann, 1938). This group of cells exerts its critical patterning functions during gastrulation, a process that defines the endodermal, mesodermal and ectodermal germlayers of the embryo. During gastrulation, the neurectoderm is induced by vertical signals from the underlying mesoderm and signals that act within the plane of the newly formed neurectoderm (planar signals) impose an anterior-to-posterior polarity (Ruiz i Altaba, 1994). The resulting neurectoderm forms the neural plate that subsequently undergoes a dramatic morphological transformation, during neurulation, to form the hollow neural tube which is bilaterally symmetrical but has distinct dorsal–ventral (D–V) and anterior–posterior (A–P) polarity. Cells at the ventral midline still overlie notochordal, or prechordal plate, mesoderm and the lateral edges of the neural plate come together at the dorsal midline, from which the neural crest cells develop and migrate.

The brain develops from the anterior neural tube, whilst the posterior forms the spinal cord. The first distinctive changes in the brain involve the formation of three primary vesicles, the prosencephalon, the mesencephalon and the rhombencephalon, that will go on to form the forebrain, midbrain and hindbrain regions respectively. The prosencephalon then becomes further subdivided to the telencephalon, from which the cerebral hemispheres will develop, and to the diencephalon, from which the thalamic and hypothalamic regions will develop.

In recent years considerable advances have been made in understanding the genetics and mechanisms of early vertebrate brain development. In essence these advances have come from:

(i) The identification of a large number of genes with developmental and putative regulatory functions.

Molecular Biology of the Neuron, edited by R.W. Davies and B.J. Morris.
© 1997 BIOS Scientific Publishers Ltd, Oxford.

(ii) The use of comparative genetic and developmental systems in mice, *Xenopus*, chick and zebrafish, to study gene functions.

(iii) Elaboration of mechanistic models of brain development.

In this chapter the main focus will be on genes involved in the early patterning mechanisms of forebrain development, considering mice in particular.

Although the anatomical changes that the neural tube undergoes can be simply described, one of the major problems for the developmental biologist is to describe in molecular terms how this happens. Essentially, central nervous system (CNS) development is initiated by establishing a blueprint of patterning information in the form of longitudinal and horizontal domains of gene expression (*Figure 11.1*). Much of our understanding of patterning mechanisms comes from studying development in the fruitfly *Drosophila melanogaster*. In *Drosophila*, development proceeds through a process of segmentation along the A–P axis of the embryo, resulting in a progressive restriction of cell fate within the embryonic anlage. In the egg, A–P polarity is established by anteriorly and posteriorly localized morphogens. Interpretation of these morphogenetic gradients leads to the activation of embryonic gap genes which divide the embryo into broad domains. Further subdivision then occurs through the activation of pair-rule genes, which divide the syncytial blastoderm into a series of repeat-

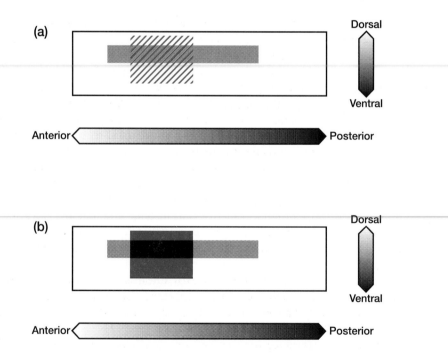

Figure 11.1. Two gene expression domains can define three developmental regions in the neural tube. (a) The schematic shows the expression patterns of two imaginary neural patterning genes in a lateral view. Both *graybox* and *orangehatch* are expressed with respect to A–P and D–V patterning cues. (b) The patterns of these genes define three developmental regions. One domain is set up by the presence of both *graybox* and *orangehatch* (shown in black). Another corresponds to the regions in which *graybox* only is expressed (gray), and the third where only *orangehatch* is present (orange). Furthermore, the other cells of the neural tube (white) receive some patterning information in that neither *graybox* nor *orangehatch* is present.

ing segments, which retain A–P positional information. These segments then become divided into parasegments through the action of segment-polarity genes, and finally segment identities become defined by the action of homeotic genes. In addition, information that specifies position along the A–P axis is superimposed on D–V positional information.

The knowledge gained from studies in *Drosophila* is of fundamental importance to understanding neural development, crucially because the high evolutionary conservation of the segmentation genes and other regulatory genes has allowed large families of homologous genes to be cloned and studied in vertebrates (including the principal model organisms for vertebrate developmental studies, mice, *Xenopus*, chicks and zebrafish). Secondly, evolutionary conservation of the genes themselves has naturally led to the speculation that some of the basic developmental mechanism might also be conserved.

11.2 Segmental development of the vertebrate nervous system

The segmental nature of *Drosophila* development has led investigators to determine whether such a paradigm may also exist in vertebrate brain development.

11.2.1 The hindbrain

The first evidence that segmental development was conserved in the CNS of vertebrates came from studies in the hindbrain (Lumsden and Keynes, 1989). Indeed hindbrain segmentation now provides a paradigm for evolutionary conservation of gene function and developmental mechanisms. The segmental units of the developing hindbrain are the rhombomeres, and were first recognized over a century ago. They develop as repeating bulges along the A–P axis of the hindbrain neuroepithelium. However the true nature of the rhombomeres as developmental compartments has been demonstrated only recently in that they are defined by domains of gene expression and act as reiterated compartments that restrict cell lineage and cell mixing (Fraser *et al.*, 1990). The organization of the rhombomeres is reminiscent of parasegments in *Drosophila* in that pairs of rhombomeres form functional units. Neurons that arise in each pair of rhombomeres innervate one adjacent branchial arch, for example the trigeminal branchiomotor nerve originates from rhombomeres r2/r3 and innervates derivatives of the first branchial arch, the facial nerve from r4/r5 innervates derivatives of the second and the glossopharyngeal nerve from r6/r7 innervates the third branchial arch.

The underlying molecular basis for hindbrain segmentation involves the spatially restricted expression of the *Hox* genes and other genes such as *Krox-20* (Schneider-Maunoury *et al.*, 1993). The *Hox* genes are homologs of genes in the *Drosophila* homeotic selector gene complex HOM-C. As in *Drosophila Hox* genes are thought to control segment identity along the A–P axis. The strongest evidence for this conserved function is homeotic transformation in segment identity in *Hox* mutants made by gene-targeting or by ectopic gene expression in transgenic mice (Krumlauf, 1994). In vertebrates, *Hox* genes exist in four paralogous clusters, *Hoxa-Hoxd*. In most cases these genes are expressed from the posterior end of the neural tube to a specific limit in the rhombencephalon that coincides with a boundary between two rhombomeres. Therefore, *Hoxb-1* is expressed in rhombomere 4 (r4) and *Hoxb-2*, *Hoxb-3*, and *Hoxb-4* are expressed with a two-segment polarity and have limits at the r2/r3, r4/r5 and r6/r7 boundaries respectively. A distinguishing feature of *Hox* gene regulation is the colinearity that exists between the positions of each gene within its cluster on the chromosome and their distinct A–P boundaries of expression. The highly conserved structure of the *Hox* clusters suggests that the genes are coordinately regulated and this may provide the mechanism that determines the segmental boundaries of gene expression (for reviews see Keynes and Krumlauf, 1994, and Guthrie 1996).

11.2.2 The midbrain

Anterior to the eight rhombomeres of the hindbrain are the isthmus and mesencephalon–midbrain segments. Significant studies have focused on structures developing from the midbrain–hindbrain boundary region, notably the cerebellum, pons, colliculi and isthmic nuclei. This region of the mesencephalon is characterized by the expression of several genes including vertebrate homologs of the *Drosophila* segment polarity genes *engrailed* (*En-1* and *En-2*), *paired* (*Pax-2*, *Pax-5* and *Pax-8*) and *wingless* (some *Wnt* family members). The importance of some of these genes have been shown by gene-targeting, for example *En-1* and *Wnt-1* null mutants each develop with similar deletions of the cerebellum and other midbrain–hindbrain boundary structures. For extensive reviews on the functions and interactions of these genes, and their parallels in *Drosophila* development see Hatten and Heintz (1995), and Millen *et al.* (1995).

11.2.3 The forebrain

The forebrain is separated from the hindbrain by the isthmus and mesencephalon–midbrain segments. *Figure 11.2* shows a schematic of the developing mouse brain on day 12.5 of gestation, illustrating the major brain subdivisions and distinctive nuclei, and should be used in reference to gene expression patterns shown in *Figures 11.3–11.6*.

In the forebrain, segmentation defined as a reiteration of similar compartments, is less evident. Indeed, strict criteria for a metameric system are violated, for instance, cell mixing can occur at intertelencephalic but not interdiencephalic boundaries (Figdor and Stern, 1993; Fishell *et al.*, 1993). However Puelles and Rubenstein, (1993), and Figdor and Stern (1993) have recently developed neuromeric models for the early organization of the forebrain. Boundaries between forebrain neuromeres, termed prosomeres, can be seen histologically as constrictions in the neuroepithelium of the prosencephalon. Puelles and Rubenstein (1993) propose that the forebrain initially becomes segmented transversely to form six prosomeres (p1–p6), that encompass the diencephalon (p1–p3) and telencephalon (p4–p6). The strongest evidence for this organization is that several genes have expression boundaries at borders between prosomeres, indicating that prosomeres may represent segments with distinct molecular identities. While the six prosomeres demarcate transverse segments along the A–P axis of the prosencephalon, gene expression patterns also reveal patterning along the D–V axis, such that the differentiating neuroepithelium is also subdivided into longitudinal domains. Thus regulation of gene expression transversely and longitudinally subdivides the forebrain neurectoderm into domains with distinct identities.

Prosomeres have two important functions. First, they are transient structures that demarcate zones of subsequent regional differentiation. Second, cell interactions at interneuromeric boundaries may define the paths of the initial fiber tracts in the

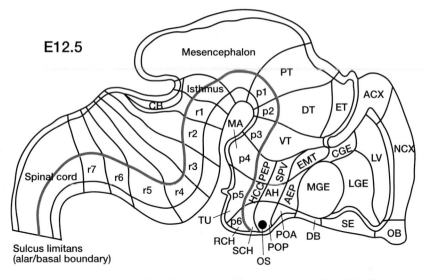

Figure 11.2. Sagittal section showing the anatomy of mouse brain at day 12.5 of gestation. Rhombomeres and prosomeres are noted by 'r' and 'p' respectively. Other abbreviations: ACX, archicortex; AEP, anterior entopeduncular area; AH, anterior hypothalamus; CB, cerebellum; CGE, caudal ganglionic eminence; DB, diagonal band; DT, dorsal thalamus; EMT, eminentia thalami; ET, epithalamus; HCC, hypothalamic cell cord; LGE, lateral ganglionic eminence; LV, lateral ventricle; MA, mammillary area; MGE, medial ganglionic eminence; NCX, neocortex; OB, olfactory bulb; OS, optic stalk; PEP, posterior entopeduncular area; POA, anterior preoptic area; POP, posterior preoptic area; PT, pretectum; RCH, retrochiasmatic area; SE, septum; SCH, suprachiasmatic area; TU, tuberal hypothalamus; VT, ventral thalamus; ZLI, zona limitans intrathalamica.

brain, providing a scaffold for subsequent anatomical development. This can account for the high degree of evolutionary conservation observed in the patterns of axonal tracts and commissures seen in vertebrates (Easter *et al.*, 1993). The history of these interneuromeric borders can be seen in the adult brain, at least in derivatives of the diencephalon, where the p1/p2 border separates the pretectum from the dorsal thalamus and the p2/p3 boundary separates the dorsal thalamus from the ventral thalamus. The latter border is delineated by the zona limitans intrathalamica, and later by the medullary lamina, while the former border is outlined by the habenulo–interpeduncular tract and habenular commissure. The border between the midbrain mesencephalon and prosomere p1 is marked by the posterior commissure.

11.2.4 Forebrain patterning genes

Given the importance of the *Hox* genes in hindbrain segmentation, initial studies focused on the identification and analysis of other homeobox-containing genes expressed in the forebrain. The homeobox encodes the homeodomain, a 60 amino acid motif with a three helix–turn–helix structure that in most cases binds DNA and acts as a regulator of gene transcription. The importance of the homeodomain was recognized early on as it is a common sequence motif in developmental regulatory genes, not only being present in genes of the *HOM-C* complex but also in a number of other putative regulatory genes. The high conservation of this motif also meant that it could be used as a probe at low stringencies to screen for novel or related homeobox-containing genes. In a recent compilation of published vertebrate homeobox-containing genes around 170 different loci were listed which fell into 40 families (Stein *et al.*, 1996). Of these, 139 were cloned in the mouse and of those 105 were expressed in parts of the nervous system. The major families with members expressed in the developing forebrain include *Dlx*, *Emx*, *Gbx*, *Gsh*, *Gtx*, *Hes*, *Dbx*, *Nkx-2*, *Nkx-5*, *otp*, *Otx*, *Pax*, *Lim*, *Pou* (*Brn*), and *Prox* and it is likely that this list will continue to grow.

Otx *and* Emx *genes.* Amongst the first forebrain homeobox-containing genes to be identified were *Otx-1*, *Otx-2*, *Emx-1* and *Emx-2* (*Figure 11.3*) which are homologs of the *Drosophila* genes *orthodenticle* (*otd*) and *empty spiracles* (*ems*) (Simeone *et al.*, 1992a,b; reviewed in Finklestein and Boncinelli, 1994). In *Drosophila*, *otd* and *ems*, together with a third gene *buttonhead* (*btd*) act as anterior gap genes, being expressed in overlapping domains at the anterior pole of the cellular blastoderm that gives rise to head structures. These genes are under the control of high levels of the graded morphogen bicoid. Null mutations in *ems* and *otd* result in loss of anterior structures and they are therefore required to specify progressively anterior regions of the head. Later in development *otd* and *ems* are also involved in fly brain segmentation. The brain of *Drosophila* develops from three neuromeres. Recently, mutations in *otd* and *ems* have been found to produce distinct segmental phenotypes in the developing brain (Hirth *et al.*, 1995). Analysis using weak mutant alleles shows that *otd* is specifically required for the formation of the most anterior neuromere b1, and *ems* is required for the development of the two more posterior neuromeres b2 and b3. The transverse borders between neuromeres are defined by expression of the segment polarity gene *engrailed*. As in vertebrates, it is proposed that the neuromeric boundaries could constitute a structural scaffold for major axonal pathways. The pre-oral embryonic brain commissure forms at the site of the first *engrailed* expression domain, the antennal nerve root forms at the second and the tritocerebral commissure forms at the third. Although it appears that *otd* and *ems* have postzygotic functions in neuromeric segmentation, it is not yet known which genes act to define these segment identities in the fly brain.

In the mouse, a striking feature of the *Otx* and *Emx* genes is that they occupy nested domains of expression within the forebrain and midbrain at midgestation (Simeone *et al.*, 1992a). *Otx-2* is expressed most broadly, occupying the majority of the forebrain and midbrain with a sharp boundary at the midbrain–hindbrain junction. *Otx-1* and *Emx-2* have successively nested anterior boundaries of expression within the *Otx-2* domain and finally *Emx-1* is expressed in the smallest domain, being restricted to the

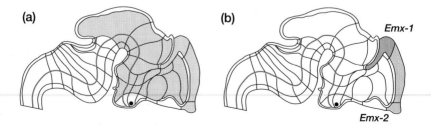

Figure 11.3. Guide to expression of (a) *Otx* and (b) *Emx* group genes. Orange areas in (a) show *Otx-1* plus *Otx-2* expression, gray shows *Otx-2* only.

dorsal telencephalon. For *Otx-2*, expression is first detected very early, throughout the epiblast at day 5.5 of gestation. It then becomes more localized to the anterior pole of the primitive streak during gastrulation, to cells fated to become prechordal meso-derm as well as to cells of the presumptive anterior neurectoderm. By contrast, *Otx-1*, *Emx 2* and *Emx-1* are first expressed between days 8.5 and 9.5 of gestation.

The function of *Otx-2* has been studied by gene targeting in mouse embryonic stem cells (Acampora *et al.*, 1995; Matsuo *et al.*, 1995). *Otx-2 –/–* embryos die around midgestation. However a significant variation in phenotype was observed possibly as a consequence of segregating genetic background effects. Most importantly, in all embryos head structures anterior to the level of the hindbrain were deleted, and in a proportion of embryos hindbrain morphology was also affected. Loss of these ante-rior structures results from a failure to specify anterior neurectoderm during gastru-lation. These observations suggest that *Otx-2* has conserved the anterior gap gene function of *otd*.

Despite the early death of *Otx-2 –/–* embryos, later functions of *Otx-2* could be seen in heterozygotes. Interestingly, phenotypes in heterozygotes were significantly affected by genetic background. Gene-targeting was performed in 129*sv* strain embry-onic stem cells, and when crossed to CBA mice heterozygous mice developed quite well and could be reared to adulthood. However when crossed to C57Bl/6 strain mice the majority died neonatally with severe head abnormalities affecting both the skull and brain. Indeed 3.2% of mice developed without head structures at all. However in less severely affected mice several defects were seen in the CNS, the cranial peripheral nervous system and in craniofacial development (which depends on cranial neural crest). Although the range of phenotypes observed in the nervous system was quite variable, all abnormalities were in the fore- and midbrains as would be predicted from the *Otx-2* expression pattern. However, the most severely affected regions included the most caudal and rostral regions of *Otx-2* expression where neither *Otx-1*, *Emx-1* or *Emx-2* are expressed, possibly implying some redundancy in *Otx-2* gene function. There was a general retardation in the development of the rostral brain, the neurecto-derm was thinner, with fewer mitotic cells, and anatomical landmarks were ill defined. This is notable at the midbrain–hindbrain boundary where *Otx-2* expression from the remaining active allele actually spread beyond the isthmus into the hind-brain. In mildly affected mice, specific defects were noted in the development of the mesencephalic trigeminal neurons and the mesencephalic trigeminal nerve root that derive from the mesencephalic neural crest, but no significant abnormalities were seen in structures derived from the diencephalon. In other mice (holoprosencephalic) the third ventricle did not develop to form a pair of lateral ventricles but remained fused as a single median ventricle. One further consistent phenotype was deformity or loss of the posterior and sometimes anterior lobes of the hypophysis. Defects were also seen in the developing eye and olfactory system.

Given the enormous variation in haploinsufficient phenotype associated with *Otx-2* heterozygosity it is difficult to assess particular functions of the gene in particular neuronal systems. It is possible that the later functions of *Otx-2* could be addressed in specific parts of the head by designing conditional mutants. It is of particular interest that the phenotypic variations are associated with genetic background effects, since mapping strain-specific modifiers' effects could provide a way to identify additional genes that interact with *Otx-2* in development.

While there is a strong case for a conserved gap-like function of *Otx-2* in head development, such a conserved function for *Otx-1* and the *Emx* genes is less likely. Instead, expression data suggest that these genes might be involved in regulating both neuroblast proliferation and cell migration to the different cortical layers, and in imparting positional identity to cells of the dorsal telencephalon. *Emx-2* expression is confined to the ventricular zones throughout development, being active in all proliferating cells of the germinal layers, but is turned off in postmitotic neurons. In contrast to *Emx-2*, *Emx-1* is expressed throughout the dorsal telencephalon, in all neurons of the presumptive cerebral cortex, including the ventricular zone, transitional field and the cortical plate, but it is not detected in the basal zone (Gulisano *et al.*, 1996). The basal and dorsal zones are subdivided early in development and become established as compartments with distinct cellular identities that prevent cell mixing (Fishell *et al.*, 1993). Given the role of homeobox-containing genes in conferring positional identity to cells, and particularly given the function of its fly homolog, it is possible that *Emx-1* has a similar function in the dorsal telencephalon. However, unlike the situation that prevails in the hindbrain in which positional information leads to determination of cell fate (permanent cell memory), positional information in the cortex appears to be instructive, in that cells transplanted from the basal region of the telencephalon acquire a dorsal fate by responding to local positional cues (Fishel, 1995; Fraser *et al.*, 1990).

Development of the cerebral neocortex proceeds in late gestation and postnatally to form a hexalaminar structure, while the hippocampus and olfactory bulbs are trilaminar. At these later stages *Emx-1* expression is confined to neurons, but it is expressed in all layers except layer 1. This contrasts with *Otx-1* expression which occurs predominately in layers 5 and 6 and the ventricular zone. At present no functional data on *Otx-1* or the *Emx* genes is available from knock-out or transgenic experiments in the mouse. However a recent screen of human disorders that affect cerebral cortex development has revealed that mutations in *EMX-2* (the human cognate of *Emx-2*) show haplo-insufficiency and give rise to a condition called schizencephaly (Brunelli *et al.*, 1996). In severe cases of this condition large regions of the cerebral hemispheres may be missing and replaced by cerebrospinal fluid. In others a cleft forms within the cerebral hemispheres characterized by an infolding of gray matter where the cortical pia mater and ventricular ependyma become fused. In four patients, four different loss of function mutations of *EMX-2* were found. The phenotypes in schizencephaly are consistent with a failure of cortical neuroblast proliferation. Further examination of null mutations of *Emx-1*, *Emx-2* and *Otx-1* in mice will be very informative.

BF-1 *genes.* *BF-1* is another gene with dramatic consequences for development of the dorsal telencephalon (Xuan *et al.*, 1995). *BF-1* is a member of the *forkhead* winged helix–loop–helix family of transcription factors. *BF-1* is expressed throughout the dorsal telencephalon, and extends ventrally into the developing ganglionic eminence (*Figure 11.4*; Tao and Lai, 1992; Tole and Patterson, 1995). The *BF-1* expression domain is adjacent to that of a related gene, *BF-2*, which is expressed in the rostral diencephalon and the temporal half of the retina and optic stalk. These expression patterns are established early, before the telencephalon/diencephalon boundary is apparent, and suggest a role in forebrain patterning. The importance of *BF-1* has been shown by gene targeting (Xuan *et al.*, 1995). *BF-1* –/– null mutants die at birth with a dramatic 95% reduction in the development of the cerebral hemispheres and olfactory

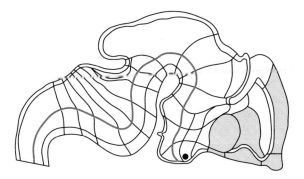

Figure 11.4. Guide to expression of *BF 1*.

bulbs. Analysis of day 9.5 gestation mutant embryos showed that the deficit was not in the initial patterning of the telencephalon but in proliferation of cells in the telencephalic neuroepithelium after day 10.5 of gestation. Further analysis showed that the ventral telencephalon was more severely affected since ventral markers such as *Pax-6*, *Dlx-1* and *Dlx-2* were not detected; in contrast dorsal markers including *Emx-1* and *Emx-2* were still expressed. A second phenotype was a precocious differentiation of neurons, seen as an increase in the proportion of cells that had exited from the cell cycle and expressed the pre-plate marker MAP2. This suggests a premature withdrawal of cells from the ventricular zone in the mutants and a depletion of the progenitor cell population. In this analysis the *Otx* genes were not examined, but expression of the *Emx* genes in the dorsal telencephalon suggests that they may function in a different pathway. In contrast to *BF-1*, *BF-2* disruption only causes subtle anomalies, in the forebrain. Instead, homozygotes died neonatally with severe kidney defects resulting from poor growth and differentiation of the mesenchyme stromal cell lineage (Hatini *et al.*, 1996).

Pax *genes*. *Pax* genes are one of the most extensively studied group of regulatory genes expressed in the CNS. There are nine murine *Pax* genes, which all share the conserved sequence of the 128 amino acid paired box which is common to the *Drosophila* segmentation genes *paired, gooseberry distal* and *gooseberry proximal*. In addition, *Pax-3*, *Pax-6* and *Pax-7* have a paired-type 61 amino acid homeodomain, whereas *Pax-1*, *Pax-2* and *Pax-8* have only the first helix of this domain. Temporal analysis of expression suggests that the *Pax* genes can be split into two classes. *Pax-3*, *Pax-6* and *Pax-7* are expressed in the neural tube from about E8–8.5, that is before cellular differentiation, whilst the *Pax-2*, *Pax-5* and *Pax-8* genes are not expressed until about E10 and are expressed in postmitotic cells only.

The *Pax-3*, *Pax-6* and *Pax-7* genes may have a primary function in neural patterning, which is particularly evident in the developing spinal cord where gene expression is spatially restricted on the D–V axis (Stuart *et al.*, 1994). *Pax-3* is expressed in the ventricular zone of the alar plate and in the roof plate along the entire A–P axis of the neural tube. *Pax-7* (defined as a paralogous gene to *Pax-3*) has a similar expression pattern but is excluded from the roof plate. In contrast *Pax-6* is expressed in the ventricular zone of the basal plate.

At midgestation in the brain, the rostral limit of *Pax-2*, *Pax-8* and *Pax-5* delineates the hindbrain–midbrain boundary. *Pax-3*, *Pax-6* and *Pax-7* are expressed more rostrally, in the diencephalon, and are found to respect proposed prosomeric boundaries; in the adult, *Pax* gene expression is maintained in structures that respect the history of their neuromeric territories (Stoykova and Gruss, 1994). At 12.5 days of gestation, *Pax-3* and *Pax-7* have overlapping expression in the epithalamus and pretectum, whereas *Pax-6* is expressed in the ventral thalamus and epithalamus (dorsal to the fasciculus retroflexus). No *Pax* gene is expressed in the dorsal thalamus (*Figure 11.5*). *Pax-6* is also expressed in the dorsal and lateral parts of the telencephalon and in the developing olfactory and optic epithelia. Since the regional expression of these genes is initiated before overt segmentation can be identified, they may be involved in establishing regional identities and in the development of axonal pathways at the borders of their expression domains. However at present the targets of *Pax* gene regulation are largely unknown.

Natural mutations have been found in three *Pax* genes, *Pax-1*, *Pax-3* and *Pax-6*. *Pax-1* is mutated in the *undulated* mouse mutant, though this gene is not expressed in the CNS. *Pax-3* is mutated in *splotch* mice, for which there are six different mutant alleles. Homozygous *splotch* mice die at about day 14 of gestation and have a number of neural tube, neural crest and brain defects (Epstein *et al.*, 1991). Mutations in *HuP2*, the human homolog of *Pax-3*, are also seen in humans, and result in Waardenburg's syndrome type I, an important genetic cause of sensorineural deafness (Tassabehji *et al.*, 1992)

Pax-6 mutations have also been found in mice and humans, as well as in rats. In each case similar phenotypes are observed. In humans, heterozygous mutations in *Pax-6* cause aniridia, a semidominant disorder that disrupts development of the eye. The equivalent mouse and rat mutants are *small eye* (*Sey*) (Hill *et al.*, 1991; Matsuo *et al.*, 1993) for which a number of alleles exist. Heterozygous animals have microphthalmia, and homozygotes die at birth with disrupted eye development as well as lack of nasal cavities and olfactory bulbs, and abnormalities in cortical plate formation. Widespread *Pax-6* expression in the anterior neural plate might give patterning information that imparts competence to form the eyes and olfactory epithelia. The optic and olfactory placodes form through interaction between the neural ectoderm and the surface ectoderm which then undergo a process of invagination to form the eyes and

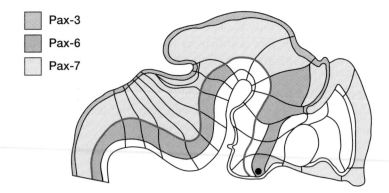

Figure 11.5. Guide to expression of *Pax-3*, *-6* and *-7*.

nasal epithelia. The function of *Pax-6* in this morphogenetic process is unclear, but analysis of *Sey/Sey* cells in chimeric fetuses has shown that *Pax-6* acts cell autonomously to control the fate of lens and nasal neurectoderm (Quinn *et al.*, 1996). It is also likely that *Pax-6* may be required to maintain cell proliferation.

Interestingly, a homolog of *Pax-6* called *eyeless* (*ey*) has recently been identified in *Drosophila* (Quiring *et al.*, 1994). The conservation between *Pax-6* and *ey* is exceptional at 95% amino acid identity and has led to the proposal that *Pax-6* represents an evolutionary conserved master gene that determines the fate of photoreceptive cells. In *Drosophila*, *ey* is expressed in the ventral nerve cord and brain of the larva, and then in the imaginal disk of the eye where it may have an early determinative function. The conservation of *Pax-6* function in eye determination has been demonstrated in *Drosophila*, where ectopic expression of *Pax-6* or *ey* can respecify imaginal disk cells to form ectopic eyes, for example on legs, wings or antennae (Halder *et al.*, 1995). This conserved function is particularly remarkable given the extreme differences in structure and function of the vertebrate eye and of the compound eye of insects, and has led to a re-evaluation of eye evolution (reviewed by Macdonald and Wilson, 1996).

11.2.5 Dlx *and* Nkx *genes*

While the dorsal telencephalon forms a laminar structure the basal telencephalon and diencephalon form structures composed of discrete nuclei. The development of basal structures is associated with different sets of homeobox-containing genes, which include *Dlx-1*, *Dlx-2*, *Nkx-2.1*, *Nkx-2.2* and *Gbx-2* (Bulfone *et al.*, 1993a,b; Price *et al.*, 1992). Extensive *in situ* hybridization analysis has revealed highly complex patterns of gene expression.

Dlx *genes*. *Dlx-1* and *Dlx-2* are members of the highly conserved *distal-less* family of genes that have been implicated in the specification of positional information in the head in a number of species, including *Drosophila*, *Xenopus*, newt, zebrafish and mice (Akimenko *et al.*, 1994; Papalopulu and Kintner 1993; Porteus *et al.*, 1991; Price *et al.*, 1991). In *Drosophila*, *distal-less* (*dll*), the founder member of this family, is required for the development of sensory organs in the larva and the distal components of appendages in the adult (Cohen and Jürgens, 1989). In mice six *distal-less* related genes have now been cloned and analyzed, four of which, *Dlx-1*, *Dlx-2*, *Dlx-5* and *Dlx-6* (Simeone *et al.*, 1994) have major sites of expression in the developing ventral forebrain (as well as other regions, including cranial neural crest). A role for these genes in patterning the brain was proposed from the observation that expression appears to respect prosomeric boundaries in the basal forebrain. Expression of individual genes is not restricted to single segments (*Figure 11.6*). Rather, expression is seen in longitudinal domains that encompass more than one segment, furthermore there is considerable overlap in the expression of these different genes. For example at day 13 of gestation, *Dlx-1* and *Dlx-2* are expressed above the alar/basal boundary in prosomeres p3 to p6 of the diencephalon and telencephalon, in regions fated to become the ventral thalamus, the posterior and anterior entopeduncular areas, the anterior preoptic area, the medial and lateral ganglionic eminences and the septum (Bulfone *et al.*, 1993a,b). But expression is excluded from the presumptive anterior hypothalamus supraoptic/paraventricular area, the eminentia thalami, the posterior preoptic area and the caudal ganglionic eminence.

Functional analysis of the *Dlx* genes was put underway by gene-targeting in the mouse (Qui *et al.*, 1995). *Dlx-2* null mutants are viable at birth but die shortly after-

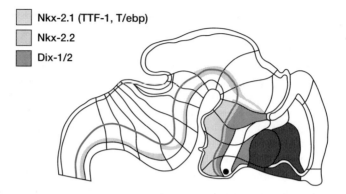

Figure 11.6. Guide to expression of *Dlx* and *Nkx* group genes.

wards. The main phenotypes observed are associated with abnormal development of the cranial neural crest cells contributing to the first and second branchial arches, which results in abnormal craniofacial morphologies. Despite a proposed role for the *Dlx* genes in regional specification in the forebrain, no overt changes in brain development were observed. The expression patterns of other markers, including *Dlx-1*, *Dlx-5*, *Nkx-2.1* and *Emx-1*, that are co-expressed with or share boundaries of gene expression with *Dlx-2* were unaltered in the *Dlx-2* null mutants. One exceptional phenotype was loss of tyrosine hydroxylase (TH) expression in the periglomerular neurons of the olfactory bulb. Although loss of TH expression in these neurons could reflect an immature state of differentiation or altered identity it is also possible that the loss of TH expression reflects poor or inappropriate contact of olfactory receptor neurons in the olfactory bulb since this is known to determine TH expression.

The lack of more extensive neuronal phenotypes implies genetic redundancy in *Dlx* function which would not be too surprising given the co-expression of *Dlx-2* with *Dlx-1* in all domains in the forebrain. Furthermore, although not yet fully reported, it is implied in the report by Rubenstein and colleagues that *Dlx-2/Dlx-1* double mutant animals do exhibit phenotypes that are not present in the single gene mutants (Qui *et al.*, 1995).

Nkx-2 *genes*. The *Nkx-2* genes constitute one of the most widely conserved families of homeobox-containing genes. They are related to the *Drosophila NK-2* gene, and may have conserved functions. Homologs have been identified in several species including mice, zebrafish and *Xenopus* (Barth and Wilson, 1995; Price *et al.*, 1992; Saha *et al.*, 1993). These genes have a highly conserved 60 amino acid homeodomain and downstream a conserved 17 amino acid region known as the NK box. In addition, the mouse *Nkx-2* genes have a conserved decapeptide near the N-terminus (Rudnick *et al.*, 1994). In the mouse *Nkx-2.2* and *Nkx-2.1* are two of six *Nkx-2* genes that have so far been identified and are expressed in the developing brain.

The *Drosophila NK-2* gene is one of the earliest to be expressed in the ventrolateral neurogenic anlage in the procephalic region of *Drosophila*, and has recently been shown to be the gene responsible for the *ventral nervous system defective* (*vnd*) phenotype (Jimenez *et al.*, 1995). *NK-2* is expressed in horizontal stripes of the developing neuroepithelium and is regulated by D–V patterning mechanisms (reviewed in

Nirenberg *et al.*, 1995). Analysis of *vnd* mutant flies shows that *NK-2* is required for the development of specific neuroblasts (Skeath *et al.*, 1994). Neuroblasts are progenitors of all the neurons and glia that make up the nervous system. In development, neuroblasts become individually specified from proneural cell clusters within the neuroepithelium (reviewed by Doe and Skeath, 1996). The specification of each proneural cell cluster is precisely determined and depends upon both positional and temporal cues provided by pair-rule segmentation genes and D–V patterning genes that activate the expression of distinct 'proneural genes' such as members of the *achaete-scute* complex. The currently favored model proposes that following activation of the proneural genes, the cell with the highest levels of proneural gene expression within each proneural cell cluster goes on to become a neuroblast. Neuroblast commitment of the selected cell within a cluster is initiated by activation of 'neurogenic genes' that mediate a process of 'lateral inhibition' that leads to repression of proneural gene expression (and loss of neuronal competency) in adjacent cells within the proneural cell cluster.

Since in *vnd* mutants selected neuroblasts fail to delaminate from the neuroepithelium, *NK-2* may give critical patterning information to confer D–V identity to proneural cell clusters (possibly by activation of proneural genes). In addition, the spatial regulation of *NK-2* expression is itself of paramount importance and has been determined by studying its expression on different mutant backgrounds (Mellerick and Nirenberg, 1995). In wild-type embryos *NK-2* is expressed in the ventrolateral neurogenic anlage and part of the procephalic region to form two longitudinal stripes of expressing cells. Expression of *NK-2* is activated in the ventral half of the embryo by the *Dorsal* gene in conjunction with *twist*, but the precise domain of expression is determined by repression in the mesodermal and mesectodermal anlage by the *snail* and *single minded* genes respectively, while in the lateral neurectoderm and dorsal epidermal anlagen *NK-2* repression is mediated via *decapentaplagic* signaling (Mellerick and Nirenberg, 1995).

In vertebrates, analysis of *Nkx-2.2* loss and gain of function mutants will be particularly interesting. In the mouse, *Nkx-2.2* is first expressed in the rostral neural plate of the 1-somite stage embryo (Price *et al.*, 1992). Subsequently, by day 10.5 of gestation *Nkx-2.2* is expressed in two ventrolateral stripes of cells along the length of the neural tube and extending into the forebrain, ventral to the boundary between the alar and basal plates and adjacent to the longitudinal stripe of cells expressing the signaling molecule *Sonic hedgehog* (Shimamura *et al.*, 1995). This pattern is continuous apart from a deflection in the diencephalon, where a narrow band of expressing cells demarcate the future zona limitans intrathalamica, a boundary between the dorsal and ventral thalami. There are also small discontinuities in expression at rhombomere boundaries in the hindbrain. This pattern of expression is established by the ventralizing actions of *Shh* and possibly dorsalizing signals that determine the D–V axis of the neural tube. Following the definition of a longitudinal domain of gene expression, *Nkx-2.2* expression in the forebrain is maintained in narrow bands in the developing thalami and hypothalamus. The early expression patterns of the *Xenopus* (*XeNK-2*) and zebrafish (*nk2.2*) homologs are essentially the same.

The *Nkx-2.2* expression pattern is notable for retaining its D–V position from the earliest stages. In the spinal cord, *Nkx-2.2* is expressed in the ventrolateral domain in which motor neurons develop. It is possible that *Nkx-2.2* provides the patterning information required for the regulation of motor neuron-specific differentiation genes such as *Islet-1* (*Isl-1*; Appel *et al.*, 1995) a member of the LIM domain family of homeobox-containing transcription factors. Recent gene-targeting of *Isl-1* in mice shows that it is essential for motor neuron development but does not affect D–V patterning within the neural tube (Pfaff *et al.*, 1996). In *Isl1 –/–* mutants the expression domains of regionally expressed markers including *Nkx-2.2*, *Pax3*, *Msx1/2*, *HNF3β* and *Shh* were unaffected. Interestingly in *Isl1 –/–* mutants a secondary phenotype was observed on the fate of a class of interneurons that express the marker *engrailed-1*. This observation demonstrates that cell differentiation involves sequential cell–cell interactions and that differentiation is not solely dependent on cell position.

In the forebrain *Nkx-2.2* might also provide patterning information (*Figure 11.6*). One important function of its expression may be to help define the longitudinal axis of the CNS below the alar/basal plate boundary. Of particular interest, the development of the first longitudinal axonal tracts in the forebrain have been mapped by whole mount immunohistochemistry with markers such as αN-catenin or class III β-tubulin (Easter *et al.*, 1993; Mastick and Easter 1996). The first major tracts originate in the anterobasal nucleus, ventral to the optic chiasma and project back as the postoptic commissure following the longitudinal domain defined by the ventral band of *Nkx-2.2* expression. Establishment of longitudinal domains throughout the CNS may be a common feature; dorsal to *Nkx-2.2* the *Dbx-2* gene is expressed in a longitudinal domain that overlaps the alar/basal plate border (Shoji *et al.*, 1996).

Nkx-2.1 *gene.* In the forebrain, *Nkx-2.1* is expressed ventrally in the anterior neuroepithelium, partially overlapping *Nkx-2.2* in the hypothalamic area. *Nkx-2.1* is also expressed more anteriorly in the basal ganglia primordium of the floor of the telencephalic vesicles (*Figure 11.6*). Unlike *Nkx-2.2*, *Nkx-2.1* expression does not extend caudally into the midbrain region (Kimura *et al.*, 1996; Lazarro *et al.*, 1991).

The function of *Nkx-2.1* has been studied by gene-targeting in embryonic stem cells. Analysis of *Nkx-2.1* null mutant fetuses showed that *Nkx-2.1* has an essential function in the development of the ventral forebrain. Severe defects were seen throughout most ventral structures in which *Nkx-2.1* is normally expressed. For example the tuberal hypothalamus and the ventromedial and dorsomedial nuclei were reduced in size and fused in the midline. The arcuate and premammillary nuclei were missing, as were the mammillary and supramammillary nuclei in the posterior hypothalamus. An additional striking phenotype is absence of the pituitary.

The abnormalities were mostly seen as a failure of the development of particular structures rather than a field defect in patterning. This would be consistent with a conserved *NK-2* family transcription factor function in cell commitment, in response to given patterning cues. It is particularly consistent with the loss of specific subsets of neuroblasts in the *NK-2* mutant of *Drosophila*. Outside of the brain *Nkx-2.1* is expressed in the lung and thyroid (*Nkx-2.1* is also known as *TTF-1*, thyroid transcription factor; or thyroid-specific enhancer-binding protein *T/ebp*; Guazzi *et al.*, 1990) and mutation of the gene results in complete loss of these organs in development. Although in the brain the downstream targets for *Nkx-2.1* transcriptional regulation are unknown, there are considerable molecular data on its role in the activation of thyroid- and lung-specific genes. Overall, it seems that members of the *Nkx-2* family may be involved in commitment and differentiation of neurons in a region-specific manner. The proposed role of *Nkx-2* genes is summarized in *Figure 11.7*.

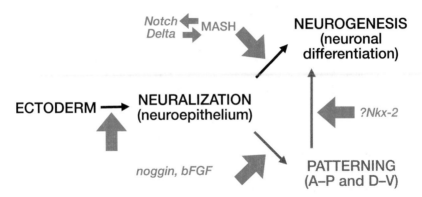

Figure 11.7. Neuronal differentiation pathway. Ectoderm is neuralized in response to inducing factors such as noggin and bFGF which probably also impart patterning information on the A–P axis. Differentiation of neurons within the neuroepithelium depends on proneural (such as mammalian *achaete-scute* homologs; MASH) and neurogenic (*Notch* and *Delta* homologs) genes (Chitnis and Kintner, 1996). The observation that vertebrate forebrain neurons develop later than those in the remainder of the CNS has led to speculation that A–P patterning is also a necessary prerequisite for neurogenesis (shown as gray arrows). *Nkx-2* group genes may have a role in this process.

11.2.6 Dorsal–ventral patterning: the role of the notochord as a ventral organizer

D–V patterning of the neural tube is initiated very early in development as a consequence of polarizing signals from nonneuronal tissue (mesoderm) that juxtaposes the neurectoderm. These signals initiate the process of neurogenesis and involve the complex action of both positive and negative regulators of neural fate (reviewed by Simpson, 1995). The mesodermal cells which comprise the notocord, that underlies the neural keel, are responsible for providing ventralizing signals to the neural tube. The first organizing function of the notochord is to induce the differentiation of floor plate cells in the ventral midline of most of the neural tube. Floor plate cells are a distinctive set of nonneuronal cells which exert critical developmental functions (*Figure 11.8*). Firstly, they act as a secondary ventral organizing center within the neural tube. Secondly, floor plate cells play a key role in axonal guidance mechanisms at later stages of development. Requirement of the notochord to induce floorplate development has been shown by embryological transplantation or extirpation experiments.

HNF3β *gene.* The importance of the notochord has also been shown genetically in mutant embryos that lack expression of the gene *HNF3β*, which is a member of the *forkhead* family of winged helix–loop–helix transcription factors (Kaufmann and Knöchel, 1996). *HNF3β* is one of a number of regulatory genes expressed in the node (a group of cells with organizing activity located at the anterior end of the primitive streak) and is subsequently expressed in the notochord and ventral midline of the entire neural tube (Monaghan *et al.*, 1993). Lack of *HNF3β* disrupts the D–V patterning of the neural tube with the primary effect being failure of floor plate differentiation (Ang and Rossant, 1994). Cells that normally develop adjacent to the floor plate, and express early motor neuron markers such as the LIM domain transcription factor Islet-

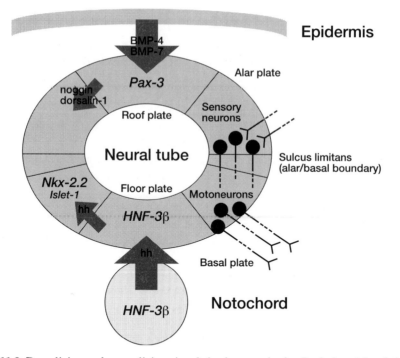

Figure 11.8. Dorsalizing and ventralizing signals in the neural tube. Both dorsal (roof plate) and ventral (floor plate) centers are present on this schematic cross-section of the developing spinal cord, which is the best characterized part of the neural tube. (Left) Interaction between these systems probably defines the boundaries of expression of genes such as *Nkx-2.2* which show restricted domains on the D–V axis. Putative signaling molecules are shown in roman, and transcription factors in italics. It is not certain that the signaling molecules diffuse as implied by the arrows (see text).

1, are also missing. Interestingly, in the absence of normal differentiation of ventral structures the expression domains of dorsal genes were expanded ventrally. For example *Pax-3* expression extended beyond the alar boundary and sometimes encompassed the whole neural tube in mutant embryos. The fact that dorsal markers are expanded ventrally implies that ventralizing signals also act to restrict the spread of dorsalizing signals as well as more straightforward ventral specification, and that the fate of lateral cells is dependent on the combined action of dorsalizing and ventralizing signals.

While the notochord and floor plate have crucial organizing functions for most of the neural tube, they do not extend to the most anterior regions of the developing forebrain, ending at the caudal mammillary area. Instead, the most anterior neuroepithelium develops over prechordal plate mesoderm. Mesodermal cells in this region, although not organized into a discrete structure like the notochord, nevertheless retain similar properties to notochordal cells. Importantly, they too express *HNF3β* and act to induce *HNF3β* in the overlying ventral neuroepithelium of the prosencephalon. Thus the ventral midline of the neural tube is extended from the anterior end of the floor plate up to the optochiasmatic region.

Although prechordal plate mesoderm has similar functions to the notochord in this regard, its development is under different control. One of the most dramatic gene targeting experiments that has been performed was at the *Lim-1* locus (Shawlot and

Behringer, 1995). *Lim-1 –/–* mutant fetuses develop to late gestation but completely lack head structures. This shows that head and trunk development are regulated by different organizing activities. In *Lim-1 –/–* embryos at E7.5 the node was disorganized and embryos lacked prechordal mesoderm and a head process.

HNF3β probably exerts its effects by activating the transcription of ventralizing signaling molecules that then act to differentiate naive progenitor cells in the neuroepithelium. Ectopic expression of *HNF3β* can induce ventral structures but only at selected ectopic sites, for example in the dorsal region of the hindbrain (Sasaki and Hogan, 1994). These studies suggest that *HNF3β* can only exert its ventralizing effects in competent, or regionally specified tissues. In the notochord and floor plate a major gene that is activated is the signaling molecule sonic hedgehog (*Shh*).

Sonic hedgehog gene. *Shh* is a member of the *hedgehog* family of signaling molecules related to the *Drosophila hh* gene (Echelhard *et al.*, 1993; Krauss *et al.*, 1993). In *Drosophila* just one *hh* gene has been found, although in vertebrates this has been expanded to form a family of related signaling molecules. HH proteins are secreted molecules and are proposed to act as either short- or long-range morphogens in different systems. In the notochord and ventral neural tube *Shh* is induced by *HNF3β*, and is the strongest candidate for directly exerting the ventralizing functions of the notochord. The mechanism by which HH proteins function is uncertain since receptors for *hedgehog* signaling have not been identified. The picture is also complicated since IIH proteins undergo autoproteolytic cleavage and hence different moieties of the protein may have different functions. *Shh* is synthesized as a 45 kDa precursor protein but cleaves itself to produce an active 20 kDa N-terminal product (SHH-N), which remains largely cell associated and is the major signaling component. SHH-C may be diffusible and have longer range effects, although no activity of the C-terminal cleavage product has yet been shown. Interestingly, studies with recombinant peptides *in vitro* show the effects on differentiation of progenitor cells to be concentration dependent which supports the notion that SHH-N could act as a diffusible morphogen; at high concentrations floor plate markers are induced, and at low concentrations motor neuron development is induced. However, although SHH is secreted, analysis of SHH distribution by immunohistochemistry showed that SHH is not present as a gradient away from its expression source, and may remain cell-associated, raising the possibility that *in vivo* Shh just acts as a short range signaling molecule and is an intermediate in a signaling cascade (Marti *et al.*, 1995).

Shh is expressed in an almost continuous stripe (together with *HNF3β*) down the length of the neural tube, so it may therefore act as a common ventralizing signal for both caudal and anterior CNS development (Ericson *et al.*, 1995). There are two notable exceptions to the continuity of *Shh* expression. First, expression deviates from the midline in the diencephalon and skirts the paramedian plate, the presumptive hypothalamic region, and second, expression is expanded dorsally into the zona limitans intrathalamica (Barth and Wilson, 1995; Shimamura *et al.*, 1995). This later expression may be of particular importance for forebrain patterning as it provides a transverse band of cells with potential polarizing activity.

Candidate target genes for *Shh* signaling are regulatory genes expressed in cell domains that run adjacent to cells that express *Shh*. Ectopic expression of *Shh* is able to induce the expression of floor plate markers at ectopic sites. In the floor plate *Shh* induces an autoregulatory loop by activating *HNF3β* expression that goes on to further activate *Shh*, thereby providing a local source of ventralizing signal. In addition, in zebrafish a second *hedgehog* gene *tiggywinkle hedgehog* is induced, which could represent a cascade of *hedgehog* signaling molecule gene expression. Cells adjacent to the floor plate, in the ventrolateral part of the neural tube are induced by *Shh* to express the homeobox gene *Nkx-2.2* and the LIM domain gene *Islet-1* (Barth and Wilson, 1995). For a function in regulating D–V patterning, possible regulation of *Nkx-2.2* by *Shh in vivo* is particularly interesting. *Nkx-2.2* is expressed in two longitudinal stripes of cells dorsal to cells that express *Shh*. If the function of *Shh* is to induce *Nkx-2.2*, the result is to define a domain of cells in the ventrolateral position on the D–V axis in the basal plate.

In zebrafish, *hh* expression in the ventral midline of the diencephalon is also required for proper eye development. An effect of ectopic *hh* expression is the downregulation of *Pax-6* and up-regulation of *Pax-2* (Ekker *et al.*, 1995b). A role for vertebrate *hh* genes in patterning the eye is also consistent with a similar function in *Drosophila* in which *hh* is involved in ommatidia development

The signaling pathways by which HH proteins mediate their effects are not yet clear. In *Drosophila* a number of genes are implicated, including the cAMP-dependent serine/threonine protein kinase (PKA), the transmembrane protein *patched* (*ptc*), the transcription factor *cubitus interruptus* (*ci*), a serine/threonine kinase *fused* (*fu*) and three additional genes, *costal-2* (*Cos²*), *smoothened* (*smo*) and *Suppressor of fused* [*Su(fu)*] (Perrimon, 1995). Of these genes, the function of PKA has gained considerable interest since it was identified in a screen for reagents that antagonize the effects of HH in the imaginal disks of *Drosophila*. Following an extracellular stimulus, binding of cAMP activates the catalytic kinase subunits of PKA to modulate the activities of downstream proteins. The precise relationship between HH and PKA activity remains to be determined; they could act through the same intracellular signaling pathway or converge on the same downstream targets. In vertebrates the relationship between *hh* signaling and PKA activity has been explored further by studying the induction of midbrain dopaminergic neurons in rat embryos (Hynes *et al.*, 1995). When the midbrain region of E9 rat embryos were cultured in the presence of agents that activate cAMP signaling pathways (e.g. forskolin), no cells were detected that expressed either TH or floor plate markers. In contrast, agents that manipulated the activities of protein kinase C, cGMP-dependent protein kinase or protein tyrosine kinases had no effect on floor plate or dopaminergic cell induction.

Other hedgehog *genes.* Although most attention has been paid to *Shh* other *hh* genes have been identified and are implicated in patterning the neural tube. *Hedgehog* genes include zebrafish *tiggywinkle* (Ekker *et al.*, 1995b), *indian* and *desert hedgehog* in the mouse (Echelhard *et al.*, 1993), and in *Xenopus*, *banded* and *cephalic hedgehog* (*X-bhh*, *X-chh*; Ekker *et al.*, 1995). *X-bhh* and *X-chh* in addition to *X-Shh* are expressed in anterior and neural ectoderm where they have profound patterning activities. These genes can induce cement gland formation (an anterior structure in *Xenopus*) and induce forebrain and pituitary markers such as *X-OtxA* and *XANF-2* respectively and reduce the expression of posterior markers such as *Krox-20* and *XlHbox-6*. *X-bhh* was also found to have a synergistic effect on neural induction in activin-treated animal cap assays (Lai *et al.*, 1995). Therefore the *hh* gene can be considered as a neural inducing gene (along with *noggin* and *follistatin*) in addition to exerting patterning influences.

Dorsalizing signals. Patterning of the neural tube is achieved through an interaction of ventralizing and dorsalizing signals (*Figure 11.8*; reviewed by Roelink, 1996). Transplantation studies have shown that dorsalizing signals emanate from epidermal ectoderm that lies adjacent to the lateral edges of the neural plate and that eventually come together at the dorsal midline following neurulation (Dickinson *et al.*, 1995). In such grafts, the dorsal markers *Wnt-1* and *Wnt-3a*, and early neural crest markers *slug*, and HNK-1 are induced, but only once the neural ectoderm has reached a certain level of competence. Thus neural ectoderm from stage 8–10 chick embryos can be induced but younger (stage 4) neural ectoderm can not.

A screen for dorsalizing molecules expressed in nonneural ectoderm has identified members of the *TGFβ* superfamily of signaling molecules, the bone morphogenetic proteins *BMP-4* and *BMP-7* (Liem *et al.*, 1995; see Hogan, 1996 for review). These two proteins can induce dorsal cell types, neural crest cells and commissural neurons in neural plate explants *in vitro*. As SHH induces a ventralizing center in the floor plate, the BMPs induce a dorsalizing center in the roof plate. BMPs increase the expression of the transcription factors *Pax-3* and *Msx-1* and a third dorsalizing gene, *Dorsalin-1*, is induced in the roof plate. *Dorsalin-1* is also a *TGFβ* family member and can induce the expression of dorsal genes in competent neurectoderm. The roof plate is also characterized by *Pax-3* expression which extends into the forebrain.

A second secreted molecule that is expressed in the roof plate is noggin which is of particular interest, as in the mouse at E10, its expression extends the length of the neural tube right to the end of the prosencephalic plate (Shimamura *et al.*, 1995; Valenzuela *et al.*, 1995). From studies in *Xenopus*, noggin has a clear neural-inducing activity (Sharpe, 1994). *Noggin* expression in the dorsal midline may be involved in signaling specific cell fates. Early in *Xenopus* development noggin has more pleiotropic functions. It is first involved in dorsal fate specification of mesoderm, and subsequently acts as a neural inducer. When tested for neural inducing activity by adding it to animal cap explant cultures, noggin induces neural differentiation with the expression of anterior fate markers such as *XOtx2*. In contrast the neural inducer bFGF induces neural tissue expressing posterior markers such as *Hox-B9*. When neural tissue is induced by noggin together with bFGF in early gastrula ectoderm, the explants develop with distinct A–P polarity, marked by *XOtx2* expression at one end and *Hox-B9* at the other. However, more interestingly these explants also express the hindbrain/midbrain markers *Krox-20* and *En-2*, that are not expressed by either noggin or bFGF alone (Lamb and Harland, 1995). Thus neural fate is determined by the combination of factors present, and as has also been shown, by the age and competence of the responding ectoderm.

11.3 Future prospects

We have reviewed some of the advances made in recent years in understanding mechanisms and some selected genes involved in the early patterning of the CNS. The prospects for future studies are enormous and fairly daunting. In addition to those genes discussed here, there are hundreds of others that have been cloned, and for which expression data and some functional data are available. Putative transcription factors include additional homeobox-containing genes (Stein *et al.*, 1996), and families of genes with the *POU* domain (Sharp and Morgan, 1996), helix–loop–helix motifs (Kageyama *et al.*, 1995), LIM domain (Sánchez-García and Rabbitts, 1994), leucine zippers and a large number of zinc finger-containing genes (Struhl, 1989), additional *forkhead* genes (Kaufmann and Knöchel, 1996) and others. Secondly, the list of genes involved in the intercellular signaling is also growing rapidly. This includes molecules such as members of the Wnt family (Shimamura *et al.*, 1994), the hedgehog genes, and genes involved in regulating retinoic acid (Sucov and Evans, 1995), as well as cell receptors such as the *Eph* family of receptor tyrosine kinase genes (Friedman and O'Leary, 1996) and receptor tyrosine phosphatases (Chiang and Flanagan, 1996).

Clearly, given the diverse gene products listed above, a major task for the forthcoming years is to study how these different genes interact to achieve normal development; for example to establish the hierarchies of gene expression in the embryological contexts of cell interactions and positional information. In the mouse this will be partly achieved by the continued use of gene targeting and the development of conditional mutation strategies (Kilby *et al.*, 1993). Conventional routes of transgenesis will also be important to dissect the regulation of key genes.

One important advance has been the development of the prosomeric model of forebrain development which has provided a framework upon which the huge volume of data on gene expression patterns can be interpreted. Despite this volume of data our current knowledge is very descriptive. Therefore the future emphasis will be to assign functions to the various genes that have temporally and spatially restricted expression patterns. Many of the genes characterized are transcription factors and presumably function within regulatory cascades. Identification and analysis of downstream 'effector' genes will give insights into how patterning and neural inducing activities are translated into the differentiation of specific types of neuron and the generation of neural networks.

Acknowledgments

N.D.A. is a BBSRC advanced fellow. J.N.P. is on the University of Cambridge Clinical School MB/PhD Programme.

References

Acampora D, Mazan S, Lallemand Y, Avantaggiato V, Maury M, Simeone A, Brulet P. (1995) Forebrain and midbrain regions are deleted in *Otx2–/–* mutants due to a defective anterior neurectoderm specification during gastrulation. *Development* 121: 3279–3290.

Akimenko M-A, Ekker M, Wegner J, Lin W, Westerfield M. (1994) Combinatorial expression of three zebrafish genes related to *Distal-less*: part of a homeobox gene code for the head. *J. Neurosci.* 14: 3475–3486.

Ang S-L, Rossant J. (1994) *HNF3β* is essential for node and notochord formation in mouse development. *Cell* 78: 561–574.

Appel B, Korzh V, Glasgow E, Thor S, Edlund T, Dawid IB, Eisen JS. (1995) Motorneuron fate specification revealed by patterned LIM homeobox gene expression in embryonic zebrafish. *Development* 121: 4117–4125.

Barth KA, Wilson SW. (1995) Expression of zebrafish Nk2.2 is influenced by sonic hedgehog/vertebrate hedgehog-1and demarcates a zone of neuronal differentiation in the embryonic forebrain. *Development*, 121: 1755–1768.

Beddington RSP. (1994) Induction of a second neural axis by the mouse node. *Development* 120: 613–620.

Brunelli S, Faiella A, Capra V, Nigro V, Simeone A, Cama A, Boncinelli E. (1996) Germline mutations in the homeobox gene *EMX-2* in patients with severe schizencephaly. *Nature Genetics* 12: 94–96.

Bulfone A, Kim H-J, Puelles L, Porteus MH, Grippo JF, Rubenstein JLR. (1993a) The mouse *Dlx-2* (*Tes-1*) gene is expressed in spatially restricted domains of the forebrain, face, limbs in midgestation mouse embryos. *Mech. Dev.* **40**: 129–140.

Bulfone A, Puelles. L, Porteus MH, Frohman MA, Martin GR, Rubenstein JLR. (1993b) Spatially restricted expression of *Dlx-1, Dlx-2(Tes-1), Gbx-2,* and *Wnt-3*, in the embryonic day 12.5 mouse forebrain defines potential transverse and longitudinal segmental boundaries. *J. Neurosci.* **13**: 3155–3172.

Chiang M-K, Flanagan JG. (1996) PTP-NP, a new member of the receptor protein tyrosine phosphatase family, implicated in development of nervous system and pancreatic endocrine cells. *Development* **122**: 2239–2250.

Chitnis A, Kintner C. (1996) Sensitivity of proneural genes to lateral inhibition affects the pattern of primary neurons in *Xenopus* embryos. *Development* **122**: 2295–2301.

Cohen SM, Jürgens G. (1989) Proximal-distal pattern formation in *Drosophila*: cell autonomous requirement for *distal-less* gene activity in limb development. *EMBO J.* **8**: 2045–2055.

Dickinson ME, Selleck MAJ, McMahon AP, Bronner-Fraser M. (1995) Dorsalization of the neural tube by non-neural ectoderm. *Development* **121**: 2099–2106.

Doe CQ, Skeath JB. (1996) Neurogenesis in the insect central nervous system. *Curr. Opin. Neurobiol.* **6**: 18–24.

Easter SS, Ross LS, Frankfurter A. (1993) Initial tract formation in the mouse brain. *J. Neurosci.* **13**: 285–299.

Echelhard Y, Epstein DJ, St-Jacques B, Shen L, Mohler J, McMahon J, McMahon AP. (1993) Sonic hedgehog, a member of a family of putative signaling molecules, is implicated in the regulation of CNS polarity. *Cell* **75**: 1417–1430.

Ekker SC, McGrew LL, Lai C-J, Lee JJ, von Kessler DP, Moon RT, Beachy PA. (1995a) Distinct expression and shared activities of members of the hedgehog gene family in *Xenopus laevis*. *Development* **121**: 2337–2347.

Ekker SC, Ungar AR, Greenstein P, von Kessler DP, Porter JA, Moon RT, Beachy PA. (1995b) Patterning activities of vertebrate hedgehog proteins in the developing eye and brain. *Curr. Biol.* **5**: 944–955.

Epstein DJ, Vekemans M, Gros P. (1991) *Splotch(Sp^{2H})*, a mutation affecting development of the mouse neural tube, shows a deletion within the paired homeodomain of *Pax-3*. *Cell* **67**: 767–774.

Ericson J, Muhr J, Placzek M, Lints T, Jessel TM, Edlund T. (1995) *Sonic hedgehog* induces the differentiation of ventral forebrain neurons: a common signal for ventral patterning within the neural tube. *Cell* **81**: 747–756.

Figdor MC, Stern CD. (1993) Segmental organization of the embryonic diencephalon. *Nature* **363**: 630–634.

Finkelstein R, Bonncinelli E. (1994) From fly head to mammalian forebrain: the story of *otd* and *Otx*. *Trends Genet.* **10**: 310–315.

Fishell G. (1995) Striatal precursors adopt identities in response to local cues. *Development* **121**: 803–812.

Fishell G, Mason CA, Hatten ME. (1993) Dispersion of neural progenitors within the germinal zones of the forebrain. *Nature* **362**: 636–638.

Fraser SE, Keynes R, Lumsden A. (1990) Segmentation in the chick embryo hindbrain is defined by cell lineage restrictions. *Nature* **344**: 431–435.

Friedman GC, O'Leary DDM. (1996) Eph receptor tyrosine kinases and their ligands in neural development. *Curr. Opin. Neurobiol.* **6**: 127–133.

Guazzi S, Price M, De Felice M, Damante G, Mattei M-G, Di Lauro R. (1990) Thyroid nuclear factor (*TTF-1*) contains a homeodomain and displays a novel DNA binding specificity. *EMBO J.* **9**: 3631–3639.

Gulisano M, Brocoli V, Pardini C, Boncinelli E. (1996) *Emx-1* and *Emx-2* show different patterns of expression during proliferation and differentiation of the developing cerebral cortex in the mouse. *Eur. J. Neurosci.* **8**: 1037–1050.

Guthrie S. (1996) Patterning the hindbrain. *Curr. Opin. Neurobiol.* **6**: 41–48.

Halder G, Callaerts P, Gehring WJ. (1995) Induction of ectopic eyes by targeted expression of the *eyeless* gene in *Drosophila*. *Science* **267**: 1788–1792.

Hatini V, Huh SO, Herzlinger D, Soares VC, Lai E. (1996) Essential role of stromal mesenchyme revealed by targeted disruption of winged helix transcription factor *BF-2*. *Genes Dev.* **10**: 1467–1478.

Hatten ME, Heintz N. (1995) Mechanisms of neural patterning and specification in the developing cerebellum. *Annu. Rev. Neurosci.* **18**: 385–408.

Hill RE, Favor J, Ton CC et al. (1991) Mouse small eye results from mutations in a paired-like homeobox-containing gene. *Nature* **354**: 522–525.

Hirth F, Stavros T, Loop T, Gehring WJ, Reichert H, Furukuba-Tokunaga. (1995), Developmental defects in brain segmentation caused by mutations of the homeobox genes *orthodenticle* and *empty spiracles* in *Drosophila*. *Neuron* **15**: 769–778.

Hogan BLM. (1996) Bone morphogenetic proteins: multifunctional regulators of vertebrate development. *Genes Dev.* **10**: 1580–1594.

Hynes M, Porter JA, Chiang C, Chang D, Tessier-Levigne M, Beachy PA, Rosenthal A. (1995) Induction of midbrain dopaminergic neurons by sonic hedgehog. *Neuron* **15**: 35–44.

Jiménez F, Martin-Morris LE, Velasco L, Chu H, Sierra J, Rosen DR, White K. (1995) *vnd*, a gene required for early neurogenesis of *Drosophila*, encodes a homeodomain protein. *EMBO J.* **14**: 3487–3495.

Kageyama R, Sasai Y, Akazawa C, Ishibashi M, Takebayashi K, Shimizu C, Tomita K, Nakanishi S. (1995) Regulation of mammalian neural development by helix-loop-helix transcription factors. *Crit. Rev. Neurobiol.* **9**: 177–188.

Kaufmann E, Knöchel W. (1996) Five years on the wings of *forkhead*. *Mech. Dev.* **57**: 3–20.

Keynes R, Krumlauf R. (1994) *Hox* genes and the regionalisation of the nervous system. *Annu. Rev. Neurosci.* **17**: 109–132.

Kilby NJ, Snaith MR, Murray JAH. (1993) Site-specific recombinases – tools for genome engineering. *Trends Genet.* **9**: 413–421.

Kimura S, Hara Y, Pineau T, Fernandez-Salguero P, Fox CH, Ward JM, Gonzalez FJ. (1996) The *T/ebp* null mouse: thyroid-specific enhancer-binding protein is essential for the organogenesis of the thyroid, lung, ventral forebrain and pituitary. *Genes Dev.* **10**: 60–69.

Krauss S, Concordet J-P, Ingham PW. (1993) A functionally conserved homolog of the *Drosophila* segment polarity gene *hh* is expressed in tissues with polarizing activity in zebrafish embryos. *Cell* **75**: 1431–1444.

Krumlauf R. (1994) *Hox* genes in vertebrate development. *Cell* **78**: 191–201.

Lai C-J, Ekker SC, Beachy PA, Moon RT. (1995) Patterning of the neural ectoderm of *Xenopus laevis* by the amino-terminal product of hedgehog autoproteolytic cleavage. *Development* **121**: 2349–2360.

Lamb TM, Harland RM. (1995) Fibroblast growth factor is a direct neural inducer, which combined with noggin generates anterior–posterior neural pattern. *Development* **121**: 3627–3636.

Lazzaro D, Price M, De Felice M, Di Lauro R. (1991) The transcription factor *TTF-1* is expressed at the onset of thyroid and lung morphogenesis and in restricted regions of the fetal brain. *Development* **13**: 1093–1104.

Liem KFJ, Tremml G, Roelink H, Jessell TM. (1995) Dorsal differentiation of neural plate cells induced by BMP-mediated signals from the epidermal ectoderm. *Cell* **82**: 969–979.

Lumsden A, Keynes R. (1989) Segmental pattern of neuronal development in the chick hindbrain. *Nature* **337**: 424–428.

Macdonald R, Wilson SW. (1996) *Pax* proteins and eye development. *Curr. Opin. Neurobiol.* **6**: 49–56.

Marti E, Takada R, Bumcrot DA, Sasaki H, McMahon AP. (1995) Distribution of *sonic hedgehog* peptides in the developing chick and mouse embryo. *Development* **121**: 2537–2547.

Mastick GS, Easter SS. (1996) Initial organisation of neurons and tracts in the embryonic mouse fore- and midbrain. *Devel. Biol.* **173**: 79–94.

Matsuo I, Osumi-Yamashita N, Noji S et al. (1993) A mutation in the Pax-6 gene in rat small eye is associated with impaired migration of midbrain crest cells. *Nature Genetics* **3**: 299–304.

Matsuo I, Kuratani S, Kimura C, Takeda N, Aizawa S. (1995) Mouse *Otx2* functions in the formation and patterning of the rostral head. *Genes Dev.* **9**: 2646–2658.

Mellerick DM, Nirenberg M. (1995) Dorsal–ventral patterning genes restrict *NK-2* homeobox gene expression of the ventral half of the central nervous system of *Drosophila* embryos. *Devel. Biol.* **171**: 306–316.

Millen KJ, Hui CC, Joyner AL. (1995) A role for En-2 and other murine homologues of Drosophila segment polarity genes in regulating positional information in the developing cerebellum. *Development* **121**: 3935–3945.

Monaghan AP, Kaestner KH, Grau E, Schütz G. (1993) Postimplantation expression patterns indicate a role for the mouse *forkhead/HNF3α, β, γ* gene in determination of the definitive endoderm, chordamesoderm and neuroectoderm. *Development*, **119**: 567–578.

Nirenberg M, Nakayama K, Nakayama N, Kim Y, Mellerick D, Wang L-H, Webber KO, Lad R. (1995) The *NK-2* homeobox gene and the early development of the central nervous system of *Drosophila*. *Ann. N.Y. Acad. Sci.* 224–242.

Papalopulu N, Kintner C. (1993) *Xenopus Distal-less* related homeobox genes are expressed in the developing forebrain and are induced by planar signals. *Development* 117: 961–975.

Perrimon N. (1995) Hedgehog and beyond. *Cell* 80: 517–520.

Pfaff SL, Mendelsohn M, Stewart CL, Edlund T, Jessel TM. (1996) Requirement for LIM homeobox gene *Isl1* in motor neuron generation reveals a motor neuron-dependent step in interneuron differentiation. *Cell* 84: 309–320.

Porteus MH, Bulfone A, Ciaranello RD, Rubenstein JLR. (1991) Isolation and characterisation of a novel cDNA clone encoding a homeodomain that is developmentally regulated in the ventral forebrain. *Neuron* 7: 221–229.

Price M, Lemaistre ML, Pischetola M, Di Lauro R, Duboule D. (1991) A mouse gene related to *Distal-less* shows a restricted expression in the developing forebrain. *Nature* 351: 748–750.

Price M, Lazzaro D, Pohl T, Mattei M-G, Rüther U, Oliv J-C, DuBoule D, DiLauro R. (1992) Regional expression of the homeobox gene *Nkx-2.2* in the developing mammalian forebrain. *Neuron* 8: 241–255.

Puelles L, Rubenstein JLR. (1993) Expression patterns of homeobox and other putative regulatory genes in the embryonic mouse forebrain suggest a neuromeric organisation. *Trends Neurosci.* 16: 472–479.

Qui M, Bulfone A, Martinez S, Meneses JJ, Shimamura K, Pedersen RA, Rubenstein JLR. (1995) Null mutation of *Dlx-2* results in abnormal morphogenesis of proximal first and second branchial arch derivatives and abnormal differentiation in the forebrain. *Genes Dev.* 9: 2523–2538.

Quinn JC, West JD, Hill RE. (1996) Multiple functions for *Pax6* in mouse eye and nasal development. *Genes Dev.* 10: 435–446.

Quiring R, Walldorf U, Kloter U, Gehring WJ. (1994) Homology of the *eyeless* gene of *Drosophila* to the *small eye* gene in mice and *aniridia* in humans. *Science* 265: 785–789.

Roelink H. (1996) Tripartite signaling of pattern: interactions between hedgehogs, BMPs and Wnts in the control of vertebrate development. *Curr. Opin. Neurobiol.* 6: 33–40.

Rudnick A, Ling TY, Odagiri H, Rutter WJ, German MS. (1994) Pancreatic beta cells express a diverse set of homeobox genes. *Proc. Natl Acad. Sci. USA* 91: 12 203–12 207.

Ruiz i Altaba A. (1994) Pattern formation in the vertebrate neural plate. *Trends Neurosci.* 17: 233–243.

Saha MS, Michel RB, Gulding KM, Grainger RM. (1993) A *Xenopus* homeobox gene defines dorsal–ventral domains in the developing brain. *Development* 118: 193–202.

Sánchez-García I, Rabbitts TH. (1994) The Lim domain: a new structural motif found in zinc-finger-like proteins. *Trends Genet.* 10: 315–320.

Sasaki H, Hogan BL. (1994) *HNF3 beta* as a regulator of floor plate development. *Cell* 76: 103–115.

Schneider-Maunoury S, Topilko P, Seitandou T, Levi G, Cohen-Tannoudji M, Pournin S, Babinet C, Charnay P. (1993) Disruption of Krox-20 results in alteration of rhombomeres 3 and 5 in the developing hindbrain. *Cell* 75:1199–214.

Sharp ZD, Morgan WW. (1996) Brain POU-er. *Bioessays* 18: 347–350.

Sharpe C. (1994) Noggin – the neural inducer or a modifier of neural induction? *Bioessays* 16: 159–160.

Shawlot W, Behringer RR. (1995) Requirement for *Lim1* in head-organizer function. *Nature* 374: 425–430.

Shimamura K, Hirano S, McMahon AP, Takeichi M. (1994) Wnt-1-dependent regulation of local E-cadherin and alpha N-catenin expression in the embryonic mouse brain. *Development* 120: 2225–2234.

Shimamura K, Hartigan DJ, Martinez S, Puelles L, Rubenstein JLR. (1995) Longitudinal organisation of the anterior neural plate and neural tube. *Development* 121: 3923–3933.

Shoji H, Ito T, Wakamatsu Y, Hayasaka N, Ohsaki K, Oyanagi M, Kominami R, Kondoh H, Takahashi N. (1996) Regionalized expression of the *Dbx* family homeobox genes in the embryonic CNS of the mouse. *Mech. Dev.* 56: 25–39.

Simeone A, Acampora D, Gulisano M, Stornaiuolo A, Boncinelli E. (1992a) Nested expression domains of four homeobox genes in the developing rostral brain. *Nature* 358: 687–690.

Simeone A, Gulisano M, Acampora D, Stornaiuolo A, Rambaldi M, Boncinelli E. (1992b) Two vertebrate homeobox genes related to the *Drosophila empty spiracles* gene are expressed in the embryonic cerebral cortex. *EMBO J.* 11: 2541–2550.

Simeone A, Acampora D, Pannese M *et al.* (1994) Cloning and characterization of two members of the vertebrate Dlx genefamily. *Proc. Natl Acad. Sci. USA* 91: 2250–2254.

Simpson P. (1995) Positive and negative regulators of neural fate. *Neuron* 15: 739–742.

Skeath JB, Panganiban GF, Carroll SB. (1994) The *ventral nervous system defective* gene controls proneural gene expression at two distinct steps during neuroblast formation in *Drosophila*. *Development* **120**: 1517–1524.

Spemann H. (1938) *Embryonic Development and Induction.* Yale University Press/ Garland Publishing, New Haven, CT.

Stein S, Fritsch R, Lemaire L, Kessel M. (1996) Checklist: vertebrate homeobox genes. *Mech. Dev.* **55**: 91–108.

Stoykova A, Gruss P. (1994) Roles of *Pax*-genes in developing and adult brain as suggested by expression patterns. *J. Neurosci.* **14**: 1395–1412.

Struhl K. (1989) Helix-turn-helix, zinc-finger, and leucine-zipper motifs for eukaryotic transcriptional regulatory proteins. *Trends Biochem. Sci.* **14**: 137–140.

Stuart ET, Kioussi C, Gruss P. (1994) Mammalian *Pax* genes. *Annu. Rev. Genet.* **28**: 219–236.

Sucov HM, Evans RM. (1995) Retinoic acid and retinoic acid receptors in development. *Mol. Neurobiol.* **10**: 169–184.

Tao W, Lai E. (1992) Telencephalon-restricted expression of BF-1, a new member of the *HNFβ /fork head* gene family, in the developing rat brain. *Neuron* **8**: 957–969.

Tassabehji M, Read AP, Newton VE, Harris R, Balling R, Gruss P, Strachan T. (1992) Waardenburg's syndrome patients have mutations in the human homologue of the *Pax-3* paired box gene. *Nature* **355**: 635–636.

Tole S, Patterson. (1995) Regionalization of the developing forebrain: a comparison of FORSE-1, Dlx-2 and BF-1. *J. Neurosci.* **15**: 970–980.

Valenzuela DM, Economides AN, Rojas E et al. (1995) Identification of mammalian *noggin* and its expression in the adult nervous system. *J. Neurosci* **15**: 6077–6084.

Xuan S, Baptista CA, Balas G, Tao W, Soares VC, Lai E. (1995) Winged helix transcription factor BF-1 is essential for the development of the cerebral hemispheres. *Neuron* **14**: 1141–1152.

Yuebing L, Allende ML, Finkelstein R, Weinberg ES. (1994) Expression of two zebrafish *orthodenticle*-related genes in the embryonic brain. *Mech. Dev.* **48**: 229–244

Neuronal plasticity

Brian J. Morris

12.1 Introduction

Neurons possess the ability to alter certain aspects of their biochemical and morphological character in response to changes in their local environment or their level of activity. This plasticity presumably allows them to adapt and survive in their altered circumstances, or to assume a different functional role. Neurons are far from being unique in this respect, and many, perhaps the majority, of different cell types in the body show some degree of plasticity. However, it can be argued that neurons have brought this particular part of the repertoire of cellular response to its highest level of sophistication. The plastic changes observed in neurons following a stimulus can be short or long-lasting, subtle or dramatic. A large number of different mechanisms can be invoked, and the changes that are induced can occur in isolation or be part of a complex, coordinated response.

Perhaps the simplest approach to discussing the large number of different processes which can contribute to neuronal plasticity is to separate two distinct temporal components of the altered sensitivity (a rapid phase, apparent within a few milliseconds and lasting up to around 3 h, and a later phase, sustained by entirely different cellular mechanisms, and lasting from 2–3 h up to a number of weeks). These distinct temporal phases are clearly observed in the various experimental models of functional neuronal plasticity, and have been characterized most extensively in the paradigm of hippocampal long-term potentiation (LTP)

12.2 Experimental models of neuronal plasticity

12.2.1 Hippocampal LTP

LTP was first observed in the hippocampal formation, a brain region with a role in the processes of learning and memory. While it has since become clear that LTP can be detected in many different brain regions, the likelihood remains that the phenomenon provides a basis for a learning-like change in the properties of networks of neurons (Bliss and Collingridge, 1993). Activity-dependent changes in the efficiency of synaptic transmission are observed in particular pathways: typically a brief high-frequency burst of stimulation results in a potentiation of transmission that can last for many days *in vivo*. During this time a number of temporal components can be identified, each caused by the activation of distinct intracellular mechanisms (Bliss and Collingridge, 1993).

Molecular Biology of the Neuron, edited by R.W. Davies and B.J. Morris.
© 1997 BIOS Scientific Publishers Ltd, Oxford.

At the synapses of two of the major hippocampal pathways – the perforant path/dentate gyrus synapses, and the Schaffer collateral/CA1 synapses – the induction of LTP is dependent on activation of the N-methyl-D-aspartate (NMDA) class of glutamate receptor (see Chapter 8). This receptor has the unique property of allowing Ca^{2+} influx in a manner that is subject to a voltage-dependent block by Mg^{2+} ions. If high-frequency afferent stimulation results in sufficient release of glutamate from the presynaptic terminals, there will be enough postsynaptic depolarization (mediated by nonNMDA glutamate receptors) to remove the Mg^{2+} blockade, and the NMDA receptor will allow influx of Ca^{2+} ions (*Figure 12.1a*).

At another major hippocampal synapse – the mossy fiber/CA3 synapse – induction of LTP is not dependent on NMDA receptor activation, and it has been suggested that metabotropic glutamate receptors (Conquet *et al.*, 1994) or opioid receptors (Morris and Johnston, 1995) may be involved. Peptide neurotransmitters would appear to be particularly convenient mediators of synaptic plasticity, since there is a great deal of evidence, from both the peripheral and central nervous systems, that peptides which coexist with conventional neurotransmitters may only be released by high frequency nerve activity. It is easy to imagine opioid peptides, which are present in the mossy fibers, playing a role in the LTP that follows high frequency mossy fiber firing (*Figure 12.1b*). At this synapse, the intracellular pathways transducing the stimulus for plasticity may involve primarily cAMP elevations, rather than Ca^{2+} (Huang *et al.*, 1994).

The mechanisms involved in hippocampal LTP are unlikely to be unique to that brain region or experimental paradigm. Indeed, there is a great deal of evidence that similar mechanisms operate in many of the other forms of neuronal plasticity that have been studied, such as LTP in the basal ganglia (Kombian *et al.*, 1994), long-term depression (LTD) in the hippocampus, cerebellum, or basal ganglia (Kombian and Malenka, 1994; Nakazawa *et al.*, 1993), or the sensitization to excitatory stimuli that occurs during limbic system 'kindling'.

12.2.2 Limbic system kindling

In limbic system kindling, electrodes are chronically implanted in regions of the limbic system such as the hippocampus or amygdala. A daily or twice-daily stimulus is then applied, at a constant level which initially has no overt behavioral effect. Over a

---

Figure 12.1. Schematic diagram of two cellular mechanisms where high frequency firing of afferent fibers leads to a sustained enhancement in synaptic efficiency. (a) Under normal (low) rates of firing, the Mg^{2+} block of the NMDA receptor (NR) prevents any Ca^{2+} influx into the postsynaptic spine. Synaptic transmission is mediated by Na^+ influx through AMPA receptors (AR). Higher firing rates produce sufficient depolarization to relieve the Mg^{2+} block, and the ensuing Ca^{2+} influx through the NMDA receptor activates calcium-dependent enzymes in the spine to alter synaptic properties. The induction of LTP in the CA1 region of the hippocampus is thought to follow such a mechanism. (b) Neuropeptides (for example opioid peptides), stored in a separate population of vesicles, coexist with glutamate in the afferent fibers. Under normal (low) rates of firing, only glutamate is released, and AMPA (or kainate) receptors mediate synaptic transmission). Higher rates of firing result in peptide release as well, and the postsynaptic (or presynaptic) peptide receptors (PR) then activate G proteins (G) and alter the activity of cAMP-dependent enzymes to affect synaptic properties. The induction of LTP in the CA3 region of the hippocampus is thought partially to follow such a mechanism.

period of weeks, this same stimulus starts to produce a behavioral response, eventually leading to a generalized seizure. Once this sensitization phenomenon, or kindling, has occurred, the same stimulation will continue to produce a seizure whenever it is given, even if no stimulation has been given for a number of days or weeks. The sensitivity of the kindling procedure to blockade by antagonists of the NMDA receptor, along with the ability of NMDA and related agonists to precipitate seizure activity, both *in vivo* and *in vitro*, has provided strong evidence that NMDA receptors are involved at some stage in the plastic process.

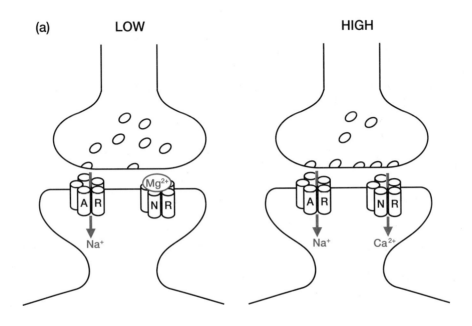

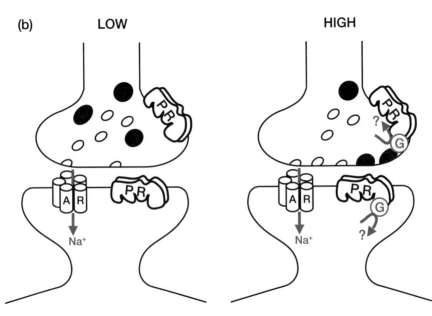

procedure is widely used as an experimental model for epilepsy, and
l and morphological changes observed in the hippocampi from kin-
e similar to those detected in the brains of patients with temporal lobe

12.2.3 Cerebellar LTD

Purkinje cells in the cerebellum receive synaptic input from both climbing fibers and
parallel fibers. Simultaneous stimulation of both inputs results in a long-lasting
depression of transmission at the parallel fiber synapses, and the phenomenon has
been suggested to form the basis of cerebellar motor learning and memory. In this
case, NMDA receptors are not involved: rather, it is the D,L-amino-3-hydroxy-5-
methyl-4-isoxalone propionic acid (AMPA) class of glutamate receptor, most likely in
association with metabotropic receptors (Conquet *et al.*, 1994) and nitric oxide release
(Nakazawa *et al.*, 1993), that provides the initial stimulus.

12.2.4 Invertebrate models

The marine snail *Aplysia* has been exploited to study the cellular mechanisms underlying plastic phenomena because of the relatively large size of its neurons and the
simplicity of the nervous system which they form. A simple reflex, where a gill is
withdrawn following a stimulus to its body, is enhanced by an unconditioned stimulus to another part of the body. Serotonin released from an interneuron by the unconditioned stimulus raises cAMP levels and protein kinase A (PKA) activity in the sensory neuron involved in the reflex. Morphological changes, including presynaptic
varicosity outgrowth, also seem to play a role in the consolidation of the synaptic plasticity (Glanzman *et al.*, 1990). As with hippocampal LTP, the slower, sustained phase
of the plastic response (which can last for days) is dependent on the synthesis of new
proteins, while the rapid phase is not (Barzilai *et al.*, 1989).

Studies of *Drosophila melanogaster* (fruitfly) with learning deficits in simple behavioral tasks (i.e. avoiding flying towards odors associated with electric shocks) have
identified various gene mutations which are presumably affecting memory processes
and the associated synaptic plasticity. Once more, this type of learning can be shown
to have a rapid phase which is not dependent on protein synthesis, followed by a
slower, protein synthesis-dependent phase.

12.3 Ca²⁺ as the trigger

The involvement of NMDA receptors in many forms of neuronal plasticity suggests
that Ca^{2+} influx may be the initial stimulus that activates the intracellular processes contributing to neuronal plasticity. This is consistent with the fact that many of the intracellular mechanisms thought to be important for neuronal plasticity are dependent on
elevations in intracellular Ca^{2+} (see below). However, the spatial and temporal pattern of
Ca^{2+} influx may be critical for determining the changes that occur. Influx of Ca^{2+}
through voltage-gated channels in hippocampal neurons, for example, produces a different series of responses compared to NMDA receptor activation (Bading *et al.*, 1993)
Furthermore, several different strands of evidence also suggest a role for increased
intracellular cAMP levels. In both mammalian and invertebrate models, those forms of
neuronal plasticity which are not dependent on NMDA receptors are frequently
observed to involve adenylyl cyclase (Alberini *et al.*, 1994; Huang *et al.*, 1994).

12.4 Rapid, transient plasticity

Events at the plasma membrane can trigger rapid alterations in the function of various molecules within the cell by activating a number of different enzymes. In particular, the action of protein kinases, which phosphorylate their various substrate proteins, dominates this type of response. This phosphorylation can, in many cases, markedly alter the characteristics of the protein's function, although, in general, the effects of phosphorylation are relatively short-lived, and the original properties of the protein are later restored by dephosphorylation (through the action of protein phosphatases).

Determination of the molecular structures of neurotransmitter receptors has, in all cases, revealed potential sites for phosphorylation (see Chapters 7 and 8). In many studies using G protein-coupled receptors, it has become clear that receptor phosphorylation is associated with a decreased responsiveness, providing a likely mechanism for the well-characterized phenomenon of desensitization (Chapter 7). Here then is a clear example of how activation of protein kinases can give rise to an altered neuronal sensitivity that outlasts the original stimulus. Phosphorylation of cytoskeletal components is known to result in plasticity in neuronal morphology (see Chapter 4). The rapid rearrangements of synaptic architecture which have been detected during hippocampal LTP may therefore be driven by the activation of kinases.

Two major classes of protein kinases have been identified – the eponymous serine/threonine kinases and the tyrosine kinases – which differ in the amino acid which they phosphorylate on their target protein. In all cases, the target serine, threonine or tyrosine which is phosphorylated is contained within a short sequence of amino acids which forms a consensus recognition site for the kinase. The recognition sequence requirements have been identified with some confidence for many of the serine/threonine kinases, although less is known in the case of the tyrosine kinases (Pearson and Kemp, 1991).

In many cases, not unique to neurons, the kinases function in cascades, where the phosphorylation of the several kinases in sequence broadens and prolongs the functional consequences of the original stimulus. Such cascades can involve serine/threonine kinases, tyrosine kinases, or both. The intracellular control of the phosphorylation state of vast numbers of different proteins must therefore be seen as a dynamic and extraordinarily complex regulatory process. Further details on the role of these kinases in neuronal function can be found in Chapter 9.

The widespread effects in a number of different cell types of activation of cAMP-dependent protein kinase (PKA), cGMP-dependent protein kinase (PKG), mitogen-activated protein kinase (MAP kinase) and protein kinase C (PKC) have been well described. One particular serine/threonine kinase – calcium/calmodulin-dependent protein kinase II (CaMKII) – is found only in the CNS, where it is expressed in neurons.

Mutant mice lacking functional type I (Ca^{2+}-stimulated) adenylyl cyclase show deficits in memory tests and in hippocampal LTP (Wu et al., 1995), suggesting that the convergence of Ca^{2+} and cAMP signaling by this enzyme has an important function in hippocampal plasticity. The induction of hippocampal LTP can also be prevented by selectively inhibiting the action of PKA, PKG, PKC or CaMKII (Bliss and Collingridge, 1993). Inhibition of protein tyrosine kinases also attenuates the induction of hippocampal LTP (O'Dell et al., 1991). These studies have been more or less confirmed by the generation of null recombinant mice lacking the corresponding kinases (Abeliovich *et al.*, 1993; Huang *et al.*, 1995; Silva *et al.*, 1992). This suggests that all of these kinases play a role both in sustaining the earliest phases of LTP, and also in triggering the changes which give rise to the slower, more sustained phases. The fact that LTP can be more or less completely blocked by inhibition of an individual kinase suggests that they each fulfill some critical role in synaptic potentiation.

The molecular structure of CaMKII makes it ideally suited as a switch to convert transient ion fluxes into more enduring changes in neuronal function. Activation of CaMKII by Ca^{2+}/calmodulin, following NMDA receptor activation, results in autophosphorylation of the enzyme, and the consequent generation of a Ca^{2+}-independent form that can maintain the phosphorylating activity in the absence of any further stimulation (Fukuraga *et al.*, 1995). The extraordinarily high concentrations of CaMKII in the synaptic area suggest that the subsequent effects should be dramatic.

Activation of PKA is also essential for synaptic facilitation in *Aplysia* neurons, while in *Drosophila*, the mutants *dunce* and *rutabaga*, isolated in a behavioral screen for associative learning deficits, are deficient in the function of a cAMP-dependent phosphodiesterase and a Ca^{2+}/calmodulin-activated adenylyl cyclase, respectively (Levin *et al.*, 1992; Qui *et al.*, 1991). The actions of adenylyl cyclase and PKA therefore assume a central role in a wide variety of different models of synaptic plasticity.

The target proteins for plasticity-associated phosphorylation in these models have yet to be conclusively identified, but, at least in the mammalian hippocampus, the glutamate receptor subunits are attractive candidates, since phosphorylation by CaMKII, PKC or PKA, and possibly PKG, is known to increase their responsiveness (Dev and Morris, 1994; McGlade-McCulloh *et al.*, 1993; Raymond *et al.*, 1993).

It follows from this clear role of protein kinases in initiating plastic changes in neuronal function that protein phosphatases will be similarly important in regulating the changes that occur. Evidence has been obtained that neuronal phosphatases are essential for normal LTP to occur, and also that the induction of hippocampal LTD may be primarily due to the activation of neuronal phosphatases, with consequent effects on synaptic function opposite to the effects of kinase activation. However, PKA is also required for hippocampal LTD (Brandon *et al.*, 1995).

Other protein modifications apart from phosphorylation are also likely to play a role in rapid neuronal plasticity. Nitric oxide has been suggested to play a role in hippocampal LTP (Böhme *et al.*, 1991). Direct nitrosylation or indirect ADP-ribosylation of proteins by nitric oxide can alter their functional properties (Stammler, 1994), and altered ADP-ribosylation of hippocampal proteins has in fact been detected following induction of LTP (Duman *et al.*, 1993). Also, protein glycosylation may be regulated by neuronal activity. The neuronal cell adhesion molecule NCAM is extensively modified by addition of sialic acid polymers, and the properties of the NCAM molecules are affected by the degree of polysialylation (Doherty *et al.*, 1995). The extent of polysialylation is reported to vary during development and, in the hippocampus, during learning (Doherty *et al.*, 1995; Doyle *et al.*, 1992).

It is generally accepted that a component of hippocampal LTP is expressed presynaptically – that is, the increased efficiency of synaptic transmission is partially due to enhanced neurotransmitter release from the presynaptic terminal (A in *Figure 12.3*). This is likely to result from the action of a retrograde messenger – possibly nitric oxide and/or arachidonic acid – released from the postsynaptic dendrite and acting on the presynaptic terminal. Assuming this to be correct, then it can be assumed that the mechanism leading to increased transmitter release involves phosphorylation or some other covalent modification of presynaptic target proteins (Herrero *et al.*, 1992; Meffert *et al.*, 1994)

12.5 Slower, sustained plasticity

In contrast to these earlier phases of neuronal plasticity, which rely heavily on modifications to existing proteins, there is abundant evidence that the later, most sustained phases of LTP are dependent on the synthesis of new proteins (Bliss and Collingridge, 1993). The later phases of plasticity therefore involve mechanisms to increase the rate of synthesis of specific proteins. Since, for perhaps the majority of cellular proteins, mRNA availability is the rate-limiting step in protein synthesis (Hargrave and Schmidt, 1989), attention has focused on changes in mRNA levels which can be detected in association with plastic phenomena.

12.5.1 Transcription factor families

One group of genes which show increased transcription relatively rapidly (15–45 min) after the stimulus encode transcription factors (TFs) (Sheng and Greenberg, 1990). These genes are classified as immediate-early genes (IEGs), in that their increased expression is fast, and is not dependent on the synthesis of other proteins.

A large number of TFs have been identified, and many of these have been shown to be expressed in neurons. These various TFs can be divided into a number of families with closely related structures. In relation to neuronal plasticity, much interest has centered on a group of TFs which contain within their protein sequence a region of basic amino acids and also a region containing regularly spaced leucine residues (*Figure 12.2a*). There is evidence that this latter structure forms a 'leucine zipper' to dimerize with another TF of the same structural family, and hence the group of TFs have become known as the bZIP family. While the leucine zipper allows the formation of functional homo- or heterodimers, the basic region is the part of the molecule that interacts with the promoter region of the target DNA. The dimer adopts a three-dimensional conformation reminiscent of a pair of scissors, with the basic region (the blades of the scissors) gripping the DNA (Glover and Harrison, 1995). An impression of the structure is shown in *Figure 12.2b*).

This family includes the widely studied *c-fos* gene, along with other related genes (*fos B*, *fos-related antigen*) and the jun proteins (c-jun, junB, junD). A major target of protein dimers formed from these TFs is the AP1 site on genomic DNA, which has the typical sequence TGAGTCA. However, a closely related sequence, TGACGTCA, is known as the cAMP-response element (CRE), and is involved in the transcriptional activation of many genes in response to elevated intracellular cAMP levels. The so-called CRE-binding protein (CREB) can be a component of the dimers that can bind to the CRE, and also has a bZIP structure (Ziff, 1990). A number of 'activating transcription factors' with homology to CREB also belong to this family. One bZIP protein, known commonly as C/EBP, may have a particularly important role in neuronal plasticity (see below).

Another family of TFs adopt a three-dimensional structure with finger-like processes, and also contain zinc. Of these 'zinc finger' TFs, zif/268 (Milbrandt, 1987), also known as egr1, NGF-IA and Krox24, has been widely studied, and binds to a target sequence of the form GCGGGGGCG. Other members of this family include Krox20 and egr3.

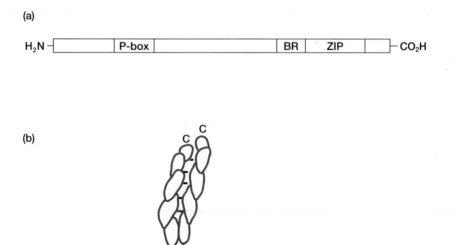

Figure 12.2. (a) Structural motifs common to the bZIP family of transcription factor genes. P box, region containing the phosphorylation sites targeted by protein kinases. BR, basic region (DNA recognition domain). ZIP, region containing regularly spaced leucine residues, responsible for dimerization. (b) Model of the binding of activated bZIP dimers to the target DNA sequence, resulting in the activation of polymerase II, and subsequent transcription of the gene.

Other TF families with a possible but as yet incompletely explored role in neuronal plasticity include those TFs with a basic helix–loop–helix structure, those with a so-called POU domain, which recognize a DNA sequence of the form $(A/T)_{4-5}$ T(A/T)TGCAT, and the rel family related to the inflammatory cell TF NF-κB.

12.5.2 Induction of transcription factors

An increased level of the mRNA encoding junB is observed within a few minutes of induction of LTP in the perforant path synapses on to the hippocampal dentate gyrus (Cole *et al.*, 1989; Wisden *et al.*, 1990). The evidence for other members of the fos/jun family is less clear, but a supramaximal LTP-inducing stimulus, which it has been suggested produces a longer-lasting LTP, results also in increased c-fos expression

(Jeffery *et al.*, 1990). Elevated expression of c-jun has also been observed during hippocampal LTP. The c-fos knockout mouse has failed to confirm an important role for fos in hippocampal plasticity.

The closest correlation between TF expression and LTP induction has been observed for zif/268. High frequency stimulation of perforant path synapses on to dentate granule cells, and of Schaffer collaterals on to CA1 pyramidal cells, results in dramatic increases in zif/268 mRNA levels in the postsynaptic neuron (Cole *et al.*, 1989; Roberts *et al.*, 1996; Wisden *et al.*, 1990). However, even then, there are situations when LTP is clearly expressed without any induction of zif/268, and also cases where zif/268 is induced in the absence of any LTP (Johnston and Morris, 1994a; Wisden *et al.*, 1990). In the former case, this may be related to the fact that other TFs of this family are likely to be involved in hippocampal plasticity. For example, egr3 is also induced by LTP (Yamagata *et al.*, 1994a).

Induction of these TFs is not restricted to the hippocampal LTP model of neuronal plasticity, since induction of cerebellar LTD produces increased levels of zif/268, c-fos and junB mRNA in the postsynaptic Purkinje cells (Nakazawa *et al.*, 1993).

In invertebrate neurons, activation of TFs also appears to be important for sustained plasticity. Proteins of the CREB family are essential for long-term memory in *Drosophila* (Yin *et al.*, 1994). Furthermore, CREB-related proteins, in particular C/EBP, are required for the expression of long-term facilitation in *Aplysia* neurons (Alberini *et al.*, 1994). The complexity of the transcriptional control is emphasized by the finding that ATF4 (CREB2) appears to function as a constitutive repressor of synaptic facilitation in *Aplysia* neurons (Bartsch *et al.*, 1995), possibly by forming an inactive dimer with C/EBP or CREB. Activation of CREB family members has yet to be demonstrated in hippocampal LTP, but a potential role for these proteins is supported by evidence that mice with a targeted disruption of the *CREB* gene lacked the late phase of LTP, and were severely compromised in several tests of associative learning (Bourtchuladze *et al.*, 1994).

A working hypothesis of synaptic plasticity, which incorporates many of the above observations (Alberini *et al.*, 1994), proposes that brief activation of protein kinases results in a local phosphorylation of target proteins (B in *Figure 12.3*). Stronger stimulation results in the translocation of the activated kinase to the nucleus, where it phosphorylates CREB-like TFs. Upon phosphorylation, these TFs then activate other TF genes, such as *zif/268* or *c-fos*, and after transcription and translation have occurred, the pattern of downstream gene expression can be altered (C in *Figure 12.3*).

12.5.3 Induction of other immediate-early genes

Apart from these putative TFs, a number of other genes are also reported to be rapidly induced in hippocampal neurons following high-frequency stimulation (*Table 12.1*). These include the growth factor β-activin (Andreasson and Worley, 1995), the spectrin-like 'arc', the protease tissue plasminogen activator (tPA, Qian *et al.*, 1993), and the prostaglandin synthetic enzyme cyclooxygenase II (cox-2, Yamagata *et al.*, 1993). Each of these genes also appears to be induced during limbic system kindling, which may strengthen the idea that they play some significant role in the plasticity process. However, as with the transcription factors, direct evidence that these proteins are necessary for synaptic plasticity has yet to be obtained. The cox-2 knockout mouse shows no clear symptoms of altered hippocampal function, although it may be relevant

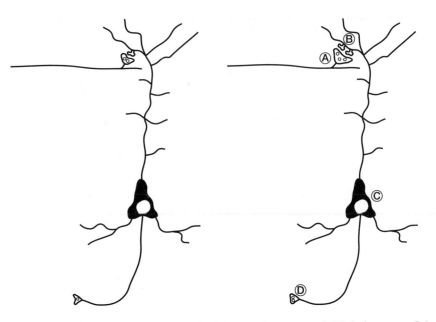

Figure 12.3. Cellular sites where neuronal plasticity may be expressed. High-frequency firing in an afferent fiber on the left of the figure induces a number of sustained changes in the presynaptic terminal and the postsynaptic neuron. A: A retrograde messenger from the postsynaptic cell enhances the amount of neurotransmitter released from the presynaptic terminal by subsequent action potentials. B: Transient activation of postsynaptic protein kinases alters the sensitivity of the synapse to subsequent stimulation, partly by phosphorylating receptor proteins. Also, more slowly, morphological changes in the structure of the dendrite occur in the region of the potentiated synapse, most likely an increase in the number and/or shape of the dendritic spines (Moser *et al.*, 1994). C: Changes in the activity of second messenger systems, may be restricted to the vicinity of the potentiated synapse or to the cell nucleus, maybe extending throughout the cytoplasm. More slowly, an activation of TFs, leading to an altered pattern of gene expression. D: An increase in the efficiency of the next synapse 'in series' ('domino' plasticity), due to elevated expression of presynaptic terminal proteins in the neuron postsynaptic to the original stimulus.

that the tPA knockout mouse is hyporesponsive to seizure stimuli (Tsirka *et al.*, 1995), which implies that tPA may increase the excitability of hippocampal neurons. In addition, recent evidence suggests that there are deficits in LTP induction in the CA1 region of the hippocampus from tPA knockout mice (Frey *et al.*, 1996)

The extent to which these effects are unique to the hippocampus, or even to particular groups of neurons within the hippocampus, remains to be explored, but it has been shown that tPA is also induced in association with cerebellar LTD (Seeds *et al.*, 1995). Evidence is therefore accumulating to suggest that tPA may play some quite fundamental role in the plasticity process.

12.5.4 Induction of late-response genes

The mRNA encoding an IEG is typically induced within 15–45 min of the initial stimulus, and then in most cases the level of mRNA expression has returned to normal within a few hours. A number of genes are induced (or suppressed) with a slower time course, the mRNA levels being altered perhaps 2–3 h after the stimulus, and remaining

Table 12.1. Changes in gene expression in hippocampal LTP

Gene	Function	Direction of change in expression	Time (h)	Reference
c-fos	Transcription factor	Increased	<2	Jeffery et al. (1990), Worley et al. (1993)
c-jun	Transcription factor	Increased	<2	Demmer et al. (1993), Worley et al. (1993)
junB	Transcription factor	Increased	<2	Cole et al. (1989), Wisden et al. (1990)
zif/268	Transcription factor	Increased	<2	Cole et al. (1989), Wisden et al. (1990)
egr3	Transcription factor	Increased	<4	Yamagata et al. (1994a)
rheb	G-protein subunit?	Increased	2	Yamagata et al. (1994b)
CaMKII-α	Protein kinase subunit	Increased	2	Mackler et al. (1992)
		Decreased	24	Thomas et al. (1994a), Johnston and Morris (1995) Roberts et al. (1996)
PKC-γ	Protein kinase subunit	Increased	2–24	Thomas et al. (1994a),
		Decreased		Meberg et al. (1993)
PKC-β	Protein kinase subunit	Unchanged	48–72	Thomas et al. (1994a),
		Decreased		Meberg et al. (1993)
ERK-2	Protein kinase	Increased	24	Thomas et al. (1994a)
raf-B	Protein kinase	Increased	24	Thomas et al. (1994a)
activin	Growth factor	Increased	<2	Andreasson and Worley (1995)
NGF	Growth factor	Increased	3	Castren et al. (1993)
		Unchanged	4	Patterson et al. (1992)
BDNF	Growth factor	Increased	4	Patterson et al. (1992), Castren et al. (1993)
NT3	Growth factor	Increased	4	Patterson et al. (1992)
		Decreased		Castren et al. (1993)
cpg1	Growth factor?	Increased	6	Nedivi et al. (1993)
syntaxin	Vesicle-associated protein	Increased	2–5	Smirnova et al. (1993)
GAP43	Presynaptic, growth-associated protein	Decreased	72	Meberg et al. (1993)
proenkephalin	Peptide neurotransmitter	Increased	24	Morris et al. (1988) Johnston and Morris (1994b)
prodynorphin	Peptide neurotransmitter	Decreased	24	Morris et al. (1988) Johnston and Morris (1994b)
arc	Cytoskeletal protein?	Increased	<2	Link et al. (1995), Lyford et al. (1995)
MAP2	Dendritic cytoskeletal protein	Increased	24	Johnston and Morris (1994c),
		Unchanged		Meberg et al (1993)
tPA	Protease	Increased	<2	Qian et al. (1993) Chen et al. (1995)
neuropsin	Protease?	Decreased	4–24	Chen et al. (1995)
TIMP	Protease inhibitor	Increased	6	Nedivi et al. (1993)
cyclooxygenase 2	Synthetic enzyme	Increased	<2	Yamagata et al. (1993)
NMDA receptor R1	Receptor subunit	Increased	48	Thomas et al. (1994a)

affected for up to 48 h. The lag period before induction/suppression presumably reflects the action of induced TFs, which need to be synthesized and modified before returning to the nucleus to alter the transcription of their target genes. These 'late-response' genes belong to various functional classes, including protein kinases, peptide neurotransmitters, growth factors and proteases (*Table 12.1*).

Considering the function of these different late-response genes, it is clear that a number of genes are affected where the protein will be expressed in the presynaptic terminal of the neuron involved. Such genes include the vesicle-associated protein syntaxin, thought to play a role in exocytosis, and the peptide neurotransmitters. Other presynaptic proteins apart from syntaxin, such as synapsin, are also likely to be induced at the transcriptional level during synaptic plasticity (Lynch *et al.*, 1994). The postsynaptic induction of those genes with a presynaptic function has some interesting functional implications. Induction of the presynaptic proteins and the peptide transmitters suggests a kind of 'domino' plasticity (Morris and Johnston, 1995), where potentiation of a synapse in the hippocampus results, via these changes in gene expression, in potentiation, some hours or days later, of the next synapse 'in series' (*Figure 12.3*). Such a phenomenon has yet to be demonstrated.

Evidence is accumulating to suggest that growth factors have an important acute function in modulating hippocampal excitability (Lo, 1995). However, a number of growth factor genes are modulated at the transcriptional level following the induction of hippocampal LTP, raising the possibility that the subsequent changes in protein levels may exert a long-lasting effect on neurotransmission. Mice lacking a functional brain-derived neurotrophic factor gene show an impaired ability to express hippocampal LTP (Korte *et al.*, 1995), and reduced sensitivity to limbic system kindling (Kokala *et al.*, 1995). In addition, it has recently been suggested that nerve growth factor is involved in the morphological changes in the hippocampus associated with kindling and temporal lobe epilepsy (Van der Zee *et al.*, 1995).

It is clear from *Table 12.1* that increased expression of various protein kinase genes has been detected following induction of LTP. Considering the importance of phosphorylation reactions for the most rapid phase of synaptic plasticity (Section 12.4 above), altered expression of these genes is likely to have a prolonged effect on the earlier responses to subsequent stimulation, and possibly on the later responses as well. Markedly reduced expression of the *CaMKIIα* gene is observed 24 h after hippocampal NMDA receptor stimulation (Johnston and Morris, 1995), and mice carrying a mutation in this gene show spontaneous epileptiform seizures (Butler *et al.*, 1995). This provides strong evidence that a reduction in *CaMKIIα* gene expression following plastic change in the hippocampus leads to a prolonged elevation in hippocampal excitability. A picture emerges of functional plasticity that lasts for days, and includes a component affecting the likelihood of further plastic change. Such alterations may be consolidated by morphological changes, involving the conformation of synapses (*Figure 12.3b*, Moser *et al.*, 1994). The altered expression of proteases and their inhibitors (*Table 12.1*) may be a part of this structural remodeling process.

A small group of genes has been identified, where the time course of induction following the generation of hippocampal LTP is exceptionally slow. It is reported that the levels of the mRNA encoding GAP43 (a protein thought to be involved in the function of the presynaptic terminal) are decreased 3 days after the stimulus, but not earlier (Meburg *et al.*, 1993). Similarly, the levels of mRNA encoding certain splice variants of the NR1 subunit of the NMDA receptor are first found to be increased 48 h after LTP induction (Thomas *et al.*, 1994b).

12.5.5 The relationship between early and late responses

It has not proved possible to link the induction of the above TFs with any of these changes in late-response gene expression. Experiments using transfected cell lines had suggested a possible causal relationship between c-fos induction and increased transcription of the proenkephalin gene, but this has proved not to be the case in CNS neurons (Johnston and Morris, 1994b; Konradi *et al.*, 1993). Induction of zif/268 also does not seem to be involved in regulating hippocampal proenkephalin, prodynorphin or CaMKII expression (Johnston and Morris, 1994c). The best evidence to date linking TF and late-response gene induction suggests that c-fos may regulate nerve growth factor expression (Hengerer *et al.*, 1990), and that zif/268 may regulate synapsin expression (Thiel *et al.*, 1994). The possible role of the various bZIP family members remains an important target for investigation.

12.6 Unanswered questions

Apart from identifying the various TFs or combinations of TFs that produce the altered pattern of late-response gene activation observed in hippocampal LTP (*Table 12.1*), a number of other crucially important issues remain unresolved:

(i)   To what extent are these long-term changes common to other forms of neuronal plasticity? Are there other genes affected uniquely in other paradigms or in other brain areas?

(ii) What other genes are affected in the hippocampus? Clearly the data summarized in *Table 12.1* are unlikely to be complete.

(iii) How important are the various genes recorded in *Table 12.1* for the processes of hippocampal plasticity? Experiments are still largely at the stage of recording the phenomena, rather than directly manipulating the expression of these genes individually and recording the effect on neuronal function. Some progress is starting to be made in this area (Pettit *et al.*, 1994).

(iv) The concept of LTP in the hippocampus is built around the potentiation of transmission at a single synapse. Activating gene transcription in the nucleus of the neuron would appear to lose that exquisite anatomical specificity. Are the gene products then selectively transported back out to the region of the stimulated synapse, or are they then ubiquitously expressed within the neuron to cause a widespread and spatially unrestricted increase in sensitivity?

(v)   How important are post-transcriptional processes in regulating gene expression at the mRNA level during functional plasticity?

(vi) Does 'domino' plasticity actually occur?

An understanding of the molecular mechanisms that combine to generate neuronal plasticity is going to be vital for all aspects of neurobiology. Progress so far has been rapid, and already many of the ingredients have been identified. The challenge is to discover the ones that are missing from the list, and to find out how they are mixed together to produce the final dish.

References

Abeliovich A, Chen C, Goda Y, Silva A, Stevens CF, Tonegawa S. (1993) Modified hippocampal LTP in PKC-γ-deficient mice. *Cell* 75: 1253–1262.

Alberini CM, Ghiradi M, Metz R, Kandel ER. (1994) C/EBP is an immediate-early gene required for the consolidation of long-term facilitation in *Aplysia*. *Cell* 75: 1099–1114.

Andreasson K, Worley PF. (1995) Induction of β-activin expression by synaptic activity and during neocortical development. *Neuroscience* **69**: 781–796.

Bading H, Ginty DD, Greenberg ME. (1993) Regulation of gene expression in hippocampal neurons by distinct calcium signalling pathways. *Science* **260**: 181–185.

Bartsch D, Ghiradi M, Skehel PA, Karl KA, Herder SP, Chen M, Bailey CH, Kandel ER. (1995) *Aplysia* CREB2 represses long-term facilitation: relief of repression converts transient facilitation into long-term functional and structural change. *Cell* **83**: 979–992.

Barzilai A, Kennedy TE, Sweatt JD, Kandel ER. (1989) 5HT modulates protein synthesis and the expression of specific proteins during long-term facilitation in *Aplysia* neurons. *Neuron* **2**: 1577–1586.

Bliss TVP, Collingridge GL. (1993) A synaptic model of memory: long-term potentiation in the hippocampus. *Nature* **361**: 31–39.

Böhme GA, Bon C, Stutzman JM, Doble A, Blanchard JC. (1993) Possible involvement of nitric oxide in LTP. *Eur. J. Pharmacol.* **199**: 379–381.

Bourtchuladze R, Frenguelli B, Blendy J, Cioffi D, Schutz G, Silva AJ. (1994) Deficient long-term memory in mice with a targeted mutation of the cAMP response element binding protein. *Cell* **79**: 59–68.

Brandon EP, Zhuo M, Huang Y-Y, Qi M, Gerhold KA, Burton KA, Kandel ER, McKnight S, Idzerda RL. (1995) Hippocampal long-term depression and depotentiation are defective in mice carrying a targeted disruption of the gene encoding the RIβ subunit of cAMP-dependent protein kinase. *Proc. Natl Acad. Sci. USA* **92**: 8851–8855.

Butler LS, Silva AJ, Abeliovich A, Watanabe Y, Tonegawa S, McNamara JO. (1995) Limbic epilepsy in transgenic mice carrying a CaMKII α-subunit mutation. *Proc. Natl Acad. Sci. USA* **92**: 6852–6855.

Castren E, Pitkanen M, Sirvio J, Parsadanian A, Lindholm D, Thoenen H, Riekkinen PJ. (1993) The induction of long-term potentiation increases BDNF and NGF mRNA but decreases NT-3 mRNA in the dentate gyrus. *Neuroreport* **4**: 895–898.

Chen Z-L, Yoshida S, Kato K et al. (1995) Expression and activity-dependent changes of a novel limbic-serine protease gene in the hippocampus. *J. Neurosci.* **15**: 5088–5097.

Cole AJ, Saffen DW, Baraban JM, Worley PF. (1989) Rapid increase of an immediate-early gene mRNA in hippocampal neurons by synaptic NMDA receptor activation. *Nature* **340**: 474–479.

Conquet F, Bashir Z, Davies C et al. (1994) Motor deficit and impairment of synaptic plasticity in mice lacking mGluR1. *Nature* **372**: 237–243.

Demmer J, Dragunow M, Lawlor PA, Mason SE, Leah JD, Abraham WC, Tate WP. (1993) *Mol. Brain. Res.* **17**: 279–286.

Dev KK, Morris BJ. (1994) Modulation of AMPA binding sites by nitric oxide *J. Neurochem.* **63**: 946–952.

Doherty P, Fazeli MS, Walsh FS. (1995) The neural cell adhesion molecule and synaptic plasticity. *J. Neurobiol.* **26**: 437–446.

Doyle E, Nolan PM, Bell R, Regan CM. (1992) Hippocampal NCAM180 transiently increases sialylation during the acquisition and consolidation of a passive avoidance response in the adult rat. *J. Neurosci. Res.* **31**: 513–523.

Duman RS, Terwilliger RZ, Nestler EJ. (1993) Alterations in nitric oxide stimulated ADP-ribosylation associated with long-term potentiation in rat hippocampus. *J. Neurochem.* **61**: 1542–1545.

Frey U, Mueller M, Kuhl D. (1996) A different form of long-lasting potentiation revealed in tissue plasminogen activator mutant mice. *J. Neurosci.* **16**: 2057–2063.

Fukuraga K, Muller D, Miyamoto E. (1995) Increased phosphorylation of Ca/calmodulin-dependent protein kinase II and its endogenous substrates in the induction of LTP *J. Biol. Chem.* **270**: 6119–6124.

Glanzman DL, Kandel ER, Scacher S. (1990) Target-dependent structural changes accompanying long-term synaptic facilitation in *Aplysia* neurons. *Science* **249**: 799–802.

Glover JNM, Harrison SC. (1995) Crystal structure of the heterodimeric bZIP transcription factor c-fos–c–jun bound to DNA. *Nature* **373**: 257–260.

Hargrave JL, Schmidt FH. (1989) The role of mRNA and protein stability in gene expression. *FASEB J.* **3**: 2360–2378.

Hengerer B, Lindholm D, Heumann R, Ruether U, Wagner EF, Thoenen H. (1990) Lesion-induced increase in nerve growth factor mRNA is mediated by c-fos. *Proc. Natl Acad. Sci. USA* **87**: 3899–3910.

Herrero I, Miras-Portugal T, Sanchez-Prieto J. (1992) Positive feedback of glutamate exocytosis by metabotropic presynaptic stimulation. *Nature* **360**: 163–166.

Huang Y-Y, Li X-C, Kandel ER. (1994) cAMP contributes to mossy fiber LTP by initiating both a covalently mediated early phase and macromolecular synthesis-dependent late phase. *Cell* **79**: 69–79.

Huang Y-Y, Kandel ER, Varshavsky L, Brandon EP, Qi M, Idzerda RJ, McKnight GS, Bourtchouladze R. (1995) A genetic test of the effects of mutations in PKA on mossy fiber LTP and its relation to spatial and contextual learning Cell **83**: 1211–1222.

Jeffery KJ, Abraham WC, Dragunow M, Mason SE. (1990) Induction of c-fos-like immunoreactivity and the maintenance of LTP in the dentate gyrus of unanaesthetised rats. *Mol. Brain. Res.* **8**: 267–274.

Johnston HM, Morris BJ. (1994a) zif/268 does not mediate increases in proenkephalin mRNA levels after NMDA receptor stimulation. *Neuroreport* **5**: 1498–1500.

Johnston HM, Morris BJ. (1994b) Induction of c-fos is not responsible for increased proenkephalin mRNA levels in the hippocampal dentate gyrus following NMDA receptor stimulation. *Mol. Brain. Res.* **25**: 147–150.

Johnston HM, Morris BJ. (1994c) NMDA and nitric oxide increase microtubule-associated protein 2 gene expression in hippocampal granule cells. *J. Neurochem* **63**: 379–382.

Johnston HM, Morris BJ. (1995) *N*-methyl-D-aspartate and nitric oxide regulate the expression of calcium/calmodulin-dependent kinase II in the hippocampal dentate gyrus. *Mol. Brain Res.* **31**: 141–151.

Kokala M, Ernfors P, Kokala Z, Elmer E, Jaenisch R, Lindvall O. (1995) Suppressed epileptogenesis in BDNF mutant mice. *Exp. Neurol.* **133**: 215–224.

Kombian SB, Malenka RC. (1994) Simultaneous LTP of non-NMDA and LTD of NMDA-receptor mediated responses in the nucleus accumbens. *Nature* **368**: 242–244.

Konradi C, Kobierski LA Nguyen TV, Heckers S, Hyman SE. (1993) The cAMP-response element binding protein interacts, but fos does not interact, with the proenkephalin enhancer in rat striatum. *Proc. Natl Acad. Sci. USA* **90**: 7005–7009.

Korte M, Carroll P, Wolf E, Benn G, Thoenen H, Bonheffer T. (1995) Hippocampal LTP is impaired in mice lacking BDNF *Proc. Natl. Acad. Sci. USA* **92**: 8856–8860.

Levin LR, Han P-L, Hwaung PM, Feinstein PG, Davis RL, Reed RR. (1992) Characterisation of the *Drosophila* learning and memory gene *rutabaga* encodes a Ca/calmodulin-responsive adenylyl cyclase. *Cell* **68**: 479–489.

Link W, Konietzo U, Kauselmann G, Krug M, Schwanke B, Frey U, Kuhl D. (1995) Somatodendritic expression of an immediate-early gene is regulated by synaptic activity. *Proc. Natl Acad. Sci. USA* **92**: 5734–5738.

Lo DC. (1995) Neurotrophic factors and synaptic plasticity. *Neuron* **15**: 979–981.

Lyford GL, Yamagata K, Kaufmann WE *et al.* (1995) *Arc*, a growth factor and activity-regulated gene, encodes a novel cytoskeleton-associated protein that is enriched in neuronal dendrites. *Neuron* **14**: 433–445.

Lynch MA, Voss KI, Rodriguez J, Bliss TVP. (1994) Increase in synaptic vesicle proteins accompanies long-term potentiation in the dentate gyrus. *Neuroscience* **60**: 1–4.

Mackler SA, Brooks BP, Eberwine JH. (1992) Stimulus-induced coordinate changes in mRNA abundance in single post-synaptic hippocampal neurons. *Neuron* **9**: 539.

McGlade-McCulloh E, Yamamoto H, Tan S-E, Brickey DA, Söderling TR. (1993) Phosphorylation and regulation of glutamate receptors by CAMKII. *Nature* **362**: 640–643.

Meberg PJ, Barnes CA, McNaughton BL, Routtenberg A. (1993) Protein kinase C and F1/GAP43 gene expression in hippocampus inversely related to synaptic enhancement lasting 3 days. *Proc. Natl Acad. Sci. USA* **90**: 12050–12054.

Meffert MK, Premack BA, Schulman H. (1994) Nitric oxide stimulates Ca-independent synaptic vesicle release *Neuron* **12**: 1235–1244.

Milbrandt J. (1987) A nerve-growth factor-induced gene encodes a possible transcription regulatory factor. *Science* **238**: 797.

Morris BJ, Johnston HM. (1995) A role for hippocampal opioid peptides in long-term functional plasticity. *Trends Neurosci.* **18**: 350–355.

Morris BJ, Feasey KJ, ten Bruggencate G, Herz A, Höllt V. (1988) Electrical stimulation *in vivo* increases the expression of proenkephalin mRNA and decreases the expression of prodynorphin mRNA in rat hippocampal granule cells. *Proc. Natl Acad. Sci. USA* **85**: 3226–3230.

Moser M-B, Trommald M, Andersen P. (1994) An increase in dendritic spine density on hippocampal CA! pyramidal cells following spatial learning in adult rats suggests the formation of new synapses. *Proc. Natl Acad. Sci. USA.* **91**: 12673–12675.

Nakazawa K, Karachot L, Nakabeppu Y, Yamamori T. (1993) The conjunctive stimuli that cause long-term desensitisation also predominantly induce c-fos and junB in cerebellar Purkinje cells. *Neuroreport* **4**: 1275–1278.

Nedivi E, Hevroni D, Naot D, Israeli D, Citri Y. (1993) Numerous candidate plasticity-related genes revealed by differential cDNA cloning. *Nature* **363**: 718–722.

Patterson SL, Grover LM, Schwartzkroin PA, Bothwell M. (1992) Neurotrophin expression in rat hippocampal slices: a stimulus paradigm inducing LTP in CA1 evokes increases in BDNF and NT3 mRNAs. *Neuron* **9**: 1081–1088.

Pearson RB, Kemp BE. (1991) Protein kinase phosphorylation sequences and consensus specificity motifs: tabulations. *Meth. Enzymol.* **200**: 62–81.

Pettit DL, Perlman S, Malinow R. (1994) Potentiated transmission and prevention of further LTP by increased CaMKII activity in postsynaptic hippocampal slice neurons. *Science* **266**: 1881–1886.

Qian Z, Gilbert ME, Colicos MA, Kandel ER, Kuhl D. (1993) Tissue plasminogen activator is induced as an immediate-early gene during seizure, kindling and long-term potentiation. *Nature* **361**: 453–456.

Qui Y, Chen C-N, Malone T, Richter L, Beckendorf SK, Davis RL. (1991) Characterisation of the memory gene dunce of *Drosophila melanogaster*. *J. Mol. Biol.* **222**: 553–565.

Raymond LA, Blackstone CD, Huganir RL. (1993) Phosphorylation of amino-acid neurotransmitter receptors in synaptic plasticity. *Trends Neurosci.* **16**: 147–152.

Roberts LA, Higgins MJ, O'Shaughnessy CT, Stone TW, Morris BJ. (1996) Changes in hippocampal gene expression associated with the induction of long-term potentiation. *Mol. Brain Res.*, in press.

Seeds NW, Williams BL, Bickford PC. (1995) Tissue plasminogen activator induction in purkinje neurons after cerebellar motor learning. *Science* **270**: 1992–1995.

Sheng M, Greenberg ME. (1990) The regulation and function of c-fos and other immediate-early genes in the nervous system. *Neuron* **4**: 477–480.

Silva AJ, Stevens CF, Tonegawa S, Wang Y. (1992) Deficient hippocampal long-term potentiation in CaMKII mutant mice. *Science* **257**: 201–206.

Smirnova T, Laroche S, Errington ML, Hicks A, Bliss TVP, Mallet J. (1993) Trans-synaptic expression of a presynaptic glutamate receptor during hippocampal long-term potentiation. *Science* **262**: 433–437.

Stammler JS. (1994). Redox signalling: nitrosylation and related target interactions of nitric oxide. *Cell* **78**: 931–936.

Thiel G, Schoch S, Petersohn D. (1994) Regulation of synapsin I gene expression by the zinc finger transcription factor zif/268/egr1. *J. Biol. Chem.* **269**. 15 294–15 298.

Thomas KL, Laroche S, Errington ML, Bliss TVP, Hunt SP. (1994a) Spatial and temporal changes in signal transduction pathways during LTP. *Neuron* **13**: 737–745.

Thomas KL, Davis S, Laroche S, Hunt SP. (1994b) Regulation of the expression of NR1 NMDA glutamate receptor subunits during hippocampal LTP. *Neuroreport* **6**: 119–123.

Tsirka SE, Gualandris A, Amaral DG, Strickland S. (1995) Excitotoxin-induced neuronal degeneration and seizure are mediated by tissue plasminogen activator. *Nature* **377**: 340–343.

Van der Zee CEEM, Rashid K, Le K, Moore KA, Stanisz J, Diamond J, Racine RJ, Fahnestock M. (1995) Intraventricular administration of antibodies to nerve growth factor retards kindling and blocks mossy fiber sprouting in adult rats. *J. Neurosci.* **15**: 5316–5323.

Wisden W, Errington ML, Williams S, Dunnett SB, Waters C, Hitchcock D, Evan G, Bliss TVP, Hunt SP. (1990) Differential expression of immediate-early genes in the hippocampus and spinal cord. *Neuron* **4**: 603–614.

Worley PF, Bhat RV, Baraban JM, Erickson CA, McNaughton BL, Barnes CA. (1993) Thresholds for synaptic activation of transcription factors in hippocampus. *J. Neurosci.* **13**: 4776–4788.

Wu Z-L, Thomas SA, Villacres EC, Xia Z, Simmons ML, Chavkin C, Palmiter RD, Storm DR. (1995) Altered behaviour and long-term potentiation in type I adenylyl cyclase mutant mice. *Proc. Natl Acad. Sci. USA* **92**: 220–224.

Yamagata K, Andreasson KI, Kaufmann WE, Barnes CA, Worley PF. (1993) Expresssion of a mitogen-inducible cyclooxygenase in brain neurons: regulation by synaptic activity and glucocorticoids. *Neuron* **11**: 371–379.

Yamagata K, Kaufmann WE, Lanahan A, Papavlou M, Barnes CA, Andreasson KI, Worley PF. (1994a) Egr3/pilot, a zinc finger transcription factor, is rapidly regulated by synaptic activity in brain neurons and colocalises with egr1/zif268. *Learn. Mem.* **1**: 141–152.

Yamagata K, Sanders LK, Kaufmann WE, Yee W, Barnes CA, Nathans D, Worley PF. (1994b) *rheb*, a growth factor and synaptic activity-regulated gene, encodes a novel ras-related protein. *J. Biol. Chem.* **269**: 16 333–16 339.

Yin JCP, Wallach JS, Del Vecchio M, Wilder EL, Zhou H, Quinn WG, Tully T. (1994) Induction of a dominant negative CREB transgene specifically blocks long-term memory in *Drosophila*. *Cell* **79**: 49–58.

Ziff EB. (1990) Transcription factors: a new family gathers at the cAMP response site. *Trends Genet.* **6**: 69–72.

Neurotrophic factors and the regulation of neuronal survival in the developing peripheral nervous system

Alun M. Davies

13.1 Introduction

The occurrence of extensive neuronal death is a prominent feature of the developing vertebrate nervous system. Neurons are generated in excess, and those that are superfluous to requirements die shortly after their axons reach their targets. To survive, each neuron must procure an adequate supply of one or more neurotrophic factors. These specialized proteins are generally produced in the targets of the neurons that require them, and the limited supply of these factors governs the number of neurons that survive. An increasing number of proteins have been shown to promote the survival of specific kinds of neurons. The most extensively characterized group of neurotrophic factors are the neurotrophins, a highly homologous family of proteins that includes nerve growth factor (NGF), brain-derived neurotrophic factor (BDNF), neurotrophin-3 (NT3), neurotrophin-4/5 (NT4/5) and neurotrophin-6 (NT6). A group of more distantly related proteins that promote neuronal survival includes ciliary neurotrophic factor (CNTF), growth promoting activity, leukemia inhibitory factor (LIF), oncostatin-M (OSM), cardiotrophin-1 (CT-1) and interleukin-6 (IL-6). In addition, several other proteins also promote neuronal survival. These include glia cell line-derived neurotrophic factor (GDNF) and basic fibroblast growth factor.

Neurotrophic factors have several other functions in the nervous system in addition to promoting neuronal survival. These include regulating neuroblast proliferation, enhancing neuronal differentiation, promoting axonal branching and influencing synaptic function. It is becoming apparent that several neurotrophic factors have a diversity of effects on a variety of different cell types outside of the nervous system. These actions are beyond the scope of this article which will focus on the regulation of neuronal survival by neurotrophic factors in development. Because neuronal death and the function of neurotrophic factors have been most extensively and comprehensively analyzed in the peripheral nervous system (PNS), this article will summarize the salient details of the extensive body of work on the regulation of neuronal survival in the periphery.

Molecular Biology of the Neuron, edited by R.W. Davies and B.J. Morris.
© 1997 BIOS Scientific Publishers Ltd, Oxford.

13.2 Neurotrophins

The purification of the first two neurotrophins, NGF and BDNF, was based on the ability of these proteins to promote the survival of embryonic neurons in culture (Barde *et al.*, 1982; Levi-Montalcini, 1987). The molecular cloning of BDNF (Leibrock *et al.*, 1989) revealed that NGF and BDNF share a 50% amino acid sequence homology. This important finding paved the way for the molecular cloning of additional members of the neurotrophin family by polymerase chain reaction using degenerate oligonucleotides to highly conserved domains within NGF and BDNF (Berkemeier *et al.*, 1991; Ernfors *et al.*, 1990; Gotz *et al.*, 1994; Hallbook *et al.*, 1991; Hohn *et al.*, 1990; Ip *et al.*, 1992; Jones and Reichardt, 1990; Maisonpierre *et al.*, 1990; Rosenthal *et al.*, 1990). All members of this family are basic, homodimeric, secreted proteins that have molecular weights in the region of 25–27 kDa. They are derived by proteolytic cleavage from larger precursor proteins that are necessary for correct folding of the mature, functional proteins. X-ray crystallography and analysis of mutated neurotrophins (Ibanez *et al.*, 1992, 1993; McDonald *et al.*, 1991) have revealed the three-dimensional structure of these proteins and indicated those parts of the molecules responsible for homodimerization and for receptor binding and discrimination.

13.2.1 Neurotrophins and the neurotrophic hypothesis

The discovery of NGF led to the formulation of the neurotrophic hypothesis which provides an explanation for how neuronal target fields influence the size of the neuronal populations that innervate them (Levi-Montalcini, 1987). This hypothesis proposes that target fields produce NGF or other neurotrophic factors which the innervating neurons require for their survival. Because the supply of these factors is thought to be limiting, only a proportion of the neurons are able to obtain enough trophic factor to survive. Thus, the level of trophic factor production in the target field directly influences the size of the innervating populations of neurons. In addition to obtaining trophic support from their targets, there is also evidence that the afferent innervation of some neurons plays a role in promoting survival (Okado and Oppenheim, 1984).

The most important evidence for the neurotrophic hypothesis is the demonstration that developing neurons whose survival is promoted by NGF *in vitro*, namely sympathetic and certain sensory neurons, also depend on NGF *in vivo*. Anti-NGF antibodies eliminate these neurons during the early stages of target field innervation whereas exogenous NGF rescues neurons that would otherwise die (Levi-Montalcini, 1987). Likewise, targeted null mutations in the NGF gene (Crowley *et al.*, 1994) or the NGF receptor tyrosine kinase gene (Smeyne *et al.*, 1994) eliminate NGF-dependent sensory and sympathetic neurons.

Studies of NGF synthesis and NGF uptake have provided additional support for the neurotrophic hypothesis. NGF synthesis begins in the target fields of NGF-dependent sensory and sympathetic neurons with the arrival of the earliest axons and is synthesized in proportion to final innervation density in developing cutaneous territories (Harper and Davies, 1990). NGF is subsequently conveyed by rapid axonal transport from its sites of synthesis in the periphery to the cell bodies of the innervating sensory and sympathetic neurons (Hendry *et al.*, 1974).

The purification of BDNF (Barde *et al.*, 1982) extended the generality of the neurotrophic theory to a second neurotrophin. BDNF promotes the survival of subsets of embryonic sensory neurons *in vitro* and prevents loss of these neurons *in vivo* when administered to embryos during the phase of naturally occurring neuronal death (Hofer and Barde, 1988). Targeted null mutations in the BDNF gene (Ernfors *et al.*, 1994a; Jones *et al.*, 1994) or the BDNF receptor tyrosine kinase gene (Klein *et al.*, 1993) eliminate these neurons. Targeted null mutations in the NT3 gene (Ernfors *et al.*, 1994b; Farinas *et al.*, 1994) or the NT3 receptor tyrosine kinase gene (Klein *et al.*, 1994) likewise eliminate the kinds of sensory neurons that survive in response to NT3 *in vitro*.

13.2.2 Neurotrophin receptors

Neurotrophin-responsive neurons possess two classes of binding sites: a common low-affinity binding site to which NGF, BDNF and NT3 bind with similar dissociation constants in the range of 0.8×10^{-9}M to 1.7×10^{-9}M and specific high-affinity binding sites that have dissociation constants in the region of 2×10^{-11} M (Rodriguez-Tebar and Barde, 1988; Rodriguez-Tebar *et al.*, 1990, 1992; Sutter *et al.*, 1979). Two kinds of cell surface receptors have been described: the common neurotrophin receptor p75 (Chao, 1994) and members of the Trk family of receptor tyrosine kinases which are receptors for different neurotrophins (Barbacid, 1994; Klein, 1994).

Trk receptor tyrosine kinases. Trk receptor tyrosine kinases are essential for neurotrophin signal transduction (Barbacid, 1994; Klein, 1994) and initiate a cascade of protein phosphorylations in cells following ligand binding (Kaplan and Stephens, 1994). Expression studies in cell lines have shown that TrkA is the receptor for NGF (Kaplan *et al.*, 1991; Klein *et al.*, 1991a), TrkB is the receptor for BDNF and NT4/5 (Berkemeier *et al.*, 1991; Glass *et al.*, 1991; Klein *et al.*, 1991b, 1992; Soppet *et al.*, 1991; Squinto *et al.*, 1991) and TrkC is the receptor for NT3 (Lamballe *et al.*, 1991).

In addition to these preferred receptor–ligand interactions, studies of Trk receptor tyrosine kinases expressed in fibroblasts have shown that NT3 is also able to signal through TrkA and TrkB (Lamballe *et al.*, 1991; Soppet *et al.*, 1991; Squinto *et al.*, 1991) and that NT4/5 is able to signal through TrkA (Berkemeier *et al.*, 1991). The demonstration that NT3 can promote the *in vitro* survival of NGF-dependent and BDNF-dependent sensory neurons from embryos that have a null mutation in the *trk*C gene and that NT3 responsiveness is abolished by additional null mutations in the *trk*A and *trk*B genes show that NT3 can also signal through TrkA and TrkB in developing neurons (Davies *et al.*, 1995). Such signaling may explain why the phenotype of NT3–/– mice (Ernfors *et al.*, 1994b; Farinas *et al.*, 1994) is more severe than that of trkC–/– mice (Klein *et al.*, 1994; Schimmang *et al.*, 1995). The ligand specificities of the Trk receptor tyrosine kinases are illustrated in *Figure 13.1*.

The ability of NT3 to signal via TrkA and TrkB decreases markedly in the late fetal stages of development whereas NGF and BDNF responsiveness is little changed (Davies *et al.*, 1995). There are at least two possible reasons for these selective changes in ligand specificities of TrkA and TrkB during development. Other molecules could affect the ligand specificity of Trks such as p75. Function-perturbing antibodies to p75 potentiate the response of PC12 cells to NT3 (Clary and Reichardt, 1994), and sympathetic neurons from postnatal mice that have a null mutation in the *p75* gene are more sensitive to NT3 than sympathetic neurons from wild-type animals (Lee *et al.*, 1994b). However, an increase in p75 expression does not necessarily lead to a selective decrease

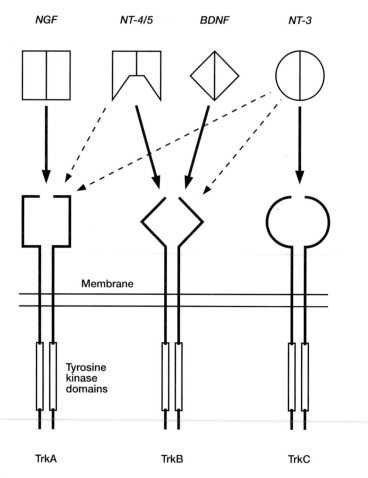

Figure 13.1. Illustration of the binding preferences of homodimeric neurotrophins to Trk receptor tyrosine kinases. The preferred interactions are illustrated by thick arrows and the nonpreferred interactions by dashed lines. Ligand binding is thought to bring two Trk receptors together in the plane of the membrane, resulting in transphosphorylation of the juxtaposed kinase domains (Jing *et al.*, 1992). Reproduced from Davies (1994b) with permission from Macmillan Magazines Ltd.

in NT3 signaling via TrkA. Whereas the level of p75 increases markedly in mouse sympathetic neurons between late fetal and postnatal stages (Wyatt and Davies, 1995), there is no selective decrease in ability of NT3 to promote neuronal survival in TrkC-deficient neurons (Davies *et al.*, 1995). An alternative explanation for the selective changes in ligand specificities of TrkA and TrkB during development could be due to structural variations in the ligand binding domains of Trk receptor tyrosine kinases. For example, a TrkA variant that contains an 18 bp exon in the extracellular region (Barker *et al.*, 1993) shows significantly higher activation by NT3 in PC12 cells compared with a variant that lacks this exon (Clary and Reichardt, 1994). Interestingly, there exist TrkB variants that also possess or lack the equivalent part of the extracellular region (Strohmaier *et al.*, 1996). Although both of these TrkB variants are activated to a similar extent by BDNF, the longer variant is activated more effectively by NT3 and NT4/5 than the shorter variant. Thus, these variants potentially play an important role in discriminating between different TrkB ligands. There are similar variants of TrkC (Shelton *et al.*, 1995), although their functional significance is not clear.

The extracellular region of Trk receptor kinases consists of several different domains: two cysteine-rich domains, three leucine-rich motifs and two immunoglobulin-like domains (Schneider and Schweiger, 1991). Mutation analysis has shown that the second immunoglobulin-like domain (Perez *et al.*, 1995; Urfer *et al.*, 1995) and the leucine-rich motifs (Windisch *et al.*, 1995a,b,c) play important roles in ligand discrimination. Several TrkB variants are expressed in the developing nervous system that differ in the number of leucine-rich motifs (N. Ninkina, M. Grashchuk, V. Buchman and A.M. Davies, unpublished data), although the functional significance of these variants is unclear. The arrangement of the structural domains of the Trk receptor tyrosine kinases is illustrated in *Figure 13.2*.

Alternative splicing also generates TrkB and TrkC variants that lack a tyrosine kinase domain (Klein *et al.*, 1990a,b; Lamballe *et al.*, 1993; Tsoulfas *et al.*, 1993). It is

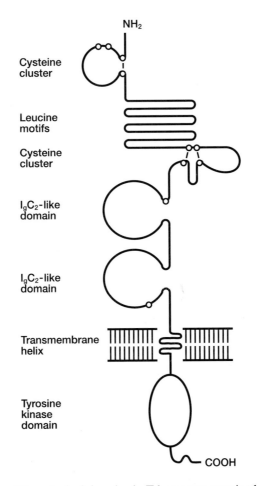

NH₂

Cysteine cluster

Leucine motifs

Cysteine cluster

I$_g$C$_2$-like domain

I$_g$C$_2$-like domain

Transmembrane helix

Tyrosine kinase domain

COOH

Figure 13.2. Drawing of the principal domains in Trk receptor tyrosine kinases. Redrawn from Schneider and Schweiger (1991).

possible that these kinase-deficient variants may have at least two different functions: restricting the diffusion of their corresponding ligands in the nervous system and acting as negative modulators of neurotrophin signaling in neurons.

The widespread expression of truncated TrkB by astrocytes in the adult central nervous system (CNS) (Frisen et al., 1993; Klein et al., 1990a; Rudge et al., 1994) together with the limited spread of injected BDNF in the brain parenchyma compared with NGF (Morse et al., 1993) raises the possibility that truncated TrkB may play an important role in limiting the diffusion of BDNF in the mature CNS. The demonstration that truncated TrkB receptors on leptomeningeal cells bind BDNF with high affinity and rapidly internalize bound BDNF (Biffo et al., 1995) suggests that selective uptake limits the spread of BDNF from its sites of synthesis in the CNS. In the chicken embryo, truncated TrkB is expressed early by nonneuronal cells that abut regions of BDNF synthesis, suggesting that in these locations truncated TrkB may form a boundary that restricts the diffusion of BDNF. For example, truncated TrkB is expressed by the mesenchymal cells that surround the otic vesicle which contains cells that express BDNF mRNA (Biffo et al., 1995). A similar role was previously suggested for p75 in restricting the diffusion of NGF in developing skin because p75 is expressed by the mesenchymal cells (Wyatt et al., 1990) that lie beneath cutaneous epithelium which expresses high levels of NGF (Davies et al., 1987).

The demonstration that full-length and kinase-deficient TrkB variants are co-expressed in developing trigeminal neurons and that the expression of kinase-deficient variants increases as the neurons lose responsiveness to BDNF during development (Ninkina et al., 1996) raises the possibility that these noncatalytic variants may be negative modulators of the BDNF survival response. This effect on the BDNF survival response was directly demonstrated by co-expressing noncatalytic and full-length TrkB variants alone and in combination in sympathetic neurons and studying the response of these neurons to BDNF (Ninkina et al., 1996).

p75. The role of p75 is complex and controversial. Expression studies in some cell lines suggest that both p75 and TrkA need to be present for the formation of high-affinity NGF receptors (Berg et al., 1991; Hempstead et al., 1991; Pleasure et al., 1990). The demonstration that PC12 cells transfected with a chimeric receptor consisting of the extracellular domain of the epidermal growth factor (EGF) receptor and the transmembrane and intracellular domains of p75 extend neurites in response to EGF also suggests that p75 plays a role in NGF signaling (Yan et al., 1991). In contrast, PC12 cells expressing chimeric receptors consisting of the extracellular domain of the tumor necrosis factor (TNF) receptor and the transmembrane and intracellular domains of TrkA extend neurites in response to TNF, suggesting that TrkA alone is sufficient for this response (Rovelli et al., 1993). Likewise, fibroblasts expressing TrkA, TrkB or TrkC proliferate in response to neurotrophins (Cordon-Cardo et al., 1991; Glass et al., 1991; Klein et al., 1992; Lamballe et al., 1991) in the absence of p75. Furthermore, specific inhibition of NGF binding to p75 by either anti-p75 antiserum (Weskamp and Reichardt, 1991) or mutations of the NGF protein (Drinkwater et al., 1991; Ibanez et al., 1992) does not affect the response of PC12 cells and sympathetic neurons to NGF, indicating that p75 is not essential for NGF signaling in these cells. Although NGF can elicit a mitogenic response in fibroblasts expressing TrkA alone, co-expression of TrkA and p75 in fibroblasts results in the formation of a class of high-affinity receptors that is not apparently present in cells expressing TrkA alone

(Battleman *et al.*, 1993), and expression of high levels of p75 in MAH cells enhances NGF-induced TrkA phosphorylation compared with cells expressing TrkA alone (Verdi *et al.*, 1994).

To clarify the physiological significance of p75, mice carrying a null mutation of the *p75* gene were generated by gene targeting (Lee *et al.*, 1992). Homozygous null mutants have decreased pain sensitivity and have a marked decrease in calcitonin gene-related peptide (CGRP)- and substance P-immunoreactive nerve fibers in the skin (Lee *et al.*, 1992) combined with loss of sympathetic innervation to the pineal gland and the sweat glands of some foot pads (Lee *et al.*, 1994a). In culture, sensory and sympathetic neurons from *p75–/–* embryos respond normally to saturating concentrations of NGF, BDNF, NT3 and NT4/5, showing that p75 is not essential for neurotrophin signaling. The dose responses of embryonic sympathetic and visceral sensory neurons from *p75–/–* embryos are also normal. However, embryonic trigeminal and DRG neurons and postnatal sympathetic neurons isolated from *p75–/–* animals display a consistent displacement in the NGF dose response. Compared with wild-type neurons, the concentration of NGF that promotes half-maximal survival is three- to four-fold higher for p75-deficient neurons (Davies *et al.*, 1993a; Lee *et al.*, 1994b). These findings indicate that p75 enhances the sensitivity of NGF-dependent embryonic sensory and postnatal sympathetic neurons to NGF. The explanation for the age-related differences in the effect of the *p75* mutation on NGF-dependent neurons may lie in the relative levels of p75 and TrkA expressed by sensory and sympathetic neurons during development. The *p75* and *trkA* mRNA levels are similar in embryonic trigeminal sensory (Wyatt and Davies, 1993) and postnatal sympathetic (Wyatt and Davies, 1995) neurons, but in embryonic sympathetic neurons the level of p75 mRNA is much lower than *trkA* mRNA (Wyatt and Davies, 1995). How p75 enhances the survival response of NGF-dependent neurons to NGF is not clear. The finding that the binding of NGF to TrkA is reduced by disrupting the binding of NGF to p75 by an anti-p75 antibody or by excess BDNF suggests that p75 enhances the binding of NGF to TrkA (Barker and Shooter, 1994). Furthermore, p75 accelerates TrkA-mediated signaling (Canossa *et al.*, 1996) and forms a complex with TrkA on the cell surface (Ross *et al.*, 1996; Wolf *et al.*, 1995).

In addition to selectively enhancing the response of NGF-dependent neurons to NGF, there is evidence that p75 may play a role in mediating neuronal death. In a neuron-like cell line and in PC12 pheochromocytoma cells grown in the absence of serum and NGF, expression of p75 increases the rate of cell death (Rabizadeh *et al.*, 1993). Antisense p75 oligonucleotides that reduce p75 expression promote the survival of postnatal rat dorsal root ganglion (DRG) neurons grown in the absence of NGF, suggesting that at this stage of development unoccupied p75 provides a constitutive death signal (Barrett and Bartlett, 1994). In the fetal period antisense p75 oligonucleotides do not rescue DRG neurons grown in the absence of NGF but do reduce the survival-promoting effects of NGF, suggesting that there is a developmental switch in the role of p75 from its participation in mediating the survival-promoting action of NGF in the fetal period to promoting neuronal death in the postnatal period. This apparent dual role of p75 in developing neurons resembles the function of two other members of the p75 family of receptors, Fas and the p70 TNF receptor. These transmembrane glycoproteins are also able to promote cell death or cell growth depending on the cells in which they are expressed (Heller *et al.*, 1992; Itoh *et al.*, 1991).

13.2.3 Timing of neurotrophin dependence

Sensory and sympathetic neurons initially survive and extend axons independently of neurotrophins and become dependent on neurotrophins when their axons reach their targets (Buchman and Davies, 1993; Coughlin and Collins, 1985; Davies and Lumsden, 1984; Ernsberger and Rohrer, 1988; Ernsberger et al., 1989; Vogel and Davies, 1991; Wright et al., 1992). The control of the timing of neurotrophin dependence has been extensively studied using cranial sensory neurons. The neurons of the vestibulocochlear, geniculate, petrosal and nodose ganglia are derived from thickened regions of head ectoderm termed neurogenic placodes, are born over the same period of development and start extending axons towards their peripheral and central targets at approximately the same time, but differ in the distances their axons have to grow to reach these targets. When cultured at low density at the stage when their axons are starting to grow towards their targets, vestibulocochlear neurons, which have the closest targets, survive without neurotrophins for only a short time before becoming dependent on BDNF for survival. Nodose neurons, which have the most distant targets, survive for the longest time in the absence of neurotrophins before becoming BDNF dependent. Geniculate and petrosal neurons, which have intermediate target distances, survive for intermediate times before becoming BDNF dependent (Vogel and Davies, 1991). This suggests that the duration of neurotrophin independence and the onset of the BDNF survival response is controlled by an intrinsic timing mechanism in the early neurons. This mechanism appears to be programmed in the progenitor cells of the corresponding neurogenic placodes because the neurons that differentiate in cultures of these placodes exhibit characteristic differences in the duration of neurotrophin independence (Vogel and Davies, 1991). Heterotopic grafting experiments have shown that the presumptive placodal ectoderm is not yet specified to differentiate into neurons but that signals acting in the vicinity of this ectoderm commit the cells to a particular neuronal fate (Vogel and Davies, 1993).

13.2.4 Developmental changes in neurotrophin survival requirements

Evidence that some neurons switch their neurotrophin survival requirements during the early stages of target field innervation has come from studying embryonic mouse trigeminal ganglion neurons in vitro (Buchman and Davies, 1993; Davies et al., 1993b). When these neurons are grown at very low density in defined medium at the stage when their axons normally reach their peripheral targets in vivo, all of the neurons die unless BDNF, NT3 or NT4/5, but not NGF, are present in the culture medium. In cultures set up over the next few days of development, the neurons acquire a survival response to NGF while, at the same time, losing responsiveness to BDNF, NT3 and NT4/5. Early trigeminal neurons do not acquire a long-term survival response to NGF in vitro no matter how long they are cultured with BDNF, NT3 or NT4/5 before being switched to NGF (Paul and Davies, 1995). However, neurons that are switched from BDNF, NT3 or NT4/5 to NGF in cultures set up at stages throughout the switchover period exhibit an NGF survival response that improves with age. Moreover, the ability of NGF to promote the long-term survival also increases with embryonic age (Paul and Davies, 1995). These results show that, unlike the onset of BDNF dependence which is controlled by an intrinsic timing mechanism in early sensory neurons, the switch to NGF dependence relies on extrinsic signals acting on the neurons during the switchover period and that in vivo signals are also required for the maturation of the

NGF survival response from a transient to a long-term response. The onset of the BDNF survival response is correlated with the expression of kinase-containing TrkB receptors (Ninkina et al., 1996; Robinson et al., 1996), and the loss of the BDNF survival response is associated with a marked increase in the expression of trkB transcripts encoding noncatalytic receptors (Ninkina et al., 1996) and a marked shift in the BDNF dose response to higher concentrations (Buj-Bello et al., 1994).

The physiological relevance of the early in vitro responses of trigeminal neurons to BDNF and NT3 has been strengthened by analysis of mice with null mutations in genes encoding neurotrophins and their receptors. The finding that BDNF−/− mice (Ernfors et al., 1994a; Jones et al., 1994), but not NT4/5−/− mice (Conover et al., 1995; Liu et al., 1995), have marked reductions of the numbers of neurons in the trigeminal ganglion, suggests that BDNF, but not NT4/5, is important for maintaining the survival of trigeminal neurons in vivo. The finding that there is a marked increase in the number of dying neurons in the trigeminal ganglia of trkB−/− embryos at the early stage of development when these neurons are supported by BDNF in culture and that the increase in neuronal death that takes place in the trigeminal ganglia of trkA−/− embryos occurs later in development demonstrates that neurotrophin switching takes place in vivo (Pinon et al., 1996).

In addition to trigeminal sensory neurons, there is in vitro evidence that cells of the sympathetic lineage change their survival requirements early in development. Although many sympathetic neuroblasts survive in the absence of neurotrophins (Ernsberger et al., 1989), there is evidence that NT3, but not NGF or BDNF, enhances the survival of these cells (Birren et al., 1993; Dechant et al., 1993; DiCicco et al., 1993). Later in development, the survival of sympathetic neurons is promoted by NGF, but only much higher concentrations of NT-3 are effective in promoting survival (Dechant et al., 1993). The physiological relevance of the early survival response of sympathetic neuroblasts to NT3 observed in vitro is strengthened by the finding that increased cell death takes place in the superior cervical sympathetic ganglia of NT3−/− embryos at an early stage of their development (ElShamy et al., 1996).

Not all neurons switch their survival requirements from one set of neurotrophins to another during the early stages of target field innervation. For example, the BDNF-dependent ventrolateral trigeminal neurons of the chicken embryo do not show early survival responses to either NGF or NT3, and the BDNF-responsive and NT3-responsive nodose neurons of the chicken embryo do not show an early response to NGF (Buj-Bello et al., 1994). Whether these neurons are supported by different neurotrophic factors at an early stage in their development is not known.

Later in development, during the phase of naturally occurring neuronal death, different populations of neurons in the PNS have distinctive neurotrophin requirements. For example, nociceptive neurons are supported by NGF and proprioceptive neurons are supported by BDNF and NT3. [For a recent review of neurotrophin specificity in the PNS see Davies (1994a).] In the adult, administration of anti-NGF antibodies has little effect on the number of neurons in sympathetic and dorsal root ganglia, suggesting that these neurons no longer require NGF for survival (Levi-Montalcini and Angeletti, 1968). Furthermore, adult DRG neurons survive in culture in the absence of added neurotrophic factors, suggesting that mature sensory neurons do not require any exogenous neurotrophic factors for survival at this stage (Lindsay, 1988). However, the demonstration that antisense BDNF oligonucleotides cause the death of about 40% of adult DRG neurons grown in single-cell cultures suggests that

BDNF may act by an autocrine loop to maintain the survival of a proportion of these neurons during maturity (Acheson et al., 1995). The extent to which neurotrophic factor autocrine loops operate in other populations of neurons to promote survival has yet to be examined.

13.3 CNTF, LIF, OSM, CT-1 and IL-6

CNTF, LIF, OSM, CT-1 and IL-6 comprise a family of cytokines that have multiple actions on cells of the nervous system and several other tissues (Sendtner et al., 1994; Stahl and Yancopoulos, 1994). Although there is less than 15% amino acid sequence identity between these factors, they share several characteristic structural features (Bazan, 1991; McDonald et al., 1995; Robinson et al., 1994) and signal via oligomeric receptor complexes that have one or more components in common. The current view (Stahl and Yancopoulos, 1994; Wollert et al., 1996) is that the gp130 transmembrane glycoprotein is a common component of the receptor complex for these factors. Two gp130 molecules form part of the IL-6 receptor, and one gp130 molecule together with another transmembrane glycoprotein termed the LIF receptor β subunit (LIFRβ) are components of the receptors for CNTF, LIF, OSM and CT-1. The CNTF and IL-6 receptor complexes are additionally comprised of α subunits: CNTFRα and IL-6Rα, respectively. CNTFRα is unusual in that it lacks cytoplasmic and transmembrane domains, but is anchored to the plasma membrane by a glycosyl-phosphatidylinositol (GPI) linkage (Davis et al., 1993). Interestingly, CNTFRα released from the plasma membrane by enzymatic disruption of the GPI linkage can combine with CNTF to form a heterodimeric factor that is capable of eliciting responses in cells expressing gp130 and LIFRβ (Davis et al., 1993). It is not known, however, whether this heterodimeric complex is physiologically relevant. The demonstration that CNTFRα null mice (DeChiara et al., 1995), unlike CNTF null mice (Masu et al., 1993), die in the perinatal period and have severe motoneuron deficits suggests that a second, developmentally important ligand exists for CNTFRα. The receptors for CNTF and related factors are illustrated schematically in Figure 13.3.

CNTF was originally identified and purified by its ability to promote the in vitro survival of the parasympathetic neurons of the ciliary ganglion (Barbin et al., 1984). Unlike neurotrophins, CNTF is an acidic cytosolic protein that lacks a leader sequence and is released poorly from cultured cells that express high levels of CNTF (Lin et al., 1989; Stockli et al., 1989). Whereas neurotrophin expression begins in neuronal target fields prior to the onset of naturally occurring neuronal death (Buchman and Davies, 1993; Davies et al., 1987; Korsching and Thoenen, 1988), CNTF synthesis commences in myelinating Schwann cells in the postnatal period, well after neuronal death has taken place (Dobrea et al., 1992; Stockli et al., 1991). Accordingly, neurotrophins start exerting their survival-promoting effects on cultured neurons when they begin innervating their targets, whereas the survival-promoting effects of CNTF are observed in sympathetic neurons and most populations of sensory neurons at later stages of neuronal development (Barbin et al., 1984; Kotzbauer et al., 1994; A.R. Horton, P.F. Bartlett, D. Pennica and A.M. Davies, unpublished observations). Taken together, these findings suggest that CNTF is not a target-derived neurotrophic factor involved in regulating the size of neuronal populations during the phase of neuronal death. Accordingly, neuronal deficiencies have not been observed in CNTF–/– mice during embryonic development, but these mice lose a small number of

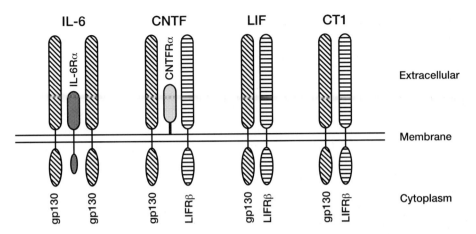

Figure 13.3. Illustration of known components of the IL-6, CNTF, LIF and CT1 receptors. All components are transmembrane proteins except for CNTFRα which is linked to the cell membrane by a GPI linkage. It is not known whether there are α subunits for the LIF and CT1 receptors.

motoneurons by 28 weeks (22% reduction in the facial nucleus) (Masu *et al.*, 1993). Although the administration of CNTF to chicken embryos rescues about half of the motoneurons that would otherwise die (Oppenheim *et al.*, 1991), this simply demonstrates that these embryonic motoneurons are capable of responding to CNTF, not that CNTF normally regulates their survival *in ovo*. Indeed the substantial loss of motoneurons occurring in *CNTFRα* null mice (DeChiara *et al.*, 1995) suggests that a novel CNTF-related ligand is required for motoneuron survival *in vivo*. Exogenous CNTF has no effect on the survival of sensory, sympathetic or parasympathetic neurons in chicken embryos (Oppenheim *et al.*, 1991) and there is no apparent decrease in volume of DRG, superior cervical sympathetic ganglion (SCG) and trigeminal ganglia in *CNTFRα* null mice (DeChiara *et al.*, 1995).

LIF also promotes the survival of sensory neurons in culture. The number of mouse DRG neurons supported by LIF increases from 20% at E16 to 90% postnatally, at which stage the neurons are supported equally well by LIF and NGF (Murphy *et al.*, 1993). There is a significant reduction in the number of DRG neurons in *LIFRβ–/–* mice (S.S. Cheema and P. Bartlett, personal communication), suggesting that the *in vitro* response of DRG neurons to LIF may be physiologically relevant. The expression of LIF mRNA in skin and gut from E15 onwards (Murphy *et al.*, 1993) and the retrograde transport of iodinated LIF from the periphery (Hendry *et al.*, 1992) raises the possibility that LIF may function as a target-derived neurotrophic factor for late fetal and newborn DRG. However, LIF mRNA is also expressed within fetal DRG, suggesting that it may also act locally on the neuron cell bodies (Murphy *et al.*, 1993). Although it is not clear whether the neurons or satellite cells in the ganglia express LIF mRNA, nonneuronal cells cultured from fetal ganglia secrete a factor that is neutralized by anti-LIF antiserum (Fan and Katz, 1993). In addition to DRG neurons, fetal nodose ganglion neurons (Thaler *et al.*, 1994) and trigeminal ganglion neurons (Horton *et al.*, 1996) also survive in culture in the presence of LIF.

OSM, IL-6 and CT-1 also support the survival of embryonic nodose and late trigeminal ganglion neurons, although IL-6 is much less effective than OSM and LIF

(Horton *et al.*, 1996). CT-1 has also recently been shown to be a potent survival factor for motoneurons (Pennica *et al.*, 1996).

13.4 GDNF

GDNF is a distantly related member of the transforming growth factor-β family that was isolated from the B49 glial cell line (Lin *et al.*, 1993). It is a potent survival factor for midbrain dopaminergic neurons (Lin *et al.*, 1993) and motoneurons (Henderson *et al.*, 1994; Oppenheim *et al.*, 1995; Yan *et al.*, 1995) and protects midbrain dopaminergic neurons from 1-methyl-4-phenyl-1,2,3,6-tetrahydropyridine toxicity (Tomac *et al.*, 1995) and axotomy-induced degeneration (Beck *et al.*, 1995). In the PNS, GDNF promotes the *in vitro* survival of embryonic sympathetic, parasympathetic and sensory neurons and is expressed in a wide variety of tissues in development (Buj-Bello *et al.*, 1995; Trupp *et al.*, 1995). With increasing developmental age, sympathetic, parasympathetic and proprioceptive neurons become less responsive to GDNF, whereas enteroceptive and cutaneous sensory neurons become more responsive. These developmental changes in GDNF responsiveness are mirrored by corresponding changes in GDNF mRNA expression in several of the tissues innervated by GDNF-responsive neurons (Buj-Bello *et al.*, 1995). These studies suggest that GDNF plays a role in regulating the survival of multiple populations of PNS and CNS neurons at different stages of their development. The physiological relevance of these *in vitro* findings has been confirmed by the appreciable reduction in the number of sensory and sympathetic neurons in *GDNF* null mice (Moore *et al.*, 1996). *GDNF* null mice also have a reduced number of lumbar motoneurons and absence of the enteric nervous system, but interestingly, apparently normal numbers of midbrain dopaminergic neurons (Moore *et al.*, 1996; Pichel *et al.*, 1996; Sanchez *et al.*, 1996).

Two receptors for GDNF have recently been identified: the Ret receptor tyrosine kinase (Durbec *et al.*, 1996a; Trupp *et al.*, 1996) and a novel GPI-linked protein designated GDNFR-α (Treanor *et al.*, 1996). Ret and GDNFRα are expressed by populations of known GDNF-responsive neurons as well as in several other locations (Durbec *et al.*, 1996a,b; Schuchardt *et al.*, 1994, 1995; Treanor *et al.*, 1996; Trupp *et al.*, 1996). GDNF binds to Ret with high affinity (K_d of approximately 2×10^{-10} M) (Trupp *et al.*, 1996), promotes tyrosine phosphorylation of Ret (Treanor *et al.*, 1996) and causes a variety of responses in cells in which Ret is experimentally expressed (Durbec *et al.*, 1996a; Treanor *et al.*, 1996). GDNFRα appears to be required for the survival-promoting effects of GDNF because treatment of neurons with a phospho-inositide-specific phospholipase C, an enzyme that specifically cleaves GPI linkages, causes a substantial reduction in the number of neurons surviving with GDNF but does not affect the neurotrophin survival response (Treanor *et al.*, 1996). Interestingly, soluble GDNFRα can combine with GDNF to form a functional heterodimeric complex (Treanor *et al.*, 1996) in much the same way as soluble CNTFRα and CNTF (Davis *et al.*, 1993). Immunoprecipitation studies also indicate that GDNF, GDNFRα and Ret can, in the presence of GDNF, form a complex on the cell surface (Treanor *et al.*, 1996). A schematic illustration of the GDNF receptor complex is shown in *Figure 13.4*.

In agreement with the loss of the enteric nervous system in *GDNF* null mice (Moore *et al.*, 1996), the enteric neurons of the midgut and hindgut are absent in *ret* null embryos (Durbec *et al.*, 1996b; Schuchardt *et al.*, 1994). This is not due, however,

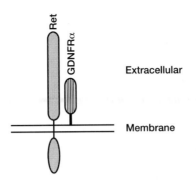

Figure 13.4. Illustration of the GDNF receptor complex consisting of the GPI-linked GDNFRα component and the Ret receptor tyrosine kinase. GDNF is unusual among members of the TGFβ (transforming growth factor) superfamily in that it signals through a receptor tyrosine kinase, whereas all receptors for other members of this superfamily that have been characterized so far are serine/threonine kinases (Attisano *et al.*, 1996; Derynck, 1994).

to the death of differentiated neurons but to a failure of neurogenesis (Durbec *et al.*, 1996b). The SCG, but not the more caudal ganglia of the sympathetic chain, is also absent in *ret* null embryos (Durbec *et al.*, 1996b). Although the SCG anlagen forms in Ret-deficient embryos, it is eliminated at a very early stage, suggesting that Ret is required for the proliferation or survival of SCG neuroblasts. Interestingly, the sympathetic and enteric neurons that are absent in *ret* null embryos are derived from the vagal neural crest, suggesting that Ret signaling is required for the genesis of at least a subset of neurons from this region of the neural crest. Accordingly, many Ret-positive post-migratory neural crest cells isolated from the fetal rat gut are capable of differentiating into neurons in culture (Lo and Anderson, 1995).

References

Acheson A, Conover JC, Fandl JP, DeChiara TM, Russell M, Thadani A, Squinto SP, Yancopoulos GD, Lindsay RM. (1995) A BDNF autocrine loop in adult sensory neurons prevents cell death. *Nature* **374**: 450–453.

Attisano L, Wrana JL, Montalvo E, Massague J. (1996) Activation of signalling by the activin receptor complex. *Mol. Cell. Biol.* **16**: 1066–1073.

Barbacid M. (1994). The Trk family of neurotrophin receptors. *J. Neurobiol.* **25**: 1386–1403.

Barbin G, Manthorpe M, Varon S. (1984) Purification of the chick eye ciliary neuronotrophic factor. *J. Neurochem.* **43**: 1468–1478.

Barde YA, Edgar D, Thoenen H. (1982) Purification of a new neurotrophic factor from mammalian brain. *EMBO J.* **1**: 549–553.

Barker PA, Shooter EM. (1994) Disruption of NGF binding to the low affinity neurotrophin receptor p75LNTR reduces NGF binding to TrkA on PC12 cells. *Neuron* **13**: 203–215.

Barker PA, Lomen-Hoerth C, Gensch EM, Meakin SO, Glass DJ, Shooter EM. (1993) Tissue-specific alternative splicing generates two isoforms of the *trk*A receptor. *J. Biol. Chem.* **268**: 15150–15157.

Barrett GL, Bartlett PF. (1994) The p75 nerve growth factor receptor mediates survival or death depending on the stage of sensory neuron development. *Proc. Natl Acad. Sci. USA* **91**: 6501–6505.

Battleman DS, Geller AI, Chao MV. (1993) HSV-1 vector-mediated gene transfer of the human nerve growth factor receptor p75hNGFR defines high-affinity NGF binding. *J. Neurosci.* **13**: 941–951.

Bazan JF. (1991) Neuropoietic cytokines in the hematopoietic fold. *Neuron* **7**: 197–208.

Beck KD, Valverde J, Alexi T, Poulsen K, Moffat B, Vandlen RA, Rosenthal A, Hefti F. (1995) Mesencephalic dopaminergic neurons protected by GDNF from axotomy-induced degeneration in the adult brain. *Nature* **373**: 339–341.

Berg MM, Sternberg DW, Hempstead BL, Chao MV. (1991) The low-affinity p75 nerve growth factor (NGF) receptor mediates NGF-induced tyrosine phosphorylation. *Proc. Natl Acad. Sci. USA* **88**: 7106–7110.

Berkemeier LR, Winslow JW, Kaplan DR, Nikolics K, Goeddel DV, Rosenthal A. (1991) Neurotrophin-5: a novel neurotrophic factor that activates trk and trkB. *Neuron* **7**: 857–866.

Biffo S, Offenhauser N, Carter BD, Barde YA. (1995) Selective binding and internalisation by truncated receptors restrict the availability of BDNF during development. *Development* **121**: 2461–2470.

Birren SJ, Lo L, Anderson DJ. (1993) Sympathetic neurons undergo a developmental switch in trophic dependence. *Development* **119**: 597–610.

Buchman VL, Davies AM. (1993) Different neurotrophins are expressed and act in a developmental sequence to promote the survival of embryonic sensory neurons. *Development* **118**: 989–1001.

Buj-Bello A, Pinon LG, Davies AM. (1994) The survival of NGF-dependent but not BDNF-dependent cranial sensory neurons is promoted by several different neurotrophins early in their development. *Development* **120**: 1573–1580.

Buj-Bello A, Buchman VL, Horton A, Rosenthal A, Davies AM. (1995) GDNF is an age-specific survival factor for sensory and autonomic neurons. *Neuron* **15**: 821–828.

Canossa M, Twiss JL, Verity AN, Shooter EM. (1996) p75NGFR and TrkA receptors collaborate to rapidly activate a p75NGFR-associated protein kinase. *EMBO J.* **15**: 3369–3376.

Chao M. (1994) The p75 neurotrophin receptor. *J. Neurobiol.* **25**: 1373–1385.

Clary DO, Reichardt LF. (1994) An alternatively spliced form of the nerve growth factor receptor TrkA confers an enhanced response to neurotrophin-3. *Proc. Natl Acad. Sci. USA* **91**: 11 133–11 137.

Conover JC, Erickson JT, Katz DM *et al.* (1995) Neuronal deficits, not involving motor neurons, in mice lacking BDNF and NT4. *Nature* **375**: 235–238.

Cordon-Cardo C, Tapley P, Jing SQ *et al.* (1991) The trk tyrosine protein kinase mediates the mitogenic properties of nerve growth factor and neurotrophin-3. *Cell* **66**: 173–183.

Coughlin MD, Collins MB. (1985) Nerve growth factor-independent development of embryonic mouse sympathetic neurons in dissociated cell culture. *Devel. Biol.* **110**: 392–401.

Crowley C, Spencer SD, Nishimura MC *et al.* (1994) Mice lacking nerve growth factor display perinatal loss of sensory and sympathetic neurons yet develop basal forebrain cholinergic neurons. *Cell* **76**: 1001–1011.

Davies AM. (1994a) Role of neurotrophins in the developing nervous system. *J. Neurobiol.* **25**: 1334–1348.

Davies AM. (1994b) Tracking neurotrophin function. *Nature* **368**: 193–194.

Davies AM, Lumsden AGS. (1984) Relation of target encounter and neuronal death to nerve growth factor responsiveness in the developing mouse trigeminal ganglion. *J. Comp. Neurol.* **223**: 124–137.

Davies AM, Bandtlow C, Heumann R, Korsching S, Rohrer H, Thoenen H. (1987) Timing and site of nerve growth factor synthesis in developing skin in relation to innervation and expression of the receptor. *Nature* **326**: 353–358.

Davies, AM, Lee, KF, Jaenisch R. (1993a) p75-deficient trigeminal sensory neurons have an altered response to NGF but not to other neurotrophins. *Neuron* **11**: 565–574.

Davies AM, Horton A, Burton LE, Schmelzer C, Vandlen R, Rosenthal A. (1993b) Neurotrophin-4/5 is a mammalian-specific survival factor for distinct populations of sensory neurons. *J. Neurosci.* **13**: 4961–4967.

Davies AM, Minichiello L, Klein R. (1995) Developmental changes in NT3 signalling via TrkA and TrkB in embryonic neurons. *EMBO J.* **14**: 4482–4489.

Davis S, Aldrich TH, Ip NY *et al.* (1993) Released form of CNTF receptor alpha component as a soluble mediator of CNTF responses. *Science* **259**: 1736–1739.

Dechant G, Rodriguez TA, Kolbeck R, Barde YA. (1993) Specific high-affinity receptors for neurotrophin-3 on sympathetic neurons. *J. Neurosci.* **13**: 2610–2616.

DeChiara TM, Vejsada R, Poueymirou WT *et al.* (1995) Mice lacking the CNTF receptor, unlike mice lacking CNTF, exhibit profound motor neuron deficits at birth. *Cell* **83**: 313–322.

Derynck R. (1994) TGF-beta-receptor-mediated signaling. *Trends Biochem. Sci.* **19**: 548–553.

DiCicco BE, Friedman WJ, Black IB. (1993) NT-3 stimulates sympathetic neuroblast proliferation by promoting precursor survival. *Neuron* **11**: 1101–1111.

Dobrea GM, Unnerstall JR, Rao MS. (1992) The expression of CNTF message and immunoreactivity in the central and peripheral nervous system of the rat. *Dev. Brain Res.* **66**: 209–219.

Drinkwater CC, Suter U, Angst C, Shooter EM. (1991) Mutation of tryptophan-21 in mouse nerve growth factor (NGF) affects binding to the fast NGF receptor but not induction of neurites on PC12 cells. *Proc. R. Soc. Lond.* **246:** 307–313.

Durbec P, Marcos-Gutierrez CV, Kilkenny C *et al.* (1996a) GDNF signalling through the Ret receptor tyrosine kinase. *Nature* **381:** 789–793.

Durbec PL, Larsson-Blomberg LB, Schuchardt A, Costantini F, Pachnis V. (1996b) Common origin and developmental dependence on c-ret of subsets of enteric and sympathetic neuroblasts. *Development* **122:** 349–358.

ElShamy WM, Linnarsson S, Lee KF, Jaenisch R, Ernfors P. (1996) Prenatal and postnatal requirements of NT-3 for sympathetic neuroblast survival and innervation of specific targets. *Development* **122:** 491–500.

Ernfors P, Ibanez CF, Ebendal T, Olson L, Persson H. (1990) Molecular cloning and neurotrophic activities of a protein with structural similarities to nerve growth factor: developmental and topographical expression in the brain. *Proc. Natl Acad. Sci. USA* **87:** 5454–5458.

Ernfors P, Lee KF, Jaenisch R. (1994a) Mice lacking brain-derived neurotrophic factor develop with sensory deficits. *Nature* **368:** 147–150.

Ernfors P, Lee KF, Kucera J, Jaenisch R. (1994b) Lack of neurotrophin-3 leads to deficiencies in the peripheral nervous system and loss of limb proprioceptive afferents. *Cell* **77:** 503–512.

Ernsberger U, Rohrer H. (1988) Neuronal precursor cells in chick dorsal root ganglia: differentiation and survival *in vitro. Devel. Biol.* **126:** 420–432.

Ernsberger U, Edgar D, Rohrer H. (1989) The survival of early chick sympathetic neurons *in vitro* is dependent on a suitable substrate but independent of NGF. *Devel. Biol.* **135:** 250–262.

Fan G, Katz DM. (1993) Non-neuronal cells inhibit catecholaminergic differentiation of primary sensory neurons: role of leukemia inhibitory factor. *Development* **118:** 83–93.

Farinas I, Jones KR, Backus C, Wang XY, Reichardt LF. (1994) Severe sensory and sympathetic deficits in mice lacking neurotrophin-3. *Nature* **369:** 658–661.

Frisen J, Verge VM, Fried K, Risling M, Persson H, Trotter J, Lindholm D. (1993) Characterisation of glia trkB receptors: differential response to injury in the central and peripheral nervous systems. *Proc. Natl Acad. Sci. USA* **90:** 4971–4975.

Glass DJ, Nye SH, Hantzopoulos P, Macchi MJ, Squinto SP, Goldfarb M, Yancopoulos GD. (1991) TrkB mediates BDNF/NT-3-dependent survival and proliferation in fibroblasts lacking the low affinity NGF receptor. *Cell* **66:** 405–413.

Gotz R, Koster R, Winkler C, Raulf F, Lottspeich F, Schartl M, Thoenen H. (1994) Neurotrophin-6 is a new member of the nerve growth factor family. *Nature* **372:** 266–269.

Hallbook F, Ibanez CF, Persson H. (1991) Evolutionary studies of the nerve growth factor family reveal a novel member abundantly expressed in *Xenopus* ovary. *Neuron* **6:** 845–858.

Harper S, Davies AM. (1990) NGF mRNA expression in developing cutaneous epithelium related to innervation density. *Development* **110:** 515–519.

Heller RA, Song K, Fan N, Chang DJ. (1992) The p70 tumor necrosis factor receptor mediates cytotoxicity. *Cell* **70:** 47–56.

Hempstead BL, Martin ZD, Kaplan DR, Parada LF, Chao MV. (1991) High-affinity NGF binding requires coexpression of the trk proto-oncogene and the low-affinity NGF receptor. *Nature* **350:** 678–683.

Henderson CE, Phillips HS, Pollock RA *et al.* (1994) GDNF: a potent survival factor for motoneurons present in peripheral nerve and muscle. *Science* **266:** 1062–1064.

Hendry IA, Stoeckel K, Thoenen H, Iversen LL. (1974) Retrograde transport of nerve growth factor. *Brain Res.* **68:** 103–121.

Hendry IA, Murphy M, Hilton DJ, Nicola NA, Bartlett PF. (1992) Binding and retrograde transport of leukemia inhibitory factor by the sensory nervous system. *J. Neurosci.* **12:** 3427–3434.

Hofer MM, Barde YA. (1988) Brain-derived neurotrophic factor prevents neuronal death *in vivo. Nature* **331:** 261–262.

Hohn A, Leibrock J, Bailey K, Barde YA. (1990) Identification and characterization of a novel member of the nerve growth factor/brain-derived neurotrophic factor family. *Nature* **344:** 339–341.

Ibanez CF, Ebendal T, Barbany G, Murray RJ, Blundell TL, Persson H. (1992) Disruption of the low affinity receptor-binding site in NGF allows neuronal survival and differentiation by binding to the trk gene product. *Cell* **69:** 329–341.

Ibanez CF, Ilag LL, Murray RJ, Persson H. (1993) An extended surface of binding to Trk tyrosine kinase receptors in NGF and BDNF allows the engineering of a multifunctional pan-neurotrophin. *EMBO J.* **12:** 2281–2293.

Ip NY, Ibanez CF, Nye SH *et al.* (1992) Mammalian neurotrophin-4: structure, chromosomal localization, tissue distribution, and receptor specificity. *Proc. Natl Acad. Sci. USA* **89:** 3060–3064.

Itoh N, Yonehara S, Ishii A, Yonehara M, Mizushima S, Sameshima M, Hase A, Seto Y, Nagata S. (1991) The polypeptide encoded by the cDNA for human cell surface antigen Fas can mediate apoptosis. *Cell* **66:** 233–243.

Jing S, Tapley P, Barbacid M. (1992) Nerve growth factor mediates signal transduction through trk homodimer receptors. *Neuron* **9:** 1067–1079.

Jones KR, Reichardt LF. (1990) Molecular cloning of a human gene that is a member of the nerve growth factor family. *Proc. Natl Acad. Sci. USA* **87:** 8060–8064.

Jones KR, Farinas I, Backus C, Reichardt LF. (1994) Targeted disruption of the BDNF gene perturbs brain and sensory neuron development but not motor neuron development. *Cell* **76:** 989–999.

Kaplan DR, Stephens RM. (1994) Neurotrophin signal transduction by the Trk receptor. *J. Neurobiol.* **25:** 1404–1417.

Kaplan DR, Martin ZD, Parada LF. (1991) Tyrosine phosphorylation and tyrosine kinase activity of the trk proto-oncogene product induced by NGF. *Nature* **350:** 158–160.

Klein R. (1994) Role of neurotrophins in mouse neuronal development. *FASEB J.* **8:** 738–744.

Klein R, Conway D, Parada LF, Barbacid M. (1990a) The trkB tyrosine protein kinase gene codes for a second neurogenic receptor that lacks the catalytic kinase domain. *Cell* **61:** 647–656.

Klein R, Martin ZD, Barbacid M, Parada LF. (1990b) Expression of the tyrosine kinase receptor gene trkB is confined to the murine embryonic and adult nervous system. *Development* **109:** 845–850.

Klein R, Jing SQ, Nanduri V, O'Rourke E, Barbacid M. (1991a) The trk proto-oncogene encodes a receptor for nerve growth factor. *Cell* **65:** 189–197.

Klein R, Nanduri V, Jing SA *et al.* (1991b) The trkB tyrosine protein kinase is a receptor for brain-derived neurotrophic factor and neurotrophin-3. *Cell* **66:** 395–403.

Klein R, Lamballe F, Bryant S, Barbacid M. (1992) The trkB tyrosine protein kinase is a receptor for neurotrophin-4. *Neuron* **8:** 947–956.

Klein R, Smeyne RJ, Wurst W, Long LK, Auerbach BA, Joyner AL, Barbacid M. (1993) Targeted disruption of the trkB neurotrophin receptor gene results in nervous system lesions and neonatal death. *Cell* **75:** 113–122.

Klein R, Silos SI, Smeyne RJ, Lira SA, Brambilla R, Bryant S, Zhang L, Snider WD, Barbacid M. (1994) Disruption of the neurotrophin-3 receptor gene trkC eliminates la muscle afferents and results in abnormal movements. *Nature* **368:** 249–251.

Korsching S, Thoenen H. (1988) Developmental changes of nerve growth factor levels in sympathetic ganglia and their target organs. *Devel. Biol.* **126:** 40–46.

Kotzbauer PT, Lampe PA, Estus S, Milbrandt J, Johnson EJ. (1994) Postnatal development of survival responsiveness in rat sympathetic neurons to leukemia inhibitory factor and ciliary neurotrophic factor. *Neuron* **12:** 763–773.

Lamballe F, Klein R, Barbacid M. (1991) trkC, a new member of the trk family of tyrosine protein kinases, is a receptor for neurotrophin-3. *Cell* **66:** 967–979.

Lamballe F, Tapley P, Barbacid M. (1993) trkC encodes multiple neurotrophin-3 receptors with distinct biological properties and substrate specificities. *EMBO J.* **12:** 3083–3094.

Lee KF, Li E, Huber LJ, Landis SC, Sharpe AH, Chao MV, Jaenisch R. (1992) Targeted mutation of the gene encoding the low affinity NGF receptor p75 leads to deficits in the peripheral sensory nervous system. *Cell* **69:** 737–749.

Lee KF, Bachman K, Landis S, Jaenisch R. (1994a) Dependence on p75 for innervation of some sympathetic targets. *Science* **263:** 1447–1449.

Lee KF, Davies AM, Jaenisch R. (1994b) p75-deficient embryonic dorsal root sensory and neonatal sympathetic neurons display a decreased sensitivity to NGF. *Development* **120:** 1027–1033.

Leibrock J, Lottspeich F, Hohn A, Hofer M, Hengerer B, Masiakowski P, Thoenen H, Barde YA. (1989) Molecular cloning and expression of brain-derived neurotrophic factor. *Nature* **341:** 149–152.

Levi-Montalcini R. (1987) The nerve growth factor 35 years later. *Science* **237:** 1154–1162.

Levi-Montalcini R, Angeletti P. (1968) Nerve growth factor. *Physiol. Rev.* **48:** 534–569.

Lin LF, Mismer D, Lile JD, Armes LG, Butler E3, Vannice JL, Collins F. (1989) Purification, cloning, and expression of ciliary neurotrophic factor (CNTF). *Science* **246:** 1023–1025.

Lin LH, Doherty DH, Lile JD, Bektesh S, Collins F. (1993) GDNF: a glial cell-derived neurotrophic factor for midbrain dopaminergic neurons. *Science* 260: 1130–1132.

Lindsay RM. (1988) Nerve growth factors (NGF, BDNF) enhance axonal regeneration but are not required for survival of adult sensory neurons. *J. Neurosci.* 8: 2394–2405.

Liu X, Ernfors P, Wu H, Jaenisch R. (1995) Sensory but not motor neuron deficits in mice lacking NT4 and BDNF. *Nature* 375: 238–241.

Lo L, Anderson DJ. (1995) Postmigratory neural crest cells expressing c-RET display restricted developmental and proliferative capacities. *Neuron* 15: 527–539.

Maisonpierre PC, Belluscio L, Squinto S, Ip NY, Furth ME, Lindsay RM, Yancopoulos GD. (1990) Neurotrophin-3: a neurotrophic factor related to NGF and BDNF. *Science* 247: 1446–1451.

Masu Y, Wolf E, Holtmann B, Sendtner M, Brem G, Thoenen H. (1993) Disruption of the CNTF gene results in motor neuron degeneration. *Nature* 365: 27–32.

McDonald NQ, Lapatto R, Murray RJ, Gunning J, Wlodawer A, Blundell TL. (1991) New protein fold revealed by a 2.3-Å resolution crystal structure of nerve growth factor. *Nature* 354: 411–414.

McDonald NQ, Panayotatos N, Hendrickson WA. (1995) Crystal structure of dimeric human ciliary neurotrophic factor determined by MAD phasing. *EMBO J.* 14: 2689–2699.

Murphy M, Reid K, Brown MA, Bartlett PF. (1993) Involvement of leukemia inhibitory factor and nerve growth factor in the development of dorsal root ganglion neurons. *Development* 117: 1173–1182.

Moore MW, Klein RD, Farinas I et al. (1996) Renal and neuronal abnormalities in mice lacking GDNF. *Nature* 382: 76–79.

Morse JK, Wiegand SJ, Anderson K et al. (1993) Brain-derived neurotrophic factor (BDNF) prevents the degeneration of medial septal cholinergic neurons following fimbria transection. *J. Neurosci.* 13: 4146–4156.

Ninkina N, Adu J, Fischer A, Pinon L, Buchman V, Davies AM. (1996) Expression and function of TrkB variants in developing trigeminal neurons. *EMBO J.*, in press.

Okado N, Oppenheim RW. (1984) Cell death of motoneurons in the chick embryo spinal cord. IX. The loss of motoneurons following removal of afferent inputs. *J. Neurosci.* 4: 1639–1652.

Oppenheim RW, Prevette D, Yin QW, Collins F, MacDonald J. (1991) Control of embryonic motoneuron survival *in vivo* by ciliary neurotrophic factor. *Science* 251: 1616–1618.

Oppenheim RW, Houenou LJ, Johnson JE, Lin LH, Li L, Lo AC, Newsome AL, Prevette DM, Wang S. (1995) Developing motoneurons rescued from programmed and axotomy-induced cell death by GDNF. *Nature* 373: 344–346.

Paul G, Davies AM. (1995) Trigeminal sensory neurons require extrinsic signals to switch neurotrophin dependence during the early stages of target field innervation. *Devel. Biol.* 171: 590–605.

Pennica D, Arce V, Wsanson TA et al. (1996) Cardiotrophin-1, a cytokine present in embryonic muscle, supports long-term survival of spinal motoneurons. *Neuron* 17: 63–74.

Perez P, Coll PM, Hempstead BL, Martin-Zanca D, Chao MV. (1995) NGF binding to the trk tyrosine kinase receptor requires the extracellular immunoglobulin-like domains. *Mol. Cell. Neurosci.* 6: 97–105.

Pichel JG, Shen L, Sheng HZ et al. (1996) Defects in enteric innervation and kidney development in mice lacking GDNF. *Nature* 382: 73–76.

Pinon LGP, Minichiello L, Klein R, Davies AM. (1996) Timing of neuronal death in *trkA, trkB* and *trkC* mutant embryos reveals developmental changes in sensory neuron dependence on Trk signalling. *Development* 122: 3255–3261.

Pleasure SJ, Reddy UR, Venkatakrishnan G, Roy AK, Chen J, Ross AH, Trojanowski JQ, Pleasure DE, Lee VM. (1990) Introduction of nerve growth factor (NGF) receptors into a medulloblastoma cell line results in expression of high- and low-affinity NGF receptors but not NGF-mediated differentiation. *Proc. Natl Acad. Sci. USA* 87: 8496–8500.

Rabizadeh S, Oh J, Zhong LT, Yang J, Bitler CM, Butcher LL, Bredesen DE. (1993) Induction of apoptosis by the low-affinity NGF receptor. *Science* 261: 345–348.

Robinson RC, Grey LM, Staunton D, Vankelecom H, Vernallis AB, Moreau JF, Stuart DI, Heath JK, Jones EY. (1994) The crystal structure and biological function of leukemia inhibitory factor: implications for receptor binding. *Cell* 77: 1101–1116.

Robinson M, Adu J, Davies AM. (1996) Timing and regulation of *trk*B and *BDNF* mRNA expression in placode-derived sensory neurons and their targets. *Eur. J. Neurosci.* 8: 2399–2406.

Rodriguez-Tebar A, Barde YA. (1988) Binding characteristics of brain-derived neurotrophic factor to its receptors on neurons from the chicken embryo. *J. Neurosci.* 8: 3337–3342.

Rodriguez-Tebar A, Dechant G, Barde YA. (1990) Binding of brain-derived neurotrophic factor to the nerve growth factor receptor. *Neuron* 4: 487–492.

Rodriguez-Tebar A, Dechant G, Gotz R, Barde YA. (1992) Binding of neurotrophin-3 to its neuronal receptors and interactions with nerve growth factor and brain-derived neurotrophic factor. *EMBO J.* **11:** 917–922.

Rosenthal A, Goeddel DV, Nguyen T, Lewis M, Shih A, Laramee GR, Nikolics K, Winslow JW. (1990) Primary structure and biological activity of a novel human neurotrophic factor. *Neuron* **4:** 767–773.

Ross AH, Daou MC, McKinnon CA, Condon PJ, Lachyankar MB, Stephens RM, Kaplan DR, Wolf DE. (1996) The neurotrophin receptor, gp75, forms a complex with the receptor tyrosine kinase TrkA. *J. Cell Biol.* **132:** 945–953.

Rovelli G, Heller RA, Canossa M, Shooter EM. (1993) Chimeric tumor necrosis factor-TrkA receptors reveal that ligand-dependent activation of the TrkA tyrosine kinase is sufficient for differentiation and survival of PC12 cells. *Proc. Natl Acad. Sci. USA* **90:** 8717–8721.

Rudge JS, Li Y, Pasnikowski EM, Mattsson K, Pan L, Yancopoulos GD, Wiegand SJ, Lindsay RM, Ip NY. (1994) Neurotrophic factor receptors and their signal transduction capabilities in rat astrocytes. *Eur. J. Neurosci.* **6:** 693–705.

Sanchez MP, Silos-Santiago I, Frisen J, He B, Sergio SA, Barbacid M. (1996) Renal agenesis and the absence of enteric neurons in mice lacking GDNF. *Nature* **382:** 70–73.

Schneider R, Schweiger M. (1991) A novel modular mosaic of cell adhesion motifs in the extracellular domains of the neurogenic trk and trkB tyrosine kinase receptors. *Oncogene* **6:** 1807–1811.

Schuchardt A, D'Agati V, Larsson-Blomberg L, Costantini F, Pachnis V. (1994) Defects in the kidney and enteric nervous system of mice lacking the tyrosine kinase receptor Ret. *Nature* **367:** 380–383.

Schuchardt A, Srinivas S, Pachnis V, Costantini F. (1995) Isolation and characterisation of a chicken homologue of the c-*ret* proto-oncogene. *Oncogene* **10:** 641–649.

Schimmang T, Minichiello L, Vazquez E, Joac IS, Giraldez F, Klein R, Represa J. (1995) Developing inner ear sensory neurons require TrkB and TrkC receptors for innervation of their peripheral targets. *Development* **121:** 3381–3391.

Sendtner M, Carroll P, Holtmann B, Hughes RA, Thoenen H. (1994) Ciliary neurotrophic factor. *J. Neurobiol.* **25:** 1436–1453.

Shelton DL, Sutherland J, Gripp J, Camerato T, Armanini MP, Phillips HS, Carroll K, Spencer SD, Levinson AD. (1995) Human trks: molecular cloning, tissue distribution, and expression of extracellular domain immunoadhesions. *J. Neurosci.* **15:** 477–491.

Smeyne RJ, Klein R, Schnapp A, Long LK, Bryant S, Lewin A, Lira SA, Barbacid M. (1994) Severe sensory and sympathetic neuropathies in mice carrying a disrupted Trk/NGF receptor gene. *Nature* **368:** 246–249.

Soppet D, Escandon E, Maragos J et al. (1991) The neurotrophic factors brain-derived neurotrophic factor and neurotrophin-3 are ligands for the trkB tyrosine kinase receptor. *Cell* **65:** 895–903.

Squinto SP, Stitt TN, Aldrich TH et al. (1991) trkB encodes a functional receptor for brain-derived neurotrophic factor and neurotrophin-3 but not nerve growth factor. *Cell* **65:** 885–893.

Stahl N, Yancopoulos GD. (1994) The tripartite CNTF receptor complex: activation and signalling involves components shared with other cytokines. *J. Neurobiol.* **25:** 1454–1466.

Stockli KA, Lottspeich F, Sendtner M, Masiakowski P, Carroll P, Gotz R, Lindholm D, Thoenen H. (1989) Molecular cloning, expression and regional distribution of rat ciliary neurotrophic factor. *Nature* **342:** 920–923.

Stockli KA, Lillien LE, Naher NM, Breitfeld G, Hughes RA, Raff MC, Thoenen H, Sendtner M. (1991) Regional distribution, developmental changes, and cellular localization of CNTF-mRNA and protein in the rat brain. *J. Cell Biol.* **115:** 447–459.

Strohmaier C, Carter BD, Urfer R, Barde YA, Dechant G. (1996) A splice variant of the neurotrophin receptor trkB with increased specificity for brain-derived neurotrophic factor. *EMBO J.* **15:** 3332–3337.

Sutter A, Riopelle RJ, Harris-Warrick RM, Shooter EM. (1979) Nerve growth factor receptors. Characterization of two distinct classes of binding sites on chick embryo sensory ganglia. *J. Biol. Chem.* **254:** 5972–5982.

Thaler CD, Suhr L, Ip N, Katz DM. (1994) Leukemia inhibitory factor and neurotrophins support overlapping populations of rat nodose sensory neurons in culture. *Devel. Biol.* **161:** 338–344.

Tomac A, Lindqvist E, Lin LH, Ogren SO, Young D, Hoffer BJ, Olson L. (1995) Protection and repair of the nigrostriatal dopaminergic system by GDNF *in vivo. Nature* **373:** 335–339.

Treanor J, Goodman L, de Sauvage F et al. (1996) Characterization of a receptor for glial cell line-derived neurotrophic factor. *Nature* **382:** 80–83.

Trupp M, Ryden M, Jornvall H, Funakoshi H, Timmusk T, Arenas E, Ibanez CF. (1995) Peripheral expression and biological activities of GDNF, a new neurotrophic factor for avian and mammalian peripheral neurons. *J. Cell Biol.* **130**: 137–148.

Trupp M, Arenas E, Fainzilber M *et al.* (1996) Functional receptor for GDNF encoded by the *c-ret* proto-oncogene. *Nature* **381**: 785–789.

Tsoulfas P, Soppet D, Escandon E, Tessarollo L, Mendoza RJ, Rosenthal A, Nikolics K, Parada LF. (1993) The rat trkC locus encodes multiple neurogenic receptors that exhibit differential response to neurotrophin-3 in PC12 cells. *Neuron* **10**: 975–990.

Urfer R, Tsoulfas P, O'Connell L, Shelton DL, Parada LF, Presta LG. (1995) An immunoglobulin-like domain determines the specificity of neurotrophin receptors. *EMBO J.* **14**: 2795–2805.

Verdi JM, Birren SJ, Ibanez CF, Persson H, Kaplan DR, Benedetti M, Chao MV, Anderson DJ. (1994) p75LNGFR regulates Trk signal transduction and NGF-induced neuronal differentiation in MAH cells. *Neuron* **12**: 733–745.

Vogel KS, Davies AM. (1991) The duration of neurotrophic factor independence in early sensory neurons is matched to the time course of target field innervation. *Neuron* **7**: 819–830.

Vogel KS, Davies AM. (1993) Heterotopic transplantation of presumptive placodal ectoderm influences the fate of sensory neuron precursors. *Development* **119**: 263–277.

Weskamp G, Reichardt LF. (1991) Evidence that biological activity of NGF is mediated through a novel subclass of high affinity receptors. *Neuron* **6**: 649–663.

Windisch JM, Auer B, Marksteiner R, Lang ME, Schneider, R. (1995a) Specific neurotrophin binding to leucine-rich motif peptides of TrkA and TrkB. *FEBS Lett.* **374**: 125–129.

Windisch JM, Marksteiner R, Lang ME, Auer B, Schneider R. (1995b) Brain-derived neurotrophic factor, neurotrophin-3, and neurotrophin-4 bind to a single leucine-rich motif of TrkB. *Biochemistry* **34**: 11 256–11 263.

Windisch JM, Marksteiner R, Schneider R. (1995c) Nerve growth factor binding site on TrkA mapped to a single 24-amino acid leucine-rich motif. *J. Biol. Chem.* **270**: 28 133–28 138.

Wolf DE, McKinnon CA, Daou MC, Stephens RM, Kaplan DR, Ross AH. (1995) Interaction with TrkA immobilizes gp75 in the high affinity nerve growth factor receptor complex. *J. Biol. Chem.* **270**: 2133–2138.

Wollert KC, Taga T, Saito M *et al.*, (1996) Cardiotrophin-1 activates a distinct form of cardiac muscle cell hypertrophy. Assembly of sarcomeric units in series via gp130/leukemia inhibitory factor receptor-dependent pathways. *J. Biol. Chem.* **271**: 9535–9545.

Wright EM, Vogel KS, Davies AM. (1992) Neurotrophic factors promote the maturation of developing sensory neurons before they become dependent on these factors for survival. *Neuron* **9**: 139–150.

Wyatt S, Davies AM. (1993) Regulation of expression of mRNAs encoding the nerve growth factor receptors p75 and trkA in developing sensory neurons. *Development* **119**: 635–648.

Wyatt S, Davies AM. (1995) Regulation of expression of p75 and *trk*A mRNAs in developing sympathetic neurons. *J. Cell Biol.* **130**: 1435–1446

Wyatt S, Shooter EM, Davies AM. (1990) Expression of the NGF receptor gene in sensory neurons and their cutaneous targets prior to and during innervation. *Neuron* **4**: 421–427.

Yan H, Schlessinger J, Chao MV. (1991) Chimeric NGF-EGF receptors define domains responsible for neuronal differentiation. *Science* **252**: 561–563.

Yan Q, Matheson C, Lopez OT. (1995) *In vivo* neurotrophic effects of GDNF on neonatal and adult facial motor neurons. *Nature* **373**: 341–344.

Genetic basis of human neuronal disease

Mark E.S. Bailey, Richard T. Moxley III and Keith J. Johnson

14.1 Introduction

Molecular neurogenetics is a relatively new field, but one which is progressing at an astonishing rate. Linkage analysis of neurological and psychiatric disorders showing straightforward Mendelian inheritance has become a routine technique by which to localize disease genes. Positional cloning or candidate gene methods, supported by the considerable progress achieved by the Human Genome Project over the last few years (*Figure 14.1*), are feasible in the majority of cases and have helped in the characterization of many disease genes. Gene cloning is a necessary prelude to functional studies designed to illuminate pathological mechanisms at the cellular level. Recent advances have also made it possible to begin to explore the causes of diseases showing complex inheritance, due either to genetic heterogeneity or to interactions between multiple predisposing genetic and environmental factors. A remarkable increase in our understanding of the genetic basis of neurological diseases has resulted from the use of these powerful approaches to the identification and investigation of genes.

In this chapter, we have summarized what is known about the genes underlying a range of human diseases where there is a clear primary effect on neurons and we have commented on other molecules also implicated in the pathology of these diseases. For reasons of limited space, we have dealt only with genes that have been cloned and with molecules that have been shown to have a proven role in neuronal pathology, as a result either of altered expression in neurons due to mutation, or of direct interactions with neurons. We have only referred to studies in animals where it has been impossible to conduct studies in man that shed light on fundamental pathological mechanisms. We have not classified diseases stringently by clinical characteristics or molecular lesion. Instead, we have made functional groupings which we feel best illustrate the diversity of genes and molecules so far shown to be involved in a variety of pathological alterations in human neuronal disease (*Table 14.1*; in the table, MIM number refers to the entry for each disease in McKusick's 'Online Mendelian Inheritance in Man' database, in which a substantial amount of clinical and molecular information is summarized and referenced. It is available over the World-Wide Web at http://www3.ncbi.nlm.nih.gov/Omim/). In the process, we have focused more attention on those gene lesions that have gained prominence in recent investigations.

Molecular Biology of the Neuron, edited by R.W. Davies and B.J. Morris.

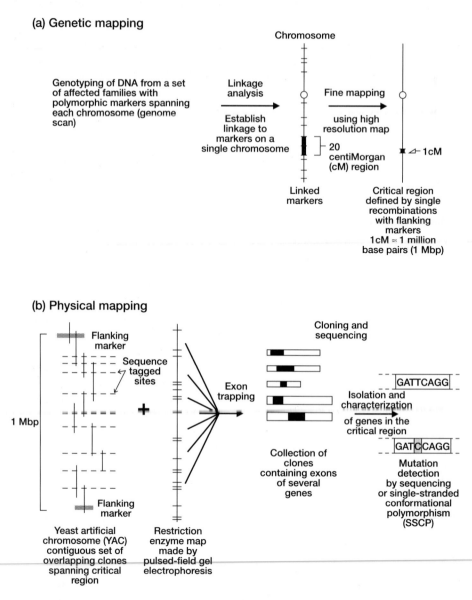

Figure 14.1. Overview of positional cloning of disease genes. Summary of the major steps involved in a typical positional cloning strategy. Reproduced in part from Johnson and Hamilton (1997) in *Principles and Practice of Medical Genetics* (ed. Connor, J.M.) with permission from Churchill Livingstone, Edinburgh.

14.2 Expanding trinucleotide repeat diseases

Recently, the group of diseases found to result from the amplification in tandem (expansion) of a trinucleotide repeat region in various genes have received special interest (see *Figure 14.2*). These trinucleotide repeat diseases vary in the identity of the expanding triplet sequence on the coding strand of the relevant gene, in the location of the repeat relative to the transcription units involved, and in the extent to

Table 14.1. Disease genes with effects mainly on neuronal phenotype

Disease group	Disease	Disease gene symbol	Gene(s) mutated, symbol	Chromosomal localization	MIM no.
Trinucleotide	Fragile X syndrome	FRAXA FRAXE	Fragile X mental retardation, FMR-1 FMR2	Xq27.3 Xq28	309550 309548
	Spinal and bulbar muscular atrophy	SBMA	Androgen receptor, AR	Xq12	313200
	Huntington's chorea	HD	IT15, huntingtin	4q16.3	143100
	Spinocerebellar ataxia type 1	SCA1	Ataxin-1	6p23	164400
	Dentatorubral-pallidoluysian atrophy	DRPLA	Atrophin-1, DRPLA	12p13.3	125370
	Machado–Joseph disease	MJD/SCA3	MJD1	14q32.1	109150
	Myotonic dystrophy	DM	Myotonin kinase, DMPK	19q13.3	160900
	Friedreich's ataxia	FRDA	STM7	9q13	229300
Prion	Creutzfeldt–Jakob disease	CJD	Prion protein, PRNP, PRP	20p12	123400
	Gerstmann–Sträussler–Scheinker syndrome	GSS	PRNP		137440
	Familial fatal insomnia	FFI	PRNP		600072
Neurodegenerative	Alzheimer's disease	AD1 AD3 AD4 AD2	β-amyloid A4 precursor protein, APP S182, Presenilin 1, PS-1 STM2, E5-1, Presenilin 2, PS-2 Apolipoprotein E, APOE Microtubule-associated protein tau, MAPT	21q21.3-q22.05 14q24.3 1q31-q42 19q13.2 17q21	104300 104311 600759 104310 157140
Oxidative damage	Amyotrophic lateral sclerosis	ALS1	Superoxide dismutase-1, SOD1	21q22.1	105400
	Ataxia with selective vitamin E deficiency	AVED	Tocopherol binding protein, TTP1	8q13.1-q13.3	277460
Channelopathies	Hyperekplexia	STHE	Glycine receptor α1-subunit, GLRA1	5q32	149400
	Autosomal dominant nocturnal frontal lobe epilepsy	ADNFLE	Nicotinic acetylcholine receptor α4-subunit, CHRNA4	20q13.2	600513
Neuronal migration	Episodic ataxia with myokimia	AEM	Potassium channel, KCNA1	12p13	160120
	Miller–Dieker lissencephaly	MDLS	Lissencephaly-1, LIS1	17p13.3	247200
	Norrie disease	ND	Norrie disease protein, NDP	Xp11.4-p11.3	310600
	Kallmann syndrome	KAL	KALIG-1	Xp22.3	308700

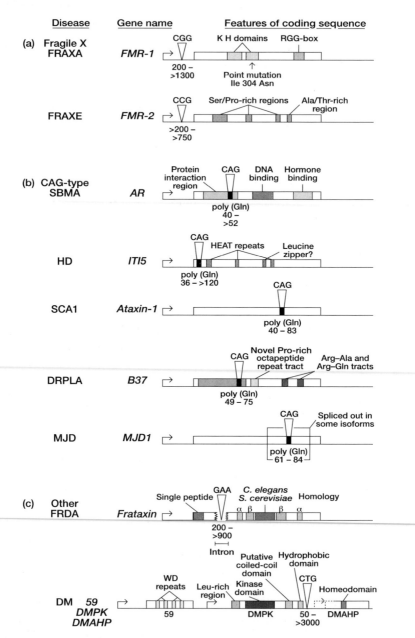

Figure 14.2. Characteristics of the trinucleotide repeat disease genes. The genes are represented as a horizontal line, not drawn to scale, with (a) a broken arrow indicating a notional transcriptional start site, followed by the 5′-UTR, (b) a box indicating the open reading frame contained in a full-length mRNA, (c) the 3′-UTR. Since three genes have been identified near the DM mutation, all are represented, but the intergenic regions are not drawn to scale. Shaded blocks within the open reading frame indicate protein homology or predicted primary or secondary structure motifs, as detailed in the text. The relative positions of the trinucleotide expansions, the amino acid tract encoded (if any) and the range in affected individuals are also shown.

which the repeat is expanded in affected individuals. Below, we discuss the disease genes individually.

14.2.1 Fragile X mental retardation syndrome

Fragile X syndrome (FRAXA) is characterized by mental retardation, macro-orchidism and a distinct facies. The syndrome segregates as an X-linked dominant disease with reduced penetrance. It is associated with a fragile site on the distal long arm of the X chromosome (cytogenetic band Xq27.3) that leads to chromosome narrowing or breakage at mitotic metaphase under folate-deficient cell growth conditions *in vitro*. This site is unstable in patients (Oberlé *et al.*, 1991) and coincides with the location of a gene, *FMR-1*, that contains a $(CGG)_n$ repeat, *n* varying from six to 54 tandem copies in the normal population (Fu *et al.*, 1991; Verkerk *et al.*, 1991). Northern blotting data indicate that the major mRNA species expressed is 4.4–4.8 kb in length. The gene is expressed widely in fetal and adult brain, with the highest levels in neurons of the nucleus basalis magnocellularis (which provides substantial cholinergic input to the cortical and limbic systems) and hippocampus, as well as in many nonneural tissues, including testis (Abitbol *et al.*, 1993; Hinds *et al.*, 1993).

The *FMR-1* gene consists of 17 exons spanning 38 kbp of genomic DNA (Eichler *et al.*, 1993). The tract of DNA containing the expanding $(CGG)_n$ repeat is located within the 5′-untranslated region (5′-UTR) of the mRNA (Ashley *et al.*, 1993a; Fu *et al.*, 1991; Verheij *et al.*, 1993). The full-length protein product is predicted to be 631 amino acids in size (approximately 67 kDa), but more than a dozen putative splice variants have been identified, largely due to alternative use of exons and 3′ acceptor splice sites in the downstream half of the gene (Ashley *et al.*, 1993a; Verkerk *et al.*, 1993). Isoforms deriving from at least five different splice products have been identified by immunoblotting studies. Their sizes range from 67 to 80 kDa, and their intracellular localization appears to be cytoplasmic (Devys *et al.*, 1993; Verheij *et al.*, 1993).

The function of the *FMR-1* gene product has not been delineated, but further investigations revealed that it acts as an RNA-binding protein. Regions of the sequence bear homology to the 'KH' domain family of ribonucleoprotein particle (RNP) proteins (Ashley *et al.*, 1993b; Siomi *et al.*, 1993) and a further subsequence lying towards the carboxyl terminus was identified by homology as an 'RGG box' (see Burd and Dreyfuss, 1994, for a review). Both of these regions are essential in RNA binding (Siomi *et al.*, 1993, 1994), and FMR-1 has been shown to bind to numerous brain mRNA species, as well as its own mRNA, with high affinity (Ashley *et al.*, 1993b). Recent reports have demonstrated that FMR-1 is attached to ribosomes, almost certainly via a direct RNA interaction, and it appears to have a role in the regulation of translation (Khandjian *et al.*, 1996; Tamanini *et al.*, 1996). The genes for two FMR-1 homologs, FXR1 and FXR2, have been cloned, and, interestingly, can interact with FMR-1 as heteromers (Zhang *et al.*, 1995).

Expansions of the $(CGG)_n$ repeat are responsible for the vast majority of cases of FRAXA, and transmission of the disease has characteristic genetic features. Expansion of the repeat into a so-called 'premutation' range of up to 200 repeats is not associated with symptoms, but further expansions to 200–1300 repeats produce the disease. Symptoms almost certainly result from a lack of expression of FMR-1 protein. This may be brought about by over-methylation of cytosine residues within a CpG island (a region rich in this rare dinucleotide combination and characteristic of the 5′-ends of approximately 60% of genes) that includes the $(CGG)_n$ repeat, leading to transcriptional silencing of the gene (Oberlé et al., 1991; Sutcliffe et al., 1992). Consistent with the idea that lack of the gene product causes the disease, deletions of the proximal part of the gene have been found (Wöhrle et al., 1992), as has a point mutation in the second KH domain (Ile367Asn) which disrupts the RNA binding capabilities of the protein (de Boulle et al., 1993; Siomi et al., 1994). The hypermethylation of the repeat-containing region may be linked to an alteration in the normal process of X-chromosome inactivation (Lyonization), whereby this region of the chromosome becomes very late-replicating in the cell cycle (Hansen et al., 1993). Variable expressivity of the disease in heterozygous females and some hemizygous males seems to depend largely on differences within affected tissues in the proportion of FMR-1 protein-deficient cells (i.e. 'mosaicism') that result from hypermethylation around the expanded $(CGG)_n$ repeat (Kruyer et al., 1994; McConkie-Rosell et al., 1993). Interestingly, gene-targeted, 'knockout' transgenic mice with no functional FMR-1 expression have a similar phenotype to that in fragile-X cases, including learning deficits and hyperactivity (The Dutch–Belgian Fragile X Consortium, 1994). Further studies using transgenic models will enable rapid progress in understanding the role of this gene in normal brain development and function.

Our ability to correlate gene defects with clinical phenotype in FRAXA is complicated by the existence of a small proportion of affected individuals exhibiting clearly X-linked mental retardation but with no evidence for involvement of the FRAXA locus. Some of these patients may have disruptions in one or more genes at nearby fragile sites. One such site is FRAXE, which lies approximately 600 kbp telomeric to FRAXA at Xq28 (Sutherland and Baker, 1992), and is characterized by an expanding $(CCG)_n$ repeat, with evidence for hypermethylation of an associated CpG island (Knight et al., 1993). Three groups have now reported the cloning of the gene, FMR-2, that appears to be disrupted by this repeat expansion (Chakrabarti et al., 1996; Gecz et al., 1996; Gu et al., 1996). The gene spans at least 650 kbp, with a huge first intron of 150 kbp. Translation of the gene probably begins approximately 330 bp downstream of the $(CCG)_n$ repeat, which is thought to lie in the 5'-UTR of the mRNA. Five exons have been identified. On Northern blots, cDNA probes have detected a 9.5 kb mRNA expressed in several fetal and adult tissues, including brain (particularly hippocampus and amygdala), with evidence for possible alternative splicing. The predicted protein of 1301 amino acids has limited homology with the product of the AF-4 (MLLT2) gene, a serine/proline-rich protein that is thought to be a transcription factor. Expansions have been observed in mentally retarded individuals from several families including some previously diagnosed as FRAXA-negative (Knight et al., 1993, 1994). It is likely that the pathological mechanism underlying most cases is underexpression of the gene due to methylation of the repeat, very much akin to the situation in FRAXA.

14.2.2 Polyglutamine tract diseases

A second major category of trinucleotide repeat diseases consists of those exhibiting expanding $(CAG)_n$ repeats located within the protein coding sequence of their associated genes. Each of these is described below.

Spinal and bulbar muscular atrophy. The first of these to yield was spinal and bulbar muscular atrophy (SBMA), or Kennedy disease, an adult onset motor neuronopathy often associated with androgen insensitivity and characterized by progressive muscle weakness and atrophy. The androgen receptor (AR) gene, *AR*, located at Xq11–q12, contains a $(CAG)_n$ repeat of 17–26 units in length, which expands to 40–52 repeats in SBMA patients (La Spada *et al.*, 1991). The androgen receptor is a member of the steroid receptor transcription factor superfamily and contains DNA binding and hormone binding domains. The $(CAG)_n$ repeat, located in the first of eight exons, encodes a polyglutamine stretch near the amino terminus that is not involved in either of these functional domains (La Spada *et al.*, 1991). Many neuronal cells express the *AR* gene, but Ogata *et al.* (1994) could find no alteration of immunoreactive protein levels in affected CNS regions in patients with SBMA. It was concluded that the phenotype is not caused by a selective deficiency of AR in neurons.

Huntington's disease. The gene for Huntington's disease (HD), a progressive neurodegenerative disorder characterized by chorea (involuntary movements), cognitive loss and, inevitably, premature death, was finally cloned in 1993 by a large consortium (HDCRG, 1993). Known as *IT15*, the gene consists of 67 exons, spanning 170 kb of genomic DNA on chromosome 4p. The expanding $(CAG)_n$ repeat is located in the first exon, less than 20 residues downstream of the initiator methionine (thus encoding a run of glutamines), and is immediately followed by an imperfect $(CCG)_n$ repeat encoding a run of proline residues.

An mRNA of approximately 10.3 kb has been detected in a fairly wide range of tissues on Northern blots. The open reading frame deduced from cDNA clones predicts a product, known as huntingtin, of 3144 amino acids and approximately 348 kDa. Alternative splicing is suspected, yielding one other isoform that contains 480 amino acids fewer (Lin *et al.*, 1994). *In situ* hybridization has revealed expression of the *IT15* gene in many parts of the brain, predominantly in neurons, but also in glia (Strong *et al.*, 1993), while the protein has been detected in a wide range of tissues, including the regions of the brain affected in HD, such as the striatum (Sharp *et al.*, 1995). Although there is some evidence for the localization of huntingtin in cell nuclei (De Rooij *et al.*, 1996; Hoogeven *et al.*, 1993), other studies have confirmed a cytoplasmic localization for huntingtin, concentrated at the perikaryon and at nerve endings and possibly around membrane-bound vesicles (DiFiglia *et al.*, 1995; Sharp *et al.*, 1995; Trottier *et al.*, 1995a). Huntingtin shares little homology with known proteins. Several copies of a loosely conserved domain, known as the HEAT repeat have been identified (Andrade and Bork, 1995). This repeat motif is probably involved in protein interactions.

As in SBMA, the pathology of HD does not appear simply to result from underexpression of the affected allele. mRNA transcribed from the expanded chromosome is not reduced compared with that from the normal allele in cortex and striatum of patients (Stine *et al.*, 1995). Trottier *et al.* (1995a), however, could not detect significant amounts of protein translated from the expanded allele transcript in HD brain regions on Western blots. Lymphoblastoid cell line extracts showed clearly defined normal and expanded products and the presence of a faint smear in the expected position on the blot in lanes containing brain extracts probably reflects somatic heterogeneity in the size of the $(CAG)_n$ repeat in brain but not lymphocytes (Telenius *et al.*, 1994). This observation is also controversial (MacDonald *et al.*, 1993).

The reasons for the specific neuropathology of the $(CAG)_n$ expansion in HD are unclear. Gene sequence and organization are highly conserved in mouse (Lin *et al.*, 1994) and the puffer fish, *Fugu rubripes* (Baxendale *et al.*, 1995). The wide expression of the gene, the characteristics of conserved promoter sequences typical of housekeeping genes (Lin *et al.*, 1995), and the lack of evidence for exceptional expression parameters in affected tissues, such as striatum (Strong *et al.*, 1993), all suggest that the restricted neuronal phenotype depends on interactions between huntingtin containing an expanded glutamine tract and other, tissue-specific factors. A recent report has described the cloning of a brain-specific gene, huntingtin-associated protein (HAP-1). The product of this gene binds specifically to huntingtin, with an affinity that is influenced by the length of the polyglutamine repeat (Li *et al.*, 1995). Other such proteins probably exist, but whether they participate in only the normal functioning of huntingtin, or play an additional role in dominant, toxic effects of repeat expansion remains to be seen. Three separate groups have now reported the results of targeted disruption of the mouse homolog of huntingtin, the *Hdh* gene (Duyao *et al.*, 1995; Nasir *et al.*, 1995; Zeitlin *et al.*, 1995). In all cases, homozygous disruption has resulted in no production of huntingtin protein and has caused embryonic lethality before about 8.5 days of gestation. These findings illustrate the necessity for expression of huntingtin in development but shed little light on the pathology in HD.

Spinocerebellar ataxia 1. Spinocerebellar ataxia type 1 (SCA1) is a progressive neurodegenerative disease characterized by ataxia and weakness, associated with degeneration of several cell types, including cerebellar Purkinje cells. The repeat has been shown to be associated with affected status in all alleles containing more than 43 repeat units (Orr *et al.*, 1993). A DNA probe made from the genomic subclone containing the repeat detected a 10.7 kb mRNA in several tissues on Northern blots, and this was later shown to correspond to a nine exon gene spanning 450 kb of genomic DNA (Banfi *et al.*, 1994). The gene, whose product is termed ataxin-1, undergoes alternative splicing in the long 5′-untranslated portion encoded by exons 1–7, the entire coding region being contained within the last two, large exons, an unusual arrangement for a mammalian gene. The $(CAG)_n$ repeat is found 588 bp downstream of the presumed start codon and encodes a run of glutamines. The predicted protein product for the commonest normal allele contains 816 amino acids, with a molecular weight of 87 kDa.

The normal function of the gene and the likely causes of its involvement in the pathology of SCA1 are not apparent from sequence analysis (Banfi *et al.*, 1994). Transcription of the gene appears to be fairly widespread, and both the normal and mutated protein are expressed in neurons in several regions of the brain in rats (Servadio *et al.*, 1995). Characteristically for proteins containing polyglutamine stretches, ataxin-1 migrates slowly on SDS-PAGE, appearing to be approximately 100 kDa in size, an effect that is likely to be indicative of an unusual polypeptide conformation. Immunohistochemically, the pattern of staining reveals nuclear expression of ataxin-1 in neurons, with additional, cytoplasmic staining in Purkinje cells of the cerebellum. These cells are badly affected by the disease, but this pattern of staining occurs both in patients and normal individuals.

The protein localization data do not in themselves reveal the cause of the pathology, but the transmission characteristics of SCA1 are similar to the other trinucleotide repeat diseases. The disease manifests when expansion of the $(CAG)_n$ stretch exceeds approximately 40 repeats and the number of repeats correlates broadly with the severity of phenotype (Orr *et al.*, 1993). Expansions are normally observed on transmission through affected males, whereas female transmission is characterized by stasis or contraction of the repeat in the majority of cases (Chung *et al.*, 1993). As in FRAXA, expansion of SCA1 alleles is associated with loss of interruptions in the repeat [e.g. tracts consisting of ... $(CAG)_n CAT(CAG)_n$ ...], which occur in most of the normal alleles. No ataxin-1 gene knockout mice have been described yet. In transgenic mice carrying a version of the human gene with an expansion, but not in those carrying the normal version, a phenotype similar to that in SCA1 was observed, suggesting that the polyglutamine tract itself is wholly responsible for neuronal degeneration in this disease (Burright et al., 1995).

Dentatorubral-pallidoluysian atrophy. Dentatorubral-pallidoluysian atrophy (DRPLA) is characterized by varying combinations of progressive myoclonus, epilepsy, ataxia and dementia. The gene underlying DRPLA is located on chromosome 12p13.3 and is identical or allelic to that underlying Haw River syndrome (Burke et al., 1994). By chance, a screening study for expressed genes containing trinucleotide repeats (Li et al., 1993) identified a cDNA clone, B37, which was later shown to be associated with expansions of a $(CAG)_n$ repeat in DRPLA (Koide et al., 1994; Nagafuchi et al., 1994b). This clone is a chimeric construct formed from two cDNAs, and the DRPLA gene itself was characterized later (Nagafuchi et al., 1994a). The gene consists of at least 10 exons, of which nine have been accurately mapped within a 9 kb genomic region. The probable initiator methionine lies in the second identified exon, with the polyglutamine tract encoded by the $(CAG)_n$ repeat starting 484 amino acids downstream in exon 5. Sequence comparisons have revealed no striking homologies with known proteins, although several notable features of the predicted protein sequence of 1184 amino acids have been discussed in the context of possible regulatory, protein–protein interactions (Nagafuchi et al., 1994a). An apparently single mRNA of approximately 4.5 kb appears to be widely expressed, and is present at relatively high levels in brain.

No clues have emerged as to the nature of the pathological mechanism in DRPLA. The neuronal cell types most prominently affected (in the dentate nucleus, rubrum, globus pallidus and Luy's body) are different from those affected in HD and SCA1. Somatic mosaicism in the extent of the expansion in genomic DNA is apparent in DRPLA, as in most of the other trinucleotide repeat diseases. This heterogeneity, although not correlating precisely with the neuropathology (Ueno et al., 1995), may account for the involvement of certain brain regions, while other regions and tissues are spared. Anti-peptide antibodies have been used to investigate the expression of the normal and mutant proteins (Yazawa et al., 1995). Both normal (apparent size 190 kDa) and mutant (210 kDa) species are present in cortex homogenates as well as other tissues, along with an additional species of approximately 100 kDa. Immunohistochemical studies with the same antiserum reveal staining in neurons in several areas of the brain, localized as granular material in cytoplasm, particularly in the perikaryon and proximal dendrites. This pattern is unaltered in sections of DRPLA brain (Ueno et al., 1995). The granular nature of the staining and the sequence motifs indicating features typical of ribonucleoprotein components have led these authors to speculate that the DRPLA gene product may be an RNP component or RNA binding protein as we have discussed above for FMR-1.

Machado–Joseph disease. Machado–Joseph disease (MJD) is characterized by cerebellar ataxia, other signs of central nervous system (CNS) dysfunction, peripheral neuropathy and bulging eyes. It maps to chromosome 14q, and has recently been shown to be identical or allelic to a previously recognized variant of spinocerebellar ataxia, SCA3 (Matilla *et al.*, 1995). As with DRPLA, the gene causing MJD was cloned by analysis of cDNAs selected by hybridization with a complementary $(CTG)_{13}$ oligonucleotide. At present the structure of the gene, *MJD1*, is not known, but a cDNA of 1.8 kb containing an open reading frame of 359 amino acids and a $(CAG)_n$ repeat encoding a polyglutamine tract near the C-terminus has been reported (Kawaguchi *et al.*, 1994). The predicted protein bears no homology to known genes. Other cDNAs that lack the CAG repeat and are divergent in sequence from the original clone in the 3' region may represent splice variants, indicating that the gene must contain at least four exons. Northern blotting data have not been presented.

Normal *MJD1* alleles contain 14–34 $(CAG)_n$ repeats, with that number increasing to 61–84 repeats in disease alleles, similar to DRPLA (Maruyama *et al.*, 1995). As with the other trinucleotide repeat diseases, MJD exhibits the phenomenon of 'anticipation', in which an earlier age of onset correlates with larger repeat expansions in patients (Kawaguchi *et al.*, 1994; Maruyama *et al.*, 1995). In addition to this phenomenon, there appears to be a relationship between the size of the expanded repeat and the subtype of disease phenotype observed (Maruyama *et al.*, 1995). The mutant allele is expressed in brain on the basis of reverse transcriptase–polymerase chain reaction (RT-PCR) experiments.

Clues to the pathological mechanism in polyglutamine tract diseases. The combined data from the $(CAG)_n$-type repeat disease genes indicate that the expanded allele is expressed as protein in the correct tissues, although quantitative experiments have not been attempted. Additionally, experiments on healthy mice that express huntingtin mRNA but not protein from expanded human transgenes suggest that translation of the expanded protein is required for the pathology (Goldberg *et al.*, 1996a). It has also been shown that homozygous null mutations that abolish expression of mature AR protein lead to testicular feminization (Griffin, 1992) rather than SBMA. These facts have led to the conclusion that a gain-of-function mechanism is most likely to underlie the pathological mechanism operating in the diseases in this group. Hints of such a mechanism are beginning to emerge. A recent paper concerning the artificial insertion of glutamine repeat tracts into proteins suggests that these tracts may subserve interactions between monomers of the same protein, or perhaps even other proteins with the same motif (Stott *et al.*, 1995). Oligomerization probably results from the β-pleated sheet-forming tendencies of these 'polar zipper'-like regions. Organization into multimers might endow these proteins with novel functions.

An alternative but similar mechanism is suggested by the cloning of unrelated proteins which bind to huntingtin, discussed above. These findings implicate a perturbation of normal regulatory interactions that results from the presence of the expanded polyglutamine tracts, but which may not involve them directly. The specificity of these regulatory interactions could account for the unique localization of the pathology in each disease, through limited cell and tissue expression of the interacting proteins. This scenario is commensurate with the idea that each of the $(CAG)_n$-type repeat disease proteins that we have discussed above serves an important regulatory function within many cell types. Two recent studies (Burke *et al.*, 1996; Koshy *et al.*, 1996) have reported an interaction between polyglutamine tract-containing proteins and the cytoplasmic, multifunctional glycolytic enzyme glyceraldehyde-3-phosphate dehydrogenase that is modulated by the length of the normal and expanded polyglutamine repeat. It has recently emerged that these proteins and their polyglutamine tracts may also be involved in the apoptotic cell death characteristic of this class of disorders. Huntingtin is specifically cleaved by the proapoptotic cysteine protease, apopain, in a manner that correlates with the onset of apoptosis (Goldberg *et al.*, 1996b). Expanded repeats in truncated MJD1 polypeptides have also been shown to cause cell death (Ikeda *et al.*, 1996).

A third possible mechanism involves an increase in liability of these proteins to undergo transglutamination and cross-linking as the polyglutamine tract expands. This would be expected to lead to a toxic build-up of the protein, or a reduction in active protein levels (Green, 1993). Polyglutamine tracts are also features of many transcription factors (Gerber *et al.*, 1994). Of the expanding $(CAG)_n$ repeat disease genes, however, only ataxin-1 and AR can reliably be said to have a nuclear localization in normal brain. $(CAG)_n$ trinucleotide expansions may also underlie other diseases showing dominant inheritance with evidence for anticipation. Tantalizing evidence for this has emerged as a result of the use of a monoclonal antibody specific against polyglutamine tracts exceeding a threshold length (Trottier *et al.*, 1995b) in any protein. On this basis, patients carrying expanded polyglutamine tracts in unknown proteins have been identified for two other dominant ataxias, SCA2 and SCA7. It has also been argued, from several points of view, that schizophrenia and bipolar disorder may share this pathological mechanism (Ross *et al.*, 1993).

14.2.3 Myotonic dystrophy

Much less is known about the pathogenetic mechanisms operating in myotonic dystrophy (DM). The primary symptoms of DM are cataract, myotonia, weakness and atrophy especially of type 1, slow, muscle fibers. Neurophysiological studies (Jamal *et al.*, 1986) have suggested direct neural involvement, as well as muscle pathology, in DM. There are indirect clinical genetic data to indicate neural dysfunction and the finding of a negative correlation in affected individuals between intelligence and age of onset, compatible with genetic anticipation (Turnpenny *et al.*, 1994), lends credence to this idea. A large DM family has been described with motor and sensory neuropathy in some of the affected individuals and there is good evidence for linkage of the combined disorder with the DM locus (Brunner *et al.*, 1991). Mental retardation is a well known characteristic of the severe, congenital form of DM. Other neurological symptoms that indicate primary CNS involvement have been reviewed by Moxley (1992).

A gene containing the mutation in DM was cloned (Brook *et al.*, 1992) as a result of the discovery of an expanded $(CTG)_n$ repeat at a locus on chromosome 19q (Aslanidis *et al.*, 1992; Buxton *et al.*, 1992; Harley *et al.*, 1992). Named, variously, DM kinase or myotonin (DMPK), the product of this gene shows amino acid homology with the cAMP-dependent, serine-threonine protein kinases (Brook *et al.*, 1992). Other domains in the 624 amino acid full length form of DMPK have high α-helical content (consistent with a 'coiled-coil' domain structure), have limited homology with a number of other neuromuscular proteins of diverse function, are rich in leucine residues, or are notably hydrophobic (Shaw *et al.* 1993; Wieringa, 1994).

The gene consists of 15 exons [the $(CTG)_n$ repeat being located in the last of these] distributed over about 13 kb of genomic DNA (Mahadevan *et al.* 1993) and is expressed in several tissues including muscle, testis and brain (Brook *et al.*, 1992; Jansen *et al.*, 1992; Roses, 1992). Alternative splicing has been observed (Jansen *et al.* 1992), but tissue-specific regulation of expression of the gene has not been clarified.

Different brain regions have recently been shown to have characteristic splice form expression and a putative brain-specific isoform lacking exon 13 has been identified (Gennarelli *et al.*, 1995). The repeat lies in the 3'-untranslated region (3'-UTR) of the mRNA in all splicing variants observed (Jansen *et al.*, 1992) and should not lead to a qualitatively different protein being produced. Quantitative changes may result from altered transcriptional rates or pre-mRNA processing, or from inhibition of translation, or from changes in mRNA stability of the expanded allele. A broad consensus exists that the $(CTG)_n$ repeat expansion reduces the steady state levels of mature mRNA transcribed from the expanded allele with little or no inhibition of primary transcript accumulation (Carango *et al.*, 1993; Fu *et al.*, 1993; Krahe *et al.*, 1995). There have been reports of a dominant negative effect of the CTG repeat expansion, whereby the mRNA transcribed from the expanded allele affects nuclear processing of pre-mRNA from the normal allele (Wang *et al.*, 1995). It is thus predicted that the levels of DMPK protein should be reduced, and indeed there is some evidence for this (Fu *et al.*, 1993). There is some doubt, however, about the identity of the protein species being detected by the antisera used in this and a number of other studies (Brewster *et al.*, 1993; Fu *et al.*, 1993; van der Ven *et al.*, 1993).

The normal function of DMPK is unclear. An immunoreactive species of approximately 52 kDa (smaller than predicted from analysis of cDNA clones) associated with membrane fractions of cell lysates (Brewster *et al.*, 1993) is concentrated at neuromuscular junctions in muscle fibers and may play a role in regeneration of muscle (van der Ven *et al.*, 1993). The same immunoreactive species occurs in several neuronal cell types in mouse brain (van der Ven *et al.*, 1993). Several other recent reports have begun to shed light on the protein isoforms that are expressed in different tissues. Whiting *et al.* (1995), using antisera that detect more predictable isoforms of 72 and 80 kDa, have suggested that one or more of the isoforms expressed in brain are localized at discrete synaptic sites in neurons in some regions. Similar isoforms have been expressed *in vitro* and shown to have serine kinase activity, as predicted from sequence homology data (Timchenko *et al.*, 1995).

Further analysis of the predicted protein sequence has revealed the existence of a sub-family of protein kinase A-related proteins that includes both DMPK and the product of a *Drosophila* gene *warts* (Justice *et al.*, 1995) that may be involved in control of cell shape and proliferation. It is also of interest that a sequence contained in the promoter region of the DM gene is capable of directing expression of a reporter transgene in mice to cells of the neural crest lineage, including some components of sensory pathways (King *et al.*, 1995).

It is conceivable that DMPK only plays a partial role in the development of symptoms in myotonic dystrophy. This may help to explain why there have been difficulties in correlating the clinical severity of DM with the measurement of quantitative changes in DMPK expression. This idea is supported by the fact that two independent gene targeting studies, in which the first half of the *DMPK* gene was disrupted in mice (Jansen *et al.*, 1996; Reddy *et al.*, 1996), have reported a phenotype of only mild myopathy. Effects of the expansion of the $(CTG)_n$ repeat on the expression of other genes in the vicinity of the DM gene cannot be ruled out. A minimally expanded block of 75 CTG repeats has been shown to promote formation of nucleosomes more strongly than any other naturally occurring sequence (Wang and Griffith, 1995). If this is the case *in vivo*, the chromatin structure of expanded alleles may be altered for some distance on either side of the *DMPK* gene. There is evidence for this in a report of the loss, from expanded alleles, of a DNase I hypersensitive site located just 3' to the $(CTG)_n$ repeat (Otten and Tapscott, 1995).

Backing up this conclusion, there is also evidence for the existence of a homeobox gene immediately downstream of the *DMPK* gene (Boucher *et al.*, 1995). This gene has been called DM-associated homeodomain protein (*DMAHP*) and is expressed in muscle and brain. A gene known as *59* (*DMR-N9* in mouse) lies immediately upstream of the *DMPK* gene (Jansen *et al.*, 1992). This gene possesses several repeated tracts with similarity to the 'WD' repeat motif found in a range of proteins with regulatory functions (Jansen *et al.*, 1995) and is expressed highly in brain and testis. Alterations in the expression of either or both of these genes may contribute to the highly variable phenotype in DM, or be responsible for the neuronal phenotype.

14.2.4 Friedreich's ataxia

Friedreich's ataxia (FRDA) is the commonest of the hereditary ataxias. Inherited as an autosomal recessive disorder, it is characterized by progressive degeneration in the central and peripheral nervous systems that causes gait and limb ataxia as well as sensory dysfunction, but without notable cerebellar involvement. Degeneration of the dorsal root ganglion sensory cells and spinocerebellar and corticospinal tracts is marked. Clinically, cardiac problems and diabetes are complicating factors. Since the first mapping of the genetic lesion to chromosome 9q13 by an early application of the genomic scanning approach (see *Figure 14.1*) to positional cloning (Chamberlain *et al.*, 1988), the search for the disrupted gene has been intense. Campuzano *et al.* (1996) initially reported the cloning of a gene they named *X25*, but it has recently emerged that this was in fact part of a larger gene now known as *STM7* (Carvajal *et al.*, 1996). The most common mutation found in this gene in patients involves the expansion of a $(GAA)_n$ repeat tract located in an intron.

The *STM7* gene spans about 450 kbp and comprises at least 24 exons. More than seven splice isoforms are thought to exist. Each is expressed at different levels in several tissues, with some isoforms showing fairly widespread expression, including in brain and heart. Transcript sizes vary between 1.3 and more than 6.5 kb. The protein products are as yet uncharacterized, but the translated open reading frame has homology with a novel human phosphatidylinositol-4-phosphate-5-kinase and two similar *S. cerevisiae* proteins. It is thought that the *STM7* gene product may function as a kinase in the inositol signaling system, and may have a role in axonal trafficking (Carvajal *et al.*, 1996).

In affected individuals, the $(GAA)_n$ tract had expanded from the normal range of 7–22 repeats up to between 200 and greater than 900 repeats. Neither the mechanism of this expansion [given the low propensity of $(GAA)_n$ for hairpin formation; Gacy *et al.*, 1995; see Section 14.2.5], nor its correlation with the phenotype, are clear. It is likely that multiple AG dinucleotides within the expanded region may form a cryptic splice acceptor site leading to aberrant mRNA processing (Campuzano *et al.*, 1996), although the evidence for this is not substantial (Carvajal *et al.*, 1996). Several individuals who are compound heterozygotes for point mutations in the *X25* gene and the expansion have also presented with typical FRDA symptoms.

14.2.5 Common characteristics of trinucleotide repeat gene diseases

As has been discussed above, there are many important differences in the molecular genetics, transmission and expression characteristics of the trinucleotide repeat diseases. Besides the fact that they all have a neurological phenotype, however, there are a number of striking similarities between them. Each of the genes studied so far is highly conserved in evolution, suggesting important and ancient functions. The repeat tracts themselves do not necessarily contribute to these functions, however (Rubinsztein et al., 1995). Nucleotide interruptions in the repeats (see Section 14.2.2) appear to reduce meiotic and mitotic instability, which is thought to occur as a result both of slippage of Okazaki fragments consisting solely of repeat units, and of hairpin loop formation (Gacy et al., 1995) during DNA replication, rather than by mispairing and recombination (Richards and Sutherland, 1994). The threshold for significant instability occurs at around 40–50 repeats in all cases. Evidence is accumulating that this lower size limit, and the high frequency of instability above this value, result from the interaction between mechanistic aspects of DNA replication and the tendency for $(CNG)_n$ repeat tracts to form hairpin loops when in single-stranded form (Chen et al., 1995; Gacy et al., 1995). Somatic heterogeneity in repeat expansion often occurs, due to continual expression of instability during mitosis. There is usually some degree of correlation between repeat expansion and pathology. In all cases, however, the genetic phenomena of anticipation (decreasing age of onset and increasing disease severity as the gene is passed from older generations to younger generations in an affected pedigree), reduced penetrance and variable expressivity are explained by the propensity of the repeats to expand or contract. This occurs both on transmission at meiosis and during mitosis. The extent and direction of the changes in repeat number vary with sex and cell type, and are possibly influenced by the orientation of the repeat tract with respect to nearby origins of replication. These features of the trinucleotide repeat diseases will undoubtedly be of use in the analysis of further, as yet unexplained, genetic diseases, with and without neuronal phenotypes.

14.3 Other disease genes with effects mainly on neuronal phenotype

14.3.1 Prion diseases

The prion diseases constitute a set of disorders in which the cellular 'prion' protein, PrP^c, exists in an abnormally stable, pathogenic, mutant form, PrP^{sc}. A prion (proteinaceous infectious particle) is capable of inducing disease by infection, wherein it appears to be made purely of protein, in contravention of the dogma that transmissible biological information with the potential for self-replication is encoded solely by nucleic acids (Prusiner, 1994). In this guise, prions are responsible for the sporadic or transmitted diseases Kuru and Creutzfeldt–Jakob disease (CJD) in humans, and scrapie (sheep) and bovine spongiform encephalopathy (cows), amongst others, in animals. In addition, mutations inherited in standard Mendelian fashion are responsible for the familial form of CJD and for the diseases Gerstmann–Sträussler–Scheinker syndrome (GSS) and fatal familial insomnia (FFI). The inherited forms make up about 10–15% of all cases of prion-related disease.

These rare diseases, together known as the subacute spongiform encephalopathies, are progressive and invariably fatal. CJD and GSS are characterized by spongiform vacuolation in the gray matter of the brain, with astrocytic proliferation and neuronal loss, with or without amyloid plaque formation. FFI, on the other hand, shows relatively specific degeneration of certain thalamic nuclei. Patients experience various neurological deficits, leading to dementia and death. CJD usually has a shorter, more severe clinical course than GSS. A wealth of clinical, biochemical and molecular information about the transmission and mechanism of these diseases has been reviewed recently by several authors (Collinge and Palmer, 1994; Prusiner, 1994).

Purification and sequencing of the mutant protein, PrP^{Sc}, enabled the cloning of a cellular gene, first in hamster (Oesch et al., 1985) then the human homolog on chromosome 20p, designated PRNP (Liao et al., 1986). The gene possesses two exons (Puckett et al., 1991), the second of which encodes the entire protein of 245 amino acids, with a predicted molecular weight of 27 kDa. It contains a signal peptide, several copies of a Gly–Pro-rich octapeptide repeat sequence, a transmembrane domain and other domains possibly involved in anchoring the protein to the exterior of the membrane via a sialoglycosyl phosphatidylinositol linkage (Prusiner, 1991). In rodents, mRNA of 2.1 kb (Oesch et al., 1985) or 2.4–2.5 kb (Chesebro et al., 1985) specific to PrP^C has been detected in various tissues, with highest levels in brain. This expression is specifically neuronal in hamster (Kretzschmar et al., 1986). In humans, PrP is detected at an apparent molecular weight of 33–35 kDa on SDS-PAGE in extracts of both normal brain and that from patients with prion diseases. On limited proteolysis, the normal PrP^C is degraded, whereas PrP^{Sc} is only partially digested to give a 27–30 kDa fragment that is resistant to further digestion. The normal function of PrP is unclear. Gene-targeted, 'knockout' mice with no copies of the PRNP gene have no obvious phenotype up to 7 months of age (Büeler et al., 1992), but there is now evidence that PrP is necessary for normal synaptic function in rodents (Collinge et al., 1994). Experiments demonstrating that this phenotype is rescued by the insertion of a human transgene into the PrP null mice (Whittington et al., 1995) have opened the way to functional studies of both normal and mutant forms of the protein.

The prion diseases in humans are due in a proportion of cases to inherited, dominant mutations of the PRNP gene. The first mutation demonstrated was an insertion of several extra copies of the octapeptide repeat region in familial CJD (Owen et al., 1989), followed closely by a report of a missense mutation in two GSS pedigrees (Hsiao et al., 1989). At present, six types of octapeptide insertion mutation and 11 different missense and nonsense mutations have been associated with familial CJD and GSS. Sporadic CJD does not seem to be caused by any of these mutations and may result from a very infrequent conversion of the wild-type protein into the PrP^{Sc} form in otherwise susceptible individuals. Intriguingly, one of the point mutations, an aspartate to asparagine substitution at codon 178 (D178N) is associated with both CJD and FFI, the phenotypic expression of the disease depending on which of two common alleles at a codon 129 polymorphism (coding for valine or methionine) is inherited on the D178N allele in the affected individual (Goldfarb et al., 1992a,b; Medori et al., 1992).

It is still unclear whether the mode of action of all the prion protein mutations mentioned is primarily a gain of function or a loss of function. It has been postulated in recent studies that the action of the PrP^{Sc} form of the mutant protein in recruitment of the wild-type PrP^C form to the pathogenic form may be simply to reduce the levels of functional, wild-type protein. If true, this suggests that a loss of function contributes to at least part of the disease phenotype (Collinge et al., 1994). This view is strengthened by the demonstration that PrP-null mice have altered circadian rhythms and sleep patterns, commensurate with an insufficiency of PrP^C leading to the pathogenesis observed in FFI (Tobler et al., 1996). The genetics and biochemistry, however, suggest a gain of function. Several lines of evidence have been adduced to support this interpretation.

Rodents lacking the PrP^C gene are not susceptible to disease through infection, cannot propagate the PrP^{Sc} form of the protein, and are not damaged by exogenous PrP^{Sc} (Brandner *et al.*, 1996; Büeler *et al.*, 1993; Sailer *et al.*, 1994). This suggests that recruitment from the pool of normal protein is an essential step in PrP^{Sc} manufacture, which is thought to occur post-translationally, possibly even outside the cell. The conversion event is likely to involve a switch from a mainly soluble, α-helical conformation to an insoluble, β-pleated sheet-rich conformation, in many cases associated with proteolysis and probably involving unfolding and refolding of the protein (Prusiner, 1991, 1994). The PrP^{Sc} form is necessary in almost all cases for the conversion of PrP^C protein to PrP^{Sc}, the accumulation of which in intracellular vesicles or as amyloid plaques may lead directly to the onset and progression of disease.

Certain combinations of sequence variants appear to be more pathogenic than others. This idea is supported by the fact that amyloid fibrils detected in some GSS patient brains contain only PrP derived from the mutant allele (Tagliavini *et al.*, 1994). Monari *et al.* (1994) have demonstrated that the conformations of the D178N mutant PrPs in cases of CJD and FFI are different, suggesting that these differences, resulting entirely from the codon 129 polymorphism (Goldfarb *et al.*, 1992b), are responsible for the very different phenotypes seen in each disease.

14.3.2 Alzheimer's disease

Alzheimer's disease (AD) is now well known as a neurodegenerative disease presenting as presenile dementia. AD has a core of symptoms (defects in memory and higher cognitive function as well as seizures in many cases) and of alterations in brain structure (including the congophilic, birefringent amyloid plaques typical of most brains in old age and after head trauma, and neurofibrillary tangles). The majority of cases are sporadic, with a small proportion that are familial, being transmitted in autosomal dominant fashion. The rapid pace of discovery of the genetic basis of the latter forms has been remarkable.

The first gene to be associated with susceptibility to AD was that encoding the major protein found in senile plaques, β-amyloid, which consists of one of a range of proteolytic products of the amyloid precursor protein (APP). The *APP* gene, located on chromosome 21q, was first cloned in 1987 (Goldgaber *et al.*, 1987; Kang *et al.*, 1987; Tanzi *et al.*, 1987). It spans 400 kbp and comprises 19 exons (Lamb *et al.*, 1993; Yoshikai *et al.*, 1990). At least four splice products exist, the longest of which covers approximately 3.5 kb, encoding a full-length protein of 770 amino acids. The APP protein has a single membrane-spanning domain near the C-terminus, with most of the N-terminal portion of the protein lying extracellularly. The latter part of the protein has several notable features (see Wasco and Tanzi, 1995), including a variably spliced domain with similarities to serine protease inhibitors (Ponte *et al.*, 1988; Yoshikai *et al.*, 1990). In addition, a short region extending from the extracellular part into the transmembrane domain has a very strong propensity for forming β-pleated sheet secondary structure and constitutes the 4–5 kDa, 28–43 amino acid protein fragment (Aβ) found in β-amyloid and neuritic plaques. The *APP* gene appears to have fairly wide, but not ubiquitous expression, including in neurons (Goldgaber *et al.*, 1987; Ponte *et al.*, 1988; Tanzi *et al.*, 1987).

The normal function of APP is far from clear. There is evidence that isoforms containing the serine protease inhibitor domain can inhibit the activity of factor IXa (Schmaier *et al.*, 1993) and secreted forms of APP point to a component of their function being independent of the known anchorage of many isoforms in the cell membrane; additionally, trophic, receptor and cell–matrix interaction functions have all been proposed (see Wasco and Tanzi, 1995, for a more detailed discussion). Overexpression of the normal full length human *APP* gene in mice has not been found to cause a phenotype resembling AD (Lamb *et al.*, 1993), although it should be noted that the development of senile plaques at an early age in Down's syndrome (trisomy 21) patients has been linked to the onset of dementia, and may occur as a result of the expression of APP at increased levels due to increased gene dosage. APP knockout mice have recently been described (Zheng *et al.*, 1995). Homozygous null mice show a mild neurological phenotype with reduced locomotor activity and reactive gliosis in the brain, suggestive of a generalized but nonlethal impairment of neuronal function.

There are several mutations in APP linked to familial AD (Goate *et al.*, 1991; Wasco and Tanzi, 1995), all being missense mutations at locations near the β-amyloid encoding region. Mutations in APP account for a tiny fraction of all AD cases, but have shed some light on the mechanism of amyloidosis. Games *et al.* (1995) have reported that mice transgenic for a human *APP* gene carrying one of the missense mutations in AD progressively develop pathology reminiscent of AD brains and a very recent study has reported that one of the isoforms expressed in brain carrying mutations found in a Swedish family causes both deposition of Aβ plaques and memory defects when overexpressed in transgenic mice (Hsiao *et al.*, 1996), making this model the closest to AD thus far generated. Several studies have shown that a number of mutations are associated with changes in levels of Aβ peptide occurring as a result of alterations in processing and/or secretion of the precursor (Citron *et al.*, 1992; Felsenstein *et al.*, 1994; Suzuki *et al.*, 1994). Overexpression of the Aβ fragment itself in neurons of transgenic mice has led to neurotoxicity, possibly through induction of apoptosis, and has caused early death of the mice (LaFerla *et al.*, 1995). Hints at the mechanism of this effect are emerging. Thomas *et al.* (1996) recently reported that β-amyloid fragments mediate overproduction of free radicals by endothelium and the cellular damage caused by this process can be prevented by treatment with superoxide dismutase (SOD; see Section 14.3.3).

Other genes have now been implicated in predisposition to AD. A substantial proportion of early onset (<60 years), nonAPP-linked, AD cases with rapid progression show linkage with markers on chromosome 14, and several missense mutations in a novel gene on chromosome 14q have recently been reported (Campion *et al.*, 1995; Sherrington *et al.*, 1995). Known at first as transcript S182, this gene has now been named presenilin 1 (*PS-1*); it spans about 75 kbp and consists of at least 12 exons, of which 10 encode parts of the open reading frame (Clark *et al.*, 1995). The encoded protein consists of 467 amino acids, featuring between seven and nine predicted hydrophobic domains and two acidic hydrophilic domains. The product may be an integral membrane receptor or channel, but the cDNA shows some similarity to two *C. elegans* proteins, SPE-4 and sel-12, that may function in cell trafficking (Levitan and Greenwald, 1995).

Very recently, two reports have identified a related gene (*STM2*, now presenilin 2, *PS-2*) at a locus on chromosome 1q, that accounts for the previously reported linkage to this locus of several families of Volga Germans with slightly later onset AD (Levy-Lahad *et al.*, 1995; Rogaev *et al.*, 1995). The structure of the *PS-2* gene, spanning at least 24 kbp (Levy-Lahed *et al.*, 1996), is very similar to that of *PS-1*, in terms of exon boundaries within the coding sequence. The proteins share 67% identity in amino acid sequence. Both genes are expressed fairly widely, both within and outside the brain, and probably undergo alternative splicing (Cruts *et al.*, 1995; Levy-Lahad *et al.*, 1996). That two genes which probably subserve similar biological roles can underlie subtly different forms of AD suggests that the function of their gene products will prove extremely enlightening in explaining how dysfunction of a common pathway can lead to the observed variability in age of onset and to the characteristics of amyloid plaques. Indeed, it has now emerged that mutations in all three familial AD genes (*APP*, and presenilin-1 and -2) act to increase the secretion of the damaging Aβ1-42(43) isoform found in AD plaques (Scheuner *et al.*, 1996).

It is as yet unclear whether these genes suffer somatic mutation, or indeed whether other functionally related genes are mutated, in the common, late onset variety of AD. Two further molecules have been implicated in the pathogenesis of AD. An allelic association between age of onset of late-onset familial/sporadic AD and the apolipoprotein E locus (APOE) on chromosome 19q (Corder *et al.*, 1993; Strittmatter *et al.*, 1993) has been reported by many groups, and it has been shown that an individual's genotype at this locus clearly influences the risk of developing AD. The ε4 allele of APOE, which confers increased risk of AD, is implicated in increased binding of APOE to Aβ in amyloid plaques, although it is not known whether this is a causal association. Other factors, such as genotype at the α1-antichymotrypsin locus, influence the interaction between APOE, APP and the onset of AD. There is also strong evidence that the microtubule-associated protein tau, found in the cores of the paired helical filaments of neurofibrillary tangles (Goedert *et al.*, 1988), is abnormally glycosylated and phosphorylated (Wang *et al.*, 1996). It is not known, however, whether this is a primary or secondary event.

14.3.3 Oxidative damage diseases

Two neurological diseases have recently provided evidence of the direct involvement of free radicals in pathological states. One is a rare, dominantly inherited form of the usually sporadic, neurodegenerative disease amyotrophic lateral sclerosis (ALS), otherwise known as motor neuron disease. This disease can in some cases result from mutations in the gene for SOD1 (*SOD1*). The second example is a very rare form of spinocerebellar degeneration that is similar to FRDA and is associated with selective vitamin E deficiency (AVED). This has been shown to be caused by mutations in the α-tocopherol transfer protein gene. Both of these neurological disorders are caused by mutations in genes whose products help to prevent oxidative damage caused by free radicals.

Mutations in the *SOD1* gene, encoding the cytosolic, Cu/Zn-containing form of the enzyme, were first demonstrated by Rosen *et al.* (1993). The gene encodes a 153 amino acid protein over five exons. Numerous point mutations, none of them truly null mutations, have been reported in the minority of ALS families that are linked to chromosome 21q (see *Figure 14.3*). In addition, mutations in *SOD1* have been reported in several sporadic ALS cases (Jones *et al.*, 1993).

Several mechanisms have been proposed to explain the relationship between the phenotype and the dominant inheritance of ALS in chromosome 21-linked families. Evidence both for active site defects (Pramatarova *et al.*, 1995) and for dominant negative effects of mutated residues in dimerization domains (Deng *et al.*, 1993; Pramatarova *et al.*, 1995) have been adduced to back up findings of reduced enzyme activity in heterozygotes. These findings point to an overall loss-of-function effect. In contradiction to the consensus on this point, a postulated dominant gain-of-function

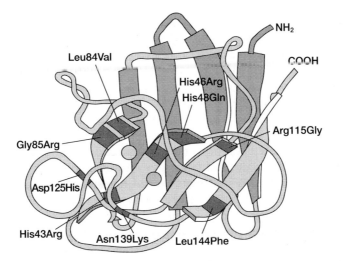

Figure 14.3. Structure of Cu,Zn-superoxide dismutase (SOD1). A diagrammatic, three-dimensional representation of SOD1 is shown based on the crystal structure of the native human enzyme. The positions of some of the mutations found in ALS that lie near or at the active site cleft are shown.

defect has been reported in a homozygous patient with normal SOD1 activity (Anderson *et al.*, 1995). Experimental manipulations have not resolved this controversy. Both inhibition of SOD1 expression (Rothstein *et al.*, 1994), and a dominant gain-of-function mutation with little effect on SOD1 activity expressed in transgenic mice (Gurney *et al.*, 1994), lead to apoptotic degeneration of spinal motor neurons. In this model, any loss of enzymatic function would be incidental to the pathological mechanism operating in *SOD1*-linked ALS [cf. the $(CAG)_n$-type trinucleotide repeat diseases discussed in Section 14.2.2 above]. It is also possible that effects on SOD1 activity and gain-of-function toxicity may interact to influence age of onset and duration in this form of the disease. SOD1 knockout mice have been generated (Reaume *et al.*, 1996), and have no pathology resembling ALS at 4–6 months of age, lending credence to a toxic, gain-of-function role for *SOD1* mutations. It was also demonstrated in this study, however, that SOD1 is required for the normal protective response to axonal injury. It should be noted that variants of neurofilament proteins have also been implicated in the ALS phenotype in a few patients and in animal models (reviewed in Brown, 1995).

AVED, a rare autosomal recessive disease, results from mutations in the α-tocopherol transfer protein (α-TTP) gene, located at 8q13 (Ouahchi *et al.*, 1995). α-TTP is a cytosolic protein of 278 amino acids expressed in liver. It mediates the loading of very low density lipoprotein particles with vitamin E. The gene encoding α-TTP comprises five exons (Hentati *et al.*, 1996). Several familial and sporadic mutations have been found, including frameshifts and premature terminations. All are thought to affect the function of the protein, thereby leading to vitamin E deficiency in peripheral tissues.

Many metabolic reactions within cells, including the normal processes of aging, lead to production of highly reactive and toxic radicals (molecules with unpaired electrons in their outer orbits) directly, such as the hydroxyl radical OH•, or to less damaging radicals such as superoxide or lipid peroxides. Because of the complex chemistry involved, it has not proved easy to link alterations in the activity of enzymes like SOD1 to the specific free radical-generating pathways most likely to be involved in the pathology of ALS. New studies are beginning to provide that link. One of the familial SOD1 mutants has been shown to have increased peroxidase activity, a toxic side-reaction also catalyzed at low levels by the wild-type enzyme (Wiedau-Pazos *et al.*, 1996). It is likely that the vitamin E deficiency of AVED is linked causally to the ataxic phenotype through disruption of the normal antioxidant properties of α-tocopherol. It has been reported that this molecule can also modulate the well-known neurotoxicity of excessive levels of glutamate in the CNS. Partial deficiency of glutamate reuptake has also been suggested to contribute to some forms of ALS. The pathway between uptake of excess glutamate mediated by *N*-methyl-D-aspartate (NMDA) or nonNMDA receptors and apoptotic neuronal cell death is not clear (although Ca^{2+} ion flux and nitric oxide (NO) synthase activity have both been implicated). It is possible that these two functions of antioxidants are not entirely unconnected, or that the two factors, glutamate neurotransmission and oxidative stress, may interact to potentiate the neurotoxic effect in a limited subset of neurons (Rothstein *et al.*, 1994).

14.3.4 Channelopathies

A number of genetic disorders are caused by mutations in genes encoding ion channels. Termed 'channelopathies', these include several neuromuscular disorders caused by mutations in muscle sodium or chloride channel genes (for example, hyperkalemic periodic paralysis and paramyotonia congenita). This category is not discussed further here. Mutations in neuronal ion channel genes, however, have recently been shown to underlie several other diseases that might also fall into the general category of channelopathies.

Hyperekplexia. Hyperekplexia, or startle disease, is a dominant disorder characterized by neonatal hypertonia and, in later life, an exaggerated response to certain sudden stimuli. Patients also have other reflex disturbances and their symptoms respond dramatically to treatment with the benzodiazepine drug, clonazepam. The disorder results from mutations in the gene for the $\alpha1$-subunit of the glycine receptor (Shiang *et al.*, 1993), a member of the ligand-gated neurotransmitter receptor superfamily. Glycine receptors probably exist as pentameric arrangements of α- and β-subunits enclosing an integral anion channel.

The gene encoding the $\alpha1$-subunit, *GLRA1*, is localized at 5q33. It is expressed from nine exons spanning at least 150 kbp, the longest mRNA product covering 1.7 kb, with an open reading frame encoding a 421 amino acid (48 kDa) protein (Grenningloh *et al.*, 1990; Shiang *et al.*, 1993, 1995). Alternative splicing has been demonstrated (Malosio *et al.*, 1991) but its significance is unknown. Several subunits of the related $GABA_A$ receptor possess splicing variants that are regulated by phosphorylation (Moss *et al.*, 1992). Several of the mutations identified thus far are concentrated in a region of the subunit close to the extracellular mouth of the predicted chloride channel. These mutations are likely to affect the gating properties of the channel or the transduction of agonist binding into ion conductance (Shiang *et al.*, 1995). Two mutations in mice, *spasmodic* (Ryan *et al.*, 1994) and *spastic* (Kingsmore *et al.*, 1994), have been localized to the α1- and β-subunit genes of the glycine receptor, respectively. Further studies are underway to characterize the correlation between mutation and phenotype at the molecular level. Recent studies have shown that a deletion within the *GLRA1* gene that abolishes production of the mature protein is not fatal in humans (Brune *et al.*, 1996) as it is in the *oscillator* mouse mutant (Buckwalter *et al.*, 1994). Instead, this defect causes a recessive form of hyperekplexia, suggesting that there is some functional redundancy in the human spinal glycinergic system.

Autosomal dominant nocturnal frontal lobe epilepsy. A recently described seizure disorder, autosomal dominant nocturnal frontal lobe epilepsy (ADNFLE; Scheffer *et al.*, 1995), results from mutations in the gene for the α4-subunit of the nicotinic acetylcholine receptor (CHRNA4; Steinlein *et al.*, 1995). In this disorder, with typical onset in mid to late childhood, tonic and tonic–clonic (grand mal) seizures occur soon after the onset of sleep or before awakening in the morning and are generated by discharges originating in frontal lobe foci. Cholinergic input has complex modulatory functions during sleep and arousal both at the cortical and thalamic levels. *CHRNA4*, located at 20q13.2, encodes a protein of 627 amino acids that is a member of the ligand-gated ion channel superfamily. The gene consists of six exons spanning at least 17 kbp (Steinlein *et al.*, 1996). It shows widespread expression in the brain and is expressed in all layers of the cortex. The only mutation described thus far alters a conserved serine residue in the second transmembrane domain of the protein, a region which contributes to the lining of the ion channel, as described in the section on hyperekplexia above. The mutation is likely to influence channel conductance, but the mechanism of seizure generation, and particularly its temporal restriction, remains a mystery.

Episodic ataxia with myokimia. Episodic ataxia with myokimia (muscle rippling) is a rare, dominant disorder in which startle or abrupt exercise can provoke the symptoms. The myokimia arises from spontaneous, repetitive discharges in peripheral nerves. Several different mutations have been observed in the gene encoding a member of the *Shaker* family of voltage-gated potassium channels, *KCNA1* (Browne *et al.*, 1994). This gene, located on chromosome 12p in a cluster of similar potassium channel genes, contains no introns and has an open reading frame spanning 1.49 kbp. The receptor comprises a tetrameric association of α-subunits, such as KCNA1, in close apposition to intracellular proteins. The α-subunits have six transmembrane domains and an intramembrane loop that does not completely span the membrane. *KCNA1* is expressed in several tissues in man, including brain and heart (Curran *et al.*, 1992), and is known to be expressed in both cerebellum and peripheral neurons in mice (Beckh and Pongs, 1990). The mutations in *KCNA1* cluster near the intracellular boundaries of transmembrane domains in several cases. Several of these mutations, all of which are present in heterozygous form, never homozygous, thus far, have been shown to alter the gating properties of mutant/wild-type heteromers. They are thought to act by delaying the regeneration of the membrane potential after an action potential has occurred (Adelman *et al.*, 1995). Possible roles for the mutations in α-subunit multimer interactions, or through altered interactions with the cytoplasmic β-subunit of the receptor, have not been ruled out, however.

As we have mentioned above, there are several other types of ion channels in which mutations result in specific neuromuscular disorders. These examples, like hyperekplexia, ADNFLE and episodic ataxia, are characterized by intermittent symptoms with apparently normal functioning between episodes. Analysis of the molecular basis of the malfunction in these diseases will shed considerable light on the processes by which neurons execute their characteristic functions of maintenance of the membrane potential and generation of the action potential.

14.3.5 Neuronal migration and maturation defects.

The characterization of mutations which specifically affect neurons during brain development and maturation has been eagerly awaited, in view of the light they may shed on the role of growth factors, guidance cues and adhesion molecules in these processes. Three findings have provided a considerable impetus to further work in this field.

Miller–Dieker lissencephaly syndrome. Miller–Dieker lissencephaly syndrome (MDLS) is characterized by microcephaly, a thickened cerebral cortex consisting of fewer layers than normal and agenesis of the corpus callosum in most cases. Neural symptoms of this disorder include retarded motor and mental development and spasticity. The consensus view holds that a general and widespread failure of neuronal migration during development is responsible for the condition. Reiner *et al.* (1993) have cloned a gene, *LIS-1*, located at 17p13.3, that has undergone partial deletion in several patients.

Several cDNA clones corresponding to *LIS-1* (and a very closely related transcript mapping to chromosome 2) have been isolated and sequence comparisons have suggested alternative splicing at both the 5′ and 3′ ends. Use of these clones as probes on Northern blots has revealed several mRNA transcripts of 2.2–7.5 kb in length. The gene is expressed in brain and a wide range of other tissues. The longest open reading frame encodes a protein of 411 amino acid residues. Much of this represents a series of repeated domains showing limited homology with the G-protein, retinal β-transducin. Reiner *et al.* isolated the *LIS-1* gene on the basis of this similarity, and they have hypothesized that LIS-1 represents a member of the 'WD' repeat family of G-protein β-subunits that are involved in signal transduction.

Neer *et al.* (1993) have pointed out, however, that the 'WD' repeat may be a general mediator of subunit interactions, since other proteins that have this repeat domain share no obvious common functions. The demonstration that human LIS-1 shows 99% identity with a noncatalytic 45 kDa subunit of bovine platelet-activating factor (PAF) acetylhydrolase (Hattori *et al.*, 1994) suggests that LIS-1 is the human homolog of this protein, which participates in the inactivation of PAF. PAF is thought to act as a neurotransmitter amongst its many other roles, and the function of LIS-1 in normal individuals may be to remove PAF from its site of action. The PAF/LIS-1 system may thus be an important regulator of migration of immature neurons in the developing brain.

Norrie disease. Norrie disease (ND) is an X-linked recessive disorder characterized by retinal degeneration and, in many cases, progressive mental disturbances and sensorineural deafness. The ND gene, which maps to Xp11.4 adjacent to the monoamine oxidase (MAO-A and -B) gene cluster, was cloned independently by two groups (Berger *et al.*, 1992; Chen *et al.*, 1992) using positional cloning techniques, aided by investigations of a number of patients carrying microdeletions of the region.

Several cDNAs have been isolated. The longest is commensurate with an mRNA of 1.9 kb that has been detected on Northern blots of retina, choroid, and fetal and adult human brain. The open reading frame contained in these cDNA clones is predicted to encode a protein (NDP) of 133 amino acids (15 kDa), which showed no striking homologies with sequences in the databases at the time the original reports were published. The predicted protein is noteworthy for the high proportion of polar, basic and cysteine residues it contains. The *NDP* gene consists of three exons spanning 27–28 kbp of genomic DNA (Chen *et al.*, 1993; Meindl *et al.*, 1992). The translation initiation site is situated in exon 2 and the coding region extends into exon 3. Promoter sequences, transcriptional start site and splice sites all conform broadly to consensus sequences.

Further investigation of the predicted amino acid sequence has revealed conserved positioning of several cysteine and other residues near the C-terminus relative to the equivalent region of a number of vertebrate mucin-like proteins and several other secreted proteins with postulated roles in cell-to-cell signaling and other interactions (Meindl *et al.*, 1992). More recently, an explanation of the functional role of these Cys-rich C-terminal domains has emerged. Molecular modeling predicts that a complex system of disulfide bridges within this domain determine a tertiary structure termed a 'cysteine knot'. This structure is characteristic of several members of the transforming growth factor (TGF$_\beta$) family and other, sequence unrelated, growth factors. Such a structure has been proposed for NDP (Meitinger *et al.*, 1993). The similarities with TGF$_\beta$ extend to a conserved Cys residue implicated in homodimer formation.

Confirmation of the role of the *NDP* gene in ND has come from the detection of a large range of point mutations, including premature stop codons yielding truncated proteins, splice site alterations and creation or deletion of specific Cys residues implicated in interactions within the knot structure (Berger *et al.*, 1992; Meindl *et al.*, 1992). Additionally, a mutation that corrupts the ATG initiation codon has been reported (Isashiki *et al.*, 1995) and appears to produce a true null phenotype in affected males.

Kallmann syndrome. Kallmann syndrome is another X-linked, multisystem disorder for which the gene has been cloned. The symptoms, which include anosmia and hypogonadotropic hypogonadism and defects in associated secondary sexual characters, are likely to arise from a much more limited primary phenotype than for MDLS and ND. They can be traced back to the failure of a specific group of neurons in the olfactory placode to migrate to their normal positions in the olfactory bulb and hypothalamus during brain development (Bick *et al.*, 1992). The gene maps to Xp22.3 and a candidate has been cloned independently by two groups on the basis of deletions present in patients, and named *KALIG-1* (Franco *et al.*, 1991) or *ADMLX* (Legouis *et al.*, 1991). Mutations in this gene have been confirmed by Hardelin *et al.* (1992), who found several patients carrying novel stop codons or frameshift mutations which would truncate the protein prematurely.

The *KALIG-1* gene encompasses between 120 and 200 kbp in the genome and consists of 14 exons, each bounded by splice sites fitting the consensus criteria (del Castillo *et al.*, 1992; Incerti *et al.*, 1992). The gene escapes inactivation upon lyonization of one of the two X chromosomes in females, along with several other loci in the same region of Xp22. Expression of the gene has been detected by RT-PCR in all tissues tested, including brain (Franco *et al.*, 1991; Legouis *et al.*, 1991). The failure to detect expression by Northern blotting suggests that transcript levels are low. The longest cDNA clone obtained has been 4.1 kb in length (Franco *et al.*, 1991), but overlapping cDNAs totaling 6.3 kb have been isolated (Legouis *et al.*, 1991), of which more than 4 kb constitute 3′-UTR. No evidence for alternative splicing has been observed. The longest open reading frame encodes a protein of 680 amino acids.

The predicted protein shows a complex system of homology with known proteins. While there is a signal peptide, there are no potential transmembrane segments internally. There are, however, several potential N-linked glycosylation sites, suggesting that KALIG-1 is a secreted protein. The positions of several cysteine residues in a Cys-rich region towards the N-terminus are similar to the four-disulfide-core domain of the so-called 'WAP' (whey acidic protein) family of proteins, which includes a number of inhibitors of serine proteases and ATPases. Further into the sequence there are four repeated domains that are characteristic of the fibronectin III family. These repeats are also found in numerous neural cell adhesion molecules, including NCAM-L1 [the protein implicated in X-linked hydrocephalus (Rosenthal *et al.*, 1992), MASA (mental retardation, aphasia, shuffling gait and adducted thumbs) syndrome and X-linked spastic paraplegia], protein kinases and tyrosine phosphatases. There is also a His-rich region of unknown significance at the C-terminus.

These sequence characteristics of the protein indicate its potential function. Fibronectin III repeats are typical of several proteins involved in axonal pathfinding by both adhesion and neurite outgrowth mechanisms. The neurons involved in the specific symptoms of Kallmann syndrome (LH-RH neurons, which migrate to the hypothalamus, and neurons of the vomeronasal and terminalis nerves of the olfactory system) originate in the same region of the developing brain. These neurons are known to fail to migrate normally, while other neural symptoms may relate to the abnormal migration or elongation of other subsets of immature neurons. The role of extracellular phosphorylation in this process, which is suggested by the homology data, is unclear. Evidence for a role for kinase/phosphatase modulation of cell adhesion is accumulating. The *KALIG-1* gene product may act in protease inhibitory processes of importance in cell–cell adhesion. The regional specificity of the symptoms is likely to be due to the more localized expression of factors which interact with KALIG-1, in view of the apparent widespread expression of the gene. A transient increase in transcript levels in the affected regions at particular stages of development cannot be ruled out, however.

14.4 Other disease genes with neuronal phenotypes

Because of space limitations, we shall not consider any of the more than 40 other diseases with neuronal phenotypes for which mutations in, or deletions encompassing, known genes have been observed. These may be divided into several categories; the metabolic, storage, peroxisomal and mitochondrial disorders, a number of which are summarized in *Table 14.2*; the myelin-associated neuropathies (showing expression in oligodendrocytes but with direct effects on the functioning of myelinated neuronal axons; *Table 14.3*); and several miscellaneous disorders including those involving cell cycle disruption or apoptosis (*Table 14.3*). All of these disorders are of interest in

Table 14.2. Disease genes with widespread expression and/or phenotype

Disease group	Disease	Disease gene symbol	Gene(s) mutated, symbol	Chromosomal localization	MIM no.
Metabolic	Lesch–Nyhan syndrome	LNS	Hypoxanthine-guanine phosphoribosyltransferase, HPRT	Xq26-q27.2	308000
	Phenylketonuria	PKU1	Phenylalanine hydroxylase	12q24.1	261600
	Maple syrup urine disease	MSUD	Branched-chain α-ketoacid dehydrogenase E1a/E2 subunits, BCKDE1A, DBT	19q13.2,1p31	248600
	Canavan disease		Aspartoacylase, ASPA	17pter-p13	271900
	Segawa syndrome (DOPA-responsive dystonia)	DRD	GTP cyclohydrolase I, GCH1	14q22.1-q22.2	128230
	Segawa syndrome, autosomal recessive		Tyrosine hydroxylase, TH	11p15.5	191290
Storage	Menke's syndrome	MNK	Cu^{2+}-transporting ATPase, ATP7A	Xq13.2-q13.3	309400
	Wilson disease	WND	Cu^{2+}-transporting ATPase, ATP7B	113q14.3	277900
	Gaucher disease	GD	Acid β-glucosidase (glucocerebrosidase), GBA	1q21	230800
	Gangliosidosis	GM-1	β-galactosidase I, GLB1	3p22-p21.3	230500
	Tay–Sachs disease	TSD, GM-2 I	Hexosaminidase A, HEXA	15q23-q24	272800
	Sandhoff disease	GM-2 II	Hexosaminidase B, HEXB	5q13	268800
	GM-2 gangliosidosis, AB variant	GM-2 III	GM-2 activator, GM2A	5q32-q33	272750
	Metachromatic leukodystrophy	MLD	Arylsulfatase A, ARSA	22q13.3-qter	250100
	Krabbe disease (globoid cell leukodystrophy)	GLD	Galactosylceramidase, GALC	14q31	245200
	Hurler and Scheie syndrome (mucopolysaccharidosis I)	MPS I	α-L-iduronidase, IDUA	4p16.3	252800
	Hunter syndrome (mucopolysaccharidosis II)	MPS II	Iduronate 2-sulfatase, IDS	Xq28	309900
Peroxisomal	Aspartylglucosaminuria	AGU	Aspartyl-glucosaminidase, AGA	4q23-q35	208400
	Niemann-Pick disease	NPD	Sphingomyelinase, SMPD1	11p15.3	257200
	Adrenoleukodystrophy	ALD	ALDP;	Xq28	300100
			Peroxisome targeting signal receptor I, PXR1	12p13	202370
	Zellweger syndrome	ZWS1	Peroxisome membrane protein, 70 kDa, PMP70	7q11.2	214100
Mitochondrial	Myoclonus epilepsy with ragged red fibers	MERRF	Mitochondrial tRNA^{lys}, MTTK	mtDNA	545000
	Leber hereditary optic neuropathy	LHON	Mitochondrial ND1, ND4 and ND6	mtDNA	535000
	Leigh syndrome	NARP	Mitochondrial ATP synthase, ATP6	mtDNA	516060

Table 14.3. Disease genes with partial or indirect neuronal phenotypic effects

Disease group	Disease	Disease gene symbol	Gene(s) mutated, symbol	Chromosomal localization	MIM no.
Neuropathies	Charcot–Marie–tooth Type 1A	CMT1A	Peripheral myelin protein-22, PMP22	17p11.2	118220
	Charcot–Marie–tooth Type 1B	CMT1B	Myelin-P(0), MPZ	1q22–q23	118200
	Charcot–Marie–tooth X-linked	CMTX1	Connexin-32, CX32	1Xq11–q13.1	302800
	Dejerine–Sottas syndrome	HMSN3	PMP22, MPZ		145900
	Hereditary neuropathy with liability to pressure palsies	HNPP	PMP22		162500
	Pelizaeus–Merzbacher disease/ X-linked spastic paraplegia	PMD/SPG2	Proteolipid protein, PLP	Xq21.3–q22	312080 312920
Cell cycle/ cell death	Neurofibromatosis I	NF1	Neurofibromin, NF1	17q11.2	162200
	Xeroderma pigmentosum I (complementation group A)	XPA	XPA	9q22.3	278700
	Spinal muscular atrophy I	SMA	Survival motor neuron/neuronal apoptosis inhibitory protein, SMN/NAIP	5q13	253300
Other	Tuberous sclerosis	TSC2	Tuberin, TSC2	16p13.3	191092
	X-linked hydrocephalus	HSAS1	L1 cell adhesion molecule, L1CAM	Xq28	307000
	Familial amyloid polyneuropathy	FAP	Transthyretin, TTR	18q11.2–q12.1	176300
	X-linked mental retardation with α-thalassemia	ATR-X	X-linked helicase 2, RAD54	Xq13	301040
	Usher syndrome, Type 1B	USH1B	Myosin VIIA, MYU7A	11q13.5	276903
	Prader-Willi/Angelman syndrome	PWS/AS	Small nuclear ribonucleoprotein N, SNRPN	15q12	176270 105830

defining the parameters of the normal functioning of many neurons, or specific subsets, in man.

Many of the disorders discussed above have yielded to the increasingly powerful techniques of positional cloning. The rapid accumulation of sequence and mapping data being generated by the Human Genome Project, particularly the development of transcript maps of the genome, will prove invaluable in future studies. These efforts are being boosted by the development of computer resources for assessing similarity between novel disease candidates and known gene and protein families. It may soon be possible to assign the domains of a newly predicted protein to the appropriate family on a first pass analysis. These advances will furnish the development of a truly reciprocal interplay between the elucidation of pathogenic processes in human CNS disease and an understanding of the role of genes whose expression in neurons underlies the development and mature functioning of the brain.

References

Abitbol M, Menini C, Delezoide A-L, Rhyner T, Vekemans M, Mallet J. (1993) Nucleus basalis magnocellularis and hippocampus are the major sites of *FMR-1* expression in the human fetal brain. *Nature Genetics* **4:** 147–153.

Adelman JP, Bond CT, Pessia M, Maylie J. (1995) Episodic ataxia results from voltage dependent potassium channels with altered functions. *Neuron* **15:** 1449–1454.

Andersen PM, Nilsson P, Alahurula V et al. (1995) Amyotrophic lateral sclerosis associated with homozygosity for an Asp90Ala mutation in CuZn superoxide dismutase. *Nature Genetics* **10:** 61–66.

Andrade MA, Bork P. (1995) HEAT repeats in the Huntington's disease protein. *Nature Genetics* **11:** 115–116.

Ashley CT, Sutcliffe JS, Kunst CB, Leiner HA, Eichler EE, Nelson DL, Warren ST. (1993a) Human and murine *FMR-1*: alternative splicing and translational initiation downstream of the CGG-repeat. *Nature Genetics* **4:** 244–251.

Ashley CT, Wilkinson KD, Reines D, Warren ST. (1993b) *FMR1* protein: conserved RNP family domains and selective RNA binding. *Science* **262:** 563–566.

Aslanidis C, Jansen G, Amemiya C et al. (1992) Cloning of the essential myotonic dystrophy region and mapping of the putative defect. *Nature* **355:** 548–551.

Banfi S, Servadio A, Chung MY et al. (1994) Identification and characterization of the gene causing type 1 spinocerebellar ataxia. *Nature Genetics* **7:** 513–520.

Baxendale S, Abdulla S, Elgar G et al. (1995) Comparative sequence analysis of the human and pufferfish Huntington's disease genes. *Nature Genetics* **10:** 67–76.

Beckh S, Pongs O. (1990) Members of the RCK potassium channel family are differentially expressed in the rat nervous system. *EMBO J.* **9:** 777–782.

Berger W, Meindl A, Vandepol TJR et al. (1992) Isolation of a candidate gene for Norrie disease by positional cloning. *Nature Genetics* **1:** 199–203.

Bick DP, Schorderet DF, Price PA, Campbell L, Huff RW, Shapiro LJ, Moore CM. (1992) Prenatal diagnosis and investigation of a fetus with chondrodysplasia punctata, ichthyosis, and Kallmann syndrome due to an Xp deletion. *Prenat. Diagn.* **12:** 19–29.

Boucher CA, King SK, Carey N et al. (1995) A novel homeodomain-encoding gene is associated with a large CpG island interrupted by the myotonic dystrophy unstable $(CTG)_n$ repeat. *Hum. Mol. Genet.* **4:** 1919–1925.

Brandner S, Isenmann S, Raeber A, Fischer M, Sailer A, Kobayashi Y, Marino S, Weissmann C, Aguzzi A. (1996) Normal host prion protein necessary for scrapie induced neurotoxicity. *Nature* **379:** 339–343.

Brewster BS, Jeal S, Strong PN. (1993) Identification of a protein product of the myotonic dystrophy gene using peptide specific antibodies. *Biochem. Biophys. Res. Commun.* **194:** 1256–1260.

Brook JD, McCurrach ME, Harley HG et al. (1992) Molecular basis of myotonic dystrophy: expansion of a trinucleotide (CTG) repeat at the 3′ end of a transcript encoding a protein kinase family member. *Cell* **68:** 799–808.

Brown RH. (1995) Amyotrophic lateral sclerosis: recent insights from genetics and transgenic mice. *Cell* **80:** 687–692.

Browne DL, Gancher ST, Nutt TG, Brunt ERP, Smith EA, Kramer P, Litt M. (1994) Episodic ataxia myokymia syndrome is associated with point mutations in the human potassium channel gene, *KCNA1. Nature Genetics* **8:** 136–140.

Brune W, Weber RG, Saul B, Doeberitz MV, Grondginsbach C, Kellermann K, Meinck HM, Becker CM. (1996) A *GLRA1* null mutation in recessive hyperekplexia challenges the functional role of glycine receptors. *Am. J. Hum. Genet.* **58:** 989–997.

Brunner HG, Spaans F, Smeets HJM, Coerwinkeldriessen M, Hulsebos T, Wieringa B, Ropers HH. (1991) Genetic-linkage with chromosome-19 but not chromosome-17 in a family with myotonic dystrophy associated with hereditary motor and sensory neuropathy. *Neurology* **41:** 80–84.

Buckwalter MS, Cook SA, Davisson MT, White WF, Camper SA. (1994) A frameshift mutation in the mouse alpha(1) glycine receptor gene (*Glra1*) results in progressive neurological symptoms and juvenile death. *Hum. Mol. Genet.* **3:** 2025–2030.

Büeler H, Fischer M, Lang Y, Bluethmann H, Lipp HP, Dearmond SJ, Prusiner SB, Aguet M, Weissmann C. (1992) Normal development and behavior of mice lacking the neuronal cell surface PRP protein. *Nature* **356:** 577–582.

Büeler H, Aguzzi A, Sailer A, Greiner RA, Autenried P, Aguet M, Weissmann C. (1993) Mice devoid of PRP are resistant to scrapie. *Cell* **73:** 1339–1347.

Burd CG, Dreyfuss G. (1994) Conserved structures and diversity of functions of RNA-binding proteins. *Science* **265:** 615–621.

Burke JR, Wingfield MS, Lewis KE, Roses AD, Lee JE, Hulette C, Pericak-Vance MA, Vance JM. (1994) The Haw River syndrome: dentatorubropallidoluysian atrophy (DRPLA) in an African American family. *Nature Genetics* **7:** 521–524.

Burke JR, Enghild JJ, Martin ME, Jou YS, Myers RM, Roses AD, Vance JM, Strittmatter WJ. (1996) Huntington and DRPLA proteins selectively interact with the enzyme GAPDH. *Nature Medicine* **2:** 347–350.

Burright EN, Clark HB, Servadio A, Matilla T, Feddersen RM, Yunis WS, Duvick LA, Zoghbi HY, Orr HT. (1995) SCA1 transgenic mice a model for neurodegeneration caused by an expanded CAG trinucleotide repeat. *Cell* **82:** 937–948.

Buxton J, Shelbourne P, Davies J et al. (1992) Detection of an unstable fragment of DNA specific to individuals with myotonic dystrophy. *Nature* **355:** 547–548.

Campion D, Flaman JM, Brice A et al. (1995) Mutations of the presenilin I gene in families with early onset Alzheimer's disease. *Hum. Mol. Genet.* **4:** 2373–2377.

Campuzano V, Montermini L, Molto MD et al. (1996) Friedreich's ataxia: autosomal recessive disease caused by an intronic GAA triplet repeat expansion. *Science* **271:** 1423–1427.

Carango P, Noble JE, Marks HG, Funanage VL. (1993) Absence of myotonic dystrophy protein kinase (DMPK) mRNA as a result of a triplet repeat expansion in myotonic dystrophy. *Genomics* **18:** 340–348.

Carvajal JJ, Pook MA, Doudney K, Hillermann R, Wilkes D, Al-Mahdawi S, Williamson R. (1995) Friedreich's ataxia: a defect in signal transduction? *Hum. Mol. Genet.* **4:** 1411–1419.

Carvajal JT, Pook MA, dos Santos M, Doudney K, Hillerman R, Minogue S, Williamson R, Hsuan JT, Chamberlain S. (1996) The Friedreich's ataxia gene encodes a novel phophatidylinositol-4-phosphate 5-kinase. *Nature Genetics* **14:** 157–162.

Chakrabarti L, Knight SJL, Flannery AV, Davies KE. (1996) A candidate gene for mild mental handicap at the FRAXE fragile site. *Hum. Mol. Genet.* **5:** 275–282.

Chamberlain S, Shaw J, Rowland A, Wallis J, South S, Nakamura Y, von Gabain A, Farrall M, Williamson R. (1988) Mapping of mutation causing Friedreich's ataxia to human chromosome 9. *Nature* **334:** 248–250.

Chen XA, Mariappan SVS, Catasti P, Ratliff R, Moyzis RK, Laayoun A, Smith SS, Bradbury EM, Gupta G. (1995) Hairpins are formed by the single DNA strands of the fragile X triplet repeats: structure and biological implications. *Proc. Natl Acad. Sci. USA* **92:** 5199–5203.

Chen ZY, Hendriks RW, Jobling MA, Powell JF, Breakefield XO, Sims KB, Craig IW. (1992) Isolation and characterization of a candidate gene for Norrie disease. *Nature Genetics* **1:** 204–208.

Chen ZY, Battinelli EM, Hendriks RW, Powell JF, Middleton-Price H, Sims KB, Breakefield XO, Craig IW. (1993) Norrie disease gene characterization of deletions and possible function. *Genomics* **16:** 533–535.

Chesebro B, Race R, Wehrly K et al. (1985) Identification of scrapie prion protein specific messenger RNA in scrapie infected and uninfected brain. *Nature* **315:** 331–333.

Chung MY, Ranum LPW, Duvick LA, Servadio A, Zoghbi HY, Orr HT. (1993) Evidence for a mechanism predisposing to intergenerational CAG repeat instability in spinocerebellar ataxia type I. *Nature Genetics* **5:** 254–258.

Citron M, Oltersdorf T, Haass C, McConlogue L, Hung AY, Seubert P, Vigo-Pelfrey C, Lieberburg I, Selkoe DJ. (1992) Mutation of the beta amyloid precursor protein in familial Alzheimer's disease increases beta protein production. *Nature* **360:** 672–674.

Clark RF, Hutton M, Fuldner RA *et al.* (1995) The structure of the presenilin 1 (S182) gene and identification of 6 novel mutations in early onset AD families. *Nature Genetics* **11:** 219–222.

Collinge J, Palmer MS. (1994) Human prion diseases. *Baillière's Clin. Neurol.* **3:** 241–255.

Collinge J, Whittington MA, Sidle KCL, Smith CJ, Palmer MS, Clarke AR, Jefferys JGR. (1994) Prion protein is necessary for normal synaptic function. *Nature* **370:** 295–297.

Corder EH, Saunders AM, Strittmatter WJ, Schmechel DE, Gaskell PC, Small GW, Roses AD, Haines JL, Pericak-Vance MA. (1993) Gene dose of apolipoprotein e type 4 allele and the risk of Alzheimer's disease in late onset families. *Science* **261:** 921–923.

Cruts M, Backhovens H, Wang S-Y *et al.* (1995) Molecular genetic analysis of familial early onset Alzheimer's disease linked to chromosome 14q24.3. *Hum. Mol. Genet.* **4:** 2363–2371.

Curran ME, Landes GM, Keating MT. (1992) Molecular cloning, characterization, and genomic localization of a human potassium channel gene. *Genomics* **12:** 729–737.

De Boulle K, Verkerk AJMH, Reyniers E *et al.* (1993) A point mutation in the *FMR-1* gene associated with fragile X mental retardation. *Nature Genetics* **3:** 31–35.

De Rooij KE, Dorsman JC, Smoor MA, Den Dunnen JT, Van Ommen G-JB. (1996) Subcellular localization of the Huntington's disease gene product in cell lines by immunofluorescence and biochemical subcellular fractionation. *Hum. Mol. Genet.* **5:** 1093–1099.

del Castillo I, Cohen-Salmon M, Blanchard S, Lutfalla G, Petit C. (1992) Structure of the X linked Kallmann syndrome gene and its homologous pseudogene on the Y chromosome. *Nature Genetics* **2:** 305–310.

Deng HX, Hentati A, Tainer JA *et al.* (1993) Amyotrophic lateral sclerosis and structural defects in Cu,Zn superoxide dismutase. *Science* **261:** 1047–1051.

Devys D, Lutz Y, Rouyer N, Bellocq J-P, Mandel J-L. (1993) The FMR-1 protein is cytoplasmic, most abundant in neurons and appears normal in carriers of a fragile X premutation. *Nature Genetics* **4:** 335–340.

DiFiglia M, Sapp E, Chase K *et al.* (1995) Huntingtin is a cytoplasmic protein associated with vesicles in human and rat brain neurons. *Neuron* **14:** 1075–1081.

The Dutch–Belgian Fragile X Consortium. (1994) *Fmr1* knockout mice: a model to study Fragile X mental retardation. *Cell* **78:** 23–33.

Duyao MP, Auerbach AB, Ryan A *et al.* (1995) Inactivation of the mouse Huntington's disease gene homolog *hdh*. *Science* **269:** 407–410.

Eichler EE, Richards S, Gibbs RA, Nelson DL. (1993) Fine structure of the human FMR1 gene. *Hum. Mol. Genet.* **2:** 1147–1153.

Felsenstein KM, Hunihan LW, Roberts SB. (1994) Altered cleavage and secretion of a recombinant beta APP bearing the Swedish familial Alzheimer's disease mutation. *Nature Genetics* **6:** 251–256.

Franco B, Guioli S, Pragliola A *et al.* (1991) A gene deleted in Kallmann's syndrome shares homology with neural cell adhesion and axonal path finding molecules. *Nature* **353:** 529–536.

Fu Y-H, Kuhl DPA, Pizzuti A *et al.* (1991) Variation of the CGG repeat at the fragile X site results in genetic instability: resolution of the Sherman paradox. *Cell* **67:** 1047–1058.

Fu YH, Friedman DL, Richards S *et al.* (1993) Decreased expression of myotonin protein-kinase messenger RNA and protein in adult form of myotonic dystrophy. *Science* **260:** 235–238.

Gacy AM, Goellner G, Juranic N, Macura S, McMurray CT. (1995) Trinucleotide repeats that expand in human disease form hairpin structures *in vitro*. *Cell* **81:** 533–540.

Games D, Adams D, Alessandrini R *et al.* (1995) Alzheimer type neuropathology in transgenic mice overexpressing V717F beta amyloid precursor protein. *Nature* **373:** 523–527.

Gecz J, Gedeon AK, Sutherland GR, Mulley JC. (1996) Identification of the gene *FMR2*, associated with *FRAXE* mental retardation. *Nature Genetics* **13:** 105–108.

Gennarelli M, Lucarelli M, Zelano G, Pizzuti A, Novelli G, Dallapiccola B. (1995) Different expression of the myotonin protein kinase gene in discrete areas of human brain. *Biochem. Biophys. Res. Commun.* **216:** 489–494.

Gerber HP, Seipel K, Georgiev O, Hofferer M, Hug M, Rusconi S, Schaffner W. (1994) Transcriptional activation modulated by homopolymeric glutamine and proline stretches. *Science* **263:** 808–811.

Goate A, Chartierharlin MC Mullan M *et al.* (1991) Segregation of a missense mutation in the amyloid precursor protein gene with familial Alzheimer's disease. *Nature* **349:** 704–706.

Goedert M, Wischik CM, Crowther RA, Walker JE, Klug A. (1988) Cloning and sequencing of the cDNA encoding a core protein of the paired helical filament of Alzheimer disease: identification as the microtubule associated protein tau. *Proc. Natl Acad. Sci. USA* **85**: 4051–4055.

Goldberg YP, Kalchman MA, Metzler M et al. (1996a) Absence of disease phenotype and intergenerational stability of the CAG repeat in transgenic mice expressing the human Huntington disease transcript. *Hum. Mol. Genet.* **5**: 177–185.

Goldberg YP, Nicholson DW, Rasper DM et al. (1996b) Cleavage of huntingtin by apopain, a proapoptotic cysteine protease, is modulated by the polyglutamine tract. *Nature Genetics* **13**: 442–449.

Goldfarb LG, Brown P, Haltia M et al. (1992a) Creutzfeldt–Jakob disease cosegregates with the codon 178^Asn PRNP mutation in families of European origin. *Ann. Neurol.* **31**: 274–281.

Goldfarb LG, Petersen RB, Tabaton M et al. (1992b) Fatal familial insomnia and familial Creutzfeldt–Jakob disease disease phenotype determined by a DNA polymorphism. *Science* **258**: 806–808.

Goldgaber D, Lerman MI, McBride OW, Saffiotti U, Gajdusek DC. (1987) Characterization and chromosomal localization of a cDNA encoding brain amyloid of Alzheimer's disease. *Science* **235**: 877–880.

Green H. (1993) Human genetic diseases due to codon reiteration: relationship to an evolutionary mechanism. *Cell* **74**: 955–956.

Grenningloh G, Schmieden V, Schofield PR, Seeburg PH, Siddique T, Mohandas TK, Becker CM, Betz H. (1990) Alpha subunit variants of the human glycine receptor: primary structures, functional expression and chromosomal localization of the corresponding genes. *EMBO J.* **9**: 771–776.

Griffin JE. (1992) Androgen resistance – the clinical and molecular spectrum. *N. Engl. J. Med.* **326**: 611–618.

Gu Y, Shen Y, Gibbs RA, Nelson DL. (1996) Identification of *FMR2*, a novel gene associated with the *FRAXE* CCG repeat and CpG island. *Nature Genetics* **13**: 109–113.

Gurney ME, Pu HF, Chiu AY et al. (1994) Motor neuron degeneration in mice that express a human Cu,Zn superoxide dismutase mutation. *Science* **264**: 1772–1775.

Hansen RS, Canfield TK, Lamb MM, Gartier SM, Laird CD. (1993) Association of the fragile X syndrome with delayed replication of the *FMR1* gene. *Cell* **73**: 1403–1409.

Hardelin JP, Levilliers J, Delcastillo I et al. (1992) X chromosome linked Kallmann syndrome stop mutations validate the candidate gene. *Proc. Natl Acad. Sci. USA* **89**: 8190–8194.

Harley HG, Brook JD, Rundle SA, Crow S, Reardon W, Buckler AJ, Harper PS, Housman DE, Shaw DJ. (1992) Expansion of an unstable DNA region and phenotypic variation in myotonic dystrophy. *Nature* **355**: 545–546.

Hattori M, Adachi H, Tsujimoto M, Arai H, Inoue K. (1994) Miller–Dieker lissencephaly gene encodes a subunit of brain platelet–activating factor. *Nature* **370**: 216–218.

HDCRC (The Huntington's Disease Collaborative Research Group). (1993) A novel gene containing a trinucleotide repeat that is expanded and unstable on Huntington's disease chromosomes. *Cell* **72**: 971–983.

Hentati A, Deng HX, Hung WY, Nayer M, Ahmed MS, He XX, Tim R, Stumpf DA, Siddique T. (1996) Human alpha tocopherol transfer protein gene: structure and mutations in familial vitamin E deficiency. *Ann. Neurol.* **39**: 295–300.

Hinds HL, Ashley CT, Sutcliffe JS, Nelson DL, Warren ST, Housman DE, Schalling M. (1993) Tissue specific expression of *FMR-1* provides evidence for a functional role in fragile X syndrome. *Nature Genetics* **3**: 36–43.

Hoogeveen AT, Willemsen R, Meyer N, de Rooij KE, Roos AC, van Ommen G-JB, Galjaard H. (1993) Characterization and localization of the Huntington disease gene product. *Hum. Mol. Genet.* **2**: 2069–2073.

Hsiao K, Baker HF, Crow TJ, Poulter M, Owen F, Terwilliger JD, Westaway D, Ott J, Prusiner SB. (1989) Linkage of a prion protein missense variant to Gerstmann–Sträussler syndrome. *Nature* **338**: 342–345.

Hsiao K, Chapman P, Nilsen S, Eckman C, Harigaya Y, Younkin S, Yang F, Cole G. (1996) Correlative memory deficits, Aβ elevation, and amyloid plaques in transgenic mice. *Science* **274**: 99–102.

Ikeda H, Yamaguchi M, Sugai S, Aze Y, Narumiya S, Kakizuka A. (1996) Expanded polyglutamine in the Machado–Joseph disease protein induces cell death *in vitro* and *in vivo*. *Nature Genetics* **13**: 196–202.

Isashiki Y, Ohba N, Yanagita T, Hokita N, Doi N, Nakagawa M, Ozawa M, Kuroda N. (1995) Novel mutation at the initiation codon in the Norrie disease gene in two Japanese families. *Hum. Genet.* **95**: 105–108.

Jamal GA, Weir AI, Hansen S, Ballantyne JP. (1986) Myotonic dystrophy – a reassessment by conventional and more recently introduced neurophysiological techniques. *Brain* **109**: 1279–1296.

Jansen G, Mahadevan M, Amemiya C et al. (1992) Characterization of the myotonic dystrophy region predicts multiple protein isoform-encoding mRNAs. *Nature Genetics* **1**: 261–266

Jansen G, Bächner D, Coerwinkel M, Wormskamp N, Hameister H, Wieringa B. (1995) Structural organization and developmental expression pattern of the mouse WD-repeat gene DMR-N9 immediately upstream of the mytonic dystrophy locus. *Hum. Mol. Genet.* **4**: 843–852.

Jansen G, Groenen PJTA, Bächner D et al. (1996) Abnormal myotonic dystrophy protein kinase levels produce only mild myopathy in mice. *Nature Genetics* **13**: 316–324.

Johnson K, Hamilton G. (1997) Genomics. In: *Principles and Practice of Medical Genetics* (ed. JM Connor). Churchill Livingstone, Edinburgh, in press.

Jones CT, Brock DJH, Chancellor AM, Warlow CP, Swingler RJ. (1993) Cu/Zn superoxide dismutase (SOD1) mutations and sporadic amyotrophic lateral sclerosis. *Lancet* **342**: 1050–1051.

Justice RW, Zilian O, Woods DF, Noll M, Bryant PJ. (1995) The Drosophila tumor-suppressor gene warts encodes a homolog of human myotonic dystrophy kinase and is required for the control of cell shape and proliferation. *Genes Dev.* **9**: 534–546.

Kang J, Lemaire HG, Unterbeck A, Salbaum JM, Masters CL, Grzeschik KH, Multhaup G, Beyreuther K, Mullerhill B. (1987) The precursor of Alzheimer's disease amyloid A4 protein resembles a cell surface receptor. *Nature* **325**: 733–736.

Kawaguchi Y, Okamoto T, Taniwaki M et al. (1994) CAG expansions in a novel gene for Machado Joseph disease at chromosome 14q32.1. *Nature Genetics* **8**: 221–228.

Khandjian EW, Corbin F, Woerly S, Rousseau F. (1996) The fragile X mental retardation protein is associated with ribosomes. *Nature Genetics* **12**: 91–93.

King SK, Wells DJ, Carey N, Bailey MES, Wells KE, Johnson KJ. (1995) Characterization of the myotonic dystrophy protein kinase (DMPK) promoter: identification of a fragment that directs neural-specific expression. *Am. J. Hum. Genet.* **57** (suppl.): A146.

Kingsmore SF, Giros B, Suh D, Bieniarz M, Caron MG, Seldin MF. (1994) Glycine receptor beta subunit gene mutation in *spastic* mouse associated with LINE-1 element insertion. *Nature Genetics* **7**: 136–142.

Knight SJL, Flannery AV, Hirst MC et al. (1993) Trinucleotide repeat amplification and hypermethylation of a CpG island in *FRAXE* mental retardation. *Cell* **74**: 127–134.

Knight SJL, Voelckel MA, Hirst MC, Flannery AV, Moncla A, Davies KE. (1994) Triplet repeat expansion at the *FRAXE* locus and X-linked mild mental handicap. *Am. J. Hum. Genet.* **55**: 81–86.

Koide R, Ikeuchi T, Onodera O et al. (1994) Unstable expansion of CAG repeat in hereditary dentatorubral pallidoluysian atrophy (DRPLA). *Nature Genetics* **6**: 9–13.

Koshy B, Matilla T, Burright EN, Merry DE, Fischbeck KH, Orr HT, Zoghbi HY. (1996) Spinocerebellar ataxia type-1 and spinobulbar muscular atrophy gene products interact with glyceraldehyde-3-phosphate dehydrogenase. *Hum. Mol. Genet.* **5**: 1311–1318.

Krahe R, Ashizawa T, Abbruzzese C, Roeder E, Carango P, Giacanelli M, Funanage VL, Siciliano MJ. (1995) Effect of myotonic dystrophy trinucleotide repeat expansion on DMPK transcription and processing. *Genomics* **28**: 1–14.

Kretzschmar HA, Prusiner SB, Stowring LE, Dearmond SJ. (1986) Scrapie prion proteins are synthesized in neurons. *Am. J. Pathol.* **122**: 1–5.

Kruyer H, Mila M, Glover G, Carbonell P, Ballesta F, Estivill X. (1994) Fragile X syndrome and the $(CGG)_n$ mutation: two families with discordant MZ twins. *Am. J. Hum. Genet.* **54**: 437–442.

LaFerla FM, Tinkle BT, Bieberich CJ, Haudenschild CC, Jay G. (1995) The Alzheimer's Aβ peptide induces neurodegeneration and apoptotic cell death in transgenic mice. *Nature Genetics* **9**: 21–30.

Lamb BT, Sisodia SS, Lawler AM, Slunt HH, Kitt CA, Kearns WG, Pearson PL, Price DL, Gearhart JD. (1993) Introduction and expression of the 400 kilobase *precursor amyloid protein* gene in transgenic mice. *Nature Genetics* **5**: 22–29.

La Spada AR, Wilson EM, Lubahn DB, Harding AE, Fischbeck KH. (1991) Androgen receptor gene mutations in X-linked spinal and bulbar muscular atrophy. *Nature* **352**: 77–79.

Legouis R, Hardelin JP, Levilliers J et al. (1991) The candidate gene for the X linked Kallmann syndrome encodes a protein related to adhesion molecules. *Cell* **67**: 423–435.

Levitan D, Greenwald I. (1995) Facilitation of *lin-12* mediated signaling by *sel-12*, a *Caenorhabditis elegans S182* Alzheimer's disease gene. *Nature* **377**: 351–354.

Levy-Lahad E, Wijsman EM, Nemens E, Anderson L, Goddard KAB, Weber JL, Bird TD, Schellenberg GD. (1995) A familial Alzheimer's disease locus on chromosome 1. *Science* **269**: 970–973.

Levy-Lahad E, Poorkaj P, Wang K, Fu YH, Oshima J, Mulligan J, Schellenberg GD. (1996) Genomic structure and expression of STM2, the chromosome 1 familial Alzheimer disease gene. *Genomics* **34**: 198–204.

Li SH, McInnis MG, Margolis RL, Antonarakis SE, Ross CA. (1993) Novel triplet repeat containing genes in human brain: cloning, expression, and length polymorphisms. *Genomics* **16**: 572–579.

Li XJ, Li SH, Sharp AH, Nucifora FC, Schilling G, Lanahan A, Worley P, Snyder SH, Ross CA. (1995) A huntingtin associated protein enriched in brain with implications for pathology. *Nature* **378**: 398–402.

Liao YCJ, Lebo RV, Clawson GA, Smuckler EA. (1986) Human prion protein cDNA: molecular cloning, chromosomal mapping, and biological implications. *Science* **233**: 364–367.

Lin B, Nasir J, Macdonald H, Hutchinson G, Graham RK, Rommens JM, Hayden MR. (1994) Sequence of the murine Huntington disease gene: evidence for conservation, alternate splicing and polymorphism in a triplet (CCG) repeat. *Hum. Mol. Genet.* **3**: 85–92.

Lin BY, Nasir J, Kalchman MA, McDonald H, Zeisler J, Goldberg YP, Hayden MR. (1995) Structural analysis of the 5' region of mouse and human Huntington disease genes reveals conservation of putative promoter region and dinucleotide and trinucleotide polymorphisms. *Genomics* **25**: 707–715.

MacDonald ME, Barnes G, Srinidhi J et al. (1993) Gametic but not somatic instability of CAG repeat length in Huntington's disease. *J. Med. Genet.* **30**: 982–986.

Mahadevan MS, Amemiya C, Jansen G et al. (1993) Structure and genomic sequence of the myotonic dystrophy (DM kinase) gene. *Hum. Mol. Genet.* **2**: 299–304.

Malosio ML, Grenningloh G, Kuhse J, Schmieden V, Schmitt B, Prior P, Betz H. (1991) Alternative splicing generates 2 variants of the alpha 1 subunit of the inhibitory glycine receptor. *J. Biol. Chem.* **266**: 2048–2053.

Maruyama H, Nakamura S, Matsuyama Z et al. (1995) Molecular features of the CAG repeats and clinical manifestation of Machado Joseph disease. *Hum. Mol. Genet.* **4**: 807–812.

Matilla T, McCall A, Subramony SH, Zoghbi HY. (1995) Molecular and clinical correlations in spinocerebellar ataxia type 3 and Machado Joseph disease. *Ann. Neurol.* **38**: 68–72.

McConkie-Rosell A, Lachiewicz AM, Spiridigliozzi GA, Tarleton J, Schoenwald S, Phelan MC, Goonewardena P, Ding X, Brown WT. (1993) Evidence that methylation of the FMR-1 locus is responsible for variable phenotypic expression of the fragile X syndrome. *Am. J. Hum. Genet.* **53**: 800–809.

Medori R, Tritschler HJ, Leblanc A et al. (1992) Fatal familial insomnia, a prion disease with a mutation at codon 178 of the prion protein gene. *N. Engl. J. Med.* **326**: 444–449.

Meindl A, Berger W, Meitinger T et al. (1992) Norrie disease is caused by mutations in an extracellular protein resembling C-terminal globular domain of mucins. *Nature Genetics* **2**: 139–143.

Meitinger T, Meindl A, Bork P, Rost B, Sander C, Haasemann M, Murken J. (1993) Molecular modeling of the Norrie disease protein predicts a cystine knot growth factor tertiary structure. *Nature Genetics* **5**: 376–380.

Monari L, Chen SG, Brown P et al. (1994) Fatal familial insomnia and familial Creutzfeldt–Jakob disease: different prion proteins determined by a DNA polymorphism. *Proc. Natl Acad. Sci. USA* **91**: 2839–2842.

Moss SJ, Doherty CA, Huganir RL. (1992) Identification of the cAMP dependent protein kinase and protein kinase C phosphorylation sites within the major intracellular domains of the beta 1 subunit, gamma 2S subunit, and gamma 2l subunit of the gamma aminobutyric acid type A receptor. *J. Biol. Chem.* **267**: 14 470–14 476.

Moxley RT III. (1992) Myotonic muscular dystrophy. In: *Myopathies* (eds LP Rowland, S DiMauro). Elsevier Science Publishers, Amsterdam, pp. 209–259.

Nagafuchi S, Yanagisawa H, Ohsaki E, Shirayama T, Tadokoro K, Inoue T, Yamada M. (1994a) Structure and expression of the gene responsible for the triplet repeat disorder, dentatorubral and pallidoluysian atrophy (DRPLA). *Nature Genetics* **8**: 177–182.

Nagafuchi S, Yanagisawa H, Sato K et al. (1994b) Dentatorubral and pallidoluysian atrophy expansion of an unstable CAG trinucleotide on chromosome 12p. *Nature Genetics* **6**: 14–18.

Nasir J, Floresco SB, Okusky JR et al. (1995) Targeted disruption of the Huntington's disease gene results in embryonic lethality and behavioral and morphological changes in heterozygotes. *Cell* **81**: 811–823.

Neer EJ, Schmidt CJ, Smith T. (1993) Lis is more. *Nature Genetics* **5**: 3–4.

Oberlé I, Rousseau F, Heitz D, Kretz C, Devys D, Hanauer A, Boue J, Bertheas MF, Mandel JL. (1991) Instability of a 550-base pair DNA segment and abnormal methylation in fragile X syndrome. *Science* **252**: 1097–1102.

Oesch B, Westaway D, Walchli M *et al.* (1985) A cellular gene encodes scrapie PRP 27–30 protein. *Cell* **40**: 735–746.

Ogata A, Matsuura T, Tashiro K, Morikawa F, Demura T, Koyanagi T, Nagashima K. (1994) Expression of androgen receptor in X-linked spinal and bulbar muscular atrophy and amyotrophic lateral sclerosis. *J. Neurol. Neurosurg. Psychiat.* **57**: 1274–1275.

Orr HT, Chung MY, Banfi S *et al.* (1993) Expansion of an unstable trinucleotide CAG repeat in spinocerebellar ataxia type 1. *Nature Genetics* **4**: 221–226.

Otten AD, Tapscott SJ. (1995) Triplet repeat expansion in myotonic dystrophy alters the adjacent chromatin structure. *Proc. Natl Acad. Sci. USA* **92**: 5465–5469.

Ouahchi K, Arita M, Kayden H *et al.* (1995) Ataxia with isolated vitamin E deficiency is caused by mutations in the alpha tocopherol transfer protein. *Nature Genetics* **9**: 141–145.

Owen F, Lofthouse R, Crow TJ *et al.* (1989) Insertion in prion protein gene in familial Creutzfeldt–Jakob disease. *Lancet* **1**: 51–52.

Ponte P, Gonzalez-DeWhitt P, Schilling J *et al.* (1988) A new A4 amyloid messenger RNA contains a domain homologous to serine proteinase inhibitors. *Nature* **331**: 525–527.

Pramatarova A, Figlewicz DA, Krizus A *et al.* (1995) Identification of new mutations in the Cu/Zn superoxide dismutase gene of patients with familial amyotrophic lateral sclerosis. *Am. J. Hum. Genet.* **56**: 592–596.

Prusiner SB. (1991) Molecular biology of prion diseases. *Science* **252**: 1515–1522.

Prusiner SB. (1994) Biology and genetics of prion diseases. *Annu. Rev. Microbiol.* **48**: 655–686.

Puckett C, Concannon P, Casey C, Hood L. (1991) Genomic structure of the human prion protein gene. *Am. J. Hum. Genet.* **49**: 320–329.

Reaume AG, Elliott JL, Hoffman EK *et al.* (1996) Motor neurons in Cu/Zn superoxide dismutase deficient mice develop normally but exhibit enhanced cell death after axonal injury. *Nature Genetics* **13**: 43–47.

Reddy S, Smith DBJ, Rich MM *et al.* (1996) Mice lacking the myotonic dystrophy protein kinase develop a late onset progressive myopathy. *Nature Genetics* **13**: 325–335.

Reiner O, Carrozzo R, Shen Y, Wehnert M, Faustinella F, Dobyns WB, Caskey CT, Ledbetter DH. (1993) Isolation of a Miller–Dieker lissencephaly gene containing G protein beta subunit-like repeats. *Nature* **364**: 717–721.

Richards RI, Sutherland GR. (1994) Simple repeat DNA is not replicated simply. *Nature Genetics* **6**: 114–116.

Rogaev EI, Sherrington R, Rogaeva EA *et al.* (1995) Familial Alzheimer's disease in kindreds with missense mutations in a gene on chromosome 1 related to the Alzheimer's disease type 3 gene. *Nature* **376**: 775–778.

Rosen DR, Siddique T, Patterson D *et al.* (1993) Mutations in Cu/Zn superoxide dismutase gene are associated with familial amyotrophic lateral sclerosis. *Nature* **362**: 59–62.

Rosenthal A, Jouet M, Kenwrick S. (1992) Aberrant splicing of neural cell adhesion molecule L1 messenger RNA in a family with X-linked hydrocephalus. *Nature Genetics* **2**: 107–112.

Roses AD. (1992) Myotonic dystrophy. *Trends Genet.* **8**: 254–255.

Ross CA, McInnis MG, Margolis RL, Li S-H. (1993) Genes with triplet repeats: candidate mediators of neuropsychiatric disorders. *Trends Neurosci.* **16**: 254–260.

Rothstein JD, Bristol LA, Hosler B, Brown RH, Kuncl RW. (1994) Chronic inhibition of superoxide dismutase produces apoptotic death of spinal neurons. *Proc. Natl Acad. Sci. USA* **91**: 4155–4159.

Rubinsztein DC, Leggo J, Coetzee GA, Irvine RA, Buckley M, Ferguson-Smith MA. (1995) Sequence variation and size ranges of CAG repeats in the Machado–Joseph disease, spinocerebellar ataxia type 1 and androgen receptor genes. *Hum. Mol. Genet.* **4**: 1585–1590.

Ryan SG, Buckwalter MS, Lynch JW *et al.* (1994) A missense mutation in the gene encoding the α_1 subunit of the inhibitory glycine receptor in the *spasmodic* mouse. *Nature Genetics* **7**: 131–135.

Sailer A, Bueler H, Fischer M, Aguzzi A, Weissmann C. (1994) No propagation of prions in mice devoid of PRP. *Cell* **77**: 967–968.

Scheffer IE, Bhatia KP, Lopescendes I *et al.* (1995) Autosomal dominant nocturnal frontal lobe epilepsy: a distinctive clinical disorder. *Brain* **118**: 61–73.

Scheuner D, Eckman C, Jensen M *et al.* (1996) Secreted amyloid β-protein similar to that in the senile plaques of Alzheimer's disease is increased *in vivo* by the presenilin 1 and 2 and *APP* mutations linked to familial Alzeimer's disease. *Nature Medicine* **2**: 864–870.

Schmaier AH, Dahl LD, Rozemuller AJM, Roos RAC, Wagner SL, Chung R, Vannostrand WE. (1993) Protease nexin 2 amyloid beta protein precursor: a tight binding inhibitor of coagulation factor IXa. *J. Clin. Invest.* **92**: 2540–2545.

Servadio A, Koshy B, Armstrong D, Antalffy B, Orr HT, Zoghbi HY. (1995) Expression analysis of the ataxin 1 protein in tissues from normal and spinocerebellar ataxia type 1 individuals. *Nature Genetics* **10:** 94–98.

Sharp AH, Loev SJ, Schilling G *et al.* (1995) Widespread expression of Huntington's disease gene (IT15) protein product. *Neuron* **14:** 1065–1074.

Shaw DJ, McCurrach M, Rundle SA *et al.* (1993) Genomic organization and transcriptional units at the myotonic dystrophy locus. *Genomics* **18:** 673–679.

Sherrington R, Rogaev EI, Liang Y *et al.* (1995) Cloning of a gene bearing missense mutations in early onset familial Alzheimer's disease. *Nature* **375:** 754–760.

Shiang R, Ryan SG, Zhu YZ, Hahn AF, Oconnell P, Wasmuth JJ. (1993) Mutations in the alpha 1 subunit of the inhibitory glycine receptor cause the dominant neurologic disorder, hyperekplexia. *Nature Genetics* **5:** 351–358.

Shiang R, Ryan SG, Zhu YZ, Fielder TJ, Allen RJ, Fryer A, Yamashita S, O'Connell P, Wasmuth JJ. (1995) Mutational analysis of familial and sporadic hyperekplexia. *Ann. Neurol.* **38:** 85–91.

Siomi H, Siomi MC, Nussbaum RL, Dreyfuss G. (1993) The protein product of the fragile X gene, *FMR1*, has characteristics of an RNA-binding protein. *Cell* **74:** 291–298.

Siomi H, Choi M, Siomi MC, Nussbaum RL, Dreyfuss G. (1994) Essential role for KH domains in RNA binding: impaired RNA binding by a mutation in the KH domain of FMR1 that causes fragile X syndrome. *Cell* **77:** 33–39.

Steinlein OK, Mulley JC, Propping P, Wallace RH, Phillips HA, Sutherland GR, Scheffer IE, Berkovic SF. (1995) A missense mutation in the neuronal nicotinic acetylcholine receptor alpha 4 subunit is associated with autosomal dominant nocturnal frontal lobe epilepsy. *Nature Genetics* **11:** 201–203.

Steinlein O, Weiland S, Stoodt J, Propping P. (1996) Exon–intron structure of the human neuronal nicotinic acetylcholine receptor a4 subunit (CHRNA4). *Genomics* **32:** 289–294.

Stine OC, Li S-H, Pleasant N, Wagster MV, Hedreen JC, Ross CA. (1995) Expression of the mutant allele of IT-15 (the HD gene) in striatum and cortex of Huntington's disease patients. *Hum. Mol. Genet.* **4:** 15–18.

Stott K, Blackburn JM, Butler PJG, Perutz M. (1995) Incorporation of glutamine repeats makes protein oligomerize: implications for neurodegenerative diseases. *Proc. Natl Acad. Sci. USA* **92:** 6509–6513.

Strittmatter WJ, Saunders AM, Schmechel D, Pericak-Vance M, Enghild J, Salvesen GS, Roses AD. (1993) Apolipoprotein E high avidity binding to beta amyloid and increased frequency of type 4 allele in late onset familial Alzheimer disease. *Proc. Natl Acad. Sci. USA* **90:** 1977–1981.

Strong TV, Tagle DA, Valdes JM, Elmer LW, Boehm K, Swaroop M, Kaatz KW, Collins FS, Albin RL. (1993) Widespread expression of the human and rat Huntington's disease gene in brain and nonneural tissues. *Nature Genetics* **5:** 259–265.

Sutcliffe JS, Nelson DL, Zhang F, Pieretti M, Caskey CT, Saxe D, Warren ST. (1992) DNA methylation represses *FMR-1* transcription in fragile X syndrome. *Hum. Mol. Genet.* **1:** 397–400.

Sutherland GR, Baker E. (1992) Characterization of a new rare fragile site easily confused with the fragile X. *Hum. Mol. Genet.* **1:** 111–113.

Suzuki N, Cheung TT, Cai XD, Odaka A, Otvos L, Eckman C, Golde TE, Younkin SG. (1994) An increased percentage of long amyloid beta protein secreted by familial amyloid beta protein precursor (beta APP(717)) mutants. *Science* **264:** 1336–1340.

Tagliavini F, Prelli F, Porro M *et al.* (1994) Amyloid fibrils in Gerstmann–Sträussler–Scheinker disease (Indiana and Swedish kindreds) express only PRP peptides encoded by the mutant allele. *Cell* **79:** 695–703.

Tamanini F, Meijer N, Verheij C, Willems PJ, Galjaard H, Oostra BA, Hoogeveen AT. (1996) FMRP is associated to the ribosomes via RNA. *Hum. Mol. Genet.* **5:** 809–813.

Tanzi RE, Gusella JF, Watkins PC *et al.* (1987) Amyloid beta protein gene cDNA, messenger RNA distribution, and genetic linkage near the Alzheimer locus. *Science* **235:** 880–884

Telenius H, Kremer B, Goldberg YP *et al.* (1994) Somatic and gonadal mosaicism of the Huntington disease gene CAG repeat in brain and sperm. *Nature Genetics* **6:** 409–414.

Thomas T, Thomas G, McLendon C, Sutton T, Mullan M. (1996) Beta amyloid mediated vasoactivity and vascular endothelial damage. *Nature* **380:** 168–171.

Timchenko L, Nastainczyk W, Schneider T, Patel B, Hofmann F, Caskey CT. (1995) Full-length myotonin protein kinase (72 kDa) displays serine kinase activity. *Proc. Natl Acad. Sci. USA* **92:** 5366–5370.

Tobler I, Gaus SE, Deboer T et al. (1996) Altered circadian activity rhythms and sleep in mice devoid of prion protein. *Nature* 380: 639–642.

Trottier Y, Devys D, Imbert G et al. (1995a) Cellular localization of the Huntington's disease protein and discrimination of the normal and mutated form *Nature Genetics* 10. 104–110.

Trottier Y, Lutz Y, Stevanin G et al. (1995b) Polyglutamine expansion as a pathological epitope in Huntington's disease and 4 dominant cerebellar ataxias. *Nature* 378: 403–406.

Turnpenny P, Clark C, Kelly K. (1994) Intelligence quotient profile in myotonic dystrophy, intergenerational deficit, and correlation with CTG amplification. *J. Med. Genet.* 31: 300–305.

Ueno S, Kondoh K, Kotani Y, Komure O, Kuno S, Kawai J, Hazama F, Sano A. (1995) Somatic mosaicism of CAG repeat in dentatorubral pallidoluysian atrophy (DRPLA). *Hum. Mol. Genet.* 4: 663–666.

van der Ven PFM, Jansen G, van Kuppevelt THMSM et al. (1993) Myotonic dystrophy kinase is a component of neuromuscular-junctions. *Hum. Mol. Genet.* 2: 1889–1894.

Verheij C, Bakker CE, de Graaff E et al. (1993) Characterization and localization of the *FMR-1* gene product associated with fragile X syndrome. *Nature* 363: 722–724.

Verkerk AJMH, Pieretti M, Sutcliffe JS et al. (1991) Identification of a gene (*FMR-1*) containing a CGG repeat coincident with a breakpoint cluster region exhibiting length variation in fragile X syndrome. *Cell* 65: 905–914.

Verkerk AJMH, de Graaff E, De Boulle K et al. (1993) Alternative splicing in the fragile X gene *FMR1*. *Hum. Mol. Genet.* 2: 399–404.

Wang J-Z, Pegoraro E, Menegazzo E, Gennarelli M, Hoop RC, Angelini C, Hoffman EP. (1995) Myotonic dystrophy: evidence for a possible dominant-negative RNA mutation. *Hum. Mol. Genet.* 4: 599–606.

Wang J-Z, Grundke-Iqbal I, Iqbal K. (1996) Glycosylation of microtubule-associated protein tau: an abnormal posttranslational modification in Alzheimer's disease. *Nature Medicine* 2: 871–875.

Wang Y-H, Griffith J. (1995) Expanded CTG triplet blocks from the myotonic dystrophy gene create the strongest known natural nucleosome positioning elements. *Genomics* 25: 570–573.

Wasco W, Tanzi RE. (1995) Molecular genetics of amyloid and apolipoprotein E in Alzheimer's disease. In: *Neurobiology of Alzheimer's disease* (eds D Dawbarn, SJ Allen). BIOS Scientific Publishers, Oxford, pp. 51–76.

Whiting EJ, Waring JD, Tamai K, Somerville MJ, Hincke M, Staines WA, Ikeda J-E, Korneluk RG. (1995) Characterization of myotonic dystrophy kinase (DMK) protein in human and rodent muscle and central nervous-tissue. *Hum. Mol. Genet.* 4: 1063–1072.

Whittington MA, Sidle KCL, Gowland I, Meads J, Hill AF, Palmer MS, Jefferys JGR, Collinge J. (1995) Rescue of neurophysiological phenotype seen in PRP null mice by transgene encoding human prion protein. *Nature Genetics* 9: 197–201.

Wiedau-Pazos M, Goto JJ, Rabizadeh S, Gralla EB, Roe JA, Lee MK, Valentine JS, Bredesen DE. (1996) Altered reactivity of superoxide dismutase in familial amyotrophic lateral sclerosis. *Science* 271: 515–518.

Wieringa B. (1994) Myotonic dystrophy reviewed: back to the future? *Hum. Mol. Genet.* 3: 1–7.

Wöhrle D, Kotzot D, Hirst MC et al. (1992) A microdeletion of less than 250kb, including the proximal part of the FMR-1 gene and the fragile site, in a male with the clinical phenotype of fragile X syndrome. *Am. J. Hum. Genet.* 51: 299–306.

Yazawa I, Nukina N, Hashida H, Goto J, Yamada M, Kanazawa I. (1995) Abnormal gene product identified in hereditary dentatorubral pallidoluysian atrophy (DRPLA) brain. *Nature Genetics* 10: 99–103.

Yoshikai S, Sasaki H, Dohura K, Furuya H, Sakaki Y. (1990) Genomic organization of the human amyloid beta protein precursor gene. *Gene* 87: 257–263.

Zeitlin S, Liu JP, Chapman DL, Papaioannou VE, Efstratiadis A. (1995) Increased apoptosis and early embryonic lethality in mice nullizygous for the Huntington's disease gene homolog. *Nature Genetics* 11: 155–163.

Zhang Y, O'Connor JP, Siomi MC, Srinivasan S, Dutra A, Nussbaum RL, Dreyfuss G. (1995) The fragile X mental retardation syndrome protein interacts with novel homologues FXR1 and FXR2. *EMBO J.* 14: 5358–5366.

Zheng H, Jiang MH, Trumbauer ME et al. (1995) Beta amyloid precursor protein deficient mice show reactive gliosis and decreased locomotor activity. *Cell* 81: 525–531.

Index

Acetylcholine receptors (nicotinic), 46, 207, 226, 259, 282
    ADNFLE, 379
    assembly, 223
    3D structure, 217
    developmental regulation, 211
    glycosylation, 215
    phosphorylation, 214–215
    synaptic clustering, 48, 212
    topology, 221
Acetylcholine, transporter, 134
Actin, 96, 126, 127
Activin, 331
Adenosine receptors, 179
Adenylyl cyclase, 177, 178, 188, 189, 242, 244, 259, 261, 326, 327
ADNFLE (autosomal dominant nocturnal frontal lobe epilepsy), 379
Adrenoceptors, 179, 182–184, 190, 193, 257, 259
Agrin, 47, 224, 272, 281–283
α-tocopherol transfer protein (αTTP), 377
Alternative splicing, 212
Alzheimer's disease, 55, 116, 117, 374
AMPA receptors, 234, 262, 325, 326
    alternative splicing, 212
    extracellular structure, 219
Amyotrophic lateral sclerosis (ALS), 40, 116, 376
Ankyrin, 98, 99, 285
Anticipation, 368, 372
Apamin, 156
Apolipoprotein E, 376
Apoptosis, 37, 39, 42
APP gene, 6, 55, 374
Arachidonic acid, 251, 261, 263, 328
Arc, 331
ARF, 250
ARIA, 212
Arrestin, 191
Ataxia, 33
Ataxin-1, 40
ATP receptors, 232–233
Atrial natriuretic peptide, 180, 244
AVED, 376
Axon pathfinding, 28
    guidance, 29
Axonal transport, 113, 114
Axonin, 285, 287
Axons, 28, 100, 101, 103, 113, 272, 287

Bcl-2, 37, 42
BF-1 gene, 306
Bone morphogenetic proteins, 25, 317
Bradykinin, 180, 260
Brain-derived neurotrophic factor (BDNF), 36, 72, 333, 334, 340–347
Brevican, 281

Ca^2/calmodulin-dependent adenylate cyclase, 55, 244, 290, 327, 328
Ca^{2+}/calmodulin-dependent protein kinase II, 104, 128, 289, 327, 333–335
Cadherins, 99, 270
Calcineurin, 256
Calcium, 127, 137, 246, 255, 256, 260, 270, 279, 289, 326
Calcium channels, 159, 177, 178, 257, 259, 261
    classification, 159
    inhibitors, 164
    openers, 165
    paralysis, 51
    phosphorylation, 214
    subunits, 161–163
Calmodulin, 97, 99, 244, 245
Calpain, 101
Cannabinoid receptors, 179
Cardiotrophin-1 (CT-1), 36, 348
CED3, CED9, 37
Cell adhesion molecules, 31, 34, 99, 285–286
Cell cycle diseases, 384
Cell death, 37–38
Cell death disease, 384
Cell fate, 23
Cerebellum, 33
Channelopathies, 378
Charybdotoxin, 154
Chloride channel, 49, 145, 207, 229, 230
Choline-acetyl transferase, 71, 73
Cholinergic receptors, *see* Muscarinic *or* Nicotinic receptors
C-kit ligand/receptor, 34
CNTF, 36, 348–350
Collapsin, 272, 274, 275
Commissureless (*comm*), 7, 29
Compartmentation, 189, 256
Connectin, 29, 32
CREB, 55, 263, 329, 331
Creutzfeldt–Jakob disease, 57, 372
Cyclic AMP, 324, 326
Cylic AMP-dependent protein kinase, *see* PKA
Cyclic AMP phosphodiesterase, 55
Cyclooxygenase, 251, 331
Cytoskeleton, 95

Delta, 23, 313
Dendrites, 113
Desensitization of receptors, 190
Development, 22–38, 269, 299, 339
    dorsal–ventral pattern, 313
    eye, 25, 309
    forebrain, 25, 302
    genetics, 22
    hindbrain, 301

Development (*continued*)
    midbrain, 302
    neurotrophins, 346–347
    polarity, 299
Differential display, 4
Dihydropyridine receptor (DHP-R), 51
Dlx gene, 309
DM-GRASP, 287
DMPK, 369–371
Dopamine
    receptors, 179, 259, 261
    transporters, 134
Dopamine-β-hydroxylase, 76
Down-regulation of receptors, 190, 196
DRPLA (dentatorubral pallidoluysian atrophy),
    367
Dynamin, 132, 137, 179
Dynein, 113

Egr3, 329, 331
Eicosanoid receptors, 179
Eicosanoids, 251
Emx genes, 304
Endocytosis, 132
Endosomes, 126, 194
Endothelin/receptor, 34
Engrailed, 302
Enhancers, 74, 87
Enteric neurons, 350–351
Eph receptor, 30
Episodic ataxia with myokimia, 379
Exocytosis, 127, 334
Expressed sequence tags (ESTs), 3
Extracellular matrix, 29, 269

F-11, 278, 285, 287
Fasciclin, 29, 31, 274
Fibrinogen, 276
Fibroblast growth factor, 289
Floor plate, 25, 29, 314
FMR-1, 363
Fodrin, 98
Forebrain development, 302
Fos, 73, 84, 329, 330, 335
Fragile X syndrome (FRAXA), 363
Friedreich's ataxia (FRDA), 371
Fugu, 2
Fyn/*fyn*, 46, 215, 289

G proteins, 177, 186, 189, 190, 242, 257
G protein-coupled receptors, 177
    regulation, 190
G-protein-receptor kinase, 191
GABA$_A$ receptors, 71, 207, 228
    assembly, 224
    genes, 209
    glycosylation, 215
    knockout mutants, 225
    phosphorylation, 214
    promoters, 211
    subunit composition, 216
    topology, 221
GABA$_B$ receptors, 189, 257
GAP43, 333, 334

Gating, ion channels, 218–219
GDNF, 350
Gene discovery, 3
Gene-trap, 7, 28
Genetic diseases, 39, 359
Genetic map (mouse), 35
Genetics, 6, 21, 359
Gephyrin, 103, 224
Gerstmann–Sträussler–Scheinker syndrome
    (GSS), 57, 372
GIRK-2, 41
Glutamate receptors, 208, 234–235
    RNA editing, 212–214
    topology, 221
Glycine receptor, 52, 207, 230
    developmental regulation, 211
    hyperekplexia, 378
Glycosylation, ion-channel receptors, 215
Growth cones, 29, 96, 99, 270, 278, 284
Guanylyl cyclase, 244

Hedgehog genes, 316
Hindbrain development, 301
Hippocampus, 262, 277, 287, 323, 324
Hirschprung's disease, 34
Histamine receptors, 179, 323–328, 330–335
HNF3-β, 313–314
Hox genes, 26–27, 301
5HT receptors, 179, 260
5HT3 receptors, 231
Human Genome Project, 1, 359
Human neuronal disease, 359
Huntington's disease, 39, 365
    huntingtin, 365, 368
Hyperekplexia, 378
Hyperkalemic periodic paralysis, 49
Hypokalemic periodic paralysis, 51

IL-6, 348
Immediate-early genes, 67, 73, 329–331
Immunoglobulins, 270, 277, 284
Induction, 28
Inositol phosphates, 248
Integrins, 99, 270, 280, 284
Interleukin-1β converting enzyme (ICE), 37
Internexin, 101
Introns, 79, 209
Inverse agonists, 187
Ion channel receptors, 205, 207
    allostery, 217, 222
    alternative splicing of mRNA, 212
    assembly, 223
    clustering, 48
    3D structure,   217
    development, 211
    editing of mRNA, 212–213
    functional domains, 222
    gating mechanisms, 218
    gene expression, 210
    gene structure, 209
    phosphorylation, 214
    topology, 221
Ion channels, 145, 205
    genetics, 46

IT15 gene, 365
Jimpy, 45
Jun, 329, 330

K⁺ channels, *see* Potassium channels
Kainate receptors (KAIN R), 235
Kallmann syndrome, 33, 381
KCNA1 gene, 379
Kennedy disease, 364
Kindling, 324, 332, 334
Kinectin, 115
Kinesin, 115
Knockouts, 22, 26, 36, 41, 55, 225, 314, 340, 350, 364
Krox-20, 28, 301
KROX 24, *see* zif/268
Kuru, 57, 372

L1 (Ng-CAM), 281, 285, 288, 289
Laminin, 29, 271, 273, 280, 282, 283, 284
Learning genetics, 210
Leptin, 53
Leucine zipper, 219, 329
LIF (leukemia inhibitory factor), 348
Limbic system-associated protein (LAMP), 287
LIM-1 (gene), 314–315
LIS-1 (gene), 380
Locus control region, 80
Long-term depression, 326, 328, 332
Long-term potentiation, 136, 262, 323–325, 330–335

Machado-Joseph disease, 367
MAP2, 104, 116, 333
MAP kinase, 252, 253, 261, 263, 327
Metabolic diseases, 383
Metabotropic receptors, 180, 205, 324, 326
Methylation, 364
Microfilaments, 96
Microtubule-associated proteins, 103–105
Microtubules, 97, 102, 284
Midbrain development, 302
Migration (neuronal), 380
    genetics, 32
Miller-Dieker lissencephaly, 380
Mitochondrial diseases, 383
Monoamine oxidases, 54
Motor endplate disease (med), 41
Mouse neurological mutations, 35
mRNA complete sequences, neuronal, 14
mRNA structure, 11–18, 213
Muscarinic acetylcholine receptors, 179, 184, 188, 189, 196, 259
Muscle-specific kinase (MuSK), 47, 224
Muscular dysgenesis (mdg), 51
Myelin
    genetics, 4
    neuropathies, 384
    structure, 43
Myelin-associated glycoprotein (MAG), 45
Myelin-basic protein (MBP), 43
Myotonia, 51
Myotonic dystrophy, 39, 369

Na⁺ channels, *see* Sodium channels
N-CAM, 281, 286–289, 328

Necrosis, 37, 42
Nerve growth factor (NGF), 34, 272, 333–335, 339–347
Nestin, 79, 100
Netrin, 29, 271, 272
Neural restrictive silencer element, 72
Neural tube, 24, 314
Neuregulin, 212
Neuro D, 24
Neurocan, 280, 281
Neurofascin, 285
Neurofilaments, 100, 101, 116
Neurogenesis, 23–24, 313
Neurokinin receptors, 180, 184, 193, 198
Neuronal apoptosis inhibitory protein (NAIP), 40, 42
Neuronal mRNA complete sequences, 14
Neuropeptide Y, 53, 257
Neuropeptide Y receptors, 180
Neurotrophic factors, 339, 341
Neurotrophic hypothesis, 340
Neurotrophin 3 (NT3), 272, 275, 333
Neurotrophin receptors, 341
Neurotrophins, 340
    timing of dependence, 346
NF-kB, 330
NgCAM, *see* L1
Nicotinic AChR, *see* Acetylcholine receptor
Nitric oxide (NO), 54, 244, 263, 326, 328
Nkx genes, 310–312
NMDA receptors, 235, 247, 251, 254, 260, 324–327, 333, 334
    extracellular domain structure, 219
    mutants, 225
    subunit composition, 216
Noggin, 317
Noradrenaline transporter, 134, 324
Notch, 23, 313
NT3, 339–347
NT4/5, 339–347
NT6, 339
NrCAM, 278, 281, 285, 287, 288

Obese, 53
Oligodendrocyte, 42
Opioid-binding cell adhesion molecule, 287
Opioid peptides, 333, 334
Opioid receptors, 180, 324
OSM, 348
Otx genes, 304
Oxidative damage disease, 376

p75, 344
PAF acetylhydrolase, 380
Parkinson's disease, 117
Pax genes, 26, 302, 307–309
P-elements, 7
Peripheral myelin protein, 22, 44
Peroxisomal disease, 383
Phospholipase A₂, 248, 251–253, 261
Phospholipase C, 177, 178, 188, 246, 248
Phospholipase D, 248–251
Phosphorylation, 242
    ion channel receptors, 214–215

Pick bodies, 117
Plasticity, 323–335
Platelet-activating factor (PAF), 252
Polyglutamine, 364
    diseases, 364–372
    pathological mechanism, 368
Positional cloning, 6, 359, 360
Post-synaptic densities, 256
Post-translational modification, 214, 215, 242
Potassium channels, 49, 150, 178, 255, 259, 261
    A-type, 150
    calcium sensitive, 150
    classification, 150
    delayed rectifiers, 145, 150
    in EA, 379
    inhibitors, 154
    inwardly rectifying, 151, 153
    openers, 158
    phosphorylation, 214
    structure, 145
    superfamily 1, 145, 152
    superfamily, 2, 146
    voltage sensitivity, 147
    weaver mutant, 41
Presenilin 1, 56, 375
Presenilin 2, 56, 375
Prion diseases, 57, 372
PRNP gene, 373
Profilin, 97, 98
Promoter structure, 67–94, 211
Prosomeres, 302
Prostaglandins, 251–253
Protein kinase A, 55, 101, 104, 191, 214, 245, 326, 327, 328
Protein kinase C, 101, 104, 132, 191, 193, 214, 248, 250, 252, 253, 255, 257, 259, 263, 284, 327, 328, 333
Protein kinase G, 214, 246, 327, 328
Protein phosphatase-1, 259
Protein zero, 44
Proteoglycans, 280–281
Proteolipid protein, 44
Purkinje cells, 39
PYK2, 255, 261

Quarterhorse channel mutant, 49

Raf, 253, 333
Rapsyn, 215, 219, 224
Receptor clustering, 48, 212, 224
Receptor tyrosine kinases, 30, 34, 341–343
Reeler, 33
Release of neurotransmitters, 127, 136, 259, 328
Repulsive axon guidance signal (RAGS), 30
Rhombomeres, 301
RNA-binding protein, 363
RNA editing, 213, 223
Ror-α nuclear receptor, 42
Roundabout (robo), 7, 29

SBMA (spinal and bulbar muscular atrophy), 39, 364
SCA1 (spino-cerebellar ataxia), 39, 365

Schwann cells, 42
Scorpion toxins, 154, 168
Second messenger signaling, 241–263
Segmentation, 24, 301–302
Semaphorins, 31, 272–275
Serotonin (5HT3) receptor, 231
    topology, 221
Shaker, 49, 152
Shiverer, 43
Signaling, 241–263
Silencers, 71
SNAP-25, 129, 130, 137
SNARE, 129, 130, 137
Sodium channels, 99, 165
    classification, 165
    inhibitors, 167
    motor endplate disease, 41
    neurodegeneration, 38
    nontoxin modulators, 170
    openers, 168
Somatostatin receptors, 180, 189
Sonic hedgehog (Shh), 24, 315
Spectrin, 97, 98
Spines, 96
Spongiform encephalopathies, 372
SR proteins, 212
Src, 289
Staggerer, 33
STM7 gene, 371
Storage diseases, 383
Subtractive hybridization, 5
Superoxide dismutase (SOD), 40, 376
Survival motor neuron (SMN) gene, 40
Synapse formation, 47, 127, 224
Synapsin, 72, 75, 99, 127, 128, 334, 335
Synaptobrevin, 129
Synaptotagmin, 129, 131, 132, 137
Syntaxin, 129, 130, 333, 334

Tau, 104, 205, 118, 376
Tenascin, 276, 277
Tetrodotoxin, 167
TGFβ family, 317, 350
Thrombospondin, 278–280
Tissue-plasminogen activator, 280, 331, 332
Transcription factors, 24, 67, 73, 329–331, 333, 335
Transport (axonal), 113, 114
Transporters
    acetylcholine, 134
    dopamine, 134
    noradrenaline, 134
    vesicular, 134
Trembler, 45
Trinucleotide repeats
    characteristics, 371
    diseases, 360–372
    genes, 362
    pathological mechanism, 368
Trk A, B, C, 341–343
Tubulin, 97, 101
Tyrosine hydroxylase, 73, 85
Tyrosine kinase/phosphorylation, 215, 250, 252, 254, 261, 263, 327

VAMP, 129, 137
Vesicles, 125
Vimentin, 100
Vinculin, 99
Voltage-dependent sodium channels, 99
Voltage-gated ion channels, 145

Weaver, 33, 41

Werdnig–Hoffmann spinal muscular atrophy
    (SMA), 40
Wnt genes, 25, 28, 302
Wobbler, 42
World Wide Web, 8

Zebrafish, 7, 23, 25, 28
Zif/268, 329, 331, 333, 335

ORDERING DETAILS

Main address for orders

BIOS Scientific Publishers Ltd
9 Newtec Place, Magdalen Road,
Oxford OX4 1RE, UK
Tel: +44 1865 726286
Fax: +44 1865 246823

Australia and New Zealand
DA Information Services
648 Whitehorse Road, Mitcham, Victoria 3132, Australia
Tel: (03) 9210 7777
Fax: (03) 9210 7788

India
Viva Books Private Ltd
4325/3 Ansari Road, Daryaganj, New Delhi 110 002, India
Tel: 11 3283121
Fax: 11 3267224

Singapore and South East Asia
(Brunei, Hong Kong, Indonesia, Korea, Malaysia, the Philippines,
Singapore, Taiwan, and Thailand)
Toppan Company (S) PTE Ltd
38 Liu Fang Road, Jurong, Singapore 2262
Tel: (265) 6666
Fax: (261) 7875

USA and Canada
BIOS Scientific Publishers
PO Box 605, Herndon, VA 20172-0605, USA
Tel: (703) 661 1500
Fax: (703) 661 1501

Payment can be made by cheque or credit card (Visa/Mastercard, quoting number and expiry date). Alternatively, a *pro forma* invoice can be sent.

Prepaid orders must include £2.50/US$5.00 to cover postage and packing
(two or more books sent post free)